Drug-Induced Nutrient Depletion Handbook

Drug-Induced Nutrient Depletion Handbook

Ross Pelton, RPh, PhD, CCN
Director of Nutrition and Anit-aging Research
Intramedicine, Inc
San Diego, California

James B. LaValle, RPh, DHM, NMD, CCN
Chief Clinical Officer
Intramedicine, Inc
Cincinnati, Ohio
Adjunct Associate Professor
University of Cincinnati, College of Pharmacy

Ernest B. Hawkins, RPh, MS
Director of Herb Research
Intramedicine, Inc
Riddle Farm, North Carolina

Daniel L. Krinsky, RPh, MS
Director, Pharmacotherapy Sales and Marketing
Lexi-Comp, Inc
Hudson, Ohio

LEXI-COMP, INC
Hudson, OH

NATURAL HEALTH RESOURCES
Cincinnati, OH

AMERICAN
PHARMACEUTICAL
ASSOCIATION **APhA**

NOTICE

This handbook is intended to serve the user as a handy quick reference and not as a complete drug or herb information resource. It does not include information on every therapeutic agent available, only selected drugs for which nutrient depletions are documented. The publication is specifically designed to present certain important aspects of drug data in a more concise format than is generally found in medical literature or product material supplied by manufacturers.

Drug information is constantly evolving because of ongoing research and clinical experience and is often subject to interpretation. While great care has been taken to ensure the accuracy of the information presented, the reader is advised that the authors, editors, reviewers, contributors, and publishers cannot be responsible for the continued currency of the information or for any errors, omissions, or the application of this information, or for any consequences arising therefrom. Therefore, the author(s) and/or the publisher shall have no liability to any person or entity with regard to claims, loss, or damage caused, or alleged to be caused, directly or indirectly, by the use of information contained herein. Because of the dynamic nature of drug information, readers are advised that decisions regarding drug therapy must be based on the independent judgment of the clinician, changing information about a drug (eg, as reflected in the literature and manufacturer's most current product information), and changing medical practices. The editors are not responsible for any inaccuracy of quotation or for any false or misleading implication that may arise due to the text or formulas as used or due to the quotation of revisions no longer official. Further, the *Drug-Induced Nutrient Depletion Handbook* is not offered as a guide to dosing. The reader, herewith, is advised that information relating to dosing is provided only as an indication of the amount of the drug typically given or taken during therapy. Actual dosing amount for any specific drug should be based on an in-depth evaluation of the individual patient's therapy requirement and strong consideration given to such issues as contraindications, warnings, precautions, adverse reactions, along with the interaction of other drugs. The manufacturers most current product information or other standard recognized references should always be consulted for such detailed information prior to drug use.

The editors and contributors have written this book in their private capacities. No official support or endorsement by any federal agency or pharmaceutical company is intended or inferred.

If you have any suggestions or questions regarding any information presented in this handbook, please contact our drug information pharmacist at

1-877-837-LEXI (5394)

This manual was produced using the FormuLex™ Program — a complete publishing service of Lexi-Comp, Inc.

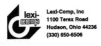

Lexi-Comp, Inc
1100 Terex Road
Hudson, Ohio 44236
(330) 650-6506

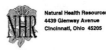

Natural Health Resources
4439 Glenway Avenue
Cincinnati, Ohio 45205

ISBN 1-930598-45-9

TABLE OF CONTENTS

ABOUT THE AUTHORS

Ross Pelton, RPh, PhD, CCN

Ross Pelton received a pharmacy degree from the University of Wisconsin in 1966 and a PhD in psychology with an emphasis in Holistic Health from the University for Humanistic Studies in San Diego, California, in 1984. In 1994, he became a Certified Clinical Nutritionist (CCN) through the International and American Association of Clinical Nutritionists (IAACN). In 1982-83, Dr. Pelton conducted cancer research at the University of California, San Diego (UCSD). Working with the world-renowned scientist, Dr Gerhard Schrauzer, Pelton's research involved studying the relationship between the trace mineral selenium and breast cancer. This research was instrumental in shifting the focus of Dr Pelton's professional interests into the direction of nutrition and natural therapies. In 1985-86, Dr Pelton worked as a consultant to The Gerson Institute, one of the oldest and most successful alternative, nontoxic cancer therapies. In 1988, Dr Pelton moved to Baja, Mexico where he became the administrator of one of the largest hospitals in the world specializing in alternative, nontoxic cancer therapies. For five and one-half years, Dr Pelton directed the inpatient and outpatient therapies for all patients. One of Dr. Pelton's books, *Alternatives in Cancer Therapy* (Simon & Schuster, 1994), was based on his experiences with alternative cancer therapies in Mexico. After returning to the United States in 1994, Dr Pelton worked part-time as a pharmacist and also developed a practice as a clinical nutritionist. In 1997, he began studying and researching drugs that cause nutrient depletions, which finally resulted in the publication of this book. Dr Pelton is the author or coauthor of several other books including *Mind Food & Smart Pills* (Doubleday, 1988), *How To Prevent Breast Cancer* (Simon & Schuster, 1995), *The Drug-Induced Nutrient Depletion Handbook* (Lexi-Comp, Inc, 1999), *The Nutritional Cost of Prescription Drugs* (Morton Publishing, 2000), and *The Natural Therapeutics Pocket Guide* (Lexi-Comp, Inc, 2000). For a number of years, Dr Pelton wrote a column on clinical nutrition for *American Druggist* magazine. Dr Pelton also frequently writes and conducts continuing education seminars for pharmacists as well as other healthcare professionals, in addition to articles on a variety of health-related topics for numerous publications. Dr Pelton is a member of the Medical Advisory Board for the Life Extension Foundation and in 1999, he was named as one of the 50 Most Influential Pharmacists in the United States by *American Druggist* magazine. Currently, Dr Pelton is Director of Nutrition and Antiaging Research for Intramedicine.

James B. LaValle, RPh, DHM, NMD, CCN

Jim has been involved with natural medicine for the past fifteen years and is a nationally recognized figure in the field of natural therapeutics. He is currently Chief Clinical Officer and cofounder of Intramedicine, Inc and is President and founder of Natural Health Resources, Inc (NHR). Jim's experience ranges from extensive clinical practice, product design and formulation, technology development, to author, educator, and media personality. Jim maintains a clinical practice at Pro Scan International. He is currently Adjunct Associate Professor at the University of Cincinnati College of Pharmacy. Jim has educated the pharmacy industry on natural products for *Drug Store News* and *Retail Pharmacy News*. He also has a featured column, the "Prescription Pad," in *Natural Pharmacy* magazine. Jim has also written and developed hundreds of articles and seminars for healthcare professionals and sales forces. He is the author of *Smart Medicine for Healthier Living* (Penguin Putnam), *Drug-Induced Nutrient Depletion Handbook* (Lexi-Comp, Inc), *The Cholestin Breakthrough* (Prima Publishing), and *Black Cohosh* (Penguin Putnam). He is the coauthor of *The Nutritional Cost of Prescription Drugs* (Morton Publishing) and *Natural Therapeutics Pocket Guide* (Lexi-Comp, Inc). Soon to be released Intramedicine titles are *Healthcare Professional's Guide to Dietary Supplements*, *Consumer's Guide to Enlightened Herb Use*, and *Cracking the Metabolic Code: Nine*

Keys to Optimal Metabolism. Jim has developed educational programs for Rite Aid, McKesson, Longs Drugs, and many others. He has trained hundreds of independent pharmacists and physicians about integrating natural medicine into pharmacy practice. Jim was named in 1998 as one of the "50 Most Influential Druggists" by *American Druggist* for his work in natural medicine. Jim is also featured regularly on radio and television programming.

Ernest B. Hawkins, MS, RPh

Ernest B. Hawkins has over 10 years of experience in hospital and retail pharmacy, as well as pharmaceutical research. Ernie has worked extensively in the herbal supplement industry, focusing on the manufacturing and quality control of herbal ingredients. Ernie is a consultant, author, and educator in the dietary supplement arena, authoring and coauthoring numerous books, articles, continuing education programs, and other educational materials. Ernie is a featured columnist for *Natural Pharmacy* magazine, and his work has appeared in other national pharmacy magazines such as *Drug Store News, Retail Pharmacy News,* and *Chain Drug Review.* He is coauthor of books such as *Natural Therapeutics Pocket Guide* (Lexi-Comp, Inc, 2000), *Drug-Induced Nutrient Depletion Handbook* (Lexi-Comp, Inc, 1999), and *Black Cohosh: Nature's Versatile Healer* (Avery Publishing, 2000). His work helps train and educate pharmacists throughout the country on the safe and proper use of nutritional supplements. Ernie is currently Director of Herb Research for Intramedicine, Inc.

Daniel L. Krinsky, MS, RPh

Dan received both his BS in Pharmacy and MS in Hospital Pharmacy from the University of Toledo. He has held positions in many areas of pharmacy practice, including community hospital, tertiary care medical center, managed care, community retail, and academia. His past experiences include Coordinator of the Clinical Pharmacokinetic Consult Service at the University of Alabama Hospital in Birmingham, Alabama from 1985-1991, and Clinical Information Specialist with the Ohio Region of Kaiser Permanente from 1991-1994. Most recently, Dan was the Vice President of Professional Services for Ritzman Pharmacies, Inc, in Wadsworth, Ohio, and Assistant Clinical Professor, Raabe College of Pharmacy, Ohio Northern University from 1994-2000. His primary responsibilities included overseeing the disease management programs, developing and delivering internal and external educational programs, overseeing quality assurance activities, answering drug information questions, and educating graduate pharmacy students. Presently, Dan is the Director of Pharmacotherapy Sales and Marketing for Lexi-Comp, Inc. His present responsibilities include directing the sales and marketing efforts of Lexi-Comp products in the community pharmacy and retail markets, directing the licensing of datasets to clients, developing partnerships with other organizations, and development and delivery of training programs for the sales staff. Dan is co-author of two Lexi-Comp, Inc. publications, *Natural Therapeutics Pocket Guide* (2000) and *Drug-Induced Nutrient Depletion Handbook* (1999). Professional interests include natural products and their use by consumers, application of medical information in the community pharmacy setting, new technologies and drug information applications, disease-state management programs, patient outcome assessments, and payment for cognitive services.

EDITORIAL ADVISORY PANEL

Wayne R. DeMott, MD
Pathologists Chartered
Overland Park, Kansas

Andrew J. Donnelly, PharmD, MBA
Clinical Pharmacist
Operating Room/Anesthesia
Assistant Director of Pharmacy
Rush-Presbyterian-St Luke's Medical Center
Chicago, Illinois

Matthew A. Fuller, PharmD, MBA
Clinical Pharmacy Specialist
Psychiatry
Cleveland Department of Veterans Affairs Medical Center
Brecksville, Ohio

Mark Geraci, PharmD, BCOP
Department of Pharmacy Practice
University of Illinois
Chicago, Illinois

Morton P. Goldman, PharmD
Assistant Director
Pharmacotherapy Services
Cleveland Clinic Foundation
Cleveland, Ohio

Harold J. Grady, PhD
Director of Clinical Chemistry
Truman Medical Center
Kansas City, Missouri

Larry D. Gray, PhD
TriHealth Clinical Microbiology Laboratory
Bethesda Oak Hospital
Cincinnati, Ohio

Martin D. Higbee, PharmD, CGP
Associate Professor
Department of Pharmacy Practice and Science
The University of Arizona
Tucson, Arizona

Jane Hurlburt Hodding, PharmD
Supervisor, Children's Pharmacy
Miller Children's Hospital at Long Beach Memorial
Long Beach, California

Rebecca T. Horvat, PhD
Assistant Professor of Pathology and Laboratory Medicine
University of Kansas Medical Center
Kansas City, Kansas

EDITORIAL ADVISORY PANEL *(Continued)*

Timothy F. Meiller, DDS, PhD
Professor
Department of Oral Medicine and Diagnostic Sciences
Baltimore College of Dental Surgery
Professor of Oncology
Greenebaum Cancer Center
University of Maryland at Baltimore
Baltimore, Maryland

Eugene S. Olsowka, MD, PhD
Pathologist
Institute of Pathology PC
Saginaw, Michigan

Thomas E. Page, MA
Drug Recognition Expert and Instructor
Pasadena, CA

Frank P. Paloucek, PharmD
Clinical Associate Professor
University of Illinois
Chicago, Illinois

Christopher J. Papasian, PhD
Director of Diagnostic Microbiology and Immunology Laboratories
Truman Medical Center
Kansas City, Missouri

Bradley G. Phillips, PharmD, BCPS
Assistant Professor
University of Iowa College of Pharmacy
Clinical Pharmacist
Veterans Affairs Medical Center
Iowa City, Iowa

Martha Sajatovic, MD
Assistant Professor of Psychiatry
Case Western Reserve University
Cleveland, Ohio

Todd P. Semla, PharmD
Associate Director of the Psychopharmacology Clinical and Research Center
Department of Psychiatry and Behavioral Sciences
Evanston Northwestern Healthcare
Evanston, Illinois
Clinical Assistant Professor of Pharmacy Practice in Medicine,
Section of Geriatric Medicine
University of Illinois at Chicago
Chicago, Illinois

Dominic A. Solimando, Jr, MA
Oncology Pharmacist
Director of Oncology Drug Information
cancer**education**.com
Arlington, VA

EDITORIAL ADVISORY PANEL *(Continued)*

INTRODUCTION

Many of the side effects from drug therapy may not be directly due to the drug itself, but rather are the result of nutritional deficiencies that are caused by the drug when taken over time. There are a number of different ways that drugs can negatively affect the status of nutrients in the body. The primary mechanisms responsible for the depletion of nutrients include inhibition of nutrient absorption, synthesis, transport, storage, metabolism, or excretion.

In the process of doing research for this book, it was amazing to uncover the large number of studies appearing in the scientific literature over the past thirty years reporting the drug-induced depletion of nutrients. Even more startling is the fact that this information has not been communicated to the patients who are taking these drugs. The importance of this book is quite simple yet powerful. Most health professionals are not aware of the fact that so many drugs are capable of causing nutritional deficiency-related health problems.

Through seminars presented by Natural Health Resources, Inc, it has been gratifying to see how enthusiastically pharmacists have embraced this material and incorporated it into their pharmacy practices. This is really a win-win situation, because the information helps to reduce potential risk of a drug's side effects, thus improving patients' health outcomes. As a positive by-product, pharmacies get to increase their sales of nutritional supplements at a time when new categories of growth are desperately needed.

It has become increasingly apparent that this information needs to get out to more people. Physicians, nurses, chiropractors, and other health professionals should be aware of drug-induced nutrient depletions. At the same time, it is important that every individual who takes medications should have access to this information.

HOW TO USE THIS BOOK

This work is intended to be used as a reference book, meaning that most people will not be interested in reading the whole book. The goal was to organize the book in such a way that individuals could easily locate the drugs and nutrients that they are specifically interested in.

This book is organized into the following six sections:

> **Section I:** Introduction and text explaining how to use this book
>
> **Section II:** Drug monographs in alphabetical order
>
> **Section III:** Alphabetical listing of nutrients and the drugs that deplete
>
> **Section IV:** Nutrient monographs in alphabetical order
>
> **Section V:** Scientific abstracts that document the drug-induced nutrient depletions
>
> **Section VI:** Appendix containing the Drug-Induced Nutrient Depletion table and several other useful reference sections
>
> **Section VII:** Alphabetical Index

Step 1: Locate the drug(s) you want to research. There are two methods of accomplishing this: 1) Look for the drug's generic name in the drug monograph section; or 2) locate the drug in the alphabetical index, which will give you the page number where the monograph is located.

Step 2: Look at the **Nutrients Depleted** field which will list the various nutrients that are depleted by that particular drug. The page numbers next to each nutrient that is depleted will direct you to the pages for the individual nutrient monographs. Use the nutritional monographs to learn about the nutrient(s) that are depleted by

INTRODUCTION *(Continued)*

the drug(s) you are interested in. In addition to reviewing the biological function and effects of a particular nutrient, be sure to read over the effects of depletion. This can help people determine if their symptoms or problems might be related to a deficiency of that nutrient. Thus, an individual can tell if he or she is taking more than one drug that can deplete the same nutrient.

Step 3: Using the scientific abstract summaries in Section V: Summaries of the abstracts are provided from the scientific studies that report the drug-induced nutrient depletions. Many physicians, pharmacists, and other healthcare professionals are often skeptical about nutritional health claims. They want to see the scientific proof. The abstracts of the published scientific studies provide the source and a summary of the study, which gives a level of validation to the claims being made. The **Studies and Abstracts** field in the drug monographs directs readers to the numerical listing of the abstracts that provide the documentation for the reported nutrient depletions.

LIMITATIONS OF THIS HANDBOOK

It would be virtually impossible to track down every single study that has been published on such a wide range of drugs and nutrients. However, we feel our team of researchers has succeeded in locating the majority of available studies on drug-induced nutrient depletions. In some cases where there is an overwhelming number of studies on a particular drug-nutrient depletion, we have limited the number of included studies to eight or ten.

We also attempted to locate and report negative or conflicting studies where they exist. We have used Medline for all of our database searches. While there are other databases available, we feel that the majority of recognized medical journals are available through Medline.

Our primary goal is to show health professionals and the general public that a large and credible body of scientific literature exists that has reported drug-induced nutrient depletions. Conflicting studies do not necessarily negate positive studies. Oftentimes there are differences in dosages, ages and health conditions of subjects, numbers of participants, etc.

This book does not suggest that drug-induced nutrient deficiencies are the source of peoples' medical problems. Many people have high stress, pollution, poor diets, and other negative influences on their health. When individuals take medications that create an additional nutrient depletion, it may be the proverbial straw that breaks the camel's back. Consequently, drug-induced nutrient depletions may become a major contributor in the development of health problems.

The possibility exists that in some cases, a nutrient depletion may be related to a drugs effectiveness. Also, the literature verifying that nutrient supplementation reverses the effects of drug-induced nutrient depletions is limited. However, it makes common sense to supplement with a nutrient to prevent or correct a nutrient depletion.

We actually believe that the problem of drug-induced nutrient depletions is substantially larger and more widespread than what is reported in this book. Our reason for saying this is that in many cases a drug's effect on various nutrients has not yet been studied. It is difficult to get funding for these kinds of studies. In the past, major drug companies have not been motivated to spend money to conduct such studies. However, with the compelling evidence offered in this book, research may be stimulated. Also, investigating a drug's effect on various nutrients is seldom part of the Food and Drug Administration's procedures for drug approval. Moreover, once a drug is on the market, it can take a significant amount of time for sufficient problems to manifest that would warrant a study evaluating a nutrient deficiency.

A PERSONAL MESSAGE FROM LEAD AUTHOR: ROSS PELTON, RPh, PhD, CCN

Writing this book gives me the opportunity to make a public statement and express my opinion on several issues that I feel very strongly about. The following cartoon is one of my favorites. But it's not just a joke. I think it makes an important statement about health and life.

POT-SHOTS NO. 1409.

LIFE IS THE ONLY GAME

IN WHICH THE OBJECT OF THE GAME

IS TO LEARN THE RULES.

Ashleigh Brilliant

© ASHLEIGH BRILLIANT 1979

When you purchase a new car, a computer, or any other piece of expensive equipment, you are given a detailed operating manual that tells you how to care for that equipment, what to do in order to keep it running smoothly, and how to trouble-shoot key problems that might develop. However, when we are born we come into this life with this amazingly complex, wonderful machine called the human body. Nobody gives us an operating manual that tells us how to care for it. And, unfortunately, many people do not think about learning these rules until something starts to break down. My life's work is to try to teach as many people as possible some of the simple, basic fundamental rules of health, which will ultimately make the Game of Life much longer, much healthier, and more enjoyable.

I would like to take this opportunity to discuss the importance of taking nutritional supplements, and I want to comment on the nutritional standards our government has promoted for many years called Recommended Dietary Allowances (RDAs).

The Food and Nutrition Board, a division of the National Academy of Sciences, first published the RDAs in 1941. Over the years, these values have been periodically revised and updated. Recently, the Food and Nutrition Board created a new set of standards called the Dietary Reference Intakes (DRIs), which consist of four separate reference ranges. These include the old RDAs, which the Board says are still to be used as the goal for individuals. Next is the Tolerable Upper Level (UL), which represents nutrient levels that could be harmful if regularly exceeded. The third value is the Estimated Average Requirement (EAR), which is an intake level that only meets the needs of approximately 50 percent of the people with that level of consumption. And last, the Adequate Intake (AI), a value similar to the

INTRODUCTION *(Continued)*

RDA that is primarily based on judgment if there is not enough scientific data to create an RDA. It is all pretty confusing, isn't it?

I want to make the following point. For over 50 years now, the government and many health professionals have promoted the RDAs as nutrient guidelines that will meet the needs of most healthy individuals. These values have been ingrained in the American psyche. The RDAs are the levels of nutrients that we have been led to believe are adequate. Adequate for what? Adequate to prevent outright nutritional deficiency diseases such as scurvy, beriberi, and pellagra, which are very serious end stage diseases. The line I have drawn below represents what I call the Health LifeLine, going from death on the one end to optimal health and wellness at the other end. On one hand, the government is telling us the truth. The RDAs are sufficient to prevent most people from getting these severe nutritional deficiency diseases, which fall on the Health LifeLine about where I have marked the X, down close to death.

Death	**X**	⇒	⇒	⇒	⇒ **Optimal Health**

HEALTH LIFELINE

However, does it make sense to consume just enough nutrients to keep you slightly beyond the X point on the Health LifeLine? This is what has been promoted for the past 50 years. It could be one of the reasons why the United States of America has the highest rate of chronic degenerative diseases in the world. We have the highest level of technology and are also one of the wealthiest nations in the world, yet we also have the highest rate of disease and spend the largest amount and percentage of our national budget on healthcare. In essence, we have not developed a sense of true "health" care. I think RDAs represent the minimum wage of nutrition. It is important for people to realize that the RDAs have nothing to do with optimal health and wellness. I am not interested in promoting minimal health. I want to promote optimal health. In most cases, nutrient intakes for optimal health are far beyond the RDAs.

In the past decade, there have been hundreds, maybe even thousands of studies published, which report that doses of nutrients substantially higher than the RDAs provide significant health benefits. The tide is already changing in the arena of scientific research. But it has traditionally taken decades for scientific research to filter down through health professionals and finally to the general public. A good example of this is the work of Dr. Kilmer McCully. Dr. McCully began publishing studies in 1969, which reported to scientific and medical professionals that elevated blood homocysteine was a major risk factor in cardiovascular disease. At the time, tremendous amounts of research dollars and large professional egos were committed to the cholesterol hypothesis. It has taken almost 30 years for Dr. McCully's message to be heard, but now we know that additional levels of folic acid, vitamin B_{12}, and vitamin B_6 will lower elevated homocysteine levels. It is now a well accepted fact that even slightly elevated levels of homocysteine represent a serious increased risk to cardiovascular disease. Dr. McCully's work is teaching us that taking three B vitamins at levels above the RDA (costing only pennies per day) may be one of the most effective ways to decrease your risk of cardiovascular disease (still the number one killer). There is no reason to wait another 30 years for the message about the importance of nutritional supplements at levels above the RDAs to gain acceptance. I believe that appropriate levels of nutritional supplements can improve the quality of life for millions of Americans now.

THE SAFETY OF NUTRITIONAL SUPPLEMENTS

The issue of safety usually comes up when nutritional supplement recommendations above the RDA are suggested, so I want to briefly address this topic. The margin of error with most nutrients is much broader than it is with prescription drugs. A case in point is the recent study published in the *Journal of the American Medical Association*, titled "Incidence of Adverse Drug Reactions in Hospitalized Patients: A Meta-analysis of Prospective Studies." The authors of this study report that in 1994, an estimated 2,216,000 hospitalized patients experienced a serious adverse drug reaction, and in the same year an estimated 106,000 hospitalized patients died, not from mistakes, but from what was believed to be the correct use of those medications. If outpatient drug-related deaths were considered, the figure would undoubtedly be much higher. I want to emphasize that this study implies that death related to medications, even when used for correct purposes, may rank among the leading causes of death in the United States.

Looking at things from a different perspective, I would like to present statistics that were first published in the *American Journal of Emergency Medicine* with data compiled from statistics from the American Association of Poison Control Centers over a period of eight years. These statistics report the number of deaths from prescription drugs, nonprescription drugs, and nutrients from 1987 through 1994. During this eight-year period, there were 4,065 deaths from all drugs (prescription and nonprescription) compared to 5 deaths from nutrients (one which was later determined to have been an error).

Fatalities from Prescription Drugs, Nonprescription Drugs, and Nutrients

	Year								
	'87	'88	'89	'90	'91	'92	'93	'94	Total
Number of centers reporting	63	64	70	72	73	68	64	65	539
Analgesics (pain killers)	93	118	126	134	190	186	172	205	1224
Antidepressants (mood elevators)	105	135	140	159	188	194	151	175	1247
Asthma therapies	16	27	34	37	39	35	27	36	251
Cardiovascular drugs[1]	52	65	70	79	87	80	74	90	597
Sedatives & hypnotics[2]	48	77	78	72	97	109	80	99	660
Deaths from amphetamines[3]	11	12	5	6	11	14	11	16	86
Deaths from all above drugs	325	434	453	487	612	618	515	621	4065
Deaths attributed to all nutrients	1*	0	0	1	2†	0	1‡	0	5

1. Includes blood pressure medications; 2. Includes sleeping pills and tranquilizers; 3. Includes stimulants

*The 1987 vitamin-related death report was later determined to be an error.

†One death was from niacin and one from vitamin A

‡Death was from niacin

Table adapted with permission from Donald Loomis (with updated information April 1999), *Townsend Letter for Doctors*, original data from the American Association of Poison Control Centers. Statistics first published in the *American Journal of Emergency Medicine*.

These studies show that drugs carry a much greater risk of death than nutritional supplements. However, improper use of nutrients can also cause problems. In my opinion, vitamin D and iron are the two nutrients that can most easily result in

INTRODUCTION *(Continued)*

problems if consumed in excessive quantities over time. In addition, vitamin A and vitamin E, which are fat-soluble, and the trace mineral selenium are examples of nutrients that can produce toxic effects when taken in excess. However, an individual would have to use gross negligence over an extended period of time in order to create a problem with these nutrients.

I think the diseases that develop, money lost, pain and suffering, and death that can result in individuals who do not ingest sufficient levels of nutrients for optimal health and wellness are much more significant than the few potential problems that result from people ingesting toxic levels of nutritional supplements.

The *American Journal of Emergency Medicine* study cited above that compares deaths from drugs versus nutrients shows that nutritional supplements are quite safe. There are many thousands of health-oriented individuals around the country who have been taking high potency nutritional supplements for years.

THE WISDOM OF TAKING NUTRITIONAL SUPPLEMENTS

In her book *New Passages*, Gail Sheehy notes that the aging process for health conscious baby boomers is quite different than it was for previous generations. Our parents were making plans for or actually retiring between the ages of 55 and 65. Ms Sheehy states that health conscious baby boomers consider themselves "in the infancy of their second adulthood." A healthy extension of both quantity and quality of life is available to everyone. One of my messages is that the judicious use of optimal levels of nutritional supplements, along with a healthy diet and life style, enables every individual to have a great deal of control over their own immune system and their own aging process. These are choices that every person makes for himself or herself. The decisions you make have enormous impact on your health, the quality of your life, and how long you will live. I would like to share a quote with you from Albert Szent-Gyorgy who was the discoverer of vitamin C. He said the following: "Active supplements are the least expensive, most effective health insurance you can buy." For many people, the term nutritional supplement means vitamins. In reality, a lack of minerals is equally problematic, if not more so, than a deficiency of vitamins. I say this because most of the huge factory farming organizations do not include trace minerals when they use chemical fertilizers. Thus, the commercial food supply throughout much of the United States is experiencing a continual decline in trace minerals, which are important essential nutrients. This is why people should be counseled to take nutritional supplements containing a wide range of both vitamins and minerals.

The message in this last cartoon does not have to happen to you. It is your option. By making some fairly simple changes in diet, nutrition, and lifestyle, individuals can literally take control of their own immune systems and their aging process. I do not have the time or space in this book to get into specifics about things like diet and exercise. However, I do feel that expressing some of my thoughts about the importance of nutritional supplements ties in nicely with the theme and content of this book.

These days most people have stressful lifestyles. The level of environmental pollutants people have been exposed to in the last 60 to 80 years is hundreds, if not thousands, of times higher than in pervious years. The nutritional content of the foods that most Americans eat is substantially below what it takes for optimal health and wellness. In addition to these problems, millions of people are taking medications that cause drug-induced depletion of nutrients. Consequently, I think the health and lives of most Americans would benefit greatly by taking well-formulated high potency multivitamin/mineral supplements every day.

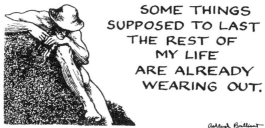

POT-SHOTS NO. 2134.

THIS IS SERIOUS:

SOME THINGS SUPPOSED TO LAST THE REST OF MY LIFE ARE ALREADY WEARING OUT.

ashleigh Brilliant

My goal, and the goal of my company, Natural Health Resources, is to provide health education, technology and services that will empower millions of Americans to have healthier, happier, longer lives. I hope this book helps each of you along this path.

Lazarou J, et al, "Incidence of Adverse Drug Reactions in Hospitalized Patients: A Meta-Analysis of Prospective Studies,' *JAMA*, 1998, 279(15):1200-5.

Loomis D, "Fatalities From Prescription Drugs, Non-prescription Drugs and Nutrients," *Townsend Letter for Doctors* 1992, 78:41.

Sheehy G, *New Passages*, 1995, New York, NY: Random House.

ACKNOWLEDGMENTS

The *Drug-Induced Nutrient Depletion Handbook* exists in its present form as the result of the concerted efforts of the following individuals: Robert D. Kerscher, publisher and president of Lexi-Comp, Inc; Lynn D. Coppinger, managing editor; Mark Bonfiglio, PharmD, director of pharmacotherapy resources; Barbara F. Kerscher, production manager; Stacy S. Robinson, project manager; Paul A. Rhine, product manager; Tracey J. Reinecke, graphic designer; David C. Marcus, director of information systems; and Julian I. Graubart, American Pharmaceutical Association (APhA), Director of Books and Electronic Products.

Much of the material contained in this book was a result of pharmacy contributors throughout the United States and Canada. Lexi-Comp has assisted many medical institutions to develop hospital-specific formulary manuals that contain clinical drug information as well as dosing. Working with clinical pharmacists, hospital pharmacy and therapeutics committees, and hospital drug information centers, Lexi-Comp has developed an evolutionary drug database that reflects the practice of pharmacy in these major institutions.

In addition, the authors wish to thank their families, friends, and colleagues who supported them in their efforts to complete this handbook.

Natural Health Resources, Inc.

The mission of NHR is to meet the challenge of providing professionals and consumers with a better awareness and understanding of the value of natural therapeutics by integrating natural therapies with traditional care. Natural Health Resources is uniquely qualified to provide natural medicine education. Its team of professionals represents a range of healthcare disciplines whose expertise can enhance the professional's knowledge base and ability to apply natural care concepts into practical working models. NHR's services include:

- Education in vitamins, minerals, herbs, and homeopathy
- Training for prevention and support for common self-care complaints
- Advanced education for an integrative approach to prevention and disease state management
- Innovative laboratory assessment and analysis

DESCRIPTION OF SECTIONS AND FIELDS IN THIS HANDBOOK

The *Drug-Induced Nutrient Depletion Handbook* is divided into seven sections.

Section I is a compilation of introductory text pertinent to the use of this book.

Section II is the drug information section of the handbook, which provides a comprehensive listing of generic drugs. Drugs which deplete nutrients are indicated with an asterisk (*). Extensive cross-referencing is provided by brand names and synonyms.

Alphabetical Listing of Drugs

Information is presented in a consistent format and provides the following:

Generic Name	U.S. adopted name
Pronunciation Guide	Phonetic pronunciation
Related Information	Cross-reference to other pertinent drug information found elsewhere in this handbook
U.S. Brand Names	Trade names found in the United States
Canadian Brand Names	Trade names found in Canada
Synonyms	Other names or accepted abbreviations for the generic drug
Pharmacologic Class	Unique systematic classification of medications
Nutrients Depleted	Listing and cross-reference to the nutrients depleted by the drug
Scientific Basis	The five study-dependent statements presented in this field include:
	1. Published scientific studies using this pharmacologic agent
	2. Published scientific studies of agents from the same pharmacologic class
	3. Published scientific studies of agents with the same mechanism of action
	4. Inferred or indirect evidence of depletion based on disruption of physiologic processes
	5. Published scientific studies of agents from the same pharmacologic class demonstrate depletion of some nutrients; however, this agent was NOT found to cause similar depletion

DESCRIPTION OF SECTIONS AND FIELDS IN THIS HANDBOOK *(Continued)*

This field is intended to allow rapid identification of the scientific basis for a drug's inclusion in the monographs. Medications are included on the basis of five designations. The most common rationales for inclusion are situations where nutrient depletions have been scientifically demonstrated for the drug in the monograph or have been demonstrated for a prototypical agent from the same pharmacologic class. In some cases, a drug has been included on the basis of a shared mechanism of action with a drug known to cause depletion by this mechanism. In addition, some drugs have been included because of inferred or indirect evidence of depletion (eg, drugs with significant impact on gastrointestinal function). Finally, in cases where specific evidence exists to document that a drug from a pharmacologic class does not deplete nutrients, despite evidence of depletion for other drugs within the class, the drug is included in the monographs to allow the identification of these exceptions. For example, there is positive evidence of nutrient depletion for some sulfonylureas, while other drugs in the same class were noted to be free of this effect. To accurately represent these observations, all of the studies of agents are included in the drug monographs section of the book, with the nondepleting agents specifically noted as exceptions. In addition to the scientific basis field in the monograph, the reader is referred within the monograph to the Studies and Abstracts section of this handbook.

Studies & Abstracts — Lists reference number(s) associated with this monograph in the Studies & Abstracts section

The summary of supporting studies included in this handbook is intended to provide a detailed, informative presentation of scientific observations which support the claims of nutrient depletion by individual pharmacologic agents and/or classes. The reader is strongly advised to review these sections. In most cases, the evidence is consistent and compelling. In other cases, there may be only a small amount of data to support an identified depletion. When possible, both positive and negative studies involving the specific agent are presented. The references and summaries are intended to identify the limits of current scientific knowledge in this field, encourage the reader to further explore these issues, and to allow interested parties to locate and critically evaluate the full article.

Additional Information — Further information concerning a particular nutrient depletion.

Section III contains an alphabetical listing of nutrients and the drugs that deplete.
Section IV contains the nutrient information.

Alphabetical Listing of Nutrient Monographs

Information is presented in a consistent format and provides the following:

Generic Name — U.S. adopted name

Synonyms	Other names or accepted abbreviations
Available Compounds	Listing (if appropriate) of the various compounds of the nutrient
Drugs That Deplete	Cross-reference to the alphabetical listing of nutrients and the drugs that deplete.
Effects of Depletion	Summary of the factors that can cause a deficiency and a review of the primary symptoms associated with a deficiency of the nutrient
Overview	Brief description of the nutrient
Biological Function & Effect	Review of the way the nutrient functions in humans
Side Effects & Toxicity	Symptoms and adverse effects associated with usual or excessive intake of the nutrient
RDA	Recommended Dietary Allowance
Dosage Range	Amount of the nutrient typically given
Dietary Sources	Listing of the best food sources for the nutrient
Forms	Information regarding available dosage forms of the nutrient

Section V comprises studies and brief abstracts that document the drug nutrient depletion issue presented and these correspond to the drug monographs.

Section VI, the Appendix section, which includes the **Drug-Induced Nutrient Depletion Table**, is a variety of tables and charts which may be helpful to the reader.

Section VII contains an alphabetical index.

ALPHABETICAL LISTING OF DRUGS

Abacavir (a BAK a veer)
U.S. Brand Names Ziagen®
Pharmacologic Class Antiretroviral Agent, Reverse Transcriptase Inhibitor (Nucleoside); Reverse Transcriptase Inhibitor
Nutrients Depleted
  Specific nutrient depletions have not been documented for this agent.

Abacavir, Lamivudine, and Zidovudine*
  (a BAK a veer, la MI vyoo deen, & zye DOE vyoo deen)
U.S. Brand Names Trizivir™
Synonyms Azidothymidine, Abacavir, and Lamivudine; AZT, Abacavir, and Lamivudine; Compound S, Abacavir, and Lamivudine; Lamivudine, Abacavir, and Zidovudine; 3TC, Abacavir, and Zidovudine; ZDV, Abacavir, and Lamivudine; Zidovudine, Abacavir, and Lamivudine
Pharmacologic Class Antiretroviral Agent, Reverse Transcriptase Inhibitor (Non-Nucleoside); Antiretroviral Agent, Reverse Transcriptase Inhibitor (Nucleoside)
Nutrients Depleted
  Carnitine *on page 316*
  Copper *on page 322*
  Vitamin B_{12} *on page 359*
  Zinc *on page 368*
Scientific Basis
  Published scientific studies using this pharmacologic agent (zidovudine)
  or
  Published scientific studies of agents from the same pharmacologic class
Studies & Abstracts 259-261

♦ **ABCD** *see* Amphotericin B Cholesteryl Sulfate Complex* *on page 33*
♦ **Abelcet™** *see* Amphotericin B (Lipid Complex)* *on page 34*
♦ **Abenol®** *see* Acetaminophen* *on page 23*
♦ **Abitrate®** *see* Clofibrate *on page 80*
♦ **ABLC** *see* Amphotericin B (Lipid Complex)* *on page 34*

Acarbose (AY car bose)
U.S. Brand Names Precose®
Pharmacologic Class Antidiabetic Agent (Miscellaneous)
Nutrients Depleted
  Specific nutrient depletions have not been documented for this agent.

♦ **Accolate®** *see* Zafirlukast *on page 269*
♦ **Accupril®** *see* Quinapril* *on page 227*
♦ **ACE** *see* Captopril* *on page 57*

Acebutolol* (a se BYOO toe lole)
Related Information
  Drug-Induced Nutrient Depletion Table *on page 498*

U.S. Brand Names Sectral®
Canadian Brand Names Monitan®; Rhotral
Synonyms Acebutolol Hydrochloride
Pharmacologic Class Antiarrhythmic Agent, Class II; Beta Blocker (with Intrinsic Sympathomimetic Activity)
Nutrients Depleted
Coenzyme Q_{10} *on page 320*
Scientific Basis
Published scientific studies using this pharmacologic agent
or
Published scientific studies of agents from the same pharmacologic class
Studies & Abstracts 348-349

♦ **Acebutolol Hydrochloride** *see* Acebutolol* *on page 22*
♦ **Aceon®** *see* Perindopril Erbumine* *on page 209*
♦ **Acephen® [OTC]** *see* Acetaminophen* *on page 23*
♦ **Aceta® [OTC]** *see* Acetaminophen* *on page 23*

Acetaminophen* (a seet a MIN oh fen)
Related Information
Drug-Induced Nutrient Depletion Table *on page 498*
U.S. Brand Names Acephen® [OTC]; Aceta® [OTC]; Apacet® [OTC]; Aspirin Free Anacin® Maximum Strength [OTC]; Children's Dynafed® Jr [OTC]; Children's Silapap® [OTC]; Extra Strength Dynafed® E.X. [OTC]; Feverall™ [OTC]; Feverall™ Sprinkle Caps [OTC]; Genapap® [OTC]; Halenol® Children's [OTC]; Infants Feverall™ [OTC]; Infants' Silapap® [OTC]; Junior Strength Panadol® [OTC]; Liquiprin® [OTC]; Mapap® [OTC]; Maranox® [OTC]; Neopap® [OTC]; Panadol® [OTC]; Redutemp® [OTC]; Ridenol® [OTC]; Tempra® [OTC]; Tylenol® [OTC]; Tylenol® Extended Relief [OTC]; Uni-Ace® [OTC]
Canadian Brand Names Abenol®; A.F. Anacin®; Atasol®; Pediatrix; Tantaphen®
Synonyms APAP; N-Acetyl-P-Aminophenol; Paracetamol
Pharmacologic Class Analgesic, Miscellaneous
Nutrients Depleted
Glutathione *on page 327*
Scientific Basis Published scientific studies using this pharmacologic agent
Studies & Abstracts 517-518

♦ **Acetaminophen and Butalbital Compound** *see* Butalbital Compound and Acetaminophen* *on page 53*

Acetaminophen and Codeine*
(a seet a MIN oh fen & KOE deen)
U.S. Brand Names Capital® and Codeine; Phenaphen® With Codeine; Tylenol® With Codeine
Canadian Brand Names Atasol® 8, 15, 30 With Caffeine; Empracet® 30, 60; Emtec-30®; Lenoltec No 1, 2, 3, 4; Novo-Gesic-C8; Novo-Gesic-C15; Novo-Gesic-C30
(Continued)

Acetaminophen and Codeine* *(Continued)*

Synonyms Codeine and Acetaminophen
Pharmacologic Class Analgesic, Narcotic
Nutrients Depleted
  Glutathione *on page 327*
Scientific Basis Published scientific studies using this pharmacologic agent (acetaminophen)
Studies & Abstracts 517-518

♦ **Acetaminophen and Hydrocodone** *see* Hydrocodone and Acetaminophen* *on page 149*

♦ **Acetaminophen and Oxycodone** *see* Oxycodone and Acetaminophen* *on page 202*

♦ **Acetazolam®** *see* Acetazolamide* *on page 24*

Acetazolamide* (a set a ZOLE a mide)

U.S. Brand Names Diamox®; Diamox Sequels®
Canadian Brand Names Acetazolam®; Apo®-Acetazolamide; Novo-Zolamide
Pharmacologic Class Anticonvulsant, Miscellaneous; Carbonic Anhydrase Inhibitor; Diuretic, Carbonic Anhydrase Inhibitor; Ophthalmic Agent, Antiglaucoma
Nutrients Depleted
  Potassium *on page 340*
  Sodium *on page 345*
Scientific Basis Inferred or indirect evidence of depletion based on disruption of physiologic processes
Studies & Abstracts 329-337
Additional Information Sodium and/or bicarbonate replacement is not recommended unless specifically instructed by the prescriber (may decrease therapeutic effect).

Acetohexamide* (a set oh HEKS a mide)

Related Information
  Drug-Induced Nutrient Depletion Table *on page 498*
U.S. Brand Names Dymelor®
Pharmacologic Class Antidiabetic Agent, Oral
Nutrients Depleted
  Coenzyme Q_{10} *on page 320*
Scientific Basis Published scientific studies using this pharmacologic agent
Studies & Abstracts 167

Acetophenazine* (a set oh FEN a zeen)

U.S. Brand Names Tindal®
Synonyms Acetophenazine Maleate
Pharmacologic Class Antipsychotic Agent, Phenothiazine, Piperazine
Nutrients Depleted
  Coenzyme Q_{10} *on page 320*

Vitamin B$_2$ *on page 353*
Scientific Basis Published scientific studies of agents from the same pharmacologic class
Studies & Abstracts 473-476

- **Acetophenazine Maleate** *see* Acetophenazine* *on page 24*
- **Acetoxymethylprogesterone** *see* Medroxyprogesterone Acetate *on page 173*
- **Acetylsalicylic Acid** *see* Aspirin* *on page 40*
- **Achromycin® Ophthalmic** *see* Tetracycline* *on page 249*
- **Achromycin® Topical** *see* Tetracycline* *on page 249*
- **Aciclovir** *see* Acyclovir *on page 25*
- **Aciphex™** *see* Rabeprazole* *on page 228*
- **ACT** *see* Dactinomycin* *on page 90*
- **Actifed® Allergy Tablet (Day) [OTC]** *see* Pseudoephedrine *on page 225*
- **Actinomycin D** *see* Dactinomycin* *on page 90*
- **Actiprofen®** *see* Ibuprofen* *on page 153*
- **Actiq® Oral Transmucosal** *see* Fentanyl *on page 125*
- **Activated Dimethicone** *see* Simethicone *on page 238*
- **Activated Methylpolysiloxane** *see* Simethicone *on page 238*
- **Activella™** *see* Estradiol and Norethindrone* *on page 115*
- **Actonel™** *see* Risedronate *on page 232*
- **Actos™** *see* Pioglitazone *on page 213*
- **Actron® [OTC]** *see* Ketoprofen* *on page 160*
- **Acutrim® 16 Hours [OTC]** *see* Phenylpropanolamine *on page 211*
- **Acutrim® II, Maximum Strength [OTC]** *see* Phenylpropanolamine *on page 211*
- **Acutrim® Late Day [OTC]** *see* Phenylpropanolamine *on page 211*
- **ACV** *see* Acyclovir *on page 25*
- **Acycloguanosine** *see* Acyclovir *on page 25*

Acyclovir (ay SYE kloe veer)
U.S. Brand Names Zovirax®
Canadian Brand Names Avirax™
Synonyms Aciclovir; ACV; Acycloguanosine
Pharmacologic Class Antiviral Agent
Nutrients Depleted
Specific nutrient depletions have not been documented for this agent.

- **Adalat®** *see* Nifedipine *on page 192*
- **Adalat® CC** *see* Nifedipine *on page 192*
- **Adalat PA®** *see* Nifedipine *on page 192*
- **Adamantanamine Hydrochloride** *see* Amantadine *on page 30*
- **Adapin® Oral** *see* Doxepin* *on page 106*
- **Adderall®** *see* Dextroamphetamine and Amphetamine *on page 96*
- **Adipex-P®** *see* Phentermine *on page 211*
- **Adlone® Injection** *see* Methylprednisolone* *on page 178*
- **ADR** *see* Doxorubicin* *on page 106*

- **Adriamycin PFS**™ *see* Doxorubicin* *on page 106*
- **Adriamycin RDF**® *see* Doxorubicin* *on page 106*
- **Adrucil® Injection** *see* Fluorouracil* *on page 130*
- **Advair**™ **Diskus**® *see* Fluticasone and Salmeterol* *on page 132*
- **Advil® [OTC]** *see* Ibuprofen* *on page 153*
- **Advil® Cold & Sinus Caplets [OTC]** *see* Pseudoephedrine and Ibuprofen* *on page 226*
- **Advil® Migraine Liqui-Gels [OTC]** *see* Ibuprofen* *on page 153*
- **AeroBid®-M Oral Aerosol Inhaler** *see* Flunisolide* *on page 129*
- **AeroBid® Oral Aerosol Inhaler** *see* Flunisolide* *on page 129*
- **Aerolate III®** *see* Theophylline* *on page 250*
- **Aerolate JR®** *see* Theophylline* *on page 250*
- **Aerolate SR®** *see* Theophylline* *on page 250*
- **Aeroseb-Dex®** *see* Dexamethasone* *on page 95*
- **Aeroseb-HC®** *see* Hydrocortisone* *on page 150*
- **A.F. Anacin®** *see* Acetaminophen* *on page 23*
- **Afrin® Tablet [OTC]** *see* Pseudoephedrine *on page 225*
- **Aggrastat®** *see* Tirofiban *on page 255*
- **Aggrenox**™ *see* Aspirin and Extended-Release Dipyridamole* *on page 40*
- **Agoral® Plain [OTC]** *see* Mineral Oil* *on page 181*
- **A-hydroCort®** *see* Hydrocortisone* *on page 150*
- **Airet®** *see* Albuterol *on page 26*
- **AK-Dex® Ophthalmic** *see* Dexamethasone* *on page 95*
- **Akineton®** *see* Biperiden *on page 48*
- **AK-Pred® Ophthalmic** *see* Prednisolone* *on page 218*
- **AKTob® Ophthalmic** *see* Tobramycin* *on page 255*
- **Ala-Cort®** *see* Hydrocortisone* *on page 150*
- **Ala-Scalp®** *see* Hydrocortisone* *on page 150*
- **Alatrofloxacin Mesylate** *see* Trovafloxacin* *on page 263*
- **Albert® Docusate** *see* Docusate *on page 104*
- **Albert® Glyburide** *see* Glyburide* *on page 139*
- **Albert® Pentoxifylline** *see* Pentoxifylline *on page 209*

Albuterol (al BYOO ter ole)

U.S. Brand Names Airet®; Proventil®; Proventil® HFA; Ventolin®; Ventolin® Rotocaps®; Volmax®

Canadian Brand Names Apo®-Salvent; Novo-Salmol; Sabulin

Synonyms Salbutamol

Pharmacologic Class Beta₂ Agonist

Nutrients Depleted

Specific nutrient depletions have not been documented for this agent.

Additional Information Although beta-agonists may cause a decrease (transient) in serum potassium, this is generally related to an intracellular shift, rather than a depletion of this ion.

- **Aldactazide®** *see* Hydrochlorothiazide and Spironolactone* *on page 148*

♦ **Aldactone**® *see* Spironolactone *on page 241*

♦ **Aldomet**® *see* Methyldopa* *on page 177*

♦ **Aldoril**® *see* Methyldopa and Hydrochlorothiazide* *on page 178*

♦ **Aldoril**®-15 *see* Methyldopa and Hydrochlorothiazide* *on page 178*

♦ **Aldoril**®-25 *see* Methyldopa and Hydrochlorothiazide* *on page 178*

Alendronate (a LEN droe nate)
U.S. Brand Names Fosamax®
Synonyms Alendronate Sodium
Pharmacologic Class Bisphosphonate Derivative
Nutrients Depleted
  Specific nutrient depletions have not been documented for this agent.
Additional Information Bisphosphonates have been (rarely) associated with hypocalcemia, as a natural extension of their therapeutic action. Correction of hypocalcemia is recommended prior to alendronate treatment. When used for osteoporosis or Paget's disease, adequate vitamin D and calcium intake should be ensured to provide for enhanced needs. Calcium administration should be separated from alendronate by at least 30 minutes.

♦ **Alendronate Sodium** *see* Alendronate *on page 27*

♦ **Alesse**™ *see* Ethinyl Estradiol and Levonorgestrel* *on page 120*

♦ **Aleve**® **[OTC]** *see* Naproxen* *on page 189*

♦ **Alkaban-AQ**® *see* Vinblastine* *on page 267*

♦ **Allegra**® *see* Fexofenadine *on page 127*

♦ **Allegra-D**™ *see* Fexofenadine and Pseudoephedrine *on page 127*

♦ **Aller-Chlor**® **[OTC]** *see* Chlorpheniramine *on page 73*

♦ **Allerdryl**® *see* Diphenhydramine *on page 102*

♦ **Allerest**® **12 Hour Capsule [OTC]** *see* Chlorpheniramine and Phenylpropanolamine *on page 73*

♦ **Allerest**® **Maximum Strength [OTC]** *see* Chlorpheniramine and Pseudoephedrine *on page 73*

♦ **AllerMax**® **Oral [OTC]** *see* Diphenhydramine *on page 102*

♦ **Allernix**® *see* Diphenhydramine *on page 102*

Allopurinol (al oh PURE i nole)
U.S. Brand Names Aloprim®; Zyloprim®
Canadian Brand Names Apo®-Allopurinol; Novo-Purol; Purinol®
Synonyms Allopurinol Sodium Injection
Pharmacologic Class Xanthine Oxidase Inhibitor
Nutrients Depleted
  Specific nutrient depletions have not been documented for this agent.

♦ **Allopurinol Sodium Injection** *see* Allopurinol *on page 27*

♦ **Aloprim**® *see* Allopurinol *on page 27*

♦ **Alor**® **5/500** *see* Hydrocodone and Aspirin* *on page 150*

♦ **Alora**® **Transdermal** *see* Estradiol* *on page 114*

♦ **Alpha-Baclofen**® *see* Baclofen *on page 44*

♦ **Alpha-Tamoxifen**® *see* Tamoxifen *on page 247*

♦ **Alphatrex**® *see* Betamethasone* *on page 46*

Alprazolam (al PRAY zoe lam)
U.S. Brand Names Xanax®
Canadian Brand Names Apo®-Alpraz; Novo-Alprazol; Nu-Alprax
Pharmacologic Class Benzodiazepine
Nutrients Depleted
  Specific nutrient depletions have not been documented for this agent.

Alprostadil (al PROS ta dill)
U.S. Brand Names Caverject® Injection; Edex® Injection; Muse® Pellet; Prostin VR Pediatric® Injection
Synonyms PGE$_1$; Prostaglandin E$_1$
Pharmacologic Class Prostaglandin
Nutrients Depleted
  Specific nutrient depletions have not been documented for this agent.

♦ **AL-R® [OTC]** *see* Chlorpheniramine *on page 73*
♦ **Altace™** *see* Ramipril* *on page 228*
♦ **ALternaGEL® [OTC]** *see* Aluminum Hydroxide* *on page 28*
♦ **Alu-Cap® [OTC]** *see* Aluminum Hydroxide* *on page 28*
♦ **Aludrox® [OTC]** *see* Aluminum Hydroxide and Magnesium Hydroxide* *on page 29*

Aluminum Hydroxide* (a LOO mi num hye DROKS ide)
Related Information
  Drug-Induced Nutrient Depletion Table *on page 498*
U.S. Brand Names ALternaGEL® [OTC]; Alu-Cap® [OTC]; Alu-Tab® [OTC]; Amphojel® [OTC]; Dialume® [OTC]; Nephrox Suspension [OTC]
Pharmacologic Class Antacid; Antidote
Nutrients Depleted
  Calcium *on page 313*
  Phosphorus *on page 339*
  Vitamin D *on page 363*
Scientific Basis Published scientific studies using this pharmacologic agent
Studies & Abstracts 1-5
Additional Information Aluminum salts may be used to prevent hyperphophatemia, therefore routine supplementation is not recommended.

Aluminum Hydroxide and Magnesium Carbonate*
  (a LOO mi num hye DROKS ide & mag NEE zhum KAR bun nate)
Related Information
  Drug-Induced Nutrient Depletion Table *on page 498*
U.S. Brand Names Gaviscon® Liquid [OTC]
Pharmacologic Class Antacid
Nutrients Depleted
  Calcium *on page 313*

Phosphorus *on page 339*
Vitamin D *on page 363*

Scientific Basis Published scientific studies of agents from the same pharmacologic class

Studies & Abstracts 1-5

Aluminum Hydroxide and Magnesium Hydroxide*

(a LOO mi num hye DROKS ide & mag NEE zhum hye DROK side)

Related Information

Drug-Induced Nutrient Depletion Table *on page 498*

U.S. Brand Names Aludrox® [OTC]; Maalox® [OTC]; Maalox® Therapeutic Concentrate [OTC]

Synonyms Magnesium Hydroxide and Aluminum Hydroxide

Pharmacologic Class Antacid

Nutrients Depleted

Calcium *on page 313*
Phosphorus *on page 339*
Vitamin D *on page 363*

Scientific Basis Published scientific studies of agents from the same pharmacologic class

Studies & Abstracts 1-5

Aluminum Hydroxide and Magnesium Trisilicate*

(a LOO mi num hye DROKS ide & mag NEE zhum trye SIL i kate)

Related Information

Drug-Induced Nutrient Depletion Table *on page 498*

U.S. Brand Names Gaviscon®-2 Tablet [OTC]; Gaviscon® Tablet [OTC]

Pharmacologic Class Antacid

Nutrients Depleted

Calcium *on page 313*
Phosphorus *on page 339*
Vitamin D *on page 363*

Scientific Basis Published scientific studies of agents from the same pharmacologic class

Studies & Abstracts 1-5

Aluminum Hydroxide, Magnesium Hydroxide, and Simethicone*

(a LOO mi num hye DROKS ide, mag NEE zhum hye DROKS ide, & sye METH i kone)

Related Information

Drug-Induced Nutrient Depletion Table *on page 498*

U.S. Brand Names Di-Gel® [OTC]; Gas-Ban DS® [OTC]; Gelusil® [OTC]; Maalox® Plus [OTC]; Magalox Plus® [OTC]; Mylanta® [OTC]; Mylanta®-II [OTC]

(Continued)

Aluminum Hydroxide, Magnesium Hydroxide, and Simethicone* *(Continued)*

Pharmacologic Class Antacid; Antiflatulent
Nutrients Depleted
  Calcium *on page 313*
  Phosphorus *on page 339*
  Vitamin D *on page 363*
Scientific Basis Published scientific studies of agents from the same pharmacologic class
Studies & Abstracts 1-5

♦ **Aluminum Sucrose Sulfate, Basic** *see* Sucralfate* *on page 242*
♦ **Alu-Tab® [OTC]** *see* Aluminum Hydroxide* *on page 28*

Amantadine (a MAN ta deen)
U.S. Brand Names Symmetrel®
Canadian Brand Names Endantadine®; PMS-Amantadine
Synonyms Adamantanamine Hydrochloride; Amantadine Hydrochloride
Pharmacologic Class Anti-Parkinson's Agent (Dopamine Agonist); Antiviral Agent
Nutrients Depleted
  Specific nutrient depletions have not been documented for this agent.

♦ **Amantadine Hydrochloride** *see* Amantadine *on page 30*
♦ **Amaphen®** *see* Butalbital Compound and Acetaminophen* *on page 53*
♦ **Amaryl®** *see* Glimepiride* *on page 139*
♦ **Ambien™** *see* Zolpidem *on page 271*
♦ **AmBisome®** *see* Amphotericin B (Liposomal)* *on page 35*
♦ **Amcort®** *see* Triamcinolone* *on page 259*
♦ **Amen® Oral** *see* Medroxyprogesterone Acetate *on page 173*
♦ **Amerge®** *see* Naratriptan *on page 189*
♦ **A-methaPred® Injection** *see* Methylprednisolone* *on page 178*
♦ **Amethopterin** *see* Methotrexate* *on page 176*
♦ **Amfepramone** *see* Diethylpropion *on page 99*

Amikacin* (am i KAY sin)
Related Information
  Drug-Induced Nutrient Depletion Table *on page 498*
U.S. Brand Names Amikin® Injection
Canadian Brand Names Amikin®
Synonyms Amikacin Sulfate
Pharmacologic Class Antibiotic, Aminoglycoside
Nutrients Depleted
  Bifidobacteria bifidum (bifidus) *on page 311*
  Biotin *on page 311*
  Calcium *on page 313*
  Inositol *on page 328*
  Lactobacillus acidophilus *on page 332*

Magnesium *on page 333*
Potassium *on page 340*
Sodium *on page 345*
Vitamin B_1 *on page 351*
Vitamin B_2 *on page 353*
Vitamin B_3 *on page 354*
Vitamin B_6 *on page 357*
Vitamin B_{12} *on page 359*
Vitamin K *on page 367*

Scientific Basis
Published scientific studies of agents from the same pharmacologic class
or
Inferred or indirect evidence of depletion based on disruption of physiologic processes

Studies & Abstracts 7-37

♦ **Amikacin Sulfate** *see* Amikacin* *on page 30*
♦ **Amikin®** *see* Amikacin* *on page 30*
♦ **Amikin® Injection** *see* Amikacin* *on page 30*

Amiloride* (a MIL oh ride)
U.S. Brand Names Midamor®
Synonyms Amiloride Hydrochloride
Pharmacologic Class Diuretic, Potassium Sparing
Nutrients Depleted
Folic Acid *on page 325*
Calcium *on page 313*
Scientific Basis Inferred or indirect evidence of depletion based on disruption of physiologic processes
Studies & Abstracts 313-319

Amiloride and Hydrochlorothiazide*
(a MIL oh ride & hye droe klor oh THYE a zide)
U.S. Brand Names Moduretic®
Canadian Brand Names Apo®-Amilzide; Moduret®; Novamilor; Nu-Amilzide
Synonyms Hydrochlorothiazide and Amiloride
Pharmacologic Class Diuretic, Combination
Nutrients Depleted
Coenzyme Q_{10} *on page 320*
Magnesium *on page 333*
Phosphorus *on page 339*
Potassium *on page 340*
Sodium *on page 345*
Zinc *on page 368*
Scientific Basis Published scientific studies using these pharmacologic agents
Studies & Abstracts 320-342
Additional Information Although thiazide diuretics deplete sodium, replacement is not recommended, as this may be directly related to
(Continued)

31

Amiloride and Hydrochlorothiazide* *(Continued)*

the therapeutic effect. Thiazides may deplete potassium; however, when combined with a potassium-sparing diuretic (amiloride), potassium loss is variable. Replacement should be guided by monitoring of serum concentrations and specific instruction by a healthcare provider.

♦ **Amiloride Hydrochloride** *see* Amiloride* *on page 31*

♦ **2-Amino-6-Trifluoromethoxy-benzothiazole** *see* Riluzole *on page 232*

♦ **5-Aminosalicylic Acid** *see* Mesalamine* *on page 174*

Amiodarone (a MEE oh da rone)

U.S. Brand Names Cordarone®; Pacerone®
Synonyms Amiodarone Hydrochloride
Pharmacologic Class Antiarrhythmic Agent, Class III
Nutrients Depleted
Specific nutrient depletions have not been documented for this agent.

♦ **Amiodarone Hydrochloride** *see* Amiodarone *on page 32*

♦ **Ami-Tex LA®** *see* Guaifenesin and Phenylpropanolamine *on page 141*

Amitriptyline* (a mee TRIP ti leen)

Related Information
Drug-Induced Nutrient Depletion Table *on page 498*
U.S. Brand Names Elavil®; Enovil®
Canadian Brand Names Apo®-Amitriptyline; Levate®; Novo-Tryptin
Synonyms Amitriptyline Hydrochloride
Pharmacologic Class Antidepressant, Tricyclic (Tertiary Amine)
Nutrients Depleted
Coenzyme Q_{10} *on page 320*
Vitamin B_2 *on page 353*
Scientific Basis Published scientific studies using this pharmacologic agent
Studies & Abstracts 467-472

♦ **Amitriptyline Hydrochloride** *see* Amitriptyline* *on page 32*

Amlodipine (am LOE di peen)

U.S. Brand Names Norvasc®
Pharmacologic Class Calcium Channel Blocker
Nutrients Depleted
Specific nutrient depletions have not been documented for this agent.

Amoxapine* (a MOKS a peen)

U.S. Brand Names Asendin®
Pharmacologic Class Antidepressant, Tricyclic (Secondary Amine)
Nutrients Depleted
Coenzyme Q_{10} *on page 320*
Vitamin B_2 *on page 353*
Scientific Basis Published scientific studies of agents from the same pharmacologic class

Studies & Abstracts 467-472

Amoxicillin* (a moks i SIL in)
Related Information
Drug-Induced Nutrient Depletion Table *on page 498*
U.S. Brand Names Amoxil®; Biomox®; Trimox®; Wymox®
Canadian Brand Names Apo®-Amoxi; Novamoxin®; Nu-Amoxi; Pro-Amox®
Synonyms Amoxicillin Trihydrate; Amoxycillin; *p*-Hydroxyampicillin
Pharmacologic Class Antibiotic, Penicillin
Nutrients Depleted
Bifidobacteria bifidum (bifidus) on page 311
Biotin *on page 311*
Inositol *on page 328*
Lactobacillus acidophilus on page 332
Potassium *on page 340*
Vitamin B$_1$ *on page 351*
Vitamin B$_2$ *on page 353*
Vitamin B$_3$ *on page 354*
Vitamin B$_6$ *on page 357*
Vitamin B$_{12}$ *on page 359*
Vitamin K *on page 367*
Scientific Basis Inferred or indirect evidence of depletion based on disruption of physiologic processes
Studies & Abstracts 7-27, 49-57

♦ **Amoxicillin Trihydrate** *see* Amoxicillin* *on page 33*
♦ **Amoxil®** *see* Amoxicillin* *on page 33*
♦ **Amoxycillin** *see* Amoxicillin* *on page 33*

Amphetamine (am FET a meen)
Synonyms Amphetamine Sulfate; Racemic Amphetamine Sulfate
Pharmacologic Class Stimulant
Nutrients Depleted
Specific nutrient depletions have not been documented for this agent.

♦ **Amphetamine Sulfate** *see* Amphetamine *on page 33*
♦ **Amphojel® [OTC]** *see* Aluminum Hydroxide* *on page 28*
♦ **Amphotec®** *see* Amphotericin B Cholesteryl Sulfate Complex* *on page 33*

Amphotericin B Cholesteryl Sulfate Complex*
(am foe TER i sin bee kole LES te ril SUL fate KOM plecks)
U.S. Brand Names Amphotec®
Synonyms ABCD; Amphotericin B Colloidal Dispersion
Pharmacologic Class Antifungal Agent, Parenteral
Nutrients Depleted
Calcium *on page 313*
Magnesium *on page 333*
Potassium *on page 340*
Sodium *on page 345*
(Continued)

Amphotericin B Cholesteryl Sulfate Complex*
(Continued)
Scientific Basis Published scientific studies using this pharmacologic agent

Studies & Abstracts 177-181

Additional Information Formulations may limit the extent of electrolyte loss. Liposomal formulations are less frequently associated with severe electrolyte disturbances.

♦ **Amphotericin B Colloidal Dispersion** *see* Amphotericin B Cholesteryl Sulfate Complex* *on page 33*

Amphotericin B (Conventional)*
(am foe TER i sin bee con VEN sha nal)

Related Information
Drug-Induced Nutrient Depletion Table *on page 498*

U.S. Brand Names Fungizone®

Synonyms Amphotericin B Desoxycholate

Pharmacologic Class Antifungal Agent, Parenteral; Antifungal Agent, Topical

Nutrients Depleted
Calcium *on page 313*
Magnesium *on page 333*
Potassium *on page 340*
Sodium *on page 345*

Scientific Basis Published scientific studies using this pharmacologic agent

Studies & Abstracts 177-181

Additional Information Formulations may limit the extent of electrolyte loss. Liposomal formulations are less frequently associated with severe electrolyte disturbances.

♦ **Amphotericin B Desoxycholate** *see* Amphotericin B (Conventional)* *on page 34*

Amphotericin B (Lipid Complex)*
(am foe TER i sin bee LIP id KOM pleks)

Related Information
Drug-Induced Nutrient Depletion Table *on page 498*

U.S. Brand Names Abelcet™

Synonyms ABLC

Pharmacologic Class Antifungal Agent, Parenteral

Nutrients Depleted
Calcium *on page 313*
Magnesium *on page 333*
Potassium *on page 340*
Sodium *on page 345*

Scientific Basis Published scientific studies using this pharmacologic agent

Studies & Abstracts 177-181

Additional Information Formulations may limit the extent of electrolyte loss. Liposomal formulations are less frequently associated with severe electrolyte disturbances.

Amphotericin B (Liposomal)*
(am foe TER i sin bee lye po SO mal)
Related Information
Drug-Induced Nutrient Depletion Table *on page 498*
U.S. Brand Names AmBisome®
Synonyms L-AmB
Pharmacologic Class Antifungal Agent, Parenteral
Nutrients Depleted
Calcium *on page 313*
Magnesium *on page 333*
Potassium *on page 340*
Sodium *on page 345*
Scientific Basis Published scientific studies using this pharmacologic agent
Studies & Abstracts 177-181
Additional Information Formulations may limit the extent of electrolyte loss. Liposomal formulations are less frequently associated with severe electrolyte disturbances.

Ampicillin* (am pi SIL in)
Related Information
Drug-Induced Nutrient Depletion Table *on page 498*
U.S. Brand Names Marcillin®; Omnipen®; Omnipen®-N; Polycillin-N®; Principen®
Canadian Brand Names Ampicin® Sodium; Apo®-Ampi Trihydrate; Jaa Amp® Trihydrate; Nu-Ampi Trihydrate; Pro-Ampi® Trihydrate; Taro-Ampicillin® Trihydrate
Pharmacologic Class Antibiotic, Penicillin
Nutrients Depleted
Bifidobacteria bifidum (bifidus) on page 311
Biotin *on page 311*
Inositol *on page 328*
Lactobacillus acidophilus on page 332
Potassium *on page 340*
Vitamin B_1 *on page 351*
Vitamin B_2 *on page 353*
Vitamin B_3 *on page 354*
Vitamin B_6 *on page 357*
Vitamin B_{12} *on page 359*
Vitamin K *on page 367*
Scientific Basis Inferred or indirect evidence of depletion based on disruption of physiologic processes
Studies & Abstracts 7-27, 49-57

♦ **Ampicin® Sodium** *see* Ampicillin* *on page 35*
♦ **Anacin® [OTC]** *see* Aspirin* *on page 40*
♦ **Anafranil®** *see* Clomipramine* *on page 80*

- **Anamine® Syrup [OTC]** *see* Chlorpheniramine and Pseudoephedrine *on page 73*
- **Anaplex® Liquid [OTC]** *see* Chlorpheniramine and Pseudoephedrine *on page 73*
- **Anaprox®** *see* Naproxen* *on page 189*
- **Anaspaz®** *see* Hyoscyamine *on page 153*
- **Anatuss® [OTC]** *see* Guaifenesin, Phenylpropanolamine, and Dextromethorphan *on page 142*
- **Anatuss® DM [OTC]** *see* Guaifenesin, Pseudoephedrine, and Dextromethorphan *on page 143*
- **Ancef®** *see* Cefazolin* *on page 61*
- **Ancobon®** *see* Flucytosine* *on page 128*
- **Ancotil®** *see* Flucytosine* *on page 128*
- **Andro/Fem® Injection** *see* Estradiol and Testosterone* *on page 115*
- **Anergan®** *see* Promethazine* *on page 222*
- **Anexsia®** *see* Hydrocodone and Acetaminophen* *on page 149*
- **Anhydron®** *see* Cyclothiazide* *on page 89*
- **Anodynos-DHC®** *see* Hydrocodone and Acetaminophen* *on page 149*
- **Anoquan®** *see* Butalbital Compound and Acetaminophen* *on page 53*
- **Ansaid® Oral** *see* Flurbiprofen* *on page 131*
- **Ansamycin** *see* Rifabutin* *on page 231*
- **Antabuse®** *see* Disulfiram *on page 103*
- **Antihist-1® [OTC]** *see* Clemastine *on page 79*
- **Antihist-D®** *see* Clemastine and Phenylpropanolamine *on page 79*
- **Antispas® Injection** *see* Dicyclomine *on page 98*
- **Anti-Tuss® Expectorant [OTC]** *see* Guaifenesin *on page 140*
- **Antivert®** *see* Meclizine *on page 172*
- **Antizol®** *see* Fomepizole *on page 133*
- **Antrizine®** *see* Meclizine *on page 172*
- **Anucort-HC® Suppository** *see* Hydrocortisone* *on page 150*
- **Anuprep HC® Suppository** *see* Hydrocortisone* *on page 150*
- **Anusol® HC 1 [OTC]** *see* Hydrocortisone* *on page 150*
- **Anusol® HC 2.5% [OTC]** *see* Hydrocortisone* *on page 150*
- **Anusol-HC® Suppository** *see* Hydrocortisone* *on page 150*
- **Anxanil®** *see* Hydroxyzine *on page 152*
- **Anzemet®** *see* Dolasetron *on page 105*
- **Apacet® [OTC]** *see* Acetaminophen* *on page 23*
- **APAP** *see* Acetaminophen* *on page 23*
- **Apo®-Acetazolamide** *see* Acetazolamide* *on page 24*
- **Apo®-Allopurinol** *see* Allopurinol *on page 27*
- **Apo®-Alpraz** *see* Alprazolam *on page 28*
- **Apo®-Amilzide** *see* Amiloride and Hydrochlorothiazide* *on page 31*
- **Apo®-Amitriptyline** *see* Amitriptyline* *on page 32*
- **Apo®-Amoxi** *see* Amoxicillin* *on page 33*

- **Apo®-Ampi Trihydrate** *see* Ampicillin* *on page 35*
- **Apo®-ASA** *see* Aspirin* *on page 40*
- **Apo®-Atenol** *see* Atenolol* *on page 41*
- **Apo® Bromocriptine** *see* Bromocriptine *on page 50*
- **Apo®-Capto** *see* Captopril* *on page 57*
- **Apo®-Carbamazepine** *see* Carbamazepine* *on page 57*
- **Apo®-Cefaclor** *see* Cefaclor* *on page 60*
- **Apo®-Cephalex** *see* Cephalexin* *on page 69*
- **Apo®-Chlordiazepoxide** *see* Chlordiazepoxide *on page 72*
- **Apo®-Chlorpromazine** *see* Chlorpromazine* *on page 74*
- **Apo®-Chlorpropamide** *see* Chlorpropamide* *on page 74*
- **Apo®-Chlorthalidone** *see* Chlorthalidone* *on page 74*
- **Apo®-Cimetidine** *see* Cimetidine* *on page 76*
- **Apo®-Clomipramine** *see* Clomipramine* *on page 80*
- **Apo®-Clonidine** *see* Clonidine* *on page 81*
- **Apo®-Clorazepate** *see* Clorazepate *on page 81*
- **Apo®-Diazepam** *see* Diazepam *on page 97*
- **Apo®-Diclo** *see* Diclofenac* *on page 97*
- **Apo®-Diflunisal** *see* Diflunisal* *on page 100*
- **Apo®-Diltiaz** *see* Diltiazem *on page 101*
- **Apo®-Dipyridamole FC** *see* Dipyridamole *on page 103*
- **Apo®-Dipyridamole SC** *see* Dipyridamole *on page 103*
- **Apo®-Doxepin** *see* Doxepin *on page 106*
- **Apo®-Doxy** *see* Doxycycline* *on page 106*
- **Apo®-Doxy Tabs** *see* Doxycycline* *on page 106*
- **Apo®-Enalapril** *see* Enalapril* *on page 110*
- **Apo®-Erythro E-C** *see* Erythromycin (Systemic)* *on page 113*
- **Apo®-Famotidine** *see* Famotidine* *on page 123*
- **Apo®-Fenofibrate** *see* Fenofibrate* *on page 124*
- **Apo®-Fluphenazine** *see* Fluphenazine* *on page 131*
- **Apo®-Flurazepam** *see* Flurazepam *on page 131*
- **Apo®-Flurbiprofen** *see* Flurbiprofen* *on page 131*
- **Apo®-Fluvoxamine** *see* Fluvoxamine *on page 133*
- **Apo®-Furosemide** *see* Furosemide* *on page 135*
- **Apo®-Gemfibrozil** *see* Gemfibrozil* *on page 137*
- **Apo®-Glyburide** *see* Glyburide* *on page 139*
- **Apo®-Hydralazine** *see* Hydralazine* *on page 146*
- **Apo®-Hydro** *see* Hydrochlorothiazide* *on page 147*
- **Apo®-Hydroxyzine** *see* Hydroxyzine *on page 152*
- **Apo®-Ibuprofen** *see* Ibuprofen* *on page 153*
- **Apo®-Imipramine** *see* Imipramine* *on page 154*
- **Apo®-Indapadmide** *see* Indapamide* *on page 154*
- **Apo®-Indomethacin** *see* Indomethacin* *on page 155*
- **Apo®-ISDN** *see* Isosorbide Dinitrate *on page 158*
- **Apo®-Keto** *see* Ketoprofen* *on page 160*
- **Apo®-Keto-E** *see* Ketoprofen* *on page 160*

- **Apo®-Lisinopril** *see* Lisinopril* *on page 166*
- **Apo®-Lorazepam** *see* Lorazepam *on page 168*
- **Apo®-Lovastatin** *see* Lovastatin* *on page 169*
- **Apo®-Methazide** *see* Methyldopa and Hydrochlorothiazide* *on page 178*
- **Apo®-Methyldopa** *see* Methyldopa* *on page 177*
- **Apo®-Metoclop** *see* Metoclopramide *on page 179*
- **Apo®-Metoprolol (Type L)** *see* Metoprolol* *on page 179*
- **Apo®-Metronidazole** *see* Metronidazole* *on page 180*
- **Apo®-Minocycline** *see* Minocycline* *on page 182*
- **Apo®-Nadol** *see* Nadolol* *on page 187*
- **Apo®-Naproxen** *see* Naproxen* *on page 189*
- **Apo®-Nifed** *see* Nifedipine *on page 192*
- **Apo®-Nitrofurantoin** *see* Nitrofurantoin* *on page 192*
- **Apo®-Nizatidine** *see* Nizatidine* *on page 193*
- **Apo®-Nortriptyline** *see* Nortriptyline* *on page 194*
- **Apo®-Oxazepam** *see* Oxazepam *on page 201*
- **Apo®-Pentoxifylline SR** *see* Pentoxifylline *on page 209*
- **Apo®-Pen VK** *see* Penicillin V Potassium* *on page 207*
- **Apo®-Perphenazine** *see* Perphenazine* *on page 210*
- **Apo®-Piroxicam** *see* Piroxicam* *on page 214*
- **Apo®-Prazo** *see* Prazosin *on page 217*
- **Apo®-Prednisone** *see* Prednisone* *on page 219*
- **Apo®-Primidone** *see* Primidone* *on page 220*
- **Apo®-Procainamide** *see* Procainamide *on page 220*
- **Apo®-Propranolol** *see* Propranolol* *on page 223*
- **Apo®-Ranitidine** *see* Ranitidine Hydrochloride* *on page 229*
- **Apo®-Salvent** *see* Albuterol *on page 26*
- **Apo®-Selegiline** *see* Selegiline *on page 236*
- **Apo®-Spirozide** *see* Hydrochlorothiazide and Spironolactone* *on page 148*
- **Apo®-Sulfamethoxazole** *see* Sulfamethoxazole* *on page 243*
- **Apo®-Sulfasalazine** *see* Sulfasalazine* *on page 244*
- **Apo®-Sulfatrim** *see* Co-Trimoxazole* *on page 86*
- **Apo®-Sulin** *see* Sulindac* *on page 245*
- **Apo®-Tamox** *see* Tamoxifen *on page 247*
- **Apo®-Temazepam** *see* Temazepam *on page 248*
- **Apo®-Tetra** *see* Tetracycline* *on page 249*
- **Apo®-Theo LA** *see* Theophylline* *on page 250*
- **Apo®-Thioridazine** *see* Thioridazine* *on page 251*
- **Apo®-Timol** *see* Timolol* *on page 254*
- **Apo®-Timop** *see* Timolol* *on page 254*
- **Apo®-Tolbutamide** *see* Tolbutamide* *on page 256*
- **Apo®-Triazide** *see* Hydrochlorothiazide and Triamterene* *on page 149*
- **Apo®-Triazo** *see* Triazolam *on page 261*

+ **Apo®-Trimip** *see* Trimipramine* *on page 262*
+ **Apo®-Verap** *see* Verapamil *on page 267*
+ **Apo®-Zidovudine** *see* Zidovudine* *on page 270*
+ **APPG** *see* Penicillin G Procaine* *on page 207*
+ **Apresazide®** *see* Hydralazine and Hydrochlorothiazide* *on page 146*
+ **Apresoline®** *see* Hydralazine* *on page 146*
+ **Aquachloral® Supprettes®** *see* Chloral Hydrate *on page 72*
+ **Aquaphyllin®** *see* Theophylline* *on page 250*
+ **Aquatag®** *see* Benzthiazide* *on page 45*
+ **Aquatensen®** *see* Methyclothiazide* *on page 177*
+ **Aqueous Procaine Penicillin G** *see* Penicillin G Procaine* *on page 207*
+ **Arabinosylcytosine** *see* Cytarabine* *on page 89*
+ **Ara-C** *see* Cytarabine* *on page 89*
+ **Aredia™** *see* Pamidronate *on page 203*

Argatroban (ar GA troh ban)
Pharmacologic Class Anticoagulant, Thrombin Inhibitor
Nutrients Depleted
Specific nutrient depletions have not been documented for this agent.

+ **Argesic®-SA** *see* Salsalate* *on page 235*
+ **Aricept®** *see* Donepezil *on page 105*
+ **Aristocort®** *see* Triamcinolone* *on page 259*
+ **Aristocort® A** *see* Triamcinolone* *on page 259*
+ **Aristocort® Forte** *see* Triamcinolone* *on page 259*
+ **Aristocort® Intralesional** *see* Triamcinolone* *on page 259*
+ **Aristospan® Intra-Articular** *see* Triamcinolone* *on page 259*
+ **Aristospan® Intralesional** *see* Triamcinolone* *on page 259*
+ **A.R.M.® Caplet [OTC]** *see* Chlorpheniramine and Phenylpropanolamine *on page 73*
+ **Armour® Thyroid** *see* Thyroid *on page 252*

Arsenic Trioxide (AR se nik tri OKS id)
U.S. Brand Names Trisenox™
Pharmacologic Class Antineoplastic Agent, Miscellaneous
Nutrients Depleted
Specific nutrient depletions have not been documented for this agent.

+ **Artha-G®** *see* Salsalate* *on page 235*
+ **Arthritis Foundation® Pain Reliever [OTC]** *see* Aspirin* *on page 40*
+ **Arthropan® [OTC]** *see* Choline Salicylate* *on page 76*
+ **Arthrotec®** *see* Diclofenac and Misoprostol* *on page 98*
+ **Articulose-50® Injection** *see* Prednisolone* *on page 218*
+ **ASA®** *see* Aspirin* *on page 40*
+ **5-ASA** *see* Mesalamine* *on page 174*
+ **Asacol® Oral** *see* Mesalamine* *on page 174*
+ **Asaphen** *see* Aspirin* *on page 40*

♦ **Ascorbic Acid and Ferrous Sulfate** *see* Ferrous Sulfate and Ascorbic Acid *on page 126*

♦ **Ascriptin® [OTC]** *see* Aspirin* *on page 40*

♦ **Asendin®** *see* Amoxapine* *on page 32*

♦ **Asmalix®** *see* Theophylline* *on page 250*

♦ **A-Spas® S/L** *see* Hyoscyamine *on page 153*

♦ **Aspergum® [OTC]** *see* Aspirin* *on page 40*

Aspirin* (AS pir in)

Related Information
Drug-Induced Nutrient Depletion Table *on page 498*

U.S. Brand Names Anacin® [OTC]; Arthritis Foundation® Pain Reliever [OTC]; A.S.A. [OTC]; Ascriptin® [OTC]; Aspergum® [OTC]; Asprimox® [OTC]; Bayer® Aspirin [OTC]; Bayer® Buffered Aspirin [OTC]; Bayer® Low Adult Strength [OTC]; Bufferin® [OTC]; Buffex® [OTC]; Cama® Arthritis Pain Reliever [OTC]; Easprin®; Ecotrin® [OTC]; Ecotrin® Low Adult Strength [OTC]; Empirin® [OTC]; Extra Strength Adprin-B® [OTC]; Extra Strength Bayer® Enteric 500 Aspirin [OTC]; Extra Strength Bayer® Plus [OTC]; Halfprin® 81® [OTC]; Regular Strength Bayer® Enteric 500 Aspirin [OTC]; St Joseph® Adult Chewable Aspirin [OTC]; ZORprin®

Canadian Brand Names Apo®-ASA; ASA®; Asaphen; Entrophen®; MSD® Enteric Coated ASA; Novasen

Synonyms Acetylsalicylic Acid; ASA

Pharmacologic Class Salicylate

Nutrients Depleted
Folic Acid *on page 325*
Iron *on page 331*
Potassium *on page 340*
Sodium *on page 345*
Vitamin C *on page 360*

Scientific Basis Published scientific studies using this pharmacologic agent

Studies & Abstracts 224-236

♦ **Aspirin and Butalbital Compound** *see* Butalbital Compound and Aspirin* *on page 54*

Aspirin and Extended-Release Dipyridamole*

(AS pir in & dye peer ID a mole)

U.S. Brand Names Aggrenox™

Pharmacologic Class Antiplatelet Agent

Nutrients Depleted
Folic Acid *on page 325*
Iron *on page 331*
Potassium *on page 340*
Sodium *on page 345*
Vitamin C *on page 360*

Scientific Basis Published scientific studies using this pharmacologic agent (aspirin)

Studies & Abstracts 224-235

- ◆ **Aspirin and Hydrocodone** *see* Hydrocodone and Aspirin* *on page 150*
- ◆ **Aspirin and Oxycodone** *see* Oxycodone and Aspirin* *on page 202*
- ◆ **Aspirin Free Anacin®️ Maximum Strength [OTC]** *see* Acetaminophen* *on page 23*
- ◆ **Asprimox®️ [OTC]** *see* Aspirin* *on page 40*
- ◆ **Astramorph™️ PF Injection** *see* Morphine Sulfate *on page 185*
- ◆ **Atacand™️** *see* Candesartan *on page 56*
- ◆ **Atacand HCT™️** *see* Candesartan and Hydrochlorothiazide* *on page 56*
- ◆ **Atarax®️** *see* Hydroxyzine *on page 152*
- ◆ **Atasol®️** *see* Acetaminophen* *on page 23*
- ◆ **Atasol®️ 8, 15, 30 With Caffeine** *see* Acetaminophen and Codeine* *on page 23*

Atenolol* (a TEN oh lole)

Related Information
Drug-Induced Nutrient Depletion Table *on page 498*
U.S. Brand Names Tenormin®️
Canadian Brand Names Apo®️-Atenol; Novo-Atenol; Nu-Atenol; Taro-Atenol®️
Pharmacologic Class Beta Blocker, Beta₁ Selective
Nutrients Depleted
Coenzyme Q₁₀ *on page 320*
Scientific Basis Published scientific studies using this pharmacologic agent
Studies & Abstracts 347-348

Atenolol and Chlorthalidone*

(a TEN oh lole & klor THAL i done)
U.S. Brand Names Tenoretic®️
Synonyms Chlorthalidone and Atenolol
Pharmacologic Class Antihypertensive Agent, Combination
Nutrients Depleted
Coenzyme Q₁₀ *on page 320*
Magnesium *on page 333*
Phosphorus *on page 339*
Potassium *on page 340*
Sodium *on page 345*
Zinc *on page 368*

Scientific Basis
Published scientific studies using these pharmacologic agents
or
Published scientific studies of agents from the same pharmacologic class

Studies & Abstracts 271-272, 347-348

- ◆ **Ativan®️** *see* Lorazepam *on page 168*
- ◆ **Atolone®️** *see* Triamcinolone* *on page 259*

Atorvastatin* (a TORE va sta tin)
Related Information
Drug-Induced Nutrient Depletion Table *on page 498*
U.S. Brand Names Lipitor®
Pharmacologic Class Antilipemic Agent (HMG-CoA Reductase Inhibitor)
Nutrients Depleted
Coenzyme Q_{10} *on page 320*
Scientific Basis Published scientific studies of agents from the same pharmacologic class
Studies & Abstracts 350-361

Atovaquone and Proguanil
(a TOE va kwone & pro GWA nil)
U.S. Brand Names Malarone™
Pharmacologic Class Antimalarial Agent
Nutrients Depleted
Specific nutrient depletions have not been documented for this agent.

- **Atridox**™ *see* Doxycycline* *on page 106*
- **Atromid-S**® *see* Clofibrate *on page 80*
- **Atrovent**® *see* Ipratropium *on page 156*
- **Avandia**® *see* Rosiglitazone *on page 234*
- **Avapro**® *see* Irbesartan *on page 157*
- **Avapro**® **HCT** *see* Irbesartan and Hydrochlorothiazide* *on page 157*
- **Avelox**™ *see* Moxifloxacin* *on page 185*
- **Aventyl**® **Hydrochloride** *see* Nortriptyline* *on page 194*
- **Avirax**™ *see* Acyclovir *on page 25*
- **Avita**® *see* Tretinoin (Topical) *on page 259*
- **Avlosulfon**® *see* Dapsone *on page 91*
- **Avonex**™ *see* Interferon Beta-1a *on page 156*
- **Axid**® *see* Nizatidine* *on page 193*
- **Axid**® **AR [OTC]** *see* Nizatidine* *on page 193*
- **Axocet**® *see* Butalbital Compound and Acetaminophen* *on page 53*
- **Ayercillin**® *see* Penicillin G Procaine* *on page 207*
- **Aygestin**® *see* Norethindrone* *on page 193*

Azathioprine (ay za THYE oh preen)
U.S. Brand Names Imuran®
Synonyms Azathioprine Sodium
Pharmacologic Class Immunosuppressant Agent
Nutrients Depleted
Specific nutrient depletions have not been documented for this agent.

- **Azathioprine Sodium** *see* Azathioprine *on page 42*
- **Azdone**® *see* Hydrocodone and Aspirin* *on page 150*
- **Azidothymidine** *see* Zidovudine* *on page 270*
- **Azidothymidine, Abacavir, and Lamivudine** *see* Abacavir, Lamivudine, and Zidovudine* *on page 22*

Azithromycin* (az ith roe MYE sin)
U.S. Brand Names Zithromax™
Synonyms Azithromycin Dihydrate
Pharmacologic Class Antibiotic, Macrolide
Nutrients Depleted
Bifidobacteria bifidum (bifidus) on page 311
Biotin *on page 311*
Inositol *on page 328*
Lactobacillus acidophilus on page 332
Vitamin B$_1$ *on page 351*
Vitamin B$_2$ *on page 353*
Vitamin B$_3$ *on page 354*
Vitamin B$_6$ *on page 357*
Vitamin B$_{12}$ *on page 359*
Vitamin K *on page 367*
Scientific Basis Inferred or indirect evidence of depletion based on disruption of physiologic processes
Studies & Abstracts 7-27

- **Azithromycin Dihydrate** *see* Azithromycin* *on page 43*
- **Azmacort™** *see* Triamcinolone* *on page 259*
- **Azo-Sulfisoxazole** *see* Sulfisoxazole and Phenazopyridine* *on page 244*
- **AZT** *see* Zidovudine* *on page 270*
- **AZT + 3TC** *see* Zidovudine and Lamivudine* *on page 271*
- **AZT, Abacavir, and Lamivudine** *see* Abacavir, Lamivudine, and Zidovudine* *on page 22*
- **Azulfidine®** *see* Sulfasalazine* *on page 244*
- **Azulfidine® EN-tabs®** *see* Sulfasalazine* *on page 244*

Bacampicillin* (ba kam pi SIL in)
Related Information
Drug-Induced Nutrient Depletion Table *on page 498*
U.S. Brand Names Spectrobid®
Synonyms Bacampicillin Hydrochloride; Carampicillin Hydrochloride
Pharmacologic Class Antibiotic, Penicillin
Nutrients Depleted
Bifidobacteria bifidum (bifidus) on page 311
Biotin *on page 311*
Inositol *on page 328*
Lactobacillus acidophilus on page 332
Potassium *on page 340*
Vitamin B$_1$ *on page 351*
Vitamin B$_2$ *on page 353*
Vitamin B$_3$ *on page 354*
Vitamin B$_6$ *on page 357*
Vitamin B$_{12}$ *on page 359*
Vitamin K *on page 367*
Scientific Basis Inferred or indirect evidence of depletion based on disruption of physiologic processes
(Continued)

Bacampicillin* *(Continued)*
Studies & Abstracts 7-27, 49-57
Additional Information Potassium depletion has been documented primarily with high dose, parenteral penicillins, mostly from the ureidopenicillin group.

♦ **Bacampicillin Hydrochloride** *see* Bacampicillin* *on page 43*

Baclofen *(BAK loe fen)*
U.S. Brand Names Lioresal®
Canadian Brand Names Alpha-Baclofen®; PMS-Baclofen
Pharmacologic Class Skeletal Muscle Relaxant
Nutrients Depleted
Specific nutrient depletions have not been documented for this agent.

♦ **Bactrim™** *see* Co-Trimoxazole* *on page 86*
♦ **Bactrim™ DS** *see* Co-Trimoxazole* *on page 86*
♦ **Baking Soda** *see* Sodium Bicarbonate* *on page 239*
♦ **Baldex®** *see* Dexamethasone* *on page 95*
♦ **Balminil® Decongestant** *see* Pseudoephedrine *on page 225*
♦ **Balminil® Expectorant** *see* Guaifenesin *on page 140*

Balsalazide* *(bal SAL a zide)*
Related Information
Drug-Induced Nutrient Depletion Table *on page 498*
U.S. Brand Names Colazal™
Synonyms Balsalazide Disodium
Pharmacologic Class 5-Aminosalicylic Acid Derivative; Anti-inflammatory Agent
Nutrients Depleted
Folic Acid *on page 325*
Scientific Basis Published scientific studies of agents with the same mechanism of action
Studies & Abstracts 237-245

♦ **Balsalazide Disodium** *see* Balsalazide* *on page 44*
♦ **Bancap HC®** *see* Hydrocodone and Acetaminophen* *on page 149*
♦ **Banophen® Oral [OTC]** *see* Diphenhydramine *on page 102*
♦ **Barbilixir®** *see* Phenobarbital* *on page 210*
♦ **Barbita®** *see* Phenobarbital* *on page 210*
♦ **Baycol®** *see* Cerivastatin* *on page 70*
♦ **Bayer® Aspirin [OTC]** *see* Aspirin* *on page 40*
♦ **Bayer® Buffered Aspirin [OTC]** *see* Aspirin* *on page 40*
♦ **Bayer® Low Adult Strength [OTC]** *see* Aspirin* *on page 40*
♦ **Bayer® Select® Pain Relief Formula [OTC]** *see* Ibuprofen* *on page 153*
♦ **BCNU** *see* Carmustine* *on page 59*
♦ **Beepen-VK®** *see* Penicillin V Potassium* *on page 207*
♦ **Belix® Oral [OTC]** *see* Diphenhydramine *on page 102*
♦ **Benadryl® Injection** *see* Diphenhydramine *on page 102*

+ **Benadryl® Oral [OTC]** *see* Diphenhydramine *on page 102*
+ **Benadryl® Topical** *see* Diphenhydramine *on page 102*
+ **Ben-Allergin-50® Injection** *see* Diphenhydramine *on page 102*

Benazepril* (ben AY ze pril)
Related Information
Drug-Induced Nutrient Depletion Table *on page 498*
U.S. Brand Names Lotensin®
Synonyms Benazepril Hydrochloride
Pharmacologic Class Angiotensin-Converting Enzyme (ACE) Inhibitors
Nutrients Depleted
Zinc *on page 368*
Scientific Basis Published scientific studies of agents from the same pharmacologic class
Studies & Abstracts 269-271

+ **Benazepril Hydrochloride** *see* Benazepril* *on page 45*
+ **Bentyl® Hydrochloride Injection** *see* Dicyclomine *on page 98*
+ **Bentyl® Hydrochloride Oral** *see* Dicyclomine *on page 98*
+ **Bentylol®** *see* Dicyclomine *on page 98*
+ **Benuryl™** *see* Probenecid *on page 220*
+ **Benylin® Cough Syrup [OTC]** *see* Diphenhydramine *on page 102*
+ **Benylin DM® [OTC]** *see* Dextromethorphan *on page 96*
+ **Benylin® Expectorant [OTC]** *see* Guaifenesin and Dextromethorphan *on page 141*
+ **Benylin® Pediatric [OTC]** *see* Dextromethorphan *on page 96*
+ **Benzathine Benzylpenicillin** *see* Penicillin G Benzathine* *on page 205*
+ **Benzathine Penicillin G** *see* Penicillin G Benzathine* *on page 205*
+ **Benzene Hexachloride** *see* Lindane *on page 166*
+ **Benzmethyzin** *see* Procarbazine* *on page 221*

Benzonatate (ben ZOE na tate)
U.S. Brand Names Tessalon® Perles
Pharmacologic Class Antitussive
Nutrients Depleted
Specific nutrient depletions have not been documented for this agent.

Benzthiazide* (benz THYE a zide)
U.S. Brand Names Aquatag®; Exna®; Hydrex®; Marazide®; Proaqua®
Pharmacologic Class Diuretic, Thiazide
Nutrients Depleted
Coenzyme Q_{10} *on page 320*
Magnesium *on page 333*
Phosphorus *on page 339*
Potassium *on page 340*
Sodium *on page 345*
Zinc *on page 368*
(Continued)

Benzthiazide* *(Continued)*

Scientific Basis Published scientific studies of agents from the same pharmacologic class

Studies & Abstracts 320-342

Additional Information Although thiazide diuretics deplete sodium, replacement is not recommended, as this may be directly related to the therapeutic effect. Thiazides may deplete potassium, however replacement should be guided by monitoring of serum concentrations and specific instruction by a healthcare provider.

Benztropine (BENZ troe peen)

U.S. Brand Names Cogentin®

Canadian Brand Names PMS-Benztropine

Synonyms Benztropine Mesylate

Pharmacologic Class Anticholinergic Agent; Anti-Parkinson's Agent (Anticholinergic)

Nutrients Depleted
Specific nutrient depletions have not been documented for this agent.

♦ **Benztropine Mesylate** *see* Benztropine *on page 46*

♦ **Benzylpenicillin Benzathine** *see* Penicillin G Benzathine* *on page 205*

♦ **Benzylpenicillin Potassium** *see* Penicillin G (Parenteral/Aqueous)* *on page 206*

♦ **Benzylpenicillin Sodium** *see* Penicillin G (Parenteral/Aqueous)* *on page 206*

♦ **Betachron E-R® Capsule** *see* Propranolol* *on page 223*

♦ **Betaloc®** *see* Metoprolol* *on page 179*

♦ **Betaloc® Durules®** *see* Metoprolol* *on page 179*

Betamethasone* (bay ta METH a sone)

Related Information
Drug-Induced Nutrient Depletion Table *on page 498*

U.S. Brand Names Alphatrex®; Betatrex®; Celestone®; Celestone® Soluspan®; Diprolene®; Diprolene® AF; Diprosone®; Maxivate®; Teladar®

Canadian Brand Names Betnesol® [Disodium Phosphate]; Diprolene® Glycol [Dipropionate]; Occlucort®; Rhoprolene; Rhoprosone; Taro-Sone; Topilene; Topisone

Synonyms Betamethasone Dipropionate; Betamethasone Dipropionate, Augmented; Betamethasone Sodium Phosphate; Betamethasone Valerate; Flubenisolone

Pharmacologic Class Corticosteroid, Oral; Corticosteroid, Parenteral; Corticosteroid, Topical

Nutrients Depleted
Calcium *on page 313*
Folic Acid *on page 325*
Magnesium *on page 333*
Potassium *on page 340*
Selenium *on page 343*

Vitamin C *on page 360*
Vitamin D *on page 363*
Zinc *on page 368*
Scientific Basis
Published scientific studies using this pharmacologic agent
or
Published scientific studies of agents from the same pharmacologic class
Studies & Abstracts 182-223

- ♦ **Betamethasone Dipropionate** *see* Betamethasone* *on page 46*
- ♦ **Betamethasone Dipropionate, Augmented** *see* Betamethasone* *on page 46*
- ♦ **Betamethasone Sodium Phosphate** *see* Betamethasone* *on page 46*
- ♦ **Betamethasone Valerate** *see* Betamethasone* *on page 46*
- ♦ **Betapace®** *see* Sotalol* *on page 240*
- ♦ **Betapace AF®** *see* Sotalol* *on page 240*
- ♦ **Betapen®-VK** *see* Penicillin V Potassium* *on page 207*
- ♦ **Betaseron®** *see* Interferon Beta-1b *on page 156*
- ♦ **Betatrex®** *see* Betamethasone* *on page 46*

Betaxolol* (be TAKS oh lol)
Related Information
Drug-Induced Nutrient Depletion Table *on page 498*
U.S. Brand Names Betoptic® Ophthalmic; Betoptic® S Ophthalmic; Kerlone® Oral
Synonyms Betaxolol Hydrochloride
Pharmacologic Class Beta Blocker, Beta$_1$ Selective; Ophthalmic Agent, Antiglaucoma
Nutrients Depleted
Coenzyme Q$_{10}$ *on page 320*
Scientific Basis
Published scientific studies using this pharmacologic agent
or
Published scientific studies of agents from the same pharmacologic class
Studies & Abstracts 348-349

- ♦ **Betaxolol Hydrochloride** *see* Betaxolol* *on page 47*

Bethanechol (be THAN e kole)
U.S. Brand Names Duvoid®; Myotonachol™; Urecholine®
Canadian Brand Names PMS-Bethanechol Chloride
Synonyms Bethanechol Chloride
Pharmacologic Class Cholinergic Agonist
Nutrients Depleted
Specific nutrient depletions have not been documented for this agent.

- ♦ **Bethanechol Chloride** *see* Bethanechol *on page 47*
- ♦ **Betimol® Ophthalmic** *see* Timolol* *on page 254*

- **Betnesol® [Disodium Phosphate]** *see* Betamethasone* *on page 46*
- **Betoptic® Ophthalmic** *see* Betaxolol* *on page 47*
- **Betoptic® S Ophthalmic** *see* Betaxolol* *on page 47*
- **Biaxin®** *see* Clarithromycin* *on page 78*
- **Biaxin® XL** *see* Clarithromycin* *on page 78*
- **Bicillin® C-R 900/300 Injection** *see* Penicillin G Benzathine and Procaine Combined* *on page 206*
- **Bicillin® C-R Injection** *see* Penicillin G Benzathine and Procaine Combined* *on page 206*
- **Bicillin® L-A** *see* Penicillin G Benzathine* *on page 205*
- **BiCNU®** *see* Carmustine* *on page 59*
- **Biocef** *see* Cephalexin* *on page 69*
- **Biomox®** *see* Amoxicillin* *on page 33*
- **Bio-Tab® Oral** *see* Doxycycline* *on page 106*

Biperiden (bye PER i den)
U.S. Brand Names Akineton®
Synonyms Biperiden Hydrochloride; Biperiden Lactate
Pharmacologic Class Anticholinergic Agent; Anti-Parkinson's Agent (Anticholinergic)
Nutrients Depleted
Specific nutrient depletions have not been documented for this agent.

- **Biperiden Hydrochloride** *see* Biperiden *on page 48*
- **Biperiden Lactate** *see* Biperiden *on page 48*
- **Bisac-Evac® [OTC]** *see* Bisacodyl* *on page 48*

Bisacodyl* (bis a KOE dil)
Related Information
Drug-Induced Nutrient Depletion Table *on page 498*
U.S. Brand Names Bisac-Evac® [OTC]; Bisacodyl Uniserts®; Bisco-Lax® [OTC]; Carter's Little Pills® [OTC]; Clysodrast®; Dacodyl® [OTC]; Deficol® [OTC]; Dulcolax® [OTC]; Fleet® Laxative [OTC]
Pharmacologic Class Laxative
Nutrients Depleted
Potassium *on page 340*
Sodium *on page 345*
Scientific Basis Published scientific studies using this pharmacologic agent
Studies & Abstracts 457-458
Additional Information Significant depletions documented only in cases of laxative abuse.

- **Bisacodyl Uniserts®** *see* Bisacodyl* *on page 48*
- **Bisco-Lax® [OTC]** *see* Bisacodyl* *on page 48*

Bisoprolol* (bis OH proe lol)
Related Information
Drug-Induced Nutrient Depletion Table *on page 498*
U.S. Brand Names Zebeta®

Synonyms Bisoprolol Fumarate
Pharmacologic Class Beta Blocker, Beta$_1$ Selective
Nutrients Depleted
Coenzyme Q$_{10}$ *on page 320*
Scientific Basis Published scientific studies of agents from the same pharmacologic class
Studies & Abstracts 348-349

♦ **Bisoprolol Fumarate** *see* Bisoprolol* *on page 48*
♦ **Blenoxane**® *see* Bleomycin* *on page 49*
♦ **Bleo** *see* Bleomycin* *on page 49*

Bleomycin* (blee oh MYE sin)
U.S. Brand Names Blenoxane®
Synonyms Bleo; Bleomycin Sulfate; BLM; NSC 125066
Pharmacologic Class Antineoplastic Agent, Antibiotic
Nutrients Depleted
See Nutrient Depletion and Cancer Chemotherapy *on page 515*.
Scientific Basis Inferred or indirect evidence of depletion based on disruption of physiologic processes

♦ **Bleomycin Sulfate** *see* Bleomycin* *on page 49*
♦ **BLM** *see* Bleomycin* *on page 49*
♦ **Blocadren**® **Oral** *see* Timolol* *on page 254*
♦ **Bonine**® **[OTC]** *see* Meclizine *on page 172*
♦ **Breonesin**® **[OTC]** *see* Guaifenesin *on page 140*
♦ **Bretylate**® *see* Bretylium *on page 49*

Bretylium (bre TIL ee um)
U.S. Brand Names Bretylol®
Canadian Brand Names Bretylate®
Synonyms Bretylium Tosylate
Pharmacologic Class Antiarrhythmic Agent, Class III
Nutrients Depleted
Specific nutrient depletions have not been documented for this agent.

♦ **Bretylium Tosylate** *see* Bretylium *on page 49*
♦ **Bretylol**® *see* Bretylium *on page 49*
♦ **Brevibloc**® **Injection** *see* Esmolol* *on page 113*
♦ **Brevicon**® *see* Ethinyl Estradiol and Norethindrone* *on page 121*
♦ **Brofed**® **Elixir [OTC]** *see* Brompheniramine and Pseudoephedrine *on page 51*
♦ **Bromaline**® **Elixir [OTC]** *see* Brompheniramine and Phenylpropanolamine *on page 50*
♦ **Bromanate**® **DC** *see* Brompheniramine, Phenylpropanolamine, and Codeine *on page 51*
♦ **Bromanate**® **Elixir [OTC]** *see* Brompheniramine and Phenylpropanolamine *on page 50*
♦ **Bromarest**® **[OTC]** *see* Brompheniramine *on page 50*
♦ **Bromatapp**® **[OTC]** *see* Brompheniramine and Phenylpropanolamine *on page 50*

♦ **Brombay®** **[OTC]** *see* Brompheniramine *on page 50*
♦ **Bromfed® Syrup [OTC]** *see* Brompheniramine and Pseudoephedrine *on page 51*
♦ **Bromfed® Tablet [OTC]** *see* Brompheniramine and Pseudoephedrine *on page 51*
♦ **Bromfenex®** *see* Brompheniramine and Pseudoephedrine *on page 51*
♦ **Bromfenex® PD** *see* Brompheniramine and Pseudoephedrine *on page 51*

Bromocriptine (broe moe KRIP teen)
U.S. Brand Names Parlodel®
Canadian Brand Names Apo® Bromocriptine
Synonyms Bromocriptine Mesylate
Pharmacologic Class Anti-Parkinson's Agent (Dopamine Agonist); Ergot Derivative
Nutrients Depleted
Specific nutrient depletions have not been documented for this agent.

♦ **Bromocriptine Mesylate** *see* Bromocriptine *on page 50*
♦ **Bromphen® [OTC]** *see* Brompheniramine *on page 50*
♦ **Bromphen® DC w/Codeine** *see* Brompheniramine, Phenylpropanolamine, and Codeine *on page 51*

Brompheniramine (brome fen IR a meen)
U.S. Brand Names Bromarest® [OTC]; Brombay® [OTC]; Bromphen® [OTC]; Brotane® [OTC]; Chlorphed® [OTC]; Cophene-B®; Diamine T.D.® [OTC]; Dimetane® Extentabs® [OTC]; Nasahist B®; ND-Stat®
Synonyms Brompheniramine Maleate; Parabromdylamine
Pharmacologic Class Antihistamine
Nutrients Depleted
Specific nutrient depletions have not been documented for this agent.

Brompheniramine and Phenylephrine
(brome fen IR a meen & fen il EF rin)
U.S. Brand Names Dimetane® Decongestant Elixir [OTC]
Pharmacologic Class Antihistamine/Decongestant Combination
Nutrients Depleted
Specific nutrient depletions have not been documented for this agent.

Brompheniramine and Phenylpropanolamine
(brome fen IR a meen & fen il proe pa NOLE a meen)
U.S. Brand Names Bromaline® Elixir [OTC]; Bromanate® Elixir [OTC]; Bromatapp® [OTC]; Bromphen® Tablet [OTC]; Cold & Allergy® Elixir [OTC]; Dimaphen® Elixir [OTC]; Dimaphen® Tablets [OTC]; Dimetapp® 4-Hour Liqui-Gel Capsule [OTC]; Dimetapp® Elixir [OTC]; Dimetapp® Extentabs® [OTC]; Dimetapp® Tablet [OTC]; Genatap® Elixir [OTC]; Tamine® [OTC]; Vicks® DayQuil® Allergy Relief 4 Hour Tablet [OTC]
Synonyms Phenylpropanolamine and Brompheniramine
Pharmacologic Class Antihistamine/Decongestant Combination
Nutrients Depleted
Specific nutrient depletions have not been documented for this agent.

Brompheniramine and Pseudoephedrine

(brome fen IR a meen & soo doe e FED rin)

U.S. Brand Names Brofed® Elixir [OTC]; Bromfed® Syrup [OTC]; Bromfed® Tablet [OTC]; Bromfenex®; Bromfenex® PD; Drixoral® Syrup [OTC]; Iofed®; Iofed® PD

Pharmacologic Class Antihistamine/Decongestant Combination

Nutrients Depleted

Specific nutrient depletions have not been documented for this agent.

♦ **Brompheniramine Maleate** *see* Brompheniramine *on page 50*

Brompheniramine, Phenylpropanolamine, and Codeine

(brome fen IR a meen, fen il proe pa NOLE a meen, & KOE deen)

U.S. Brand Names Bromanate® DC; Bromphen® DC w/Codeine; Dimetane®-DC; Myphetane DC®; Poly-Histine CS®

Synonyms Codeine, Brompheniramine, and Phenylpropanolamine; Phenylpropanolamine, Brompheniramine, and Codeine

Pharmacologic Class Antihistamine/Decongestant/Antitussive

Nutrients Depleted

Specific nutrient depletions have not been documented for this agent.

♦ **Bromphen® Tablet [OTC]** *see* Brompheniramine and Phenylpropanolamine *on page 50*

♦ **Bronalide®** *see* Flunisolide* *on page 129*

♦ **Bronkodyl®** *see* Theophylline* *on page 250*

♦ **Brotane® [OTC]** *see* Brompheniramine *on page 50*

Budesonide* (byoo DES oh nide)

U.S. Brand Names Pulmicort® Turbuhaler®; Rhinocort®; Rhinocort® Aqua™

Canadian Brand Names Entocort®; Pulmicort®

Pharmacologic Class Corticosteroid, Oral Inhaler; Corticosteroid, Nasal

Nutrients Depleted

Calcium *on page 313*
Folic Acid *on page 325*
Magnesium *on page 333*
Potassium *on page 340*
Selenium *on page 343*
Vitamin C *on page 360*
Vitamin D *on page 363*
Zinc *on page 368*

Scientific Basis

Published scientific studies using this pharmacologic agent
or
Published scientific studies of agents from the same pharmacologic class

Studies & Abstracts 182-223

- **Bufferin®** [OTC] *see* Aspirin* *on page 40*
- **Buffex®** [OTC] *see* Aspirin* *on page 40*

Bumetanide* (byoo MET a nide)
Related Information
Drug-Induced Nutrient Depletion Table *on page 498*
U.S. Brand Names Bumex®
Canadian Brand Names Burinex®
Pharmacologic Class Diuretic, Loop
Nutrients Depleted
Calcium *on page 313*
Magnesium *on page 333*
Potassium *on page 340*
Sodium *on page 345*
Vitamin B₁ *on page 351*
Vitamin B₆ *on page 357*
Vitamin C *on page 360*
Zinc *on page 368*
Scientific Basis Published scientific studies of agents from the same pharmacologic class
Studies & Abstracts 280-311
Additional Information Sodium replacement is not recommended in patients receiving loop diuretics. Potassium replacement should be guided by monitoring of serum concentrations.

- **Bumex®** *see* Bumetanide* *on page 52*
- **Bupap®** *see* Butalbital Compound and Acetaminophen* *on page 53*
- **Buprenex®** *see* Buprenorphine *on page 52*

Buprenorphine (byoo pre NOR feen)
U.S. Brand Names Buprenex®
Synonyms Buprenorphine Hydrochloride
Pharmacologic Class Analgesic, Narcotic
Nutrients Depleted
Specific nutrient depletions have not been documented for this agent.

- **Buprenorphine Hydrochloride** *see* Buprenorphine *on page 52*

Bupropion (byoo PROE pee on)
U.S. Brand Names Wellbutrin®; Wellbutrin® SR; Zyban™
Pharmacologic Class Antidepressant, Dopamine-Reuptake Inhibitor
Nutrients Depleted
Specific nutrient depletions have not been documented for this agent.

- **Burinex®** *see* Bumetanide* *on page 52*
- **BuSpar®** *see* Buspirone *on page 52*

Buspirone (byoo SPYE rone)
U.S. Brand Names BuSpar®
Synonyms Buspirone Hydrochloride
Pharmacologic Class Antianxiety Agent, Miscellaneous
Nutrients Depleted
Specific nutrient depletions have not been documented for this agent.

♦ **Buspirone Hydrochloride** *see Buspirone on page 52*

Busulfan* (byoo SUL fan)

U.S. Brand Names Myleran®

Pharmacologic Class Antineoplastic Agent, Alkylating Agent

Nutrients Depleted

See Nutrient Depletion and Cancer Chemotherapy *on page 515.*

Scientific Basis Inferred or indirect evidence of depletion based on disruption of physiologic processes

Butabarbital Sodium* (byoo ta BAR bi tal SOW dee um)

U.S. Brand Names Butalan®; Buticaps®; Butisol Sodium®

Pharmacologic Class Barbiturate

Nutrients Depleted

Biotin *on page 311*

Calcium *on page 313*

Folic Acid *on page 325*

Vitamin D *on page 363*

Vitamin K *on page 367*

Scientific Basis

Published scientific studies using this pharmacologic agent

or

Published scientific studies of agents from the same pharmacologic class

Studies & Abstracts 73-92

♦ **Butalan®** *see Butabarbital Sodium* on page 53*

Butalbital Compound and Acetaminophen*

(byoo TAL bi tal KOM pound & a seet a MIN oh fen)

U.S. Brand Names Amaphen®; Anoquan®; Axocet®; Bupap®; Endolor®; Esgic®; Esgic-Plus®; Femcet®; Fioricet®; G-1®; Medigesic®; Phrenilin®; Phrenilin® Forte; Repan®; Sedapap-10®; Triapin®; Two-Dyne®

Synonyms Acetaminophen and Butalbital Compound

Pharmacologic Class Barbiturate

Nutrients Depleted

Biotin *on page 311*

Calcium *on page 313*

Folic Acid *on page 325*

Glutathione *on page 327*

Vitamin D *on page 363*

Vitamin K *on page 367*

Scientific Basis

Published scientific studies using these pharmacologic agents

or

Published scientific studies of agents from the same pharmacologic class

Studies & Abstracts 73-92, 517-518

Butalbital Compound and Aspirin*
(byoo TAL bi tal KOM pound & AS pir in)

U.S. Brand Names Fiorgen PF®; Fiorinal®; Isollyl® Improved; Lanorinal®

Canadian Brand Names Tecnal

Synonyms Aspirin and Butalbital Compound

Pharmacologic Class Barbiturate

Nutrients Depleted

Biotin *on page 311*

Calcium *on page 313*

Folic Acid *on page 325*

Iron *on page 331*

Potassium *on page 340*

Sodium *on page 345*

Vitamin C *on page 360*

Vitamin D *on page 363*

Vitamin K *on page 367*

Scientific Basis Published scientific studies using these pharmacologic agents

Studies & Abstracts 73-92, 224-236

Butalbital Compound and Codeine*
(byoo TAL bi tal KOM pound & KOE deen)

U.S. Brand Names Fiorinal® With Codeine

Canadian Brand Names Fiorinal®-C ¼, ½; Tecnal C¼, C½

Synonyms Codeine and Butalbital Compound

Pharmacologic Class Analgesic, Combination (Narcotic); Barbiturate

Nutrients Depleted

Biotin *on page 311*

Calcium *on page 313*

Folic Acid *on page 325*

Vitamin D *on page 363*

Vitamin K *on page 367*

Scientific Basis Published scientific studies using this pharmacologic agent (butalbital)

Studies & Abstracts 73-92

♦ **Buticaps®** *see* Butabarbital Sodium* *on page 53*

♦ **Butisol Sodium®** *see* Butabarbital Sodium* *on page 53*

Butoconazole (byoo toe KOE na zole)

U.S. Brand Names Femstat®-3 [OTC]; Gynazole-1™

Synonyms Butoconazole Nitrate

Pharmacologic Class Antifungal Agent, Vaginal

Nutrients Depleted

Specific nutrient depletions have not been documented for this agent.

♦ **Butoconazole Nitrate** *see* Butoconazole *on page 54*

Butorphanol (byoo TOR fa nole)
U.S. Brand Names Stadol®; Stadol® NS
Synonyms Butorphanol Tartrate
Pharmacologic Class Analgesic, Narcotic
Nutrients Depleted
Specific nutrient depletions have not been documented for this agent.

♦ **Butorphanol Tartrate** *see* Butorphanol *on page 55*

♦ **BW-430C** *see* Lamotrigine *on page 162*

♦ **Byclomine® Injection** *see* Dicyclomine *on page 98*

♦ **Bydramine® Cough Syrup [OTC]** *see* Diphenhydramine *on page 102*

♦ **311C90** *see* Zolmitriptan *on page 271*

Cabergoline (ca BER go leen)
U.S. Brand Names Dostinex®
Pharmacologic Class Ergot Derivative
Nutrients Depleted
Specific nutrient depletions have not been documented for this agent.

♦ **Calan®** *see* Verapamil *on page 267*

♦ **Calan® SR** *see* Verapamil *on page 267*

♦ **Calcimar® Injection** *see* Calcitonin *on page 55*

Calcitonin (kal si TOE nin)
U.S. Brand Names Calcimar® Injection; Cibacalcin® Injection; Miacalcin® Injection; Miacalcin® Nasal Spray; Osteocalcin® Injection; Salmonine® Injection
Canadian Brand Names Caltine®
Synonyms Calcitonin (Human); Calcitonin (Salmon)
Pharmacologic Class Antidote
Nutrients Depleted
Specific nutrient depletions have not been documented for this agent.

♦ **Calcitonin (Human)** *see* Calcitonin *on page 55*

♦ **Calcitonin (Salmon)** *see* Calcitonin *on page 55*

Calcium Acetate (KAL see um AS e tate)
U.S. Brand Names Calphron®; PhosLo®
Pharmacologic Class Antidote; Calcium Salt; Electrolyte Supplement, Oral
Nutrients Depleted
Specific nutrient depletions have not been documented for this agent.
Additional Information Calcium acetate may be used therapeutically to limit phosphate absorption.

♦ **Calcium Disodium Versenate®** *see* Edetate Calcium Disodium* *on page 109*

♦ **Caldecort®** *see* Hydrocortisone* *on page 150*

♦ **Caldecort® Anti-Itch Spray** *see* Hydrocortisone* *on page 150*

- **Calmylin Expectorant** *see* Guaifenesin *on page 140*
- **Calphron®** *see* Calcium Acetate *on page 55*
- **Caltine®** *see* Calcitonin *on page 55*
- **Cama® Arthritis Pain Reliever [OTC]** *see* Aspirin* *on page 40*
- **Camptosar®** *see* Irinotecan* *on page 157*
- **Camptothecin-11** *see* Irinotecan* *on page 157*

Candesartan (kan de SAR tan)
U.S. Brand Names Atacand™
Synonyms Candesartan Cilexetil
Pharmacologic Class Angiotensin II Antagonists
Nutrients Depleted
Specific nutrient depletions have not been documented for this agent.

Candesartan and Hydrochlorothiazide*
(kan de SAR tan & hye droe klor oh THYE a zide)
U.S. Brand Names Atacand HCT™
Synonyms Candesartan Cilexetil and Hydrochlorothiazide
Pharmacologic Class Angiotensin II Antagonist Combination
Nutrients Depleted
Coenzyme Q_{10} *on page 320*
Magnesium *on page 333*
Phosphorus *on page 339*
Potassium *on page 340*
Sodium *on page 345*
Zinc *on page 368*
Scientific Basis Published scientific studies using this pharmacologic agent (hydrochlorothiazide)
Studies & Abstracts 320-342
Additional Information Although thiazide diuretics deplete sodium, replacement is not recommended, as this may be directly related to the therapeutic effect. Thiazides may deplete potassium, however replacement should be guided by monitoring of serum concentrations and specific instruction by a healthcare provider.

- **Candesartan Cilexetil** *see* Candesartan *on page 56*
- **Candesartan Cilexetil and Hydrochlorothiazide** *see* Candesartan and Hydrochlorothiazide* *on page 56*

Capecitabine* (ka pe SITE a been)
U.S. Brand Names Xeloda®
Pharmacologic Class Antineoplastic Agent, Antimetabolite
Nutrients Depleted
See Nutrient Depletion and Cancer Chemotherapy *on page 515*.
Scientific Basis Inferred or indirect evidence of depletion based on disruption of physiologic processes

- **Capital® and Codeine** *see* Acetaminophen and Codeine* *on page 23*
- **Capoten®** *see* Captopril* *on page 57*

Captopril* (KAP toe pril)
Related Information
Drug-Induced Nutrient Depletion Table *on page 498*
U.S. Brand Names Capoten®
Canadian Brand Names Apo®-Capto; Novo-Captopril; Nu-Capto; Syn-Captopril
Synonyms ACE
Pharmacologic Class Angiotensin-Converting Enzyme (ACE) Inhibitors
Nutrients Depleted
Zinc *on page 368*
Scientific Basis Published scientific studies using this pharmacologic agent
Studies & Abstracts 269-271

♦ **Carafate®** *see Sucralfate* on page 242*
♦ **Carampicillin Hydrochloride** *see Bacampicillin* on page 43*

Carbamazepine* (kar ba MAZ e peen)
Related Information
Drug-Induced Nutrient Depletion Table *on page 498*
U.S. Brand Names Carbatrol®; Epitol®; Tegretol®; Tegretol®-XR
Canadian Brand Names Apo®-Carbamazepine; Mazepine®; Novo-Carbamaz; Nu-Carbamazepine; PMS-Carbamazepine
Synonyms CBZ
Pharmacologic Class Anticonvulsant, Miscellaneous
Nutrients Depleted
Biotin *on page 311*
Calcium *on page 313*
Folic Acid *on page 325*
Vitamin D *on page 363*
Scientific Basis Published scientific studies using this pharmacologic agent
Studies & Abstracts 93-111

♦ **Carbatrol®** *see Carbamazepine* on page 57*

Carbenicillin* (kar ben i SIL in)
Related Information
Drug-Induced Nutrient Depletion Table *on page 498*
U.S. Brand Names Geocillin®
Canadian Brand Names Geopen®
Synonyms Carbenicillin Indanyl Sodium; Carindacillin
Pharmacologic Class Antibiotic, Penicillin
Nutrients Depleted
Bifidobacteria bifidum (bifidus) on page 311
Biotin *on page 311*
Inositol *on page 328*
Lactobacillus acidophilus on page 332
Potassium *on page 340*
Vitamin B$_1$ *on page 351*
(Continued)

Carbenicillin* *(Continued)*

Vitamin B_2 *on page 353*
Vitamin B_3 *on page 354*
Vitamin B_6 *on page 357*
Vitamin B_{12} *on page 359*
Vitamin K *on page 367*

Scientific Basis Inferred or indirect evidence of depletion based on disruption of physiologic processes

Studies & Abstracts 7-27, 49-57

- **Carbenicillin Indanyl Sodium** *see* Carbenicillin* *on page 57*
- **Carbidopa and Levodopa** *see* Levodopa and Carbidopa* *on page 164*

Carboplatin* (KAR boe pla tin)

U.S. Brand Names Paraplatin®
Synonyms CBDCA
Pharmacologic Class Antineoplastic Agent, Alkylating Agent
Nutrients Depleted
See Nutrient Depletion and Cancer Chemotherapy *on page 515*.
Scientific Basis Inferred or indirect evidence of depletion based on disruption of physiologic processes

- **Cardene®** *see* Nicardipine *on page 191*
- **Cardene® SR** *see* Nicardipine *on page 191*
- **Cardizem® CD** *see* Diltiazem *on page 101*
- **Cardizem® Injectable** *see* Diltiazem *on page 101*
- **Cardizem® SR** *see* Diltiazem *on page 101*
- **Cardizem® Tablet** *see* Diltiazem *on page 101*
- **Cardura®** *see* Doxazosin *on page 105*
- **Carindacillin** *see* Carbenicillin* *on page 57*
- **Carisoprodate** *see* Carisoprodol *on page 58*

Carisoprodol (kar i soe PROE dole)

U.S. Brand Names Soma®
Synonyms Carisoprodate; Isobamate
Pharmacologic Class Skeletal Muscle Relaxant
Nutrients Depleted
Specific nutrient depletions have not been documented for this agent.

Carisoprodol and Aspirin*

(kar i soe PROE dole & AS pir in)
U.S. Brand Names Soma® Compound
Pharmacologic Class Skeletal Muscle Relaxant
Nutrients Depleted
Folic Acid *on page 325*
Iron *on page 331*
Potassium *on page 340*
Sodium *on page 345*
Vitamin C *on page 360*

Scientific Basis Published scientific studies using this pharmacologic agent (aspirin)
Studies & Abstracts 224-236

Carisoprodol, Aspirin, and Codeine*
(kar i soe PROE dole, AS pir in, and KOE deen)
U.S. Brand Names Soma® Compound w/Codeine
Pharmacologic Class Skeletal Muscle Relaxant
Nutrients Depleted
  Folic Acid *on page 325*
  Iron *on page 331*
  Potassium *on page 340*
  Sodium *on page 345*
  Vitamin C *on page 360*
Scientific Basis Published scientific studies using this pharmacologic agent (aspirin)
Studies & Abstracts 224-236

Carmustine* (kar MUS teen)
U.S. Brand Names BiCNU®
Synonyms BCNU
Pharmacologic Class Antineoplastic Agent, Alkylating Agent
Nutrients Depleted
  See Nutrient Depletion and Cancer Chemotherapy *on page 515*.
Scientific Basis Inferred or indirect evidence of depletion based on disruption of physiologic processes

Carteolol* (KAR tee oh lole)
Related Information
  Drug-Induced Nutrient Depletion Table *on page 498*
U.S. Brand Names Cartrol® Oral; Ocupress® Ophthalmic
Synonyms Carteolol Hydrochloride
Pharmacologic Class Beta Blocker (with Intrinsic Sympathomimetic Activity); Ophthalmic Agent, Antiglaucoma
Nutrients Depleted
  Coenzyme Q_{10} *on page 320*
Scientific Basis Published scientific studies of agents from the same pharmacologic class
Studies & Abstracts 348-349

♦ **Carteolol Hydrochloride** *see* Carteolol* *on page 59*
♦ **Carter's Little Pills® [OTC]** *see* Bisacodyl* *on page 48*
♦ **Cartrol® Oral** *see* Carteolol* *on page 59*

Carvedilol* (KAR ve dil ole)
U.S. Brand Names Coreg®
Pharmacologic Class Alpha-/Beta- Blocker
Nutrients Depleted
  Coenzyme Q_{10} *on page 320*
Scientific Basis Published scientific studies of agents from the same pharmacologic class
(Continued)

Carvedilol* *(Continued)*
Studies & Abstracts 348-349

♦ **Casanthranol and Docusate** *see Docusate and Casanthranol* on page 104*
♦ **Cataflam® Oral** *see Diclofenac* on page 97*
♦ **Catapres® Oral** *see Clonidine* on page 81*
♦ **Catapres-TTS® Transdermal** *see Clonidine* on page 81*
♦ **Caverject® Injection** *see Alprostadil on page 28*
♦ **CBDCA** *see Carboplatin* on page 58*
♦ **CBZ** *see Carbamazepine* on page 57*
♦ **2-CdA** *see Cladribine* on page 78*
♦ **CDDP** *see Cisplatin* on page 78*
♦ **Ceclor®** *see Cefaclor* on page 60*
♦ **Ceclor® CD** *see Cefaclor* on page 60*
♦ **Cedax®** *see Ceftibuten* on page 67*
♦ **Cedocard®-SR** *see Isosorbide Dinitrate on page 158*

Cefaclor* (SEF a klor)
U.S. Brand Names Ceclor®; Ceclor® CD
Canadian Brand Names Apo®-Cefaclor
Pharmacologic Class Antibiotic, Cephalosporin (Second Generation)
Nutrients Depleted
Bifidobacteria bifidum (bifidus) on page 311
Biotin *on page 311*
Inositol *on page 328*
Lactobacillus acidophilus on page 332
Vitamin B_1 *on page 351*
Vitamin B_2 *on page 353*
Vitamin B_3 *on page 354*
Vitamin B_6 *on page 357*
Vitamin B_{12} *on page 359*
Vitamin K *on page 367*
Scientific Basis Inferred or indirect evidence of depletion based on disruption of physiologic processes
Studies & Abstracts 7-27

Cefadroxil* (sef a DROKS il)
U.S. Brand Names Duricef®
Synonyms Cefadroxil Monohydrate
Pharmacologic Class Antibiotic, Cephalosporin (First Generation)
Nutrients Depleted
Bifidobacteria bifidum (bifidus) on page 311
Biotin *on page 311*
Inositol *on page 328*
Lactobacillus acidophilus on page 332
Vitamin B_1 *on page 351*
Vitamin B_2 *on page 353*

Vitamin B_3 *on page 354*
Vitamin B_6 *on page 357*
Vitamin B_{12} *on page 359*
Vitamin K *on page 367*
Scientific Basis Inferred or indirect evidence of depletion based on disruption of physiologic processes
Studies & Abstracts 7-27

♦ **Cefadroxil Monohydrate** *see* Cefadroxil* *on page 60*

♦ **Cefadyl®** *see* Cephapirin* *on page 70*

Cefamandole* (sef a MAN dole)
U.S. Brand Names Mandol®
Synonyms Cefamandole Nafate
Pharmacologic Class Antibiotic, Cephalosporin (Second Generation)
Nutrients Depleted
Bifidobacteria bifidum (bifidus) on page 311
Biotin *on page 311*
Inositol *on page 328*
Lactobacillus acidophilus on page 332
Vitamin B_1 *on page 351*
Vitamin B_2 *on page 353*
Vitamin B_3 *on page 354*
Vitamin B_6 *on page 357*
Vitamin B_{12} *on page 359*
Vitamin K *on page 367*
Scientific Basis Inferred or indirect evidence of depletion based on disruption of physiologic processes
Studies & Abstracts 7-27

♦ **Cefamandole Nafate** *see* Cefamandole* *on page 61*

Cefazolin* (sef A zoe lin)
U.S. Brand Names Ancef®; Kefzol®; Zolicef®
Synonyms Cefazolin Sodium
Pharmacologic Class Antibiotic, Cephalosporin (First Generation)
Nutrients Depleted
Bifidobacteria bifidum (bifidus) on page 311
Biotin *on page 311*
Inositol *on page 328*
Lactobacillus acidophilus on page 332
Vitamin B_1 *on page 351*
Vitamin B_2 *on page 353*
Vitamin B_3 *on page 354*
Vitamin B_6 *on page 357*
Vitamin B_{12} *on page 359*
Vitamin K *on page 367*
Scientific Basis Inferred or indirect evidence of depletion based on disruption of physiologic processes
Studies & Abstracts 7-27

♦ **Cefazolin Sodium** *see* Cefazolin* *on page 61*

Cefdinir* (SEF di ner)
U.S. Brand Names Omnicef®
Synonyms CFDN
Pharmacologic Class Antibiotic, Cephalosporin (Third Generation)
Nutrients Depleted
Bifidobacteria bifidum (bifidus) on page 311
Biotin *on page 311*
Inositol *on page 328*
Lactobacillus acidophilus on page 332
Vitamin B_1 *on page 351*
Vitamin B_2 *on page 353*
Vitamin B_3 *on page 354*
Vitamin B_6 *on page 357*
Vitamin B_{12} *on page 359*
Vitamin K *on page 367*
Scientific Basis Inferred or indirect evidence of depletion based on disruption of physiologic processes
Studies & Abstracts 7-27

Cefepime* (SEF e pim)
U.S. Brand Names Maxipime®
Synonyms Cefepime Hydrochloride
Pharmacologic Class Antibiotic, Cephalosporin (Fourth Generation)
Nutrients Depleted
Bifidobacteria bifidum (bifidus) on page 311
Biotin *on page 311*
Inositol *on page 328*
Lactobacillus acidophilus on page 332
Vitamin B_1 *on page 351*
Vitamin B_2 *on page 353*
Vitamin B_3 *on page 354*
Vitamin B_6 *on page 357*
Vitamin B_{12} *on page 359*
Vitamin K *on page 367*
Scientific Basis Inferred or indirect evidence of depletion based on disruption of physiologic processes
Studies & Abstracts 7-27

♦ **Cefepime Hydrochloride** *see* Cefepime* *on page 62*

Cefixime* (sef IKS eem)
U.S. Brand Names Suprax®
Pharmacologic Class Antibiotic, Cephalosporin (Third Generation)
Nutrients Depleted
Bifidobacteria bifidum (bifidus) on page 311
Biotin *on page 311*
Inositol *on page 328*
Lactobacillus acidophilus on page 332
Vitamin B_1 *on page 351*

Vitamin B_2 *on page 353*
Vitamin B_3 *on page 354*
Vitamin B_6 *on page 357*
Vitamin B_{12} *on page 359*
Vitamin K *on page 367*
Scientific Basis Inferred or indirect evidence of depletion based on disruption of physiologic processes
Studies & Abstracts 7-27

♦ **Cefizox®** *see* Ceftizoxime* *on page 67*

Cefmetazole* (sef MET a zole)
U.S. Brand Names Zefazone®
Synonyms Cefmetazole Sodium
Pharmacologic Class Antibiotic, Cephalosporin (Second Generation)
Nutrients Depleted
Bifidobacteria bifidum (bifidus) on page 311
Biotin *on page 311*
Inositol *on page 328*
Lactobacillus acidophilus on page 332
Vitamin B_1 *on page 351*
Vitamin B_2 *on page 353*
Vitamin B_3 *on page 354*
Vitamin B_6 *on page 357*
Vitamin B_{12} *on page 359*
Vitamin K *on page 367*
Scientific Basis Inferred or indirect evidence of depletion based on disruption of physiologic processes
Studies & Abstracts 7-27

♦ **Cefmetazole Sodium** *see* Cefmetazole* *on page 63*
♦ **Cefobid®** *see* Cefoperazone* *on page 64*

Cefonicid* (se FON i sid)
U.S. Brand Names Monocid®
Synonyms Cefonicid Sodium
Pharmacologic Class Antibiotic, Cephalosporin (Second Generation)
Nutrients Depleted
Bifidobacteria bifidum (bifidus) on page 311
Biotin *on page 311*
Inositol *on page 328*
Lactobacillus acidophilus on page 332
Vitamin B_1 *on page 351*
Vitamin B_2 *on page 353*
Vitamin B_3 *on page 354*
Vitamin B_6 *on page 357*
Vitamin B_{12} *on page 359*
Vitamin K *on page 367*
Scientific Basis Inferred or indirect evidence of depletion based on disruption of physiologic processes
(Continued)

Cefonicid* *(Continued)*
Studies & Abstracts 7-27

♦ **Cefonicid Sodium** *see Cefonicid* on page 63*

Cefoperazone* (sef oh PER a zone)
U.S. Brand Names Cefobid®
Synonyms Cefoperazone Sodium
Pharmacologic Class Antibiotic, Cephalosporin (Third Generation)
Nutrients Depleted
  Bifidobacteria bifidum (bifidus) on page 311
  Biotin *on page 311*
  Inositol *on page 328*
  Lactobacillus acidophilus on page 332
  Vitamin B_1 *on page 351*
  Vitamin B_2 *on page 353*
  Vitamin B_3 *on page 354*
  Vitamin B_6 *on page 357*
  Vitamin B_{12} *on page 359*
  Vitamin K *on page 367*
Scientific Basis Inferred or indirect evidence of depletion based on disruption of physiologic processes
Studies & Abstracts 7-27

♦ **Cefoperazone Sodium** *see Cefoperazone* on page 64*
♦ **Cefotan®** *see Cefotetan* on page 64*

Cefotaxime* (sef oh TAKS eem)
U.S. Brand Names Claforan®
Synonyms Cefotaxime Sodium
Pharmacologic Class Antibiotic, Cephalosporin (Third Generation)
Nutrients Depleted
  Bifidobacteria bifidum (bifidus) on page 311
  Biotin *on page 311*
  Inositol *on page 328*
  Lactobacillus acidophilus on page 332
  Vitamin B_1 *on page 351*
  Vitamin B_2 *on page 353*
  Vitamin B_3 *on page 354*
  Vitamin B_6 *on page 357*
  Vitamin B_{12} *on page 359*
  Vitamin K *on page 367*
Scientific Basis Inferred or indirect evidence of depletion based on disruption of physiologic processes
Studies & Abstracts 7-27

♦ **Cefotaxime Sodium** *see Cefotaxime* on page 64*

Cefotetan* (SEF oh tee tan)
U.S. Brand Names Cefotan®
Synonyms Cefotetan Disodium

Pharmacologic Class Antibiotic, Cephalosporin (Second Generation)

Nutrients Depleted
Bifidobacteria bifidum (bifidus) on page 311
Biotin *on page 311*
Inositol *on page 328*
Lactobacillus acidophilus on page 332
Vitamin B$_1$ *on page 351*
Vitamin B$_2$ *on page 353*
Vitamin B$_3$ *on page 354*
Vitamin B$_6$ *on page 357*
Vitamin B$_{12}$ *on page 359*
Vitamin K *on page 367*

Scientific Basis Inferred or indirect evidence of depletion based on disruption of physiologic processes

Studies & Abstracts 7-27

♦ **Cefotetan Disodium** *see* Cefotetan* *on page 64*

Cefoxitin* (se FOKS i tin)

U.S. Brand Names Mefoxin®

Synonyms Cefoxitin Sodium

Pharmacologic Class Antibiotic, Cephalosporin (Second Generation)

Nutrients Depleted
Bifidobacteria bifidum (bifidus) on page 311
Biotin *on page 311*
Inositol *on page 328*
Lactobacillus acidophilus on page 332
Vitamin B$_1$ *on page 351*
Vitamin B$_2$ *on page 353*
Vitamin B$_3$ *on page 354*
Vitamin B$_6$ *on page 357*
Vitamin B$_{12}$ *on page 359*
Vitamin K *on page 367*

Scientific Basis Inferred or indirect evidence of depletion based on disruption of physiologic processes

Studies & Abstracts 7-27

♦ **Cefoxitin Sodium** *see* Cefoxitin* *on page 65*

Cefpodoxime* (sef pode OKS eem)

U.S. Brand Names Vantin®

Synonyms Cefpodoxime Proxetil

Pharmacologic Class Antibiotic, Cephalosporin (Third Generation)

Nutrients Depleted
Bifidobacteria bifidum (bifidus) on page 311
Biotin *on page 311*
Inositol *on page 328*
Lactobacillus acidophilus on page 332
Vitamin B$_1$ *on page 351*
Vitamin B$_2$ *on page 353*
(Continued)

Cefpodoxime* *(Continued)*

    Vitamin B_3 *on page 354*
    Vitamin B_6 *on page 357*
    Vitamin B_{12} *on page 359*
    Vitamin K *on page 367*

Scientific Basis Inferred or indirect evidence of depletion based on disruption of physiologic processes

Studies & Abstracts 7-27

♦ **Cefpodoxime Proxetil** *see* Cefpodoxime* *on page 65*

Cefprozil* (sef PROE zil)

U.S. Brand Names Cefzil®

Pharmacologic Class Antibiotic, Cephalosporin (Second Generation)

Nutrients Depleted

    Bifidobacteria bifidum (bifidus) on page 311
    Biotin *on page 311*
    Inositol *on page 328*
    Lactobacillus acidophilus on page 332
    Vitamin B_1 *on page 351*
    Vitamin B_2 *on page 353*
    Vitamin B_3 *on page 354*
    Vitamin B_6 *on page 357*
    Vitamin B_{12} *on page 359*
    Vitamin K *on page 367*

Scientific Basis Inferred or indirect evidence of depletion based on disruption of physiologic processes

Studies & Abstracts 7-27

Ceftazidime* (SEF tay zi deem)

U.S. Brand Names Ceptaz™; Fortaz®; Tazicef®; Tazidime®

Canadian Brand Names Ceptaz™

Pharmacologic Class Antibiotic, Cephalosporin (Third Generation)

Nutrients Depleted

    Bifidobacteria bifidum (bifidus) on page 311
    Biotin *on page 311*
    Inositol *on page 328*
    Lactobacillus acidophilus on page 332
    Vitamin B_1 *on page 351*
    Vitamin B_2 *on page 353*
    Vitamin B_3 *on page 354*
    Vitamin B_6 *on page 357*
    Vitamin B_{12} *on page 359*
    Vitamin K *on page 367*

Scientific Basis Inferred or indirect evidence of depletion based on disruption of physiologic processes

Studies & Abstracts 7-27

Ceftibuten* (sef TYE byoo ten)
U.S. Brand Names Cedax®
Pharmacologic Class Antibiotic, Cephalosporin (Third Generation)
Nutrients Depleted
Bifidobacteria bifidum (bifidus) on page 311
Biotin *on page 311*
Inositol *on page 328*
Lactobacillus acidophilus on page 332
Vitamin B_1 *on page 351*
Vitamin B_2 *on page 353*
Vitamin B_3 *on page 354*
Vitamin B_6 *on page 357*
Vitamin B_{12} *on page 359*
Vitamin K *on page 367*
Scientific Basis Inferred or indirect evidence of depletion based on disruption of physiologic processes
Studies & Abstracts 7-27

♦ **Ceftin® Oral** *see* Cefuroxime* *on page 68*

Ceftizoxime* (sef ti ZOKS eem)
U.S. Brand Names Cefizox®
Synonyms Ceftizoxime Sodium
Pharmacologic Class Antibiotic, Cephalosporin (Third Generation)
Nutrients Depleted
Bifidobacteria bifidum (bifidus) on page 311
Biotin *on page 311*
Inositol *on page 328*
Lactobacillus acidophilus on page 332
Vitamin B_1 *on page 351*
Vitamin B_2 *on page 353*
Vitamin B_3 *on page 354*
Vitamin B_6 *on page 357*
Vitamin B_{12} *on page 359*
Vitamin K *on page 367*
Scientific Basis Inferred or indirect evidence of depletion based on disruption of physiologic processes
Studies & Abstracts 7-27

♦ **Ceftizoxime Sodium** *see* Ceftizoxime* *on page 67*

Ceftriaxone* (sef trye AKS one)
U.S. Brand Names Rocephin®
Synonyms Ceftriaxone Sodium
Pharmacologic Class Antibiotic, Cephalosporin (Third Generation)
Nutrients Depleted
Bifidobacteria bifidum (bifidus) on page 311
Biotin *on page 311*
Inositol *on page 328*
Lactobacillus acidophilus on page 332
Vitamin B_1 *on page 351*
(Continued)

Ceftriaxone* *(Continued)*

Vitamin B$_2$ *on page 353*
Vitamin B$_3$ *on page 354*
Vitamin B$_6$ *on page 357*
Vitamin B$_{12}$ *on page 359*
Vitamin K *on page 367*

Scientific Basis Inferred or indirect evidence of depletion based on disruption of physiologic processes
Studies & Abstracts 7-27

♦ **Ceftriaxone Sodium** *see* Ceftriaxone* *on page 67*

Cefuroxime* (se fyoor OKS eem)

U.S. Brand Names Ceftin® Oral; Kefurox® Injection; Zinacef® Injection
Synonyms Cefuroxime Axetil; Cefuroxime Sodium
Pharmacologic Class Antibiotic, Cephalosporin (Second Generation)
Nutrients Depleted
Bifidobacteria bifidum (bifidus) on page 311
Biotin *on page 311*
Inositol *on page 328*
Lactobacillus acidophilus on page 332
Vitamin B$_1$ *on page 351*
Vitamin B$_2$ *on page 353*
Vitamin B$_3$ *on page 354*
Vitamin B$_6$ *on page 357*
Vitamin B$_{12}$ *on page 359*
Vitamin K *on page 367*

Scientific Basis Inferred or indirect evidence of depletion based on disruption of physiologic processes
Studies & Abstracts 7-27

♦ **Cefuroxime Axetil** *see* Cefuroxime* *on page 68*
♦ **Cefuroxime Sodium** *see* Cefuroxime* *on page 68*
♦ **Cefzil®** *see* Cefprozil* *on page 66*
♦ **Celebrex™** *see* Celecoxib* *on page 68*

Celecoxib* (ce le COX ib)

U.S. Brand Names Celebrex™
Pharmacologic Class Nonsteroidal Anti-inflammatory Drug (NSAID), COX-2 Selective
Nutrients Depleted
Folic Acid *on page 325*

Scientific Basis Inferred or indirect evidence of depletion based on disruption of physiologic processes
Studies & Abstracts 252
Additional Information Selective COX-2 inhibitors may not share potential depletions of nonselective agents.

♦ **Celestone®** *see* Betamethasone* *on page 46*
♦ **Celestone® Soluspan®** *see* Betamethasone* *on page 46*

- **Celexa**® *see* Citalopram *on page 78*
- **Celontin**® *see* Methsuximide* *on page 177*
- **Cenafed**® **[OTC]** *see* Pseudoephedrine *on page 225*
- **Cena-K**® *see* Potassium Chloride (Timed Release)* *on page 216*
- **Cenestin**™ *see* Estrogens (Conjugated A/Synthetic)* *on page 117*

Cephalexin* (sef a LEKS in)
U.S. Brand Names Biocef; Keflex®; Keftab®
Canadian Brand Names Apo®-Cephalex; Novo-Lexin; Nu-Cephalex
Synonyms Cephalexin Hydrochloride; Cephalexin Monohydrate
Pharmacologic Class Antibiotic, Cephalosporin (First Generation)
Nutrients Depleted
Bifidobacteria bifidum (bifidus) on page 311
Biotin *on page 311*
Inositol *on page 328*
Lactobacillus acidophilus on page 332
Vitamin B_1 *on page 351*
Vitamin B_2 *on page 353*
Vitamin B_3 *on page 354*
Vitamin B_6 *on page 357*
Vitamin B_{12} *on page 359*
Vitamin K *on page 367*
Scientific Basis Inferred or indirect evidence of depletion based on disruption of physiologic processes
Studies & Abstracts 7-27

- **Cephalexin Hydrochloride** *see* Cephalexin* *on page 69*
- **Cephalexin Monohydrate** *see* Cephalexin* *on page 69*

Cephalothin* (sef A loe thin)
Synonyms Cephalothin Sodium
Pharmacologic Class Antibiotic, Cephalosporin (First Generation)
Nutrients Depleted
Bifidobacteria bifidum (bifidus) on page 311
Biotin *on page 311*
Inositol *on page 328*
Lactobacillus acidophilus on page 332
Vitamin B_1 *on page 351*
Vitamin B_2 *on page 353*
Vitamin B_3 *on page 354*
Vitamin B_6 *on page 357*
Vitamin B_{12} *on page 359*
Vitamin K *on page 367*
Scientific Basis Inferred or indirect evidence of depletion based on disruption of physiologic processes
Studies & Abstracts 7-27

- **Cephalothin Sodium** *see* Cephalothin* *on page 69*

Cephapirin* (sef a PYE rin)
U.S. Brand Names Cefadyl®
Synonyms Cephapirin Sodium
Pharmacologic Class Antibiotic, Cephalosporin (First Generation)
Nutrients Depleted
  Bifidobacteria bifidum (bifidus) on page 311
  Biotin *on page 311*
  Inositol *on page 328*
  Lactobacillus acidophilus on page 332
  Vitamin B_1 *on page 351*
  Vitamin B_2 *on page 353*
  Vitamin B_3 *on page 354*
  Vitamin B_6 *on page 357*
  Vitamin B_{12} *on page 359*
  Vitamin K *on page 367*
Scientific Basis Inferred or indirect evidence of depletion based on disruption of physiologic processes
Studies & Abstracts 7-27

♦ **Cephapirin Sodium** *see Cephapirin* on page 70*

Cephradine* (SEF ra deen)
U.S. Brand Names Velosef®
Pharmacologic Class Antibiotic, Cephalosporin (First Generation)
Nutrients Depleted
  Bifidobacteria bifidum (bifidus) on page 311
  Biotin *on page 311*
  Inositol *on page 328*
  Lactobacillus acidophilus on page 332
  Vitamin B_1 *on page 351*
  Vitamin B_2 *on page 353*
  Vitamin B_3 *on page 354*
  Vitamin B_6 *on page 357*
  Vitamin B_{12} *on page 359*
  Vitamin K *on page 367*
Scientific Basis Inferred or indirect evidence of depletion based on disruption of physiologic processes
Studies & Abstracts 7-27

♦ **Ceptaz™** *see Ceftazidime* on page 66*
♦ **Cerebyx®** *see Fosphenytoin* on page 134*

Cerivastatin* (se ree va STAT in)
Related Information
  Drug-Induced Nutrient Depletion Table *on page 498*
U.S. Brand Names Baycol®
Synonyms Cerivastatin Sodium
Pharmacologic Class Antilipemic Agent (HMG-CoA Reductase Inhibitor)
Nutrients Depleted
  Coenzyme Q_{10} *on page 320*

Scientific Basis Published scientific studies of agents from the same pharmacologic class
Studies & Abstracts 350-361

♦ **Cerivastatin Sodium** *see* Cerivastatin* *on page 70*

♦ **C.E.S.**™ *see* Estrogens (Conjugated)* *on page 117*

Cetirizine (se TI ra zeen)
U.S. Brand Names Zyrtec®
Synonyms Cetirizine Hydrochloride; P-071; UCB-P071
Pharmacologic Class Antihistamine
Nutrients Depleted
Specific nutrient depletions have not been documented for this agent.

♦ **Cetirizine Hydrochloride** *see* Cetirizine *on page 71*

Cetrorelix (se troh REE liks)
U.S. Brand Names Cetrotide™
Synonyms Cetrorelix Acetate
Pharmacologic Class Antigonadotropic Agent
Nutrients Depleted
Specific nutrient depletions have not been documented for this agent.

♦ **Cetrorelix Acetate** *see* Cetrorelix *on page 71*

♦ **Cetrotide**™ *see* Cetrorelix *on page 71*

Cevimeline (se vi ME leen)
U.S. Brand Names Evoxac™
Synonyms Cevimeline Hydrochloride
Pharmacologic Class Cholinergic Agonist
Nutrients Depleted
Specific nutrient depletions have not been documented for this agent.

♦ **Cevimeline Hydrochloride** *see* Cevimeline *on page 71*

♦ **CFDN** *see* Cefdinir* *on page 62*

♦ **Cheracol® D [OTC]** *see* Guaifenesin and Dextromethorphan *on page 141*

♦ **Chibroxin**™ **Ophthalmic** *see* Norfloxacin* *on page 194*

♦ **Children's Advil® Oral Suspension [OTC]** *see* Ibuprofen* *on page 153*

♦ **Children's Dynafed® Jr [OTC]** *see* Acetaminophen* *on page 23*

♦ **Children's Hold® [OTC]** *see* Dextromethorphan *on page 96*

♦ **Children's Motrin® Oral Suspension [OTC]** *see* Ibuprofen* *on page 153*

♦ **Children's Silapap® [OTC]** *see* Acetaminophen* *on page 23*

♦ **Children's Silfedrine® [OTC]** *see* Pseudoephedrine *on page 225*

♦ **Chlo-Amine® [OTC]** *see* Chlorpheniramine *on page 73*

♦ **Chlorafed® Liquid [OTC]** *see* Chlorpheniramine and Pseudoephedrine *on page 73*

♦ **Chloral** *see* Chloral Hydrate *on page 72*

Chloral Hydrate (KLOR al HYE drate)
U.S. Brand Names Aquachloral® Supprettes®
Canadian Brand Names Novo-Chlorhydrate; PMS-Chloral Hydrate
Synonyms Chloral; Hydrated Chloral; Trichloroacetaldehyde Monohydrate
Pharmacologic Class Hypnotic, Miscellaneous
Nutrients Depleted
Specific nutrient depletions have not been documented for this agent.

Chlorambucil* (klor AM byoo sil)
U.S. Brand Names Leukeran®
Pharmacologic Class Antineoplastic Agent, Alkylating Agent
Nutrients Depleted
See Nutrient Depletion and Cancer Chemotherapy *on page 515.*
Scientific Basis Inferred or indirect evidence of depletion based on disruption of physiologic processes

♦ **Chlorate® [OTC]** *see* Chlorpheniramine *on page 73*

Chlordiazepoxide (klor dye az o POKS ide)
U.S. Brand Names Libritabs®; Librium®; Mitran® Oral; Reposans-10® Oral
Canadian Brand Names Apo®-Chlordiazepoxide; Corax®; Medilium®; Novo-Poxide; Solium®
Synonyms Methaminodiazepoxide Hydrochloride
Pharmacologic Class Benzodiazepine
Nutrients Depleted
Specific nutrient depletions have not been documented for this agent.

♦ **2-Chlorodeoxyadenosine** *see* Cladribine* *on page 78*

Chlorothiazide* (klor oh THYE a zide)
Related Information
Drug-Induced Nutrient Depletion Table *on page 498*
U.S. Brand Names Diurigen®; Diuril®
Pharmacologic Class Diuretic, Thiazide
Nutrients Depleted
Coenzyme Q_{10} *on page 320*
Magnesium *on page 333*
Phosphorus *on page 339*
Potassium *on page 340*
Sodium *on page 345*
Zinc *on page 368*
Scientific Basis Published scientific studies of agents from the same pharmacologic class
Studies & Abstracts 320-342
Additional Information Although thiazide diuretics deplete sodium, replacement is not recommended, as this may be directly related to the therapeutic effect. Thiazides may deplete potassium, however replacement should be guided by monitoring of serum concentrations and specific instruction by a healthcare provider.

Chlorotrianisene* (klor oh trye AN i seen)

U.S. Brand Names TACE®

Pharmacologic Class Estrogen Derivative

Nutrients Depleted

Magnesium *on page 333*

Vitamin B₆ *on page 357*

Scientific Basis Published scientific studies of agents from the same pharmacologic class

Studies & Abstracts 378-379

♦ **Chlorphed® [OTC]** *see* Brompheniramine *on page 50*

Chlorpheniramine (klor fen IR a meen)

U.S. Brand Names Aller-Chlor® [OTC]; AL-R® [OTC]; Chlo-Amine® [OTC]; Chlorate® [OTC]; Chlor-Pro® [OTC]; Chlor-Trimeton® [OTC]; Telachlor®; Teldrin® [OTC]

Synonyms Chlorpheniramine Maleate; CTM

Pharmacologic Class Antihistamine

Nutrients Depleted

Specific nutrient depletions have not been documented for this agent.

Chlorpheniramine and Phenylephrine

(klor fen IR a meen & fen il EF rin)

U.S. Brand Names Dallergy-D® Syrup; Ed A-Hist® Liquid; Histatab® Plus Tablet [OTC]; Histor-D® Syrup; Rolatuss® Plain Liquid; Ru-Tuss® Liquid

Synonyms Phenylephrine and Chlorpheniramine

Pharmacologic Class Antihistamine/Decongestant Combination

Nutrients Depleted

Specific nutrient depletions have not been documented for this agent.

Chlorpheniramine and Phenylpropanolamine

(klor fen IR a meen & fen il proe pa NOLE a meen)

U.S. Brand Names Allerest® 12 Hour Capsule [OTC]; A.R.M.® Caplet [OTC]; Chlor-Rest® Tablet [OTC]; Demazin® Syrup [OTC]; Genamin® Cold Syrup [OTC]; Resaid®; Rescon Liquid [OTC]; Silaminic® Cold Syrup [OTC]; Temazin® Cold Syrup [OTC]; Thera-Hist® Syrup [OTC]; Triaminic® Allergy Tablet [OTC]; Triaminic® Cold Tablet [OTC]; Triaminic® Syrup [OTC]; Tri-Nefrin® Extra Strength Tablet [OTC]; Triphenyl® Syrup [OTC]

Synonyms Phenylpropanolamine and Chlorpheniramine

Pharmacologic Class Antihistamine/Decongestant Combination

Nutrients Depleted

Specific nutrient depletions have not been documented for this agent.

Chlorpheniramine and Pseudoephedrine

(klor fen IR a meen & soo doe e FED rin)

U.S. Brand Names Allerest® Maximum Strength [OTC]; Anamine® Syrup [OTC]; Anaplex® Liquid [OTC]; Chlorafed® Liquid [OTC]; Chlor-Trimeton® 4 Hour Relief Tablet [OTC]; Co-Pyronil® 2 Pulvules® [OTC]; Deconamine® SR; Deconamine® Syrup [OTC]; Deconamine® Tablet
(Continued)

73

Chlorpheniramine and Pseudoephedrine
(Continued)

[OTC]; Fedahist® Tablet [OTC]; Hayfebrol® Liquid [OTC]; Histalet® Syrup [OTC]; Klerist-D® Tablet [OTC]; Pseudo-Gest Plus® Tablet [OTC]; Rhinosyn® Liquid [OTC]; Rhinosyn-PD® Liquid [OTC]; Ryna® Liquid [OTC]; Sudafed® Plus Tablet [OTC]

Synonyms Pseudoephedrine and Chlorpheniramine
Pharmacologic Class Antihistamine/Decongestant Combination
Nutrients Depleted
Specific nutrient depletions have not been documented for this agent.

- **Chlorpheniramine Maleate** *see* Chlorpheniramine *on page 73*
- **Chlor-Pro® [OTC]** *see* Chlorpheniramine *on page 73*
- **Chlorprom®** *see* Chlorpromazine* *on page 74*
- **Chlorpromanyl®** *see* Chlorpromazine* *on page 74*

Chlorpromazine* (klor PROE ma zeen)
Related Information
Drug-Induced Nutrient Depletion Table *on page 498*
U.S. Brand Names Ormazine; Thorazine®
Canadian Brand Names Apo®-Chlorpromazine; Chlorprom®; Chlorpromanyl®; Largactil®; Novo-Chlorpromazine
Synonyms Chlorpromazine Hydrochloride; CPZ
Pharmacologic Class Antipsychotic Agent, Phenothiazine, Aliphatic
Nutrients Depleted
Coenzyme Q_{10} *on page 320*
Vitamin B_2 *on page 353*
Scientific Basis Published scientific studies using this pharmacologic agent
Studies & Abstracts 474-477

- **Chlorpromazine Hydrochloride** *see* Chlorpromazine* *on page 74*

Chlorpropamide* (klor PROE pa mide)
U.S. Brand Names Diabinese®
Canadian Brand Names Apo®-Chlorpropamide; Novo-Propamide
Pharmacologic Class Antidiabetic Agent (Sulfonylurea)
Nutrients Depleted
Coenzyme Q_{10} *on page 320*
Scientific Basis Published scientific studies of agents from the same pharmacologic class demonstrate depletion of some nutrients; however, this agent was NOT found to cause a similar depletion
Studies & Abstracts 167

- **Chlor-Rest® Tablet [OTC]** *see* Chlorpheniramine and Phenylpropanolamine *on page 73*

Chlorthalidone* (klor THAL i done)
Related Information
Drug-Induced Nutrient Depletion Table *on page 498*
U.S. Brand Names Hygroton®; Thalitone®

Canadian Brand Names Apo®-Chlorthalidone; Novo-Thalidone; Uridon®

Pharmacologic Class Diuretic, Miscellaneous

Nutrients Depleted

Zinc *on page 368*

Scientific Basis Published scientific studies using this pharmacologic agent

Studies & Abstracts 272

Additional Information Although thiazide diuretics (and related agents such as chlorthalidone) deplete sodium, replacement is not recommended, as this may be directly related to the therapeutic effect. Thiazides may deplete potassium, however replacement should be guided by monitoring of serum concentrations and specific instruction by a healthcare provider.

♦ **Chlorthalidone and Atenolol** *see* Atenolol and Chlorthalidone* *on page 41*

♦ **Chlor-Trimeton® [OTC]** *see* Chlorpheniramine *on page 73*

♦ **Chlor-Trimeton® 4 Hour Relief Tablet [OTC]** *see* Chlorpheniramine and Pseudoephedrine *on page 73*

♦ **Chlor-Tripolon® N.D.** *see* Loratadine and Pseudoephedrine *on page 168*

Chlorzoxazone (klor ZOKS a zone)

U.S. Brand Names Flexaphen®; Paraflex®; Parafon Forte™ DSC

Synonyms Chlorzoxazone with Acetaminophen

Pharmacologic Class Skeletal Muscle Relaxant

Nutrients Depleted

Specific nutrient depletions have not been documented for this agent.

♦ **Chlorzoxazone with Acetaminophen** *see* Chlorzoxazone *on page 75*

Cholestyramine Resin* (koe LES tir a meen REZ in)

Related Information

Drug-Induced Nutrient Depletion Table *on page 498*

U.S. Brand Names Prevalite®; Questran®; Questran® Light

Canadian Brand Names PMS-Cholestyramine

Pharmacologic Class Antilipemic Agent (Bile Acid Sequestrant)

Nutrients Depleted

Beta-Carotene *on page 310*

Calcium *on page 313*

Folic Acid *on page 325*

Iron *on page 331*

Magnesium *on page 333*

Phosphorus *on page 339*

Vitamin A *on page 349*

Vitamin B_{12} *on page 359*

Vitamin D *on page 363*

Vitamin E *on page 365*

Vitamin K *on page 367*

Zinc *on page 368*

(Continued)

Cholestyramine Resin* *(Continued)*
Scientific Basis Published scientific studies using this pharmacologic agent
Studies & Abstracts 363-370

Choline Magnesium Trisalicylate*
(KOE leen mag NEE zhum trye sa LIS i late)
Related Information
Drug-Induced Nutrient Depletion Table *on page 498*
U.S. Brand Names Tricosal®; Trilisate®
Pharmacologic Class Salicylate
Nutrients Depleted
Folic Acid *on page 325*
Iron *on page 331*
Potassium *on page 340*
Sodium *on page 345*
Vitamin C *on page 360*
Scientific Basis Published scientific studies of agents from the same pharmacologic class
Studies & Abstracts 224-236

Choline Salicylate* (KOE leen sa LIS i late)
Related Information
Drug-Induced Nutrient Depletion Table *on page 498*
U.S. Brand Names Arthropan® [OTC]
Canadian Brand Names Teejel®
Pharmacologic Class Analgesic, Salicylate; Nonsteroidal Anti-Inflammatory Agent (NSAID); Salicylate
Nutrients Depleted
Folic Acid *on page 325*
Iron *on page 331*
Potassium *on page 340*
Sodium *on page 345*
Vitamin C *on page 360*
Scientific Basis Published scientific studies of agents from the same pharmacologic class
Studies & Abstracts 224-236

♦ **Cibacalcin® Injection** *see* Calcitonin *on page 55*

Cidofovir (si DOF o veer)
U.S. Brand Names Vistide®
Pharmacologic Class Antiviral Agent
Nutrients Depleted
Specific nutrient depletions have not been documented for this agent.

♦ **Ciloxan™ Ophthalmic** *see* Ciprofloxacin* *on page 77*

Cimetidine* (sye MET i deen)
Related Information
Drug-Induced Nutrient Depletion Table *on page 498*

U.S. Brand Names Tagamet®; Tagamet® HB [OTC]
Canadian Brand Names Apo®-Cimetidine; Novo-Cimetine; Nu-Cimet; Peptol®
Pharmacologic Class Histamine H₂ Antagonist
Nutrients Depleted
    Calcium *on page 313*
    Folic Acid *on page 325*
    Iron *on page 331*
    Vitamin B₁₂ *on page 359*
    Vitamin D *on page 363*
    Zinc *on page 368*
Scientific Basis Published scientific studies using this pharmacologic agent
Studies & Abstracts 484-510

♦ **Cinobac® Pulvules®** *see Cinoxacin* on page 77*

Cinoxacin* (sin OKS a sin)
U.S. Brand Names Cinobac® Pulvules®
Pharmacologic Class Antibiotic, Quinolone
Nutrients Depleted
    Bifidobacteria bifidum (bifidus) on page 311
    Biotin *on page 311*
    Inositol *on page 328*
    Lactobacillus acidophilus on page 332
    Vitamin B₁ *on page 351*
    Vitamin B₂ *on page 353*
    Vitamin B₃ *on page 354*
    Vitamin B₆ *on page 357*
    Vitamin B₁₂ *on page 359*
    Vitamin K *on page 367*
Scientific Basis Inferred or indirect evidence of depletion based on disruption of physiologic processes
Studies & Abstracts 7-27

Ciprofloxacin* (sip roe FLOKS a sin)
U.S. Brand Names Ciloxan™ Ophthalmic; Cipro® Injection; Cipro® Oral
Synonyms Ciprofloxacin Hydrochloride
Pharmacologic Class Antibiotic, Ophthalmic; Antibiotic, Quinolone
Nutrients Depleted
    Bifidobacteria bifidum (bifidus) on page 311
    Biotin *on page 311*
    Inositol *on page 328*
    Lactobacillus acidophilus on page 332
    Vitamin B₁ *on page 351*
    Vitamin B₂ *on page 353*
    Vitamin B₃ *on page 354*
    Vitamin B₆ *on page 357*
    Vitamin B₁₂ *on page 359*
    Vitamin K *on page 367*
    (Continued)

Ciprofloxacin* *(Continued)*
Scientific Basis Inferred or indirect evidence of depletion based on disruption of physiologic processes
Studies & Abstracts 7-27

+ **Ciprofloxacin Hydrochloride** *see* Ciprofloxacin* *on page 77*
+ **Cipro® Injection** *see* Ciprofloxacin* *on page 77*
+ **Cipro® Oral** *see* Ciprofloxacin* *on page 77*

Cisplatin* (SIS pla tin)
U.S. Brand Names Platinol®; Platinol®-AQ
Synonyms CDDP
Pharmacologic Class Antineoplastic Agent, Alkylating Agent
Nutrients Depleted
See Nutrient Depletion and Cancer Chemotherapy *on page 515.*
Scientific Basis Inferred or indirect evidence of depletion based on disruption of physiologic processes

Citalopram (sye TAL oh pram)
U.S. Brand Names Celexa®
Synonyms Citalopram Hydrobromide; Nitalapram
Pharmacologic Class Antidepressant, Selective Serotonin Reuptake Inhibitor
Nutrients Depleted
Specific nutrient depletions have not been documented for this agent.
Additional Information Selective serotonin reuptake inhibitors have been associated with rare, potentially severe hyponatremia. However, this is generally associated with fluid excess (SIADH), rather than a sodium deficiency. Treatment must be guided by a qualified healthcare provider.

+ **Citalopram Hydrobromide** *see* Citalopram *on page 78*
+ **CI-719** *see* Gemfibrozil* *on page 137*
+ **Cla** *see* Clarithromycin* *on page 78*

Cladribine* (KLA dri been)
U.S. Brand Names Leustatin™
Synonyms 2-CdA; 2-Chlorodeoxyadenosine
Pharmacologic Class Antineoplastic Agent, Antimetabolite
Nutrients Depleted
See Nutrient Depletion and Cancer Chemotherapy *on page 515.*
Scientific Basis Inferred or indirect evidence of depletion based on disruption of physiologic processes

+ **Claforan®** *see* Cefotaxime* *on page 64*
+ **Claripex®** *see* Clofibrate *on page 80*

Clarithromycin* (kla RITH roe mye sin)
U.S. Brand Names Biaxin®; Biaxin® XL
Synonyms Cla
Pharmacologic Class Antibiotic, Macrolide

Nutrients Depleted
Bifidobacteria bifidum (bifidus) on page 311
Biotin *on page 311*
Inositol *on page 328*
Lactobacillus acidophilus on page 332
Vitamin B$_1$ *on page 351*
Vitamin B$_2$ *on page 353*
Vitamin B$_3$ *on page 354*
Vitamin B$_6$ *on page 357*
Vitamin B$_{12}$ *on page 359*
Vitamin K *on page 367*

Scientific Basis Inferred or indirect evidence of depletion based on disruption of physiologic processes

Studies & Abstracts 7-27

- **Claritin-D® 12-Hour** *see* Loratadine and Pseudoephedrine *on page 168*
- **Claritin-D® 24-Hour** *see* Loratadine and Pseudoephedrine *on page 168*
- **Claritin® Extra** *see* Loratadine and Pseudoephedrine *on page 168*
- **Claritin® RediTabs®** *see* Loratadine *on page 168*
- **Claritin® Syrup** *see* Loratadine *on page 168*
- **Claritin® Tablets** *see* Loratadine *on page 168*
- **Clear Tussin® 30** *see* Guaifenesin and Dextromethorphan *on page 141*

Clemastine (KLEM as teen)

U.S. Brand Names Antihist-1® [OTC]; Tavist®; Tavist®-1 [OTC]
Synonyms Clemastine Fumarate
Pharmacologic Class Antihistamine
Nutrients Depleted
Specific nutrient depletions have not been documented for this agent.

Clemastine and Phenylpropanolamine

(KLEM as teen & fen il proe pa NOLE a meen)
U.S. Brand Names Antihist-D®; Tavist-D®
Pharmacologic Class Antihistamine/Decongestant Combination
Nutrients Depleted
Specific nutrient depletions have not been documented for this agent.

- **Clemastine Fumarate** *see* Clemastine *on page 79*
- **Cleocin-3®** *see* Clindamycin* *on page 80*
- **Cleocin HCl®** *see* Clindamycin* *on page 80*
- **Cleocin Pediatric®** *see* Clindamycin* *on page 80*
- **Cleocin Phosphate®** *see* Clindamycin* *on page 80*
- **Cleocin T®** *see* Clindamycin* *on page 80*
- **Climara® Transdermal** *see* Estradiol* *on page 114*
- **Clinda-Derm® Topical Solution** *see* Clindamycin* *on page 80*

Clindamycin* (klin da MYE sin)
U.S. Brand Names Cleocin-3®; Cleocin HCl®; Cleocin Pediatric®; Cleocin Phosphate®; Cleocin T®; Clinda-Derm® Topical Solution; Clindets® Pledgets; C/T/S® Topical Solution
Canadian Brand Names Dalacin® C [Hydrochloride]
Synonyms Clindamycin Hydrochloride; Clindamycin Phosphate
Pharmacologic Class Antibiotic, Miscellaneous
Nutrients Depleted
  Bifidobacteria bifidum (bifidus) on page 311
  Lactobacillus acidophilus on page 332
Scientific Basis Inferred or indirect evidence of depletion based on disruption of physiologic processes
Studies & Abstracts 7-27

♦ **Clindamycin Hydrochloride** *see* Clindamycin* *on page 80*
♦ **Clindamycin Phosphate** *see* Clindamycin* *on page 80*
♦ **Clindets® Pledgets** *see* Clindamycin* *on page 80*
♦ **Clinoril®** *see* Sulindac* *on page 245*
♦ **Clocort® Maximum Strength** *see* Hydrocortisone* *on page 150*

Clofazimine (kloe FA zi meen)
U.S. Brand Names Lamprene®
Synonyms Clofazimine Palmitate
Pharmacologic Class Leprostatic Agent
Nutrients Depleted
  Specific nutrient depletions have not been documented for this agent.

♦ **Clofazimine Palmitate** *see* Clofazimine *on page 80*

Clofibrate (kloe FYE brate)
U.S. Brand Names Atromid-S®
Canadian Brand Names Abitrate®; Claripex®; Novo-Fibrate
Pharmacologic Class Antilipemic Agent (Fibric Acid)
Nutrients Depleted
  Specific nutrient depletions have not been documented for this agent.

♦ **Clomid®** *see* Clomiphene *on page 80*

Clomiphene (KLOE mi feen)
U.S. Brand Names Clomid®; Milophene®; Serophene®
Synonyms Clomiphene Citrate
Pharmacologic Class Ovulation Stimulator
Nutrients Depleted
  Specific nutrient depletions have not been documented for this agent.

♦ **Clomiphene Citrate** *see* Clomiphene *on page 80*

Clomipramine* (kloe MI pra meen)
U.S. Brand Names Anafranil®
Canadian Brand Names Apo®-Clomipramine
Synonyms Clomipramine Hydrochloride
Pharmacologic Class Antidepressant, Tricyclic (Tertiary Amine)

Nutrients Depleted
Coenzyme Q_{10} *on page 320*
Vitamin B_2 *on page 353*
Scientific Basis Published scientific studies of agents from the same pharmacologic class
Studies & Abstracts 467-472

♦ **Clomipramine Hydrochloride** *see Clomipramine* on page 80*

Clonazepam (kloe NA ze pam)
U.S. Brand Names Klonopin™
Canadian Brand Names PMS-Clonazepam; Rivotril®
Pharmacologic Class Benzodiazepine
Nutrients Depleted
Specific nutrient depletions have not been documented for this agent.

Clonidine* (KLOE ni deen)
Related Information
Drug-Induced Nutrient Depletion Table *on page 498*
U.S. Brand Names Catapres® Oral; Catapres-TTS® Transdermal; Duraclon® Injection
Canadian Brand Names Apo®-Clonidine; Dixarit®; Novo-Clonidine; Nu-Clonidine
Synonyms Clonidine Hydrochloride
Pharmacologic Class Alpha$_2$ Agonist
Nutrients Depleted
Coenzyme Q_{10} *on page 320*
Scientific Basis Published scientific studies using this pharmacologic agent
Studies & Abstracts 274

♦ **Clonidine Hydrochloride** *see Clonidine* on page 81*

Clopidogrel (kloh PID oh grel)
U.S. Brand Names Plavix®
Synonyms Clopidogrel Bisulfate
Pharmacologic Class Antiplatelet Agent
Nutrients Depleted
Specific nutrient depletions have not been documented for this agent.

♦ **Clopidogrel Bisulfate** *see Clopidogrel on page 81*

Clorazepate (klor AZ e pate)
U.S. Brand Names Gen-XENE®; Tranxene®
Canadian Brand Names Apo®-Clorazepate; Novo-Clopate
Synonyms Clorazepate Dipotassium
Pharmacologic Class Benzodiazepine
Nutrients Depleted
Specific nutrient depletions have not been documented for this agent.

♦ **Clorazepate Dipotassium** see Clorazepate on page 81

Clotrimazole (kloe TRIM a zole)
U.S. Brand Names Femizole-7® [OTC]; Fungoid® Solution; Gyne-Lotrimin® [OTC]; Lotrimin®; Lotrimin® AF Cream [OTC]; Lotrimin® AF Lotion [OTC]; Lotrimin® AF Solution [OTC]; Mycelex®; Mycelex®-7; Mycelex®-G; Trivagizole 3™ [OTC]

Pharmacologic Class Antifungal Agent, Oral Nonabsorbed; Antifungal Agent, Topical; Antifungal Agent, Vaginal

Nutrients Depleted
Specific nutrient depletions have not been documented for this agent.

Cloxacillin* (kloks a SIL in)
Related Information
Drug-Induced Nutrient Depletion Table on page 498

U.S. Brand Names Cloxapen®; Tegopen®

Pharmacologic Class Antibiotic, Penicillin

Nutrients Depleted
Bifidobacteria bifidum (bifidus) on page 311
Biotin on page 311
Inositol on page 328
Lactobacillus acidophilus on page 332
Potassium on page 340
Vitamin B_1 on page 351
Vitamin B_2 on page 353
Vitamin B_3 on page 354
Vitamin B_6 on page 357
Vitamin B_{12} on page 359
Vitamin K on page 367

Scientific Basis Inferred or indirect evidence of depletion based on disruption of physiologic processes

Studies & Abstracts 7-27, 49-57

♦ **Cloxapen®** see Cloxacillin* on page 82

Clozapine (KLOE za peen)
U.S. Brand Names Clozaril®

Pharmacologic Class Antipsychotic Agent, Dibenzodiazepine

Nutrients Depleted
Specific nutrient depletions have not been documented for this agent.

♦ **Clozaril®** see Clozapine on page 82
♦ **Clysodrast®** see Bisacodyl* on page 48

Cocaine (koe KANE)
Synonyms Cocaine Hydrochloride

Pharmacologic Class Local Anesthetic

Nutrients Depleted
Specific nutrient depletions have not been documented for this agent.

- **Cocaine Hydrochloride** *see* Cocaine *on page 82*
- **Codafed® Expectorant** *see* Guaifenesin, Pseudoephedrine, and Codeine *on page 143*

Codeine (KOE deen)

Canadian Brand Names Codeine Contin®; Linctus Codeine Blac; Linctus With Codeine Phosphate; Paveral Stanley Syrup With Codeine Phosphate

Synonyms Codeine Phosphate; Codeine Sulfate; Methylmorphine

Pharmacologic Class Analgesic, Narcotic; Antitussive

Nutrients Depleted

Specific nutrient depletions have not been documented for this agent.

- **Codeine and Acetaminophen** *see* Acetaminophen and Codeine* *on page 23*
- **Codeine and Butalbital Compound** *see* Butalbital Compound and Codeine* *on page 54*
- **Codeine, Brompheniramine, and Phenylpropanolamine** *see* Brompheniramine, Phenylpropanolamine, and Codeine *on page 51*
- **Codeine Contin®** *see* Codeine *on page 83*
- **Codeine, Guaifenesin, and Pseudoephedrine** *see* Guaifenesin, Pseudoephedrine, and Codeine *on page 143*
- **Codeine Phosphate** *see* Codeine *on page 83*
- **Codeine Sulfate** *see* Codeine *on page 83*
- **Codoxy®** *see* Oxycodone and Aspirin* *on page 202*
- **Cogentin®** *see* Benztropine *on page 46*
- **Co-Gesic®** *see* Hydrocodone and Acetaminophen* *on page 149*
- **Cognex®** *see* Tacrine *on page 246*
- **Colace® [OTC]** *see* Docusate *on page 104*
- **Colax-C®** *see* Docusate *on page 104*
- **Colazal™** *see* Balsalazide* *on page 44*
- **ColBENEMID®** *see* Colchicine and Probenecid* *on page 84*

Colchicine* (KOL chi seen)

Related Information

Drug-Induced Nutrient Depletion Table *on page 498*

Pharmacologic Class Colchicine

Nutrients Depleted

Beta-Carotene *on page 310*

Calcium *on page 313*

Potassium *on page 340*

Sodium *on page 345*

Vitamin B_{12} *on page 359*

Scientific Basis Published scientific studies using this pharmacologic agent

Studies & Abstracts 437-448

Colchicine and Probenecid*
(KOL chi seen & proe BEN e sid)
U.S. Brand Names ColBENEMID®
Synonyms Probenecid and Colchicine
Pharmacologic Class Antigout Agent
Nutrients Depleted
Beta-Carotene *on page 310*
Potassium *on page 340*
Sodium *on page 345*
Vitamin B$_{12}$ *on page 359*
Scientific Basis Published scientific studies using this pharmacologic agent (colchicine)
Studies & Abstracts 437-448

♦ **Cold & Allergy® Elixir [OTC]** *see* Brompheniramine and Phenylpropanolamine *on page 50*
♦ **Coldlac-LA®** *see* Guaifenesin and Phenylpropanolamine *on page 141*
♦ **Coldloc®** *see* Guaifenesin, Phenylpropanolamine, and Phenylephrine *on page 142*

Colesevelam* (koh le SEV a lam)
U.S. Brand Names Welchol™
Pharmacologic Class Antilipemic Agent (Bile Acid Sequestrant)
Nutrients Depleted
Beta-Carotene *on page 310*
Folic Acid *on page 325*
Iron *on page 331*
Vitamin A *on page 349*
Vitamin B$_{12}$ *on page 359*
Vitamin D *on page 363*
Vitamin E *on page 365*
Scientific Basis Published scientific studies of agents with the same mechanism of action
Studies & Abstracts 371-373

♦ **Colestid®** *see* Colestipol* *on page 84*

Colestipol* (koe LES ti pole)
Related Information
Drug-Induced Nutrient Depletion Table *on page 498*
U.S. Brand Names Colestid®
Synonyms Colestipol Hydrochloride
Pharmacologic Class Antilipemic Agent (Bile Acid Sequestrant)
Nutrients Depleted
Beta-Carotene *on page 310*
Folic Acid *on page 325*
Iron *on page 331*
Vitamin A *on page 349*
Vitamin B$_{12}$ *on page 359*
Vitamin D *on page 363*

Vitamin E *on page 365*

Scientific Basis Published scientific studies using this pharmacologic agent

Studies & Abstracts 371-373

♦ **Colestipol Hydrochloride** *see* Colestipol* *on page 84*

♦ **CombiPatch**™ *see* Estradiol and Norethindrone* *on page 115*

♦ **Combivent**® *see* Ipratropium and Albuterol *on page 157*

♦ **Combivir**® *see* Zidovudine and Lamivudine* *on page 271*

♦ **Compazine**® *see* Prochlorperazine* *on page 221*

♦ **Compound E** *see* Cortisone Acetate* *on page 86*

♦ **Compound F** *see* Hydrocortisone* *on page 150*

♦ **Compound S** *see* Zidovudine* *on page 270*

♦ **Compound S, Abacavir, and Lamivudine** *see* Abacavir, Lamivudine, and Zidovudine* *on page 22*

♦ **Compoz**® **Gel Caps [OTC]** *see* Diphenhydramine *on page 102*

♦ **Compoz**® **Nighttime Sleep Aid [OTC]** *see* Diphenhydramine *on page 102*

♦ **Comtan**® *see* Entacapone *on page 111*

♦ **Concerta**™ *see* Methylphenidate *on page 178*

♦ **Conex**® **[OTC]** *see* Guaifenesin and Phenylpropanolamine *on page 141*

♦ **Congess**® **Jr** *see* Guaifenesin and Pseudoephedrine *on page 142*

♦ **Congess**® **Sr** *see* Guaifenesin and Pseudoephedrine *on page 142*

♦ **Congest** *see* Estrogens (Conjugated)* *on page 117*

♦ **Congestac**® *see* Guaifenesin and Pseudoephedrine *on page 142*

♦ **Conjugated Estrogen and Methyltestosterone** *see* Estrogens and Methyltestosterone* *on page 117*

♦ **Contac**® **Cough Formula Liquid [OTC]** *see* Guaifenesin and Dextromethorphan *on page 141*

♦ **Contergan**® *see* Thalidomide *on page 250*

♦ **Control**® **[OTC]** *see* Phenylpropanolamine *on page 211*

♦ **Contuss**® *see* Guaifenesin, Phenylpropanolamine, and Phenylephrine *on page 142*

♦ **Contuss**® **XT** *see* Guaifenesin and Phenylpropanolamine *on page 141*

♦ **Cophene-B**® *see* Brompheniramine *on page 50*

♦ **Coptin**® *see* Sulfadiazine* *on page 243*

♦ **Co-Pyronil**® **2 Pulvules**® **[OTC]** *see* Chlorpheniramine and Pseudoephedrine *on page 73*

♦ **Coradur**® *see* Isosorbide Dinitrate *on page 158*

♦ **Corax**® *see* Chlordiazepoxide *on page 72*

♦ **Cordarone**® *see* Amiodarone *on page 32*

♦ **Coreg**® *see* Carvedilol* *on page 59*

♦ **Corgard**® *see* Nadolol* *on page 187*

♦ **CortaGel**® **[OTC]** *see* Hydrocortisone* *on page 150*

♦ **Cortaid**® **Maximum Strength [OTC]** *see* Hydrocortisone* *on page 150*

- **Cortaid® With Aloe [OTC]** *see* Hydrocortisone* *on page 150*
- **Cort-Dome®** *see* Hydrocortisone* *on page 150*
- **Cortef®** *see* Hydrocortisone* *on page 150*
- **Cortef® Feminine Itch** *see* Hydrocortisone* *on page 150*
- **Cortenema®** *see* Hydrocortisone* *on page 150*
- **Cortifoam®** *see* Hydrocortisone* *on page 150*
- **Cortisol** *see* Hydrocortisone* *on page 150*

Cortisone Acetate* (KOR ti sone AS e tate)
Related Information
Drug-Induced Nutrient Depletion Table *on page 498*
U.S. Brand Names Cortone® Acetate
Synonyms Compound E
Pharmacologic Class Corticosteroid, Oral; Corticosteroid, Parenteral
Nutrients Depleted
Calcium *on page 313*
Folic Acid *on page 325*
Magnesium *on page 333*
Potassium *on page 340*
Selenium *on page 343*
Vitamin C *on page 360*
Vitamin D *on page 363*
Zinc *on page 368*
Scientific Basis
Published scientific studies using this pharmacologic agent
or
Published scientific studies of agents from the same pharmacologic class
Studies & Abstracts 182-223

- **Cortizone®-5 [OTC]** *see* Hydrocortisone* *on page 150*
- **Cortizone®-10 [OTC]** *see* Hydrocortisone* *on page 150*
- **Cortone® Acetate** *see* Cortisone Acetate* *on page 86*
- **Cosmegen®** *see* Dactinomycin* *on page 90*
- **Cotrim** *see* Co-Trimoxazole* *on page 86*
- **Cotrim® DS** *see* Co-Trimoxazole* *on page 86*

Co-Trimoxazole* (koe trye MOKS a zole)
Related Information
Drug-Induced Nutrient Depletion Table *on page 498*
U.S. Brand Names Bactrim™; Bactrim™ DS; Cotrim®; Cotrim® DS; Septra®; Septra® DS; Sulfatrim®
Canadian Brand Names Apo®-Sulfatrim; Novo-Trimel; Nu-Cotrimox; Pro-Trin®; Roubac®; Trisulfa®; Trisulfa-S®
Synonyms SMZ-TMP; Sulfamethoxazole and Trimethoprim; TMP-SMZ; Trimethoprim and Sulfamethoxazole
Pharmacologic Class Antibiotic, Sulfonamide Derivative
Nutrients Depleted
Bifidobacteria bifidum (bifidus) on page 311

Folic Acid *on page 325*
Lactobacillus acidophilus on page 332

Scientific Basis

Published scientific studies using this pharmacologic agent
  or
Inferred or indirect evidence of depletion based on disruption of physiologic processes

Studies & Abstracts 7-27, 69-71

Additional Information Folinic acid has been used to address hematologic toxicities. Replacement has been associated with a worse outcome in the treatment of some infections (*Pneumocystis carinii*).

♦ **Coumadin**® *see* Warfarin *on page 269*
♦ **Covera-HS**® *see* Verapamil *on page 267*
♦ **Cozaar**® *see* Losartan *on page 169*
♦ **CP-99,219-27** *see* Trovafloxacin* *on page 263*
♦ **CPM** *see* Cyclophosphamide* *on page 88*
♦ **CPT-11** *see* Irinotecan* *on page 157*
♦ **CPZ** *see* Chlorpromazine* *on page 74*
♦ **Creo-Terpin**® **[OTC]** *see* Dextromethorphan *on page 96*
♦ **Crinone**™ *see* Progesterone *on page 221*
♦ **Crixivan**® *see* Indinavir *on page 155*
♦ **Crolom**® **Ophthalmic Solution** *see* Cromolyn Sodium *on page 87*
♦ **Cromoglycic Acid** *see* Cromolyn Sodium *on page 87*

Cromolyn Sodium (KROE moe lin SOW dee um)

U.S. Brand Names Crolom® Ophthalmic Solution; Gastrocrom® Oral; Intal® Nebulizer Solution; Intal® Oral Inhaler; Nasalcrom® Nasal Solution [OTC]

Canadian Brand Names Novo-Cromolyn; Opticrom®; PMS-Sodium Cromoglycate; Rynacrom®

Synonyms Cromoglycic Acid; Disodium Cromoglycate; DSCG

Pharmacologic Class Antihistamine, Inhalation; Mast Cell Stabilizer

Nutrients Depleted

Specific nutrient depletions have not been documented for this agent.

♦ **Crystalline Penicillin** *see* Penicillin G (Parenteral/Aqueous)* *on page 206*
♦ **Crysticillin**® **A.S.** *see* Penicillin G Procaine* *on page 207*
♦ **CSA** *see* Cyclosporine* *on page 88*
♦ **CTM** *see* Chlorpheniramine *on page 73*
♦ **C/T/S**® **Topical Solution** *see* Clindamycin* *on page 80*
♦ **CTX** *see* Cyclophosphamide* *on page 88*
♦ **Cuprimine**® *see* Penicillamine* *on page 205*
♦ **Curretab**® **Oral** *see* Medroxyprogesterone Acetate *on page 173*
♦ **Cutivate**™ *see* Fluticasone* *on page 132*
♦ **CyA** *see* Cyclosporine* *on page 88*
♦ **Cyclen**® *see* Ethinyl Estradiol and Norgestimate* *on page 121*

Cyclizine (SYE kli zeen)
U.S. Brand Names Marezine® [OTC]
Synonyms Cyclizine Hydrochloride; Cyclizine Lactate
Pharmacologic Class Antihistamine
Nutrients Depleted
Specific nutrient depletions have not been documented for this agent.

♦ **Cyclizine Hydrochloride** *see* Cyclizine *on page 88*
♦ **Cyclizine Lactate** *see* Cyclizine *on page 88*

Cyclobenzaprine (sye kloe BEN za preen)
U.S. Brand Names Flexeril®
Canadian Brand Names Novo-Cycloprine
Synonyms Cyclobenzaprine Hydrochloride
Pharmacologic Class Skeletal Muscle Relaxant
Nutrients Depleted
Specific nutrient depletions have not been documented for this agent.

♦ **Cyclobenzaprine Hydrochloride** *see* Cyclobenzaprine *on page 88*

Cyclophosphamide* (sye kloe FOS fa mide)
U.S. Brand Names Cytoxan® Injection; Cytoxan® Oral; Neosar® Injection
Canadian Brand Names Procytox®
Synonyms CPM; CTX; CYT; NSC 26271
Pharmacologic Class Antineoplastic Agent, Alkylating Agent
Nutrients Depleted
See Nutrient Depletion and Cancer Chemotherapy *on page 515*.
Scientific Basis Inferred or indirect evidence of depletion based on disruption of physiologic processes

Cycloserine (sye kloe SER een)
U.S. Brand Names Seromycin® Pulvules®
Pharmacologic Class Antibiotic, Miscellaneous; Antitubercular Agent
Nutrients Depleted
Specific nutrient depletions have not been documented for this agent.

♦ **Cyclosporin A** *see* Cyclosporine* *on page 88*

Cyclosporine* (SYE kloe spor een)
U.S. Brand Names Neoral® Oral; Sandimmune® Injection; Sandimmune® Oral
Synonyms CSA; CyA; Cyclosporin A
Pharmacologic Class Immunosuppressant Agent
Nutrients Depleted
Magnesium *on page 333*
Potassium *on page 340*
Scientific Basis Published scientific studies using this pharmacologic agent
Studies & Abstracts 449-450

Additional Information Electrolyte changes may be extremely complex during immunosuppressive therapy. In particular, cyclosporine may be associated with either a decrease **OR** increase in potassium serum concentrations. Excessive levels of electrolytes may be dangerous. Potassium replacement and/or magnesium supplementation MUST be guided by a qualified healthcare practitioner based on serum level monitoring.

Cyclothiazide* (sye kloe THYE a zide)
U.S. Brand Names Anhydron®
Pharmacologic Class Diuretic, Thiazide
Nutrients Depleted
Coenzyme Q_{10} on page 320
Magnesium on page 333
Phosphorus on page 339
Potassium on page 340
Sodium on page 345
Vitamin B_6 on page 357
Zinc on page 368
Scientific Basis Published scientific studies using this pharmacologic agent
Studies & Abstracts 320-342
Additional Information Although thiazide diuretics deplete sodium, replacement is not recommended, as this may be directly related to the therapeutic effect. Thiazides may deplete potassium, however replacement should be guided by monitoring of serum concentrations and specific instruction by a healthcare provider.

♦ **Cycofed® Pediatric** see Guaifenesin, Pseudoephedrine, and Codeine on page 143
♦ **Cycrin® Oral** see Medroxyprogesterone Acetate on page 173
♦ **Cylert®** see Pemoline on page 204

Cyproheptadine (si proe HEP ta deen)
U.S. Brand Names Periactin®
Canadian Brand Names PMS-Cyproheptadine
Synonyms Cyproheptadine Hydrochloride
Pharmacologic Class Antihistamine
Nutrients Depleted
Specific nutrient depletions have not been documented for this agent.

♦ **Cyproheptadine Hydrochloride** see Cyproheptadine on page 89
♦ **Cystospaz®** see Hyoscyamine on page 153
♦ **Cystospaz-M®** see Hyoscyamine on page 153
♦ **CYT** see Cyclophosphamide* on page 88

Cytarabine* (sye TARE a been)
U.S. Brand Names Cytosar-U®
Synonyms Arabinosylcytosine; Ara-C; Cytarabine Hydrochloride; Cytosine Arabinosine Hydrochloride
Pharmacologic Class Antineoplastic Agent, Antimetabolite
(Continued)

Cytarabine* *(Continued)*
Nutrients Depleted
See Nutrient Depletion and Cancer Chemotherapy *on page 515*.
Scientific Basis Inferred or indirect evidence of depletion based on disruption of physiologic processes

♦ **Cytarabine Hydrochloride** *see* Cytarabine* *on page 89*

Cytarabine (Liposomal)*
(sye TARE a been lip po SOE mal)
U.S. Brand Names DepoCyt®
Pharmacologic Class Antineoplastic Agent, Antimetabolite
Nutrients Depleted
See Nutrient Depletion and Cancer Chemotherapy *on page 515*.
Scientific Basis Inferred or indirect evidence of depletion based on disruption of physiologic processes

♦ **Cytosar-U®** *see* Cytarabine* *on page 89*
♦ **Cytosine Arabinosine Hydrochloride** *see* Cytarabine* *on page 89*
♦ **Cytotec®** *see* Misoprostol *on page 183*
♦ **Cytovene®** *see* Ganciclovir *on page 136*
♦ **Cytoxan® Injection** *see* Cyclophosphamide* *on page 88*
♦ **Cytoxan® Oral** *see* Cyclophosphamide* *on page 88*
♦ **D-3-Mercaptovaline** *see* Penicillamine* *on page 205*
♦ **d4T** *see* Stavudine* *on page 241*

Dacarbazine* (da KAR ba zeen)
U.S. Brand Names DTIC-Dome®
Synonyms DIC; Dimethyl Triazeno Imidazol Carboxamide; Imidazole Carboxamide
Pharmacologic Class Antineoplastic Agent, Alkylating Agent
Nutrients Depleted
See Nutrient Depletion and Cancer Chemotherapy *on page 515*.
Scientific Basis Inferred or indirect evidence of depletion based on disruption of physiologic processes

♦ **Dacodyl® [OTC]** *see* Bisacodyl* *on page 48*

Dactinomycin* (dak ti noe MYE sin)
U.S. Brand Names Cosmegen®
Synonyms ACT; Actinomycin D
Pharmacologic Class Antineoplastic Agent, Antibiotic
Nutrients Depleted
See Nutrient Depletion and Cancer Chemotherapy *on page 515*.
Scientific Basis Inferred or indirect evidence of depletion based on disruption of physiologic processes

♦ **Dalacin® C [Hydrochloride]** *see* Clindamycin* *on page 80*
♦ **Dalalone®** *see* Dexamethasone* *on page 95*
♦ **Dalalone D.P.®** *see* Dexamethasone* *on page 95*

+ **Dalalone L.A.**® *see* Dexamethasone* *on page 95*
+ **Dallergy-D**® **Syrup** *see* Chlorpheniramine and Phenylephrine *on page 73*
+ **Dalmane**® *see* Flurazepam *on page 131*

Dalteparin (dal TE pa rin)
U.S. Brand Names Fragmin®
Pharmacologic Class Low Molecular Weight Heparin
Nutrients Depleted
Specific nutrient depletions have not been documented for this agent.

+ **Damason-P**® *see* Hydrocodone and Aspirin* *on page 150*

Danaparoid (da NAP a roid)
U.S. Brand Names Orgaran®
Synonyms Danaparoid Sodium
Pharmacologic Class Anticoagulant
Nutrients Depleted
Specific nutrient depletions have not been documented for this agent.

+ **Danaparoid Sodium** *see* Danaparoid *on page 91*
+ **Dantrium**® *see* Dantrolene *on page 91*

Dantrolene (DAN troe leen)
U.S. Brand Names Dantrium®
Synonyms Dantrolene Sodium
Pharmacologic Class Skeletal Muscle Relaxant
Nutrients Depleted
Specific nutrient depletions have not been documented for this agent.

+ **Dantrolene Sodium** *see* Dantrolene *on page 91*

Dapsone (DAP sone)
U.S. Brand Names Avlosulfon®
Synonyms Diaminodiphenylsulfone
Pharmacologic Class Antibiotic, Miscellaneous
Nutrients Depleted
Specific nutrient depletions have not been documented for this agent.

+ **Darvocet-N**® *see* Propoxyphene and Acetaminophen* *on page 223*
+ **Darvocet-N**® **100** *see* Propoxyphene and Acetaminophen* *on page 223*
+ **Darvon**® *see* Propoxyphene *on page 223*
+ **Darvon-N**® *see* Propoxyphene *on page 223*

Daunorubicin Citrate (Liposomal)*
(daw noe ROO bi sin SI trate lip po SOE mal)
U.S. Brand Names DaunoXome®
Pharmacologic Class Antineoplastic Agent, Antibiotic
Nutrients Depleted
See Nutrient Depletion and Cancer Chemotherapy *on page 515*.
Scientific Basis Inferred or indirect evidence of depletion based on disruption of physiologic processes

Delavirdine* (de la VIR deen)

Related Information
Drug-Induced Nutrient Depletion Table on page 498

U.S. Brand Names Rescriptor®

Synonyms U-90152S

Pharmacologic Class Antiretroviral Agent, Protease Inhibitor

Nutrients Depleted
Carnitine on page 316
Copper on page 322
Vitamin B_{12} on page 359
Zinc on page 368

Scientific Basis Published scientific studies of agents from the same
pharmacologic class

Studies & Abstracts 260-262

- **Deltadehydrocortisone** *see* Prednisone* *on page 219*
- **Deltahydrocortisone** *see* Prednisolone* *on page 218*
- **Deltasone**® *see* Prednisone* *on page 219*
- **Delta-Tritex**® *see* Triamcinolone* *on page 259*
- **Demadex**® *see* Torsemide* *on page 257*
- **Demazin**® **Syrup [OTC]** *see* Chlorpheniramine and Phenylpropanolamine *on page 73*

Demeclocycline* (dem e kloe SYE kleen)

Related Information
Drug-Induced Nutrient Depletion Table *on page 498*
U.S. Brand Names Declomycin®
Synonyms Demeclocycline Hydrochloride; Demethylchlortetracycline
Pharmacologic Class Antibiotic, Tetracycline Derivative
Nutrients Depleted
Bifidobacteria bifidum (bifidus) on page 311
Biotin *on page 311*
Calcium *on page 313*
Inositol *on page 328*
Iron *on page 331*
Lactobacillus acidophilus on page 332
Magnesium *on page 333*
Vitamin B_1 *on page 351*
Vitamin B_2 *on page 353*
Vitamin B_3 *on page 354*
Vitamin B_6 *on page 357*
Vitamin B_{12} *on page 359*
Vitamin K *on page 367*
Scientific Basis Published scientific studies of agents from the same pharmacologic class
Studies & Abstracts 7-27, 62-68
Additional Information Calcium, iron, and magnesium depletion may be minimal during brief treatments. Replacement should not be attempted unless the time of administration is separated from the dosing of the tetracycline.

- **Demeclocycline Hydrochloride** *see* Demeclocycline* *on page 93*
- **Demethylchlortetracycline** *see* Demeclocycline* *on page 93*
- **Demulen**® *see* Estradiol and Ethynodiol Diacetate* *on page 114*
- **Denavir**™ *see* Penciclovir *on page 205*
- **Depacon**™ *see* Valproic Acid and Derivatives* *on page 265*
- **Depade**® *see* Naltrexone *on page 188*
- **Depakene**® *see* Valproic Acid and Derivatives* *on page 265*
- **Depakote**® **Delayed Release** *see* Valproic Acid and Derivatives* *on page 265*
- **Depakote**® **ER** *see* Valproic Acid and Derivatives* *on page 265*
- **depAndrogyn**® **Injection** *see* Estradiol and Testosterone* *on page 115*
- **Depen**® *see* Penicillamine* *on page 205*
- **depGynogen**® **Injection** *see* Estradiol* *on page 114*

- **depMedalone® Injection** *see* Methylprednisolone* *on page 178*
- **DepoCyt®** *see* Cytarabine (Liposomal)* *on page 90*
- **Depo®-Estradiol Injection** *see* Estradiol* *on page 114*
- **Depogen® Injection** *see* Estradiol* *on page 114*
- **Depoject® Injection** *see* Methylprednisolone* *on page 178*
- **Depo-Medrol Injection** *see* Methylprednisolone* *on page 178*
- **Deponit® Patch** *see* Nitroglycerin *on page 192*
- **Depopred® Injection** *see* Methylprednisolone* *on page 178*
- **Depo-Provera® Injection** *see* Medroxyprogesterone Acetate *on page 173*
- **Depo-Testadiol® Injection** *see* Estradiol and Testosterone* *on page 115*
- **Depotestogen® Injection** *see* Estradiol and Testosterone* *on page 115*
- **Deprenyl** *see* Selegiline *on page 236*
- **Deproic** *see* Valproic Acid and Derivatives* *on page 265*
- **Deproist® Expectorant With Codeine** *see* Guaifenesin, Pseudoephedrine, and Codeine *on page 143*
- **Dermacort®** *see* Hydrocortisone* *on page 150*
- **Dermarest Dricort®** *see* Hydrocortisone* *on page 150*
- **Derma-Smoothe/FS®** *see* Fluocinolone* *on page 129*
- **DermiCort®** *see* Hydrocortisone* *on page 150*
- **Dermolate® [OTC]** *see* Hydrocortisone* *on page 150*
- **Dermtex® HC With Aloe** *see* Hydrocortisone* *on page 150*
- **DES** *see* Diethylstilbestrol* *on page 99*
- **Desiccated Thyroid** *see* Thyroid *on page 252*

Desipramine* (des IP ra meen)

Related Information
Drug-Induced Nutrient Depletion Table *on page 498*

U.S. Brand Names Norpramin®

Canadian Brand Names PMS-Desipramine

Synonyms Desipramine Hydrochloride; Desmethylimipramine Hydrochloride

Pharmacologic Class Antidepressant, Tricyclic (Secondary Amine)

Nutrients Depleted
Coenzyme Q_{10} *on page 320*
Vitamin B_2 *on page 353*

Scientific Basis Published scientific studies of agents from the same pharmacologic class

Studies & Abstracts 467-472

- **Desipramine Hydrochloride** *see* Desipramine* *on page 94*
- **Desmethylimipramine Hydrochloride** *see* Desipramine* *on page 94*
- **Desogen®** *see* Ethinyl Estradiol and Desogestrel* *on page 119*
- **Desogestrel and Ethinyl Estradiol** *see* Ethinyl Estradiol and Desogestrel* *on page 119*
- **Desoxyphenobarbital** *see* Primidone* *on page 220*

- **Desyrel®** *see* Trazodone *on page 259*
- **Detensol®** *see* Propranolol* *on page 223*
- **Detrol™** *see* Tolterodine *on page 257*
- **Dexacort® Phosphate in Respihaler®** *see* Dexamethasone* *on page 95*
- **Dexacort® Phosphate Turbinaire®** *see* Dexamethasone* *on page 95*

Dexamethasone* (deks a METH a sone)
Related Information
Drug-Induced Nutrient Depletion Table *on page 498*

U.S. Brand Names Aeroseb-Dex®; AK-Dex® Ophthalmic; Baldex®; Dalalone®; Dalalone D.P.®; Dalalone L.A.®; Decadron®; Decadron®-LA; Decadron® Phosphate; Decaject®; Decaject-LA®; Dexacort® Phosphate in Respihaler®; Dexacort® Phosphate Turbinaire®; Dexasone®; Dexasone® L.A.; Dexone®; Dexone® LA; Dexotic®; Hexadrol®; Hexadrol® Phosphate; Maxidex®; Solurex®; Solurex L.A.®

Synonyms Dexamethasone Acetate; Dexamethasone Sodium Phosphate

Pharmacologic Class Corticosteroid, Oral; Corticosteroid, Oral Inhaler; Corticosteroid, Nasal; Corticosteroid, Ophthalmic; Corticosteroid, Parenteral; Corticosteroid, Topical

Nutrients Depleted
Calcium *on page 313*
Folic Acid *on page 325*
Magnesium *on page 333*
Potassium *on page 340*
Selenium *on page 343*
Vitamin C *on page 360*
Vitamin D *on page 363*
Zinc *on page 368*

Scientific Basis
Published scientific studies using this pharmacologic agent
  or
Published scientific studies of agents from the same pharmacologic class

Studies & Abstracts 182-223

Additional Information Due to low mineralocorticoid activity, loss of electrolytes (potassium) is not likely to be significant.

- **Dexamethasone Acetate** *see* Dexamethasone* *on page 95*
- **Dexamethasone Sodium Phosphate** *see* Dexamethasone* *on page 95*
- **Dexasone®** *see* Dexamethasone* *on page 95*
- **Dexasone® L.A.** *see* Dexamethasone* *on page 95*
- **Dexatrim® Pre-Meal [OTC]** *see* Phenylpropanolamine *on page 211*
- **Dexchlor®** *see* Dexchlorpheniramine *on page 95*

Dexchlorpheniramine (deks klor fen EER a meen)
U.S. Brand Names Dexchlor®; Poladex®; Polaramine®
Synonyms Dexchlorpheniramine Maleate
(Continued)

Dexchlorpheniramine *(Continued)*
Pharmacologic Class Antihistamine
Nutrients Depleted
  Specific nutrient depletions have not been documented for this agent.

♦ **Dexchlorpheniramine Maleate** *see* Dexchlorpheniramine *on page 95*

♦ **Dexedrine®** *see* Dextroamphetamine *on page 96*

♦ **Dexone®** *see* Dexamethasone* *on page 95*

♦ **Dexone® LA** *see* Dexamethasone* *on page 95*

♦ **Dexotic®** *see* Dexamethasone* *on page 95*

Dextroamphetamine (deks troe am FET a meen)
U.S. Brand Names Dexedrine®
Synonyms Dextroamphetamine Sulfate
Pharmacologic Class Stimulant
Nutrients Depleted
  Specific nutrient depletions have not been documented for this agent.

Dextroamphetamine and Amphetamine
  (deks troe am FET a meen & am FET a meen)
U.S. Brand Names Adderall®
Pharmacologic Class Stimulant
Nutrients Depleted
  Specific nutrient depletions have not been documented for this agent.

♦ **Dextroamphetamine Sulfate** *see* Dextroamphetamine *on page 96*

Dextromethorphan (deks troe meth OR fan)
U.S. Brand Names Benylin DM® [OTC]; Benylin® Pediatric [OTC]; Children's Hold® [OTC]; Creo-Terpin® [OTC]; Delsym® [OTC]; Drixoral® Cough Liquid Caps [OTC]; Hold® DM [OTC]; Pertussin® CS [OTC]; Pertussin® ES [OTC]; Robitussin® Cough Calmers [OTC]; Robitussin® Pediatric [OTC]; Scot-Tussin DM® Cough Chasers [OTC]; Silphen DM® [OTC]; St. Joseph® Cough Suppressant [OTC]; Sucrets® Cough Calmers [OTC]; Suppress® [OTC]; Trocal® [OTC]; Vicks Formula 44® [OTC]; Vicks Formula 44® Pediatric Formula [OTC]
Pharmacologic Class Antitussive
Nutrients Depleted
  Specific nutrient depletions have not been documented for this agent.

♦ **Dextromethorphan and Guaifenesin** *see* Guaifenesin and Dextromethorphan *on page 141*

♦ **Dextromethorphan, Guaifenesin, and Phenylpropanolamine** *see* Guaifenesin, Phenylpropanolamine, and Dextromethorphan *on page 142*

♦ **Dextromethorphan, Guaifenesin, and Pseudoephedrine** *see* Guaifenesin, Pseudoephedrine, and Dextromethorphan *on page 143*

♦ **Dextropropoxyphene** *see* Propoxyphene *on page 223*

♦ **DFMO** *see* Eflornithine *on page 109*

♦ **DHAD** *see* Mitoxantrone* *on page 183*

- **DHPG Sodium** *see* Ganciclovir *on page 136*
- **Diaβeta®** *see* Glyburide* *on page 139*
- **Diabetic Tussin DM® [OTC]** *see* Guaifenesin and Dextromethorphan *on page 141*
- **Diabetic Tussin® EX [OTC]** *see* Guaifenesin *on page 140*
- **Diabinese®** *see* Chlorpropamide* *on page 74*
- **Dialose® [OTC]** *see* Docusate *on page 104*
- **Dialose® Plus Capsule [OTC]** *see* Docusate and Casanthranol* *on page 104*
- **Dialume® [OTC]** *see* Aluminum Hydroxide* *on page 28*
- **Diamine T.D.® [OTC]** *see* Brompheniramine *on page 50*
- **Diaminodiphenylsulfone** *see* Dapsone *on page 91*
- **Diamox®** *see* Acetazolamide* *on page 24*
- **Diamox Sequels®** *see* Acetazolamide* *on page 24*
- **Diar-Aid® [OTC]** *see* Loperamide *on page 167*
- **Diastat® Rectal Delivery System** *see* Diazepam *on page 97*
- **Diazemuls®** *see* Diazepam *on page 97*
- **Diazemuls® Injection** *see* Diazepam *on page 97*

Diazepam (dye AZ e pam)

U.S. Brand Names Diastat® Rectal Delivery System; Diazemuls® Injection; Diazepam Intensol®; Dizac® Injectable Emulsion; Valium® Injection; Valium® Oral

Canadian Brand Names Apo®-Diazepam; Diazemuls®; E Pam®; Meval®; Novo-Dipam; PMS-Diazepam; Vivol®

Pharmacologic Class Benzodiazepine

Nutrients Depleted
Specific nutrient depletions have not been documented for this agent.

- **Diazepam Intensol®** *see* Diazepam *on page 97*
- **Dibent® Injection** *see* Dicyclomine *on page 98*
- **DIC** *see* Dacarbazine* *on page 90*

Diclofenac* (dye KLOE fen ak)

Related Information
Drug-Induced Nutrient Depletion Table *on page 498*

U.S. Brand Names Cataflam® Oral; Voltaren® Ophthalmic; Voltaren® Oral; Voltaren®-XR Oral

Canadian Brand Names Apo®-Diclo; Novo-Difenac®; Novo-Difenac®-SR; Nu-Diclo; Voltaren Rapide®

Synonyms Diclofenac Potassium; Diclofenac Sodium

Pharmacologic Class Nonsteroidal Anti-Inflammatory Agent (NSAID)

Nutrients Depleted
Folic Acid *on page 325*

Scientific Basis Published scientific studies of agents from the same pharmacologic class

Studies & Abstracts 252

Diclofenac and Misoprostol*
(dye KLOE fen ak & mye soe PROST ole)
U.S. Brand Names Arthrotec®
Synonyms Misoprostol and Diclofenac
Pharmacologic Class Nonsteroidal Anti-Inflammatory Agent (NSAID); Prostaglandin
Nutrients Depleted
Folic Acid *on page 325*
Scientific Basis Published scientific studies of agents from the same pharmacologic class (diclofenac)
Studies & Abstracts 252

♦ **Diclofenac Potassium** *see Diclofenac* on page 97*
♦ **Diclofenac Sodium** *see Diclofenac* on page 97*

Dicloxacillin* (dye kloks a SIL in)
Related Information
Drug-Induced Nutrient Depletion Table *on page 498*
U.S. Brand Names Dycill®; Dynapen®; Pathocil®
Synonyms Dicloxacillin Sodium
Pharmacologic Class Antibiotic, Penicillin
Nutrients Depleted
Bifidobacteria bifidum (bifidus) on page 311
Biotin *on page 311*
Inositol *on page 328*
Lactobacillus acidophilus on page 332
Potassium *on page 340*
Vitamin B_1 *on page 351*
Vitamin B_2 *on page 353*
Vitamin B_3 *on page 354*
Vitamin B_6 *on page 357*
Vitamin B_{12} *on page 359*
Vitamin K *on page 367*
Scientific Basis Inferred or indirect evidence of depletion based on disruption of physiologic processes
Studies & Abstracts 7-27, 49-57

♦ **Dicloxacillin Sodium** *see Dicloxacillin* on page 98*

Dicyclomine (dye SYE kloe meen)
U.S. Brand Names Antispas® Injection; Bentyl® Hydrochloride Injection; Bentyl® Hydrochloride Oral; Byclomine® Injection; Dibent® Injection; Di-Spaz® Injection; Di-Spaz® Oral; Or-Tyl® Injection
Canadian Brand Names Bentylol®; Formulex®
Synonyms Dicyclomine Hydrochloride; Dicycloverine Hydrochloride
Pharmacologic Class Anticholinergic Agent
Nutrients Depleted
Specific nutrient depletions have not been documented for this agent.

♦ **Dicyclomine Hydrochloride** *see Dicyclomine on page 98*
♦ **Dicycloverine Hydrochloride** *see Dicyclomine on page 98*

Didanosine* (dye DAN oh seen)
Related Information
Drug-Induced Nutrient Depletion Table *on page 498*
U.S. Brand Names Videx®
Synonyms ddl
Pharmacologic Class Antiretroviral Agent, Reverse Transcriptase Inhibitor (Nucleoside)
Nutrients Depleted
Carnitine *on page 316*
Copper *on page 322*
Vitamin B_{12} *on page 359*
Zinc *on page 368*
Scientific Basis Published scientific studies of agents from the same pharmacologic class
Studies & Abstracts 260-262

♦ **Dideoxycytidine** *see Zalcitabine* on page 269*

Diethylpropion (dye eth il PROE pee on)
U.S. Brand Names Tenuate®; Tenuate® Dospan®
Canadian Brand Names Nobesine®
Synonyms Amfepramone; Diethylpropion Hydrochloride
Pharmacologic Class Anorexiant
Nutrients Depleted
Specific nutrient depletions have not been documented for this agent.

♦ **Diethylpropion Hydrochloride** *see Diethylpropion on page 99*

Diethylstilbestrol* (dye eth il stil BES trole)
U.S. Brand Names Stilphostrol®
Canadian Brand Names Honvol®
Synonyms DES; Diethylstilbestrol Diphosphate Sodium; Stilbestrol
Pharmacologic Class Estrogen Derivative
Nutrients Depleted
Magnesium *on page 333*
Vitamin B_6 *on page 357*
Scientific Basis Published scientific studies of agents from the same pharmacologic class
Studies & Abstracts 378-379

♦ **Diethylstilbestrol Diphosphate Sodium** *see Diethylstilbestrol* on page 99*

Diflorasone* (dye FLOR a sone)
U.S. Brand Names Florone®; Florone E®; Maxiflor®; Psorcon™
Synonyms Diflorasone Diacetate
Pharmacologic Class Corticosteroid, Topical
Nutrients Depleted
Calcium *on page 313*
Folic Acid *on page 325*
Magnesium *on page 333*
Potassium *on page 340*
(Continued)

Diflorasone* *(Continued)*

Selenium *on page 343*
Vitamin C *on page 360*
Vitamin D *on page 363*
Zinc *on page 368*

Scientific Basis

Published scientific studies using this pharmacologic agent
or
Published scientific studies of agents from the same pharmacologic
class

Studies & Abstracts 182-223

Additional Information Potential for depletion is limited with topical
use.

♦ **Diflorasone Diacetate** *see* Diflorasone* *on page 99*

♦ **Diflucan**® *see* Fluconazole *on page 128*

Diflunisal* (dye FLOO ni sal)

Related Information

Drug-Induced Nutrient Depletion Table *on page 498*

U.S. Brand Names Dolobid®

Canadian Brand Names Apo®-Diflunisal; Novo-Diflunisal; Nu-Diflunisal

Pharmacologic Class Nonsteroidal Anti-Inflammatory Agent
(NSAID)

Nutrients Depleted

Folic Acid *on page 325*

Scientific Basis

Published scientific studies using this pharmacologic agent
or
Published scientific studies of agents from the same pharmacologic
class

Studies & Abstracts 252

♦ **Di-Gel**® **[OTC]** *see* Aluminum Hydroxide, Magnesium Hydroxide, and
Simethicone* *on page 29*

Digoxin* (di JOKS in)

Related Information

Drug-Induced Nutrient Depletion Table *on page 498*

U.S. Brand Names Lanoxicaps®; Lanoxin®

Canadian Brand Names Novo-Digoxin

Pharmacologic Class Antiarrhythmic Agent, Class IV; Cardiac
Glycoside

Nutrients Depleted

Calcium *on page 313*
Magnesium *on page 333*
Phosphorus *on page 339*
Vitamin B_1 *on page 351*

Scientific Basis Published scientific studies using this pharmacologic
agent

Studies & Abstracts 343-347

♦ **Dihistine® Expectorant** *see* Guaifenesin, Pseudoephedrine, and Codeine *on page 143*

♦ **Dihydrohydroxycodeinone** *see* Oxycodone *on page 202*

♦ **Dihydromorphinone** *see* Hydromorphone *on page 151*

♦ **Dilacor™ XR** *see* Diltiazem *on page 101*

♦ **Dilantin®** *see* Phenytoin* *on page 212*

♦ **Dilatrate®-SR** *see* Isosorbide Dinitrate *on page 158*

♦ **Dilaudid®** *see* Hydromorphone *on page 151*

♦ **Dilaudid-5®** *see* Hydromorphone *on page 151*

♦ **Dilaudid-HP®** *see* Hydromorphone *on page 151*

Diltiazem (dil TYE a zem)

U.S. Brand Names Cardizem® CD; Cardizem® Injectable; Cardizem® SR; Cardizem® Tablet; Dilacor™ XR; Tiamate®; Tiazac™

Canadian Brand Names Apo®-Diltiaz; Novo-Diltazem; Nu-Diltiaz; Syn-Diltiazem

Synonyms Diltiazem Hydrochloride

Pharmacologic Class Calcium Channel Blocker

Nutrients Depleted
Specific nutrient depletions have not been documented for this agent.

♦ **Diltiazem Hydrochloride** *see* Diltiazem *on page 101*

♦ **Dimacol® Caplets [OTC]** *see* Guaifenesin, Pseudoephedrine, and Dextromethorphan *on page 143*

♦ **Dimaphen® Elixir [OTC]** *see* Brompheniramine and Phenylpropanolamine *on page 50*

♦ **Dimaphen® Tablets [OTC]** *see* Brompheniramine and Phenylpropanolamine *on page 50*

♦ **Dimetane®-DC** *see* Brompheniramine, Phenylpropanolamine, and Codeine *on page 51*

♦ **Dimetane® Decongestant Elixir [OTC]** *see* Brompheniramine and Phenylephrine *on page 50*

♦ **Dimetane® Extentabs® [OTC]** *see* Brompheniramine *on page 50*

♦ **Dimetapp® 4-Hour Liqui-Gel Capsule [OTC]** *see* Brompheniramine and Phenylpropanolamine *on page 50*

♦ **Dimetapp® Elixir [OTC]** *see* Brompheniramine and Phenylpropanolamine *on page 50*

♦ **Dimetapp® Extentabs® [OTC]** *see* Brompheniramine and Phenylpropanolamine *on page 50*

♦ **Dimetapp® Sinus Caplets [OTC]** *see* Pseudoephedrine and Ibuprofen* *on page 226*

♦ **Dimetapp® Tablet [OTC]** *see* Brompheniramine and Phenylpropanolamine *on page 50*

♦ **β,β-Dimethylcysteine** *see* Penicillamine* *on page 205*

♦ **Dimethyl Triazeno Imidazol Carboxamide** *see* Dacarbazine* *on page 90*

♦ **Diocto® [OTC]** *see* Docusate *on page 104*

♦ **Diocto C® [OTC]** *see* Docusate and Casanthranol* *on page 104*

- **Diocto-K®** [OTC] *see* Docusate *on page 104*
- **Diocto-K Plus®** [OTC] *see* Docusate and Casanthranol* *on page 104*
- **Dioctolose Plus®** [OTC] *see* Docusate and Casanthranol* *on page 104*
- **Dioctyl Calcium Sulfosuccinate** *see* Docusate *on page 104*
- **Dioctyl Potassium Sulfosuccinate** *see* Docusate *on page 104*
- **Dioctyl Sodium Sulfosuccinate** *see* Docusate *on page 104*
- **Dioeze®** [OTC] *see* Docusate *on page 104*
- **Diomycin** *see* Erythromycin (Systemic)* *on page 113*
- **Dioval® Injection** *see* Estradiol* *on page 114*
- **Diovan™** *see* Valsartan *on page 265*
- **Diovan HCTZ®** *see* Valsartan and Hydrochlorothiazide* *on page 265*
- **Dipentum®** *see* Olsalazine* *on page 199*
- **Diphen® Cough** [OTC] *see* Diphenhydramine *on page 102*
- **Diphenhist®** [OTC] *see* Diphenhydramine *on page 102*

Diphenhydramine (dye fen HYE dra meen)

U.S. Brand Names AllerMax® Oral [OTC]; Banophen® Oral [OTC]; Belix® Oral [OTC]; Benadryl® Injection; Benadryl® Oral [OTC]; Benadryl® Topical; Ben-Allergin-50® Injection; Benylin® Cough Syrup [OTC]; Bydramine® Cough Syrup [OTC]; Compoz® Gel Caps [OTC]; Compoz® Nighttime Sleep Aid [OTC]; Diphen® Cough [OTC]; Diphenhist® [OTC]; Dormarex® 2 Oral [OTC]; Dormin® Oral [OTC]; Genahist® Oral; Hydramyn® Syrup [OTC]; Hyrexin-50® Injection; Maximum Strength Nytol® [OTC]; Miles Nervine® Caplets [OTC]; Nytol® Oral [OTC]; Phendry® Oral [OTC]; Siladryl® Oral [OTC]; Silphen® Cough [OTC]; Sleep-eze 3® Oral [OTC]; Sleepinal® [OTC]; Sleepwell 2-nite® [OTC]; Snooze Fast® [OTC]; Sominex® Oral [OTC]; Tusstat® Syrup; Twilite® Oral [OTC]; Uni-Bent® Cough Syrup; 40 Winks® [OTC]

Canadian Brand Names Allerdryl®; Allernix®; Nytol® Extra Strength

Synonyms Diphenhydramine Hydrochloride

Pharmacologic Class Antihistamine

Nutrients Depleted

Specific nutrient depletions have not been documented for this agent.

- **Diphenhydramine Hydrochloride** *see* Diphenhydramine *on page 102*
- **Diphenylan Sodium®** *see* Phenytoin* *on page 212*
- **Diphenylhydantoin** *see* Phenytoin* *on page 212*
- **Diprolene®** *see* Betamethasone* *on page 46*
- **Diprolene® AF** *see* Betamethasone* *on page 46*
- **Diprolene® Glycol [Dipropionate]** *see* Betamethasone* *on page 46*
- **Dipropylacetic Acid** *see* Valproic Acid and Derivatives* *on page 265*
- **Diprosone®** *see* Betamethasone* *on page 46*

Dipyridamole (dye peer ID a mole)
U.S. Brand Names Persantine®
Canadian Brand Names Apo®-Dipyridamole FC; Apo®-Dipyridamole SC; Novo-Dipiradol
Pharmacologic Class Antiplatelet Agent; Vasodilator
Nutrients Depleted
Specific nutrient depletions have not been documented for this agent.

Dirithromycin* (dye RITH roe mye sin)
U.S. Brand Names Dynabac®
Pharmacologic Class Antibiotic, Macrolide
Nutrients Depleted
Bifidobacteria bifidum (bifidus) on page 311
Biotin *on page 311*
Inositol *on page 328*
Lactobacillus acidophilus on page 332
Vitamin B_1 *on page 351*
Vitamin B_2 *on page 353*
Vitamin B_3 *on page 354*
Vitamin B_6 *on page 357*
Vitamin B_{12} *on page 359*
Vitamin K *on page 367*
Scientific Basis Inferred or indirect evidence of depletion based on disruption of physiologic processes
Studies & Abstracts 7-27

- **Disalcid®** *see* Salsalate* *on page 235*
- **Disalicylic Acid** *see* Salsalate* *on page 235*
- **Disanthrol® [OTC]** *see* Docusate and Casanthranol* *on page 104*
- **Disodium Cromoglycate** *see* Cromolyn Sodium *on page 87*
- ***d*-Isoephedrine Hydrochloride** *see* Pseudoephedrine *on page 225*
- **Disonate® [OTC]** *see* Docusate *on page 104*

Disopyramide (dye soe PEER a mide)
U.S. Brand Names Norpace®
Synonyms Disopyramide Phosphate
Pharmacologic Class Antiarrhythmic Agent, Class I-A
Nutrients Depleted
Specific nutrient depletions have not been documented for this agent.

- **Disopyramide Phosphate** *see* Disopyramide *on page 103*
- **Di-Spaz® Injection** *see* Dicyclomine *on page 98*
- **Di-Spaz® Oral** *see* Dicyclomine *on page 98*
- **Distaval®** *see* Thalidomide *on page 250*

Disulfiram (dye SUL fi ram)
U.S. Brand Names Antabuse®
Pharmacologic Class Aldehyde Dehydrogenase Inhibitor
Nutrients Depleted
Specific nutrient depletions have not been documented for this agent.

- **Diucardin**® *see* Hydroflumethiazide* *on page 151*
- **Diuchlor**® *see* Hydrochlorothiazide* *on page 147*
- **Diurigen**® *see* Chlorothiazide* *on page 72*
- **Diuril**® *see* Chlorothiazide* *on page 72*
- **Divalproex Sodium** *see* Valproic Acid and Derivatives* *on page 265*
- **Dixarit**® *see* Clonidine* *on page 81*
- **Dizac**® **Injectable Emulsion** *see* Diazepam *on page 97*
- **Dizmiss**® **[OTC]** *see* Meclizine *on page 172*
- **dl-Norephedrine Hydrochloride** *see* Phenylpropanolamine *on page 211*
- **D-Med**® **Injection** *see* Methylprednisolone* *on page 178*

Docetaxel* (doe se TAKS el)

U.S. Brand Names Taxotere®

Pharmacologic Class Antineoplastic Agent, Natural Source (Plant) Derivative

Nutrients Depleted

See Nutrient Depletion and Cancer Chemotherapy *on page 515*.

Scientific Basis Inferred or indirect evidence of depletion based on disruption of physiologic processes

Docusate (DOK yoo sate)

U.S. Brand Names Colace® [OTC]; DC 240® Softgels® [OTC]; Dialose® [OTC]; Diocto® [OTC]; Diocto-K® [OTC]; Dioeze® [OTC]; Disonate® [OTC]; DOK® [OTC]; DOS® Softgel® [OTC]; D-S-S® [OTC]; Kasof® [OTC]; Modane® Soft [OTC]; Pro-Cal-Sof® [OTC]; Regulax SS® [OTC]; Sulfalax® [OTC]; Surfak® [OTC]

Canadian Brand Names Albert® Docusate; Colax-C®; PMS-Docusate Calcium; Regulex®; Selax®; SoFlax™

Synonyms Dioctyl Calcium Sulfosuccinate; Dioctyl Potassium Sulfosuccinate; Dioctyl Sodium Sulfosuccinate; Docusate Calcium; Docusate Potassium; Docusate Sodium; DOSS; DSS

Pharmacologic Class Stool Softener

Nutrients Depleted

Specific nutrient depletions have not been documented for this agent.

Docusate and Casanthranol*

(DOK yoo sate & ka SAN thra nole)

U.S. Brand Names Dialose® Plus Capsule [OTC]; Diocto C® [OTC]; Diocto-K Plus® [OTC]; Dioctolose Plus® [OTC]; Disanthrol® [OTC]; DSMC Plus® [OTC]; Genasoft® Plus [OTC]; Peri-Colace® [OTC]; Pro-Sof® Plus [OTC]; Regulace® [OTC]; Silace-C® [OTC]

Synonyms Casanthranol and Docusate; DSS With Casanthranol

Pharmacologic Class Laxative/Stool Softner

Nutrients Depleted

Potassium *on page 340*

Sodium *on page 345*

Scientific Basis Published scientific studies using this pharmacologic agent

Studies & Abstracts 451-454
Additional Information Significant depletions documented only in cases of laxative abuse.

♦ **Docusate Calcium** *see Docusate on page 104*
♦ **Docusate Potassium** *see Docusate on page 104*
♦ **Docusate Sodium** *see Docusate on page 104*

Dofetilide doe FET il ide
U.S. Brand Names Tikosyn™
Pharmacologic Class Antiarrhythmic Agent, Class III
Nutrients Depleted
  Specific nutrient depletions have not been documented for this agent.

♦ **DOK®** [OTC] *see Docusate on page 104*
♦ **Dolacet®** *see Hydrocodone and Acetaminophen* on page 149*

Dolasetron (dol A se tron)
U.S. Brand Names Anzemet®
Synonyms Dolasetron Mesylate
Pharmacologic Class Selective 5-HT$_3$ Receptor Antagonist
Nutrients Depleted
  Specific nutrient depletions have not been documented for this agent.

♦ **Dolasetron Mesylate** *see Dolasetron on page 105*
♦ **Dolene®** *see Propoxyphene on page 223*
♦ **Dolobid®** *see Diflunisal* on page 100*

Donepezil (don EH pa zil)
U.S. Brand Names Aricept®
Synonyms E2020
Pharmacologic Class Acetylcholinesterase Inhibitor (Central)
Nutrients Depleted
  Specific nutrient depletions have not been documented for this agent.

♦ **Donnamar®** *see Hyoscyamine on page 153*
♦ **Dopamet®** *see Methyldopa* on page 177*
♦ **Dopar®** *see Levodopa* on page 164*
♦ **Doral®** *see Quazepam on page 227*
♦ **Dormarex® 2 Oral** [OTC] *see Diphenhydramine on page 102*
♦ **Dormin® Oral** [OTC] *see Diphenhydramine on page 102*
♦ **Doryx®** *see Doxycycline* on page 106*
♦ **DOSS** *see Docusate on page 104*
♦ **DOS® Softgel®** [OTC] *see Docusate on page 104*
♦ **Dostinex®** *see Cabergoline on page 55*

Doxazosin (doks AYE zoe sin)
U.S. Brand Names Cardura®
Pharmacologic Class Alpha$_1$ Blockers
Nutrients Depleted
  Specific nutrient depletions have not been documented for this agent.

Doxepin* (DOKS e pin)
Related Information
Drug-Induced Nutrient Depletion Table *on page 498*
U.S. Brand Names Adapin® Oral; Sinequan® Oral; Zonalon® Topical Cream
Canadian Brand Names Apo®-Doxepin; Novo-Doxepin; Triadapin®
Synonyms Doxepin Hydrochloride
Pharmacologic Class Antidepressant, Tricyclic (Tertiary Amine); Topical Skin Product
Nutrients Depleted
Coenzyme Q_{10} *on page 320*
Vitamin B_2 *on page 353*
Scientific Basis Published scientific studies of agents from the same pharmacologic class
Studies & Abstracts 467-472

♦ **Doxepin Hydrochloride** *see* Doxepin* *on page 106*
♦ **Doxil®** *see* Doxorubicin (Liposomal)* *on page 106*

Doxorubicin* (doks oh ROO bi sin)
U.S. Brand Names Adriamycin PFS™; Adriamycin RDF®; Rubex®
Synonyms ADR; Doxorubicin Hydrochloride; Hydroxydaunomycin Hydrochloride
Pharmacologic Class Antineoplastic Agent, Antibiotic
Nutrients Depleted
See Nutrient Depletion and Cancer Chemotherapy *on page 515*.
Scientific Basis Inferred or indirect evidence of depletion based on disruption of physiologic processes

♦ **Doxorubicin Hydrochloride** *see* Doxorubicin* *on page 106*
♦ **Doxorubicin Hydrochloride (Liposomal)** *see* Doxorubicin (Liposomal)* *on page 106*

Doxorubicin (Liposomal)*
(doks oh ROO bi sin lip pah SOW mal)
U.S. Brand Names Doxil®
Synonyms Doxorubicin Hydrochloride (Liposomal)
Pharmacologic Class Antineoplastic Agent, Anthracycline; Antineoplastic Agent, Antibiotic
Nutrients Depleted
See Nutrient Depletion and Cancer Chemotherapy *on page 515*.
Scientific Basis Inferred or indirect evidence of depletion based on disruption of physiologic processes

♦ **Doxy®** *see* Doxycycline* *on page 106*
♦ **Doxychel®** *see* Doxycycline* *on page 106*
♦ **Doxycin** *see* Doxycycline* *on page 106*

Doxycycline* (doks i SYE kleen)
Related Information
Drug-Induced Nutrient Depletion Table *on page 498*

U.S. Brand Names Atridox™; Bio-Tab® Oral; Doryx®; Doxy®; Doxy-chel®; Periostat®; Vibramycin®; Vibramycin® IV; Vibra-Tabs®

Canadian Brand Names Apo®-Doxy; Apo®-Doxy Tabs; Doxycin; Doxytec; Novo-Doxylin; Nu-Doxycycline

Synonyms Doxycycline Hyclate; Doxycycline Monohydrate

Pharmacologic Class Antibiotic, Tetracycline Derivative

Nutrients Depleted
  Bifidobacteria bifidum (bifidus) on page 311
  Biotin *on page 311*
  Calcium *on page 313*
  Inositol *on page 328*
  Iron *on page 331*
  Lactobacillus acidophilus on page 332
  Magnesium *on page 333*
  Vitamin B_1 *on page 351*
  Vitamin B_2 *on page 353*
  Vitamin B_3 *on page 354*
  Vitamin B_6 *on page 357*
  Vitamin B_{12} *on page 359*
  Vitamin K *on page 367*

Scientific Basis Published scientific studies of agents from the same pharmacologic class

Studies & Abstracts 7-27, 62-68

Additional Information Calcium, iron, and magnesium depletion may be minimal during brief treatments. Replacement should not be attempted unless the time of administration is separated from the dosing of the tetracycline.

- **Doxycycline Hyclate** *see* Doxycycline* *on page 106*
- **Doxycycline Monohydrate** *see* Doxycycline* *on page 106*
- **Doxytec** *see* Doxycycline* *on page 106*
- **DPA** *see* Valproic Acid and Derivatives* *on page 265*
- **D-Penicillamine** *see* Penicillamine* *on page 205*
- **DPH** *see* Phenytoin* *on page 212*
- **Dramamine® II [OTC]** *see* Meclizine *on page 172*
- **Dristan® Sinus Caplets [OTC]** *see* Pseudoephedrine and Ibuprofen* *on page 226*
- **Drixoral® Cough & Congestion Liquid Caps [OTC]** *see* Pseudoephedrine and Dextromethorphan *on page 225*
- **Drixoral® Cough Liquid Caps [OTC]** *see* Dextromethorphan *on page 96*
- **Drixoral® Non-Drowsy [OTC]** *see* Pseudoephedrine *on page 225*
- **Drixoral® Syrup [OTC]** *see* Brompheniramine and Pseudoephedrine *on page 51*

Droperidol* (droe PER i dole)
U.S. Brand Names Inapsine®
Pharmacologic Class Antiemetic
Nutrients Depleted
  Coenzyme Q_{10} *on page 320*
  (Continued)

Droperidol* *(Continued)*

Scientific Basis Published scientific studies of agents from the same pharmacologic class
Studies & Abstracts 478

+ **Ecotrin® Low Adult Strength [OTC]** *see* Aspirin* *on page 40*
+ **Ed A-Hist® Liquid** *see* Chlorpheniramine and Phenylephrine *on page 73*
+ **Edecrin®** *see* Ethacrynic Acid* *on page 118*

Edetate Calcium Disodium*
(ED e tate KAL see um dye SOW dee um)
Related Information
Drug-Induced Nutrient Depletion Table *on page 498*
U.S. Brand Names Calcium Disodium Versenate®
Pharmacologic Class Chelating Agent
Nutrients Depleted
Calcium *on page 313*
Scientific Basis Published scientific studies using this pharmacologic agent
Studies & Abstracts 374-375

+ **Edex® Injection** *see* Alprostadil *on page 28*
+ **ED-SPAZ®** *see* Hyoscyamine *on page 153*
+ **Edstinyl®** *see* Ethinyl Estradiol* *on page 119*
+ **E.E.S.® Oral** *see* Erythromycin (Systemic)* *on page 113*
+ **Effer-Syllium® [OTC]** *see* Psyllium *on page 226*
+ **Effexor®** *see* Venlafaxine *on page 266*
+ **Effexor-XR®** *see* Venlafaxine *on page 266*
+ **Efidac/24® [OTC]** *see* Pseudoephedrine *on page 225*

Eflornithine (ee FLOR ni theen)
U.S. Brand Names Ornidyl® Injection; Vaniqa™ Cream
Synonyms DFMO; Eflornithine Hydrochloride
Pharmacologic Class Antiprotozoal; Topical Skin Product
Nutrients Depleted
Specific nutrient depletions have not been documented for this agent.

+ **Eflornithine Hydrochloride** *see* Eflornithine *on page 109*
+ **Efudex® Topical** *see* Fluorouracil* *on page 130*
+ **Elavil®** *see* Amitriptyline* *on page 32*
+ **Eldecort®** *see* Hydrocortisone* *on page 150*
+ **Eldepryl®** *see* Selegiline *on page 236*
+ **Elixomin®** *see* Theophylline* *on page 250*
+ **Elixophyllin®** *see* Theophylline* *on page 250*
+ **Elocom** *see* Mometasone Furoate* *on page 184*
+ **Elocon®** *see* Mometasone Furoate* *on page 184*
+ **Eltor®** *see* Pseudoephedrine *on page 225*
+ **Eltroxin®** *see* Levothyroxine *on page 165*
+ **Emcyt®** *see* Estramustine* *on page 116*
+ **Empirin® [OTC]** *see* Aspirin* *on page 40*
+ **Empracet® 30, 60** *see* Acetaminophen and Codeine* *on page 23*
+ **Emtec-30®** *see* Acetaminophen and Codeine* *on page 23*
+ **E-Mycin® Oral** *see* Erythromycin (Systemic)* *on page 113*

Enalapril* (e NAL a pril)
Related Information
Drug-Induced Nutrient Depletion Table *on page 498*
U.S. Brand Names Vasotec®; Vasotec® I.V.
Canadian Brand Names Apo®-Enalapril
Synonyms Enalaprilat; Enalapril Maleate
Pharmacologic Class Angiotensin-Converting Enzyme (ACE) Inhibitors
Nutrients Depleted
Zinc *on page 368*
Scientific Basis Published scientific studies using this pharmacologic agent
Studies & Abstracts 269-271

Enalapril and Diltiazem* (e NAL a pril & dil TYE a zem)
U.S. Brand Names Teczem®
Pharmacologic Class Antihypertensive Agent, Combination
Nutrients Depleted
Zinc *on page 368*
Scientific Basis Published scientific studies using this pharmacologic agent (enalapril)
Studies & Abstracts 269-271

Enalapril and Felodipine* (e NAL a pril & fe LOE di peen)
U.S. Brand Names Lexxel™
Pharmacologic Class Antihypertensive Agent, Combination
Nutrients Depleted
Zinc *on page 368*
Scientific Basis Published scientific studies using this pharmacologic agent (enalapril)
Studies & Abstracts 269-271

Enalapril and Hydrochlorothiazide*
(e NAL a pril & hye droe klor oh THYE a zide)
U.S. Brand Names Vaseretic® 10-25
Canadian Brand Names Vaseretic®
Synonyms Hydrochlorothiazide and Enalapril
Pharmacologic Class Antihypertensive Agent, Combination
Nutrients Depleted
Coenzyme Q_{10} *on page 320*
Magnesium *on page 333*
Phosphorus *on page 339*
Potassium *on page 340*
Sodium *on page 345*
Vitamin B_6 *on page 357*
Zinc *on page 368*
Scientific Basis Published scientific studies using these pharmacologic agents
Studies & Abstracts 269-271, 320-342

Additional Information Although thiazide diuretics deplete sodium, replacement is not recommended, as this may be directly related to the therapeutic effect. Thiazides may deplete potassium, however ACE-inhibitors may increase this ion. Replacement should be guided by monitoring of serum concentrations and specific instruction by a healthcare provider.

♦ **Enalaprilat** see Enalapril* on page 110

♦ **Enalapril Maleate** see Enalapril* on page 110

♦ **Enbrel®** see Etanercept on page 118

♦ **Endal®** see Guaifenesin and Phenylephrine on page 141

♦ **Endantadine®** see Amantadine on page 30

♦ **Endocet®** see Oxycodone and Acetaminophen* on page 202

♦ **Endodan®** see Oxycodone and Aspirin* on page 202

♦ **Endolor®** see Butalbital Compound and Acetaminophen* on page 53

♦ **Enduron®** see Methyclothiazide* on page 177

♦ **Enomine®** see Guaifenesin, Phenylpropanolamine, and Phenylephrine on page 142

♦ **Enovil®** see Amitriptyline* on page 32

Enoxacin* (en OKS a sin)
U.S. Brand Names Penetrex™
Pharmacologic Class Antibiotic, Quinolone
Nutrients Depleted
Coenzyme Q_{10} on page 320
Magnesium on page 333
Potassium on page 340
Vitamin B_6 on page 357
Zinc on page 368
Scientific Basis Published scientific studies using this pharmacologic agent
Studies & Abstracts 7-27

Enoxaparin (ee noks a PA rin)
U.S. Brand Names Lovenox® Injection
Synonyms Enoxaparin Sodium
Pharmacologic Class Low Molecular Weight Heparin
Nutrients Depleted
Specific nutrient depletions have not been documented for this agent.

♦ **Enoxaparin Sodium** see Enoxaparin on page 111

Entacapone (en TA ka pone)
U.S. Brand Names Comtan®
Pharmacologic Class Anti-Parkinson's Agent (COMT Inhibitor)
Nutrients Depleted
Specific nutrient depletions have not been documented for this agent.

♦ **Entex®** see Guaifenesin, Phenylpropanolamine, and Phenylephrine on page 142

♦ **Entex® LA** see Guaifenesin and Phenylpropanolamine on page 141

- **Entex® PSE** *see* Guaifenesin and Pseudoephedrine *on page 142*
- **Entocort®** *see* Budesonide* *on page 51*
- **Entrophen®** *see* Aspirin* *on page 40*
- **E Pam®** *see* Diazepam *on page 97*
- **Epimorph®** *see* Morphine Sulfate *on page 185*
- **Epipodophyllotoxin** *see* Etoposide* *on page 123*
- **Epitol®** *see* Carbamazepine* *on page 57*
- **Epivir®** *see* Lamivudine* *on page 162*
- **Epivir® HBV** *see* Lamivudine* *on page 162*

Eprosartan (ep roe SAR tan)
U.S. Brand Names Teveten®
Pharmacologic Class Angiotensin II Antagonists
Nutrients Depleted
Specific nutrient depletions have not been documented for this agent.

- **Epsom Salts** *see* Magnesium Sulfate* *on page 171*

Eptifibatide (ep TIF i ba tide)
U.S. Brand Names Integrilin®
Synonyms Intrifiban
Pharmacologic Class Antiplatelet Agent
Nutrients Depleted
Specific nutrient depletions have not been documented for this agent.

Erwinia Asparaginase* (ehr WIN ee ah a SPAIR a ji nase)
Synonyms NSC-106977; Porton Asparaginase
Pharmacologic Class Antineoplastic Agent, Miscellaneous
Nutrients Depleted
See Nutrient Depletion and Cancer Chemotherapy *on page 515*.
Scientific Basis Inferred or indirect evidence of depletion based on disruption of physiologic processes

- **Erybid™** *see* Erythromycin (Systemic)* *on page 113*
- **Eryc® Oral** *see* Erythromycin (Systemic)* *on page 113*
- **EryPed® Oral** *see* Erythromycin (Systemic)* *on page 113*
- **Ery-Tab® Oral** *see* Erythromycin (Systemic)* *on page 113*
- **Erythro-Base®** *see* Erythromycin (Systemic)* *on page 113*
- **Erythrocin® Oral** *see* Erythromycin (Systemic)* *on page 113*
- **Erythromycin Base** *see* Erythromycin (Systemic)* *on page 113*
- **Erythromycin Estolate** *see* Erythromycin (Systemic)* *on page 113*
- **Erythromycin Ethylsuccinate** *see* Erythromycin (Systemic)* *on page 113*
- **Erythromycin Gluceptate** *see* Erythromycin (Systemic)* *on page 113*
- **Erythromycin Lactobionate** *see* Erythromycin (Systemic)* *on page 113*
- **Erythromycin Stearate** *see* Erythromycin (Systemic)* *on page 113*

Erythromycin (Systemic)* (er ith roe MYE sin)

U.S. Brand Names E.E.S.® Oral; E-Mycin® Oral; Eryc® Oral; EryPed® Oral; Ery-Tab® Oral; Erythrocin® Oral; Ilosone® Oral; PCE® Oral

Canadian Brand Names Apo®-Erythro E-C; Diomycin; Erybid™; Erythro-Base®; Novo-Rythro Encap; PMS-Erythromycin

Synonyms Erythromycin Base; Erythromycin Estolate; Erythromycin Ethylsuccinate; Erythromycin Gluceptate; Erythromycin Lactobionate; Erythromycin Stearate

Pharmacologic Class Antibiotic, Macrolide

Nutrients Depleted

Bifidobacteria bifidum (bifidus) on page 311

Biotin *on page 311*

Inositol *on page 328*

Lactobacillus acidophilus on page 332

Vitamin B_1 *on page 351*

Vitamin B_2 *on page 353*

Vitamin B_3 *on page 354*

Vitamin B_6 *on page 357*

Vitamin B_{12} *on page 359*

Vitamin K *on page 367*

Scientific Basis Inferred or indirect evidence of depletion based on disruption of physiologic processes

Studies & Abstracts 7-27

♦ **Esclim® Transdermal** *see Estradiol* on page 114*

♦ **Esgic®** *see Butalbital Compound and Acetaminophen* on page 53*

♦ **Esgic-Plus®** *see Butalbital Compound and Acetaminophen* on page 53*

♦ **Esidrix®** *see Hydrochlorothiazide* on page 147*

♦ **Eskalith®** *see Lithium* on page 166*

Esmolol* (ES moe lol)

Related Information

Drug-Induced Nutrient Depletion Table *on page 498*

U.S. Brand Names Brevibloc® Injection

Synonyms Esmolol Hydrochloride

Pharmacologic Class Antiarrhythmic Agent, Class II; Beta Blocker, Beta$_1$ Selective

Nutrients Depleted

Coenzyme Q_{10} *on page 320*

Scientific Basis Published scientific studies of agents from the same pharmacologic class

Studies & Abstracts 348-349

♦ **Esmolol Hydrochloride** *see Esmolol* on page 113*

Estazolam (es TA zoe lam)

U.S. Brand Names ProSom™

Pharmacologic Class Benzodiazepine

Nutrients Depleted

Specific nutrient depletions have not been documented for this agent.

◆ **Esterified Estrogen and Methyltestosterone** *see* Estrogens and Methyltestosterone* *on page 117*

◆ **Esterified Estrogens** *see* Estrogens (Esterified)* *on page 118*

◆ **Estrace® Oral** *see* Estradiol* *on page 114*

◆ **Estraderm® Transdermal** *see* Estradiol* *on page 114*

◆ **Estra-D® Injection** *see* Estradiol* *on page 114*

Estradiol* <small>(es tra DYE ole)</small>

U.S. Brand Names Alora® Transdermal; Climara® Transdermal; Delestrogen® Injection; depGynogen® Injection; Depo®-Estradiol Injection; Depogen® Injection; Dioval® Injection; Dura-Estrin® Injection; Duragen® Injection; Esclim® Transdermal; Estrace® Oral; Estraderm® Transdermal; Estra-D® Injection; Estra-L® Injection; Estro-Cyp® Injection; Gynogen L.A.® Injection; Innofem®; Vagifem®; Vivelle® Transdermal

Synonyms Estradiol Cypionate; Estradiol Hemihydrate; Estradiol Transdermal; Estradiol Valerate

Pharmacologic Class Estrogen Derivative

Nutrients Depleted

Folic Acid *on page 325*
Magnesium *on page 333*
Vitamin B_2 *on page 353*
Vitamin B_6 *on page 357*
Vitamin C *on page 360*
Zinc *on page 368*

Scientific Basis Published scientific studies of agents from the same pharmacologic class

Studies & Abstracts 378-379

Estradiol and Ethynodiol Diacetate*

<small>(ETH in il es tra DYE ole & e thye noe DYE ole dye AS e tate)</small>

Related Information

Drug-Induced Nutrient Depletion Table *on page 498*

U.S. Brand Names Demulen®; Zovia®

Synonyms Ethynodiol Diacetate and Ethinyl Estradiol

Pharmacologic Class Contraceptive

Nutrients Depleted

Folic Acid *on page 325*
Magnesium *on page 333*
Tyrosine *on page 347*
Vitamin B_2 *on page 353*
Vitamin B_3 *on page 354*
Vitamin B_6 *on page 357*
Vitamin B_{12} *on page 359*
Vitamin C *on page 360*
Zinc *on page 368*

Scientific Basis Published scientific studies of agents from the same pharmacologic class

Studies & Abstracts 380-436

Estradiol and Norethindrone*
(es tra DYE ole & nor eth IN drone)

U.S. Brand Names Activella™; CombiPatch™

Pharmacologic Class Estrogen Derivative

Nutrients Depleted
Folic Acid *on page 325*
Magnesium *on page 333*
Vitamin B_2 *on page 353*
Vitamin B_6 *on page 357*
Vitamin B_{12} *on page 359*
Vitamin C *on page 360*
Zinc *on page 368*

Scientific Basis Published scientific studies of agents from the same pharmacologic class

Studies & Abstracts 380-436

Estradiol and Testosterone*
(es tra DYE ole & tes TOS ter one)

U.S. Brand Names Andro/Fem® Injection; Deladumone® Injection; depAndrogyn® Injection; Depo-Testadiol® Injection; Depotestogen® Injection; Duo-Cyp® Injection; Duratestrin® Injection; Valertest No.1® Injection

Synonyms Estradiol Cypionate and Testosterone Cypionate; Estradiol Valerate and Testosterone Enanthate; Testosterone and Estradiol

Pharmacologic Class Estrogen Derivative

Nutrients Depleted
Folic Acid *on page 325*
Magnesium *on page 333*
Vitamin B_2 *on page 353*
Vitamin B_6 *on page 357*
Vitamin C *on page 360*
Zinc *on page 368*

Scientific Basis Published scientific studies of agents from the same pharmacologic class

Studies & Abstracts 378-379

♦ **Estradiol Cypionate** *see* Estradiol* *on page 114*

Estradiol Cypionate and Medroxyprogesterone Acetate*
(es tra DYE ole sip pe OH nate & me DROKS ee proe JES te rone AS e tate)

U.S. Brand Names Lunelle™

Synonyms E_2C and MPA; Medroxyprogesterone Acetate and Estradiol Cypionate

Pharmacologic Class Contraceptive

Nutrients Depleted
Folic Acid *on page 325*
(Continued)

Estradiol Cypionate and Medroxyprogesterone Acetate* *(Continued)*

Magnesium *on page 333*
Vitamin B$_2$ *on page 353*
Vitamin B$_6$ *on page 357*
Vitamin C *on page 360*
Zinc *on page 368*

Scientific Basis Published scientific studies of agents from the same pharmacologic class
Studies & Abstracts 378-379

♦ **Estradiol Cypionate and Testosterone Cypionate** *see* Estradiol and Testosterone* *on page 115*
♦ **Estradiol Hemihydrate** *see* Estradiol* *on page 114*
♦ **Estradiol Transdermal** *see* Estradiol* *on page 114*
♦ **Estradiol Valerate** *see* Estradiol* *on page 114*
♦ **Estradiol Valerate and Testosterone Enanthate** *see* Estradiol and Testosterone* *on page 115*
♦ **Estra-L® Injection** *see* Estradiol* *on page 114*

Estramustine* (es tra MUS teen)

U.S. Brand Names Emcyt®
Synonyms Estramustine Phosphate Sodium
Pharmacologic Class Antineoplastic Agent, Alkylating Agent
Nutrients Depleted
See Nutrient Depletion and Cancer Chemotherapy *on page 515*.
Scientific Basis Inferred or indirect evidence of depletion based on disruption of physiologic processes

♦ **Estramustine Phosphate Sodium** *see* Estramustine* *on page 116*
♦ **Estratab®** *see* Estrogens (Esterified)* *on page 118*
♦ **Estratest®** *see* Estrogens and Methyltestosterone* *on page 117*
♦ **Estratest® H.S.** *see* Estrogens and Methyltestosterone* *on page 117*
♦ **Estro-Cyp® Injection** *see* Estradiol* *on page 114*

Estrogen and Medroxyprogesterone*

(ES troe jenz & me DROKS ee proe JES te rone)
Related Information
Drug-Induced Nutrient Depletion Table *on page 498*
U.S. Brand Names Premphase™; Prempro™
Synonyms Medroxyprogesterone and Estrogens
Pharmacologic Class Estrogen Derivative
Nutrients Depleted
Folic Acid *on page 325*
Magnesium *on page 333*
Vitamin B$_2$ *on page 353*
Vitamin B$_6$ *on page 357*
Vitamin C *on page 360*
Zinc *on page 368*

Scientific Basis Published scientific studies of agents from the same pharmacologic class
Studies & Abstracts 378-379

♦ **Estrogenic Substances, Conjugated** *see* Estrogens (Conjugated)* *on page 117*

Estrogens and Methyltestosterone*
(ES troe jenz & meth il tes TOS te rone)
U.S. Brand Names Estratest®; Estratest® H.S.; Premarin® With Methyltestosterone
Synonyms Conjugated Estrogen and Methyltestosterone; Esterified Estrogen and Methyltestosterone
Pharmacologic Class Estrogen Derivative
Nutrients Depleted
Magnesium *on page 333*
Vitamin B₆ *on page 357*
Zinc *on page 368*
Scientific Basis Published scientific studies of agents from the same pharmacologic class
Studies & Abstracts 378-379

Estrogens (Conjugated)*
(ES troe jenz KON joo gate ed, EE kwine)
Related Information
Drug-Induced Nutrient Depletion Table *on page 498*
U.S. Brand Names Premarin®
Canadian Brand Names C.E.S.™; Congest
Synonyms C.E.S.; Estrogenic Substances, Conjugated
Pharmacologic Class Estrogen Derivative
Nutrients Depleted
Magnesium *on page 333*
Vitamin B₆ *on page 357*
Scientific Basis
Published scientific studies using this pharmacologic agent
or
Published scientific studies of agents from the same pharmacologic class
Studies & Abstracts 378-379

Estrogens (Conjugated A/Synthetic)*
(ES troe jenz, KON joo gate ed, aye, sin THET ik)
U.S. Brand Names Cenestin™
Pharmacologic Class Estrogen Derivative
Nutrients Depleted
Magnesium *on page 333*
Vitamin B₆ *on page 357*
Scientific Basis Published scientific studies of agents from the same pharmacologic class
Studies & Abstracts 378-379

Estrogens (Esterified)* (ES troe jenz, es TER i fied)
Related Information
  Drug-Induced Nutrient Depletion Table *on page 498*
U.S. Brand Names Estratab®; Menest®
Canadian Brand Names Neo-Estrone®
Synonyms Esterified Estrogens
Pharmacologic Class Estrogen Derivative
Nutrients Depleted
  Magnesium *on page 333*
  Vitamin B$_6$ *on page 357*
Scientific Basis Published scientific studies of agents from the same pharmacologic class
Studies & Abstracts 378-379

Estropipate* (ES troe pih pate)
U.S. Brand Names Ogen® Oral; Ogen® Vaginal; Ortho-Est® Oral
Canadian Brand Names Estrouis®
Synonyms Piperazine Estrone Sulfate
Pharmacologic Class Estrogen Derivative
Nutrients Depleted
  Magnesium *on page 333*
  Vitamin B$_6$ *on page 357*
Scientific Basis
  Published scientific studies using this pharmacologic agent
    or
  Published scientific studies of agents from the same pharmacologic class
Studies & Abstracts 378-379

♦ **Estrostep® 21** *see* Ethinyl Estradiol and Norethindrone* *on page 121*
♦ **Estrostep® Fe** *see* Ethinyl Estradiol and Norethindrone* *on page 121*
♦ **Estrouis®** *see* Estropipate* *on page 118*
♦ **Estrovis®** *see* Quinestrol* *on page 227*

Etanercept (et a NER cept)
U.S. Brand Names Enbrel®
Pharmacologic Class Antirheumatic, Disease Modifying
Nutrients Depleted
  Specific nutrient depletions have not been documented for this agent.

♦ **Ethacrynate Sodium** *see* Ethacrynic Acid* *on page 118*

Ethacrynic Acid* (eth a KRIN ik AS id)
Related Information
  Drug-Induced Nutrient Depletion Table *on page 498*
U.S. Brand Names Edecrin®
Synonyms Ethacrynate Sodium
Pharmacologic Class Diuretic, Loop
Nutrients Depleted
  Calcium *on page 313*

Magnesium *on page 333*
Potassium *on page 340*
Sodium *on page 345*
Vitamin B$_1$ *on page 351*
Vitamin B$_6$ *on page 357*
Vitamin C *on page 360*
Zinc *on page 368*

Scientific Basis Published scientific studies of agents with the same mechanism of action

Studies & Abstracts 280-311

Additional Information Sodium replacement is not recommended in patients receiving loop diuretics. Potassium replacement should be guided by monitoring of serum concentrations.

Ethambutol* (e THAM byoo tole)

Related Information

Drug-Induced Nutrient Depletion Table *on page 498*

U.S. Brand Names Myambutol®

Canadian Brand Names Etibi®

Synonyms Ethambutol Hydrochloride

Pharmacologic Class Antitubercular Agent

Nutrients Depleted

Copper *on page 322*
Zinc *on page 368*

Scientific Basis Published scientific studies using this pharmacologic agent

Studies & Abstracts 38

♦ **Ethambutol Hydrochloride** *see* Ethambutol* *on page 119*

Ethinyl Estradiol* (ETH in il es tra DYE ole)

U.S. Brand Names Edstinyl®

Pharmacologic Class Estrogen Derivative

Nutrients Depleted

Folic Acid *on page 325*
Magnesium *on page 333*
Vitamin B$_2$ *on page 353*
Vitamin B$_6$ *on page 357*
Vitamin B$_{12}$ *on page 359*
Vitamin C *on page 360*
Zinc *on page 368*

Scientific Basis Published scientific studies of agents from the same pharmacologic class

Studies & Abstracts 380-436

Ethinyl Estradiol and Desogestrel*

(ETH in il es tra DYE ole & des oh JES trel)

Related Information

Drug-Induced Nutrient Depletion Table *on page 498*

U.S. Brand Names Desogen®; Mircette™; Ortho-Cept®

(Continued)

Ethinyl Estradiol and Desogestrel* *(Continued)*

Synonyms Desogestrel and Ethinyl Estradiol
Pharmacologic Class Contraceptive
Nutrients Depleted
Folic Acid *on page 325*
Magnesium *on page 333*
Tyrosine *on page 347*
Vitamin B_2 *on page 353*
Vitamin B_3 *on page 354*
Vitamin B_6 *on page 357*
Vitamin B_{12} *on page 359*
Vitamin C *on page 360*
Zinc *on page 368*
Scientific Basis Published scientific studies of agents from the same pharmacologic class
Studies & Abstracts 380-436

Ethinyl Estradiol and Fluoxymesterone*

(eth i nil es tra DYE ole & floo oks i MES te rone)
Synonyms Fluoxymesterone and Estradiol
Pharmacologic Class Androgen; Estrogen Derivative
Nutrients Depleted
Folic Acid *on page 325*
Magnesium *on page 333*
Vitamin B_2 *on page 353*
Vitamin B_6 *on page 357*
Vitamin B_{12} *on page 359*
Vitamin C *on page 360*
Zinc *on page 368*
Scientific Basis Published scientific studies of agents from the same pharmacologic class
Studies & Abstracts 380-436

Ethinyl Estradiol and Levonorgestrel*

(ETH in il es tra DYE ole & LEE voe nor jes trel)
U.S. Brand Names Alesse™; Levlen®; Levlite®; Levora®; Nordette®; PREVEN™; Tri-Levlen®; Triphasil®
Synonyms Levonorgestrel and Ethinyl Estradiol
Pharmacologic Class Contraceptive
Nutrients Depleted
Folic Acid *on page 325*
Magnesium *on page 333*
Tyrosine *on page 347*
Vitamin B_2 *on page 353*
Vitamin B_3 *on page 354*
Vitamin B_6 *on page 357*
Vitamin B_{12} *on page 359*
Vitamin C *on page 360*
Zinc *on page 368*

Scientific Basis Published scientific studies of agents from the same pharmacologic class
Studies & Abstracts 380-436

Ethinyl Estradiol and Norethindrone*

(ETH in il es tra DYE ole & nor eth IN drone)

Related Information
Drug-Induced Nutrient Depletion Table *on page 498*

U.S. Brand Names Brevicon®; Estrostep® 21; Estrostep® Fe; Femhrt™; Genora® 0.5/35; Genora® 1/35; Jenest-28™; Loestrin®; Modicon™; N.E.E.® 1/35; Nelova™ 0.5/35E; Nelova™ 10/11; Norethin™ 1/35E; Norinyl® 1+35; Ortho-Novum® 1/35; Ortho-Novum® 7/7/7; Ortho-Novum® 10/11; Ovcon® 35; Ovcon® 50; Tri-Norinyl®

Synonyms Norethindrone Acetate and Ethinyl Estradiol

Pharmacologic Class Contraceptive

Nutrients Depleted
Folic Acid *on page 325*
Magnesium *on page 333*
Tyrosine *on page 347*
Vitamin B_2 *on page 353*
Vitamin B_3 *on page 354*
Vitamin B_6 *on page 357*
Vitamin B_{12} *on page 359*
Vitamin C *on page 360*
Zinc *on page 368*

Scientific Basis Published scientific studies of agents from the same pharmacologic class
Studies & Abstracts 380-436

Ethinyl Estradiol and Norgestimate*

(ETH in il es tra DYE ole & nor JES ti mate)

Related Information
Drug-Induced Nutrient Depletion Table *on page 498*

U.S. Brand Names Ortho-Cyclen®; Ortho-Prefest®; Ortho Tri-Cyclen®

Canadian Brand Names Cyclen®; Tri-Cyclen®

Synonyms Norgestimate and Ethinyl Estradiol

Pharmacologic Class Contraceptive

Nutrients Depleted
Folic Acid *on page 325*
Magnesium *on page 333*
Tyrosine *on page 347*
Vitamin B_2 *on page 353*
Vitamin B_3 *on page 354*
Vitamin B_6 *on page 357*
Vitamin B_{12} *on page 359*
Vitamin C *on page 360*
Zinc *on page 368*

Scientific Basis Published scientific studies of agents from the same pharmacologic class
Studies & Abstracts 380-436

Ethinyl Estradiol and Norgestrel*
(ETH in il es tra DYE ole & nor JES trel)

Related Information
Drug-Induced Nutrient Depletion Table *on page 498*
U.S. Brand Names Lo/Ovral®; Ovral®
Synonyms Morning After Pill; Norgestrel and Ethinyl Estradiol
Pharmacologic Class Contraceptive
Nutrients Depleted
Folic Acid *on page 325*
Magnesium *on page 333*
Tyrosine *on page 347*
Vitamin B_2 *on page 353*
Vitamin B_3 *on page 354*
Vitamin B_6 *on page 357*
Vitamin B_{12} *on page 359*
Vitamin C *on page 360*
Zinc *on page 368*
Scientific Basis Published scientific studies of agents from the same pharmacologic class
Studies & Abstracts 380-436

Ethosuximide* (eth oh SUKS i mide)
U.S. Brand Names Zarontin®
Pharmacologic Class Anticonvulsant, Succinimide
Nutrients Depleted
Biotin *on page 311*
Calcium *on page 313*
Folic Acid *on page 325*
Vitamin D *on page 363*
Vitamin K *on page 367*
Scientific Basis Published scientific studies of agents with the same mechanism of action
Studies & Abstracts 72-92

♦ **Ethoxynaphthamido Penicillin Sodium** *see* Nafcillin* *on page 187*
♦ **Ethynodiol Diacetate and Ethinyl Estradiol** *see* Estradiol and Ethynodiol Diacetate* *on page 114*
♦ **Etibi®** *see* Ethambutol* *on page 119*

Etodolac* (ee toe DOE lak)
Related Information
Drug-Induced Nutrient Depletion Table *on page 498*
U.S. Brand Names Lodine®; Lodine® XL
Synonyms Etodolic Acid
Pharmacologic Class Nonsteroidal Anti-Inflammatory Agent (NSAID)
Nutrients Depleted
Folic Acid *on page 325*

Scientific Basis Published scientific studies of agents from the same pharmacologic class
Studies & Abstracts 252

♦ **Etodolic Acid** *see* Etodolac* *on page 122*

Etoposide* (e toe POE side)

U.S. Brand Names Toposar® Injection; VePesid® Injection; VePesid® Oral
Synonyms Epipodophyllotoxin; VP-16; VP-16-213
Pharmacologic Class Antineoplastic Agent, Natural Source (Plant) Derivative
Nutrients Depleted
See Nutrient Depletion and Cancer Chemotherapy *on page 515.*
Scientific Basis Inferred or indirect evidence of depletion based on disruption of physiologic processes

♦ **Eudal-SR**® *see* Guaifenesin and Pseudoephedrine *on page 142*
♦ **Euglucon**® *see* Glyburide* *on page 139*
♦ **Eulexin**® *see* Flutamide *on page 132*
♦ **Evista**® *see* Raloxifene* *on page 228*
♦ **Evoxac**™ *see* Cevimeline *on page 71*
♦ **Exelon**® *see* Rivastigmine *on page 233*
♦ **Exna**® *see* Benzthiazide* *on page 45*
♦ **Extra Action Cough Syrup [OTC]** *see* Guaifenesin and Dextromethorphan *on page 141*
♦ **Extra Strength Adprin-B**® **[OTC]** *see* Aspirin* *on page 40*
♦ **Extra Strength Bayer**® **Enteric 500 Aspirin [OTC]** *see* Aspirin* *on page 40*
♦ **Extra Strength Bayer**® **Plus [OTC]** *see* Aspirin* *on page 40*
♦ **Extra Strength Dynafed**® **E.X. [OTC]** *see* Acetaminophen* *on page 23*
♦ **Ezide**® *see* Hydrochlorothiazide* *on page 147*

Famciclovir (fam SYE kloe veer)

U.S. Brand Names Famvir™
Pharmacologic Class Antiviral Agent
Nutrients Depleted
Specific nutrient depletions have not been documented for this agent.

Famotidine* (fa MOE ti deen)

Related Information
Drug-Induced Nutrient Depletion Table *on page 498*
U.S. Brand Names Pepcid®; Pepcid® AC Acid Controller [OTC]
Canadian Brand Names Apo®-Famotidine; Novo-Famotidine; Nu-Famotidine
Pharmacologic Class Histamine H_2 Antagonist
Nutrients Depleted
Calcium *on page 313*
Folic Acid *on page 325*
Iron *on page 331*
(Continued)

Famotidine* *(Continued)*

Vitamin B$_{12}$ *on page 359*
Vitamin D *on page 363*
Zinc *on page 368*
Scientific Basis Published scientific studies of agents from the same pharmacologic class
Studies & Abstracts 484-510

♦ **Famvir™** *see Famciclovir on page 123*
♦ **Fastin®** *see Phentermine on page 211*
♦ **5-FC** *see Flucytosine* on page 128*
♦ **Fedahist® Expectorant [OTC]** *see Guaifenesin and Pseudoephedrine on page 142*
♦ **Fedahist® Expectorant Pediatric [OTC]** *see Guaifenesin and Pseudoephedrine on page 142*
♦ **Fedahist® Tablet [OTC]** *see Chlorpheniramine and Pseudoephedrine on page 73*

Felbamate *(FEL ba mate)*
U.S. Brand Names Felbatol®
Pharmacologic Class Anticonvulsant, Miscellaneous
Nutrients Depleted
Specific nutrient depletions have not been documented for this agent.

♦ **Felbatol®** *see Felbamate on page 124*
♦ **Feldene®** *see Piroxicam* on page 214*

Felodipine *(fe LOE di peen)*
U.S. Brand Names Plendil®
Canadian Brand Names Renedil®
Pharmacologic Class Calcium Channel Blocker
Nutrients Depleted
Specific nutrient depletions have not been documented for this agent.

♦ **Femcet®** *see Butalbital Compound and Acetaminophen* on page 53*
♦ **Femhrt™** *see Ethinyl Estradiol and Norethindrone* on page 121*
♦ **Femiron® [OTC]** *see Ferrous Fumarate on page 126*
♦ **Femizole-7® [OTC]** *see Clotrimazole on page 82*
♦ **Femstat®-3 [OTC]** *see Butoconazole on page 54*
♦ **Fenesin™** *see Guaifenesin on page 140*
♦ **Fenesin™ DM** *see Guaifenesin and Dextromethorphan on page 141*

Fenofibrate* *(fen oh FYE brate)*
Related Information
Drug-Induced Nutrient Depletion Table *on page 498*
U.S. Brand Names TriCor™
Canadian Brand Names Apo®-Fenofibrate
Synonyms Procetofene; Proctofene
Pharmacologic Class Antilipemic Agent (Fibric Acid)
Nutrients Depleted
Coenzyme Q$_{10}$ *on page 320*

Vitamin E *on page 365*
Scientific Basis Published scientific studies of agents from the same pharmacologic class
Studies & Abstracts 350

Fenoprofen* (fen oh PROE fen)
Related Information
Drug-Induced Nutrient Depletion Table *on page 498*
U.S. Brand Names Nalfon®
Synonyms Fenoprofen Calcium
Pharmacologic Class Nonsteroidal Anti-Inflammatory Agent (NSAID)
Nutrients Depleted
Folic Acid *on page 325*
Scientific Basis Published scientific studies of agents from the same pharmacologic class
Studies & Abstracts 252

♦ **Fenoprofen Calcium** *see* Fenoprofen* *on page 125*

Fentanyl (FEN ta nil)
U.S. Brand Names Actiq® Oral Transmucosal; Duragesic® Transdermal; Fentanyl Oralet®; Sublimaze® Injection
Synonyms Fentanyl Citrate
Pharmacologic Class Analgesic, Narcotic; General Anesthetic
Nutrients Depleted
Specific nutrient depletions have not been documented for this agent.

♦ **Fentanyl Citrate** *see* Fentanyl *on page 125*
♦ **Fentanyl Oralet®** *see* Fentanyl *on page 125*
♦ **Feosol® [OTC]** *see* Ferrous Sulfate *on page 126*
♦ **Feostat® [OTC]** *see* Ferrous Fumarate *on page 126*
♦ **Ferancee® [OTC]** *see* Ferrous Sulfate and Ascorbic Acid *on page 126*
♦ **Feratab® [OTC]** *see* Ferrous Sulfate *on page 126*
♦ **Fergon® [OTC]** *see* Ferrous Gluconate *on page 126*
♦ **Fer-In-Sol® [OTC]** *see* Ferrous Sulfate *on page 126*
♦ **Fer-Iron® [OTC]** *see* Ferrous Sulfate *on page 126*
♦ **Fero-Grad 500® [OTC]** *see* Ferrous Sulfate and Ascorbic Acid *on page 126*
♦ **Fero-Gradumet® [OTC]** *see* Ferrous Sulfate *on page 126*
♦ **Ferospace® [OTC]** *see* Ferrous Sulfate *on page 126*
♦ **Ferralet® [OTC]** *see* Ferrous Gluconate *on page 126*
♦ **Ferralyn® Lanacaps® [OTC]** *see* Ferrous Sulfate *on page 126*
♦ **Ferra-TD® [OTC]** *see* Ferrous Sulfate *on page 126*

Ferric Gluconate (FER ik GLOO koe nate)
U.S. Brand Names Ferrlecit®
Synonyms Sodium Ferric Gluconate
Pharmacologic Class Iron Salt
(Continued)

Ferric Gluconate *(Continued)*
Nutrients Depleted
Specific nutrient depletions have not been documented for this agent.

♦ **Ferrlecit**® *see Ferric Gluconate on page 125*
♦ **Ferro-Sequels**® **[OTC]** *see Ferrous Fumarate on page 126*

Ferrous Fumarate (FER us FYOO ma rate)
U.S. Brand Names Femiron® [OTC]; Feostat® [OTC]; Ferro-Sequels®
[OTC]; Fumasorb® [OTC]; Fumerin® [OTC]; Hemocyte® [OTC]; Ircon®
[OTC]; Nephro-Fer™ [OTC]; Span-FF® [OTC]
Pharmacologic Class Iron Salt
Nutrients Depleted
Specific nutrient depletions have not been documented for this agent.

Ferrous Gluconate (FER us GLOO koe nate)
U.S. Brand Names Fergon® [OTC]; Ferralet® [OTC]; Simron® [OTC]
Pharmacologic Class Iron Salt
Nutrients Depleted
Specific nutrient depletions have not been documented for this agent.

Ferrous Sulfate (FER us SUL fate)
U.S. Brand Names Feosol® [OTC]; Feratab® [OTC]; Fer-In-Sol®
[OTC]; Fer-Iron® [OTC]; Fero-Gradumet® [OTC]; Ferospace® [OTC];
Ferralyn® Lanacaps® [OTC]; Ferra-TD® [OTC]; Mol-Iron® [OTC]; Slow
FE® [OTC]
Synonyms FeSO$_4$
Pharmacologic Class Iron Salt
Nutrients Depleted
Specific nutrient depletions have not been documented for this agent.

Ferrous Sulfate and Ascorbic Acid
(FER us SUL fate & a SKOR bik AS id)
U.S. Brand Names Ferancee® [OTC]; Fero-Grad 500® [OTC]
Synonyms Ascorbic Acid and Ferrous Sulfate
Pharmacologic Class Iron Salt; Vitamin
Nutrients Depleted
Specific nutrient depletions have not been documented for this agent.

Ferrous Sulfate, Ascorbic Acid, and Vitamin B-Complex
(FER us SUL fate, a SKOR bik AS id, & VYE ta min bee KOM
pleks)
U.S. Brand Names Iberet®-Liquid [OTC]
Pharmacologic Class Iron Salt; Vitamin
Nutrients Depleted
Specific nutrient depletions have not been documented for this agent.

Ferrous Sulfate, Ascorbic Acid, Vitamin B-Complex, and Folic Acid
(FER us SUL fate, a SKOR bik AS id, VYE ta min bee KOM pleks, & FOE lik AS id)
U.S. Brand Names Iberet-Folic-500®
Pharmacologic Class Vitamin
Nutrients Depleted
Specific nutrient depletions have not been documented for this agent.

♦ FeSO₄ *see* Ferrous Sulfate *on page 126*

♦ Feverall™ [OTC] *see* Acetaminophen* *on page 23*

♦ Feverall™ Sprinkle Caps [OTC] *see* Acetaminophen* *on page 23*

Fexofenadine (feks oh FEN a deen)
U.S. Brand Names Allegra®
Synonyms Fexofenadine Hydrochloride
Pharmacologic Class Antihistamine
Nutrients Depleted
Specific nutrient depletions have not been documented for this agent.

Fexofenadine and Pseudoephedrine
(feks oh FEN a deen & soo doe e FED rin)
U.S. Brand Names Allegra-D™
Pharmacologic Class Antihistamine/Decongestant Combination
Nutrients Depleted
Specific nutrient depletions have not been documented for this agent.

♦ **Fexofenadine Hydrochloride** *see* Fexofenadine *on page 127*

♦ **Fiberall® Powder [OTC]** *see* Psyllium *on page 226*

♦ **Fiberall® Wafer [OTC]** *see* Psyllium *on page 226*

♦ **Fibrepur®** *see* Psyllium *on page 226*

Finasteride (fi NAS teer ide)
U.S. Brand Names Proscar®
Pharmacologic Class Antiandrogen
Nutrients Depleted
Specific nutrient depletions have not been documented for this agent.

♦ **Fiorgen PF®** *see* Butalbital Compound and Aspirin* *on page 54*

♦ **Fioricet®** *see* Butalbital Compound and Acetaminophen* *on page 53*

♦ **Fiorinal®** *see* Butalbital Compound and Aspirin* *on page 54*

♦ **Fiorinal®-C ¹/₄, ¹/₂** *see* Butalbital Compound and Codeine* *on page 54*

♦ **Fiorinal® With Codeine** *see* Butalbital Compound and Codeine* *on page 54*

♦ **Fisalamine** *see* Mesalamine* *on page 174*

♦ **FK506** *see* Tacrolimus* *on page 246*

♦ **Flagyl®** *see* Metronidazole* *on page 180*

♦ **Flagyl ER®** *see* Metronidazole* *on page 180*

- **Flatulex®** [OTC] *see* Simethicone *on page 238*
- **Fleet® Enema** [OTC] *see* Sodium Phosphates* *on page 239*
- **Fleet® Laxative** [OTC] *see* Bisacodyl* *on page 48*
- **Fleet® Mineral Oil Enema** [OTC] *see* Mineral Oil* *on page 181*
- **Fleet® Phospho®-Soda** [OTC] *see* Sodium Phosphates* *on page 239*
- **Flexaphen®** *see* Chlorzoxazone *on page 75*
- **Flexeril®** *see* Cyclobenzaprine *on page 88*
- **Flonase®** *see* Fluticasone* *on page 132*
- **Florone®** *see* Diflorasone* *on page 99*
- **Florone E®** *see* Diflorasone* *on page 99*
- **Flovent®** *see* Fluticasone* *on page 132*
- **Floxin®** *see* Ofloxacin* *on page 198*

Floxuridine* (floks YOOR i deen)
U.S. Brand Names FUDR®
Synonyms Fluorodeoxyuridine; FUDR
Pharmacologic Class Antineoplastic Agent, Antimetabolite
Nutrients Depleted
 See Nutrient Depletion and Cancer Chemotherapy *on page 515*.
Scientific Basis Inferred or indirect evidence of depletion based on disruption of physiologic processes

- **Flubenisolone** *see* Betamethasone* *on page 46*

Fluconazole (floo KOE na zole)
U.S. Brand Names Diflucan®
Pharmacologic Class Antifungal Agent, Oral; Antifungal Agent, Parenteral
Nutrients Depleted
 Specific nutrient depletions have not been documented for this agent.

Flucytosine* (floo SYE toe seen)
U.S. Brand Names Ancobon®
Canadian Brand Names Ancotil®
Synonyms 5-FC; 5-Flurocytosine
Pharmacologic Class Antifungal Agent, Oral
Nutrients Depleted
 Calcium *on page 313*
 Magnesium *on page 333*
 Potassium *on page 340*
 Sodium *on page 345*
Scientific Basis Inferred or indirect evidence of depletion based on disruption of physiologic processes
Studies & Abstracts 177-181

- **Fludara®** *see* Fludarabine* *on page 128*

Fludarabine* (floo DARE a been)
U.S. Brand Names Fludara®
Synonyms Fludarabine Phosphate

Pharmacologic Class Antineoplastic Agent, Antimetabolite

Nutrients Depleted

See Nutrient Depletion and Cancer Chemotherapy *on page 515.*

Scientific Basis Inferred or indirect evidence of depletion based on disruption of physiologic processes

♦ **Fludarabine Phosphate** *see* Fludarabine* *on page 128*

♦ **Flumadine®** *see* Rimantadine *on page 232*

Flunisolide* (floo NIS oh lide)

Related Information

Drug-Induced Nutrient Depletion Table *on page 498*

U.S. Brand Names AeroBid®-M Oral Aerosol Inhaler; AeroBid® Oral Aerosol Inhaler; Nasalide® Nasal Aerosol; Nasarel® Nasal Spray

Canadian Brand Names Bronalide®; Rhinalar®; Rhinaris®-F; Syn-Flunisolide

Pharmacologic Class Corticosteroid, Oral Inhaler; Corticosteroid, Nasal

Nutrients Depleted

Calcium *on page 313*
Folic Acid *on page 325*
Magnesium *on page 333*
Potassium *on page 340*
Selenium *on page 343*
Vitamin C *on page 360*
Vitamin D *on page 363*
Zinc *on page 368*

Scientific Basis

Published scientific studies using this pharmacologic agent
    or
Published scientific studies of agents from the same pharmacologic class

Studies & Abstracts 182-223

Fluocinolone* (floo oh SIN oh lone)

U.S. Brand Names Derma-Smoothe/FS®; Fluonid®; Flurosyn®; FS Shampoo®; Synalar®; Synalar-HP®; Synemol®

Canadian Brand Names Lidemol®

Synonyms Fluocinolone Acetonide

Pharmacologic Class Corticosteroid, Topical

Nutrients Depleted

Calcium *on page 313*
Folic Acid *on page 325*
Magnesium *on page 333*
Potassium *on page 340*
Selenium *on page 343*
Vitamin C *on page 360*
Vitamin D *on page 363*
Zinc *on page 368*
(Continued)

Fluocinolone* *(Continued)*

Scientific Basis
Published scientific studies using this pharmacologic agent
  or
Published scientific studies of agents from the same pharmacologic
  class
Studies & Abstracts 182-223
Additional Information Depletion from topical products is limited.

♦ **Fluocinolone Acetonide** *see* Fluocinolone* *on page 129*

Fluocinonide* *(floo oh SIN oh nide)*
U.S. Brand Names Lidex®; Lidex-E®
Canadian Brand Names Lyderm; Lydonide; Tiamol®; Topactin®;
  Topsyn®
Pharmacologic Class Corticosteroid, Topical
Nutrients Depleted
  Calcium *on page 313*
  Folic Acid *on page 325*
  Magnesium *on page 333*
  Potassium *on page 340*
  Selenium *on page 343*
  Vitamin C *on page 360*
  Vitamin D *on page 363*
  Zinc *on page 368*
Scientific Basis
Published scientific studies using this pharmacologic agent
  or
Published scientific studies of agents from the same pharmacologic
  class
Studies & Abstracts 182-223
Additional Information Depletion from topical products is limited.

♦ **Fluonid®** *see* Fluocinolone* *on page 129*
♦ **Fluorodeoxyuridine** *see* Floxuridine* *on page 128*
♦ **Fluoroplex® Topical** *see* Fluorouracil* *on page 130*

Fluorouracil* *(flure oh YOOR a sil)*
U.S. Brand Names Adrucil® Injection; Efudex® Topical; Fluoroplex®
  Topical
Synonyms 5-Fluorouracil; 5-FU
Pharmacologic Class Antineoplastic Agent, Antimetabolite
Nutrients Depleted
  See Nutrient Depletion and Cancer Chemotherapy *on page 515.*
Scientific Basis Inferred or indirect evidence of depletion based on
  disruption of physiologic processes

♦ **5-Fluorouracil** *see* Fluorouracil* *on page 130*

Fluoxetine *(floo OKS e teen)*
U.S. Brand Names Prozac®; Sarafem™
Synonyms Fluoxetine Hydrochloride

Pharmacologic Class Antidepressant, Selective Serotonin Reuptake Inhibitor

Nutrients Depleted
Specific nutrient depletions have not been documented for this agent.

Additional Information Selective serotonin reuptake inhibitors have been associated with rare, potentially severe hyponatremia. However, this is generally associated with fluid excess (SIADH), rather than a sodium deficiency. Treatment must be guided by a qualified healthcare provider.

♦ **Fluoxetine Hydrochloride** see Fluoxetine on page 130

♦ **Fluoxymesterone and Estradiol** see Ethinyl Estradiol and Fluoxymesterone* on page 120

Fluphenazine* (floo FEN a zeen)
Related Information
Drug-Induced Nutrient Depletion Table on page 498
U.S. Brand Names Permitil® Oral; Prolixin Decanoate® Injection; Prolixin Enanthate® Injection; Prolixin® Injection; Prolixin® Oral
Canadian Brand Names Apo®-Fluphenazine; Modecate®; Modecate® Enanthate; Moditen® Hydrochloride; PMS-Fluphenazine
Synonyms Fluphenazine Decanoate; Fluphenazine Enanthate; Fluphenazine Hydrochloride
Pharmacologic Class Antipsychotic Agent, Phenothiazine, Piperazine
Nutrients Depleted
Coenzyme Q_{10} on page 320
Vitamin B_2 on page 353
Scientific Basis Published scientific studies of agents from the same pharmacologic class
Studies & Abstracts 474-477

♦ **Fluphenazine Decanoate** see Fluphenazine* on page 131

♦ **Fluphenazine Enanthate** see Fluphenazine* on page 131

♦ **Fluphenazine Hydrochloride** see Fluphenazine* on page 131

Flurazepam (flure AZ e pam)
U.S. Brand Names Dalmane®
Canadian Brand Names Apo®-Flurazepam; Novo-Flupam; PMS-Flupam; Somnol®; Som Pam®
Synonyms Flurazepam Hydrochloride
Pharmacologic Class Benzodiazepine
Nutrients Depleted
Specific nutrient depletions have not been documented for this agent.

♦ **Flurazepam Hydrochloride** see Flurazepam on page 131

Flurbiprofen* (flure BI proe fen)
U.S. Brand Names Ansaid® Oral; Ocufen® Ophthalmic
Canadian Brand Names Apo®-Flurbiprofen; Froben®; Froben-SR®; Novo-Flurprofen; Nu-Flurprofen
Synonyms Flurbiprofen Sodium
(Continued)

Flurbiprofen* (Continued)

Pharmacologic Class Nonsteroidal Anti-Inflammatory Agent (NSAID)

Nutrients Depleted
Folic Acid on page 325

Scientific Basis Published scientific studies of agents from the same pharmacologic class

Studies & Abstracts 252

- ♦ **Flurbiprofen Sodium** see Flurbiprofen* on page 131
- ♦ **5-Flurocytosine** see Flucytosine* on page 128
- ♦ **Flurosyn®** see Fluocinolone* on page 129

Flutamide (FLOO ta mide)

U.S. Brand Names Eulexin®

Canadian Brand Names Novo-Flutamide

Pharmacologic Class Antiandrogen

Nutrients Depleted
Specific nutrient depletions have not been documented for this agent.

- ♦ **Flutex®** see Triamcinolone* on page 259

Fluticasone* (floo TIK a sone)

Related Information
Drug-Induced Nutrient Depletion Table on page 498

U.S. Brand Names Cutivate™; Flonase®; Flovent®

Synonyms Fluticasone Propionate

Pharmacologic Class Corticosteroid, Oral Inhaler; Corticosteroid, Nasal

Nutrients Depleted
Calcium on page 313
Folic Acid on page 325
Magnesium on page 333
Potassium on page 340
Selenium on page 343
Vitamin C on page 360
Vitamin D on page 363
Zinc on page 368

Scientific Basis
Published scientific studies using this pharmacologic agent
or
Published scientific studies of agents from the same pharmacologic class

Studies & Abstracts 182-223

Additional Information Potential for depletions is limited with topical administration.

Fluticasone and Salmeterol*
(floo TIK a sone & sal ME te role)

U.S. Brand Names Advair™ Diskus®

Synonyms Salmeterol and Fluticasone

Pharmacologic Class Beta$_2$ Agonist; Corticosteroid, Oral Inhaler
Nutrients Depleted
  Calcium *on page 313*
  Folic Acid *on page 325*
  Magnesium *on page 333*
  Potassium *on page 340*
  Selenium *on page 343*
  Vitamin C *on page 360*
  Vitamin D *on page 363*
  Zinc *on page 368*
Scientific Basis
  Published scientific studies using these pharmacologic agents
    or
  Published scientific studies of agents from the same pharmacologic
    class
Studies & Abstracts 182-223

♦ **Fluticasone Propionate** *see* Fluticasone* *on page 132*

Fluvastatin* (FLOO va sta tin)
Related Information
  Drug-Induced Nutrient Depletion Table *on page 498*
U.S. Brand Names Lescol®
Pharmacologic Class Antilipemic Agent (HMG-CoA Reductase
Inhibitor)
Nutrients Depleted
  Coenzyme Q$_{10}$ *on page 320*
Scientific Basis Published scientific studies of agents from the same
pharmacologic class
Studies & Abstracts 350-361

Fluvoxamine (floo VOKS ah meen)
U.S. Brand Names Luvox®
Canadian Brand Names Apo®-Fluvoxamine
Pharmacologic Class Antidepressant, Selective Serotonin Reuptake
Inhibitor
Nutrients Depleted
  Specific nutrient depletions have not been documented for this agent.
Additional Information Selective serotonin reuptake inhibitors have
been associated with rare, potentially severe hyponatremia. However,
this is generally associated with fluid excess (SIADH), rather than a
sodium deficiency. Treatment must be guided by a qualified healthcare
provider.

♦ **Folex® PFS** *see* Methotrexate* *on page 176*

Fomepizole (foe ME pi zole)
U.S. Brand Names Antizol®
Synonyms 4-Methylpyrazole; 4-MP
Pharmacologic Class Antidote
Nutrients Depleted
  Specific nutrient depletions have not been documented for this agent.

- **Formulex**® *see* Dicyclomine *on page 98*
- **Fortaz**® *see* Ceftazidime* *on page 66*
- **Fortovase**® *see* Saquinavir *on page 236*
- **Fosamax**® *see* Alendronate *on page 27*

Foscarnet* (fos KAR net)
Related Information
Drug-Induced Nutrient Depletion Table *on page 498*
U.S. Brand Names Foscavir® Injection
Synonyms PFA; Phosphonoformate; Phosphonoformic Acid
Pharmacologic Class Antiviral Agent
Nutrients Depleted
Calcium *on page 313*
Magnesium *on page 333*
Phosphorus *on page 339*
Potassium *on page 340*
Scientific Basis Published scientific studies using this pharmacologic agent
Studies & Abstracts 253-259

- **Foscavir® Injection** *see* Foscarnet* *on page 134*

Fosinopril* (foe SIN oh pril)
Related Information
Drug-Induced Nutrient Depletion Table *on page 498*
U.S. Brand Names Monopril®
Pharmacologic Class Angiotensin-Converting Enzyme (ACE) Inhibitors
Nutrients Depleted
Zinc *on page 368*
Scientific Basis Published scientific studies of agents from the same pharmacologic class
Studies & Abstracts 269-271

Fosphenytoin* (FOS fen i toyn)
U.S. Brand Names Cerebyx®
Synonyms Fosphenytoin Sodium
Pharmacologic Class Anticonvulsant, Hydantoin
Nutrients Depleted
Biotin *on page 311*
Calcium *on page 313*
Folic Acid *on page 325*
Vitamin B_1 *on page 351*
Vitamin B_{12} *on page 359*
Vitamin D *on page 363*
Vitamin K *on page 367*
Scientific Basis Published scientific studies using this pharmacologic agent
Studies & Abstracts 112-150
Additional Information Addition of folic acid to patients on a stable dose of phenytoin may alter serum concentrations and/or result in

breakthrough seizures. Consultation with the prescriber and careful monitoring should be instituted prior to beginning supplementation.

- **Fosphenytoin Sodium** *see* Fosphenytoin* *on page 134*
- **Fragmin**® *see* Dalteparin *on page 91*
- **Froben**® *see* Flurbiprofen* *on page 131*
- **Froben-SR**® *see* Flurbiprofen* *on page 131*
- **Frusemide** *see* Furosemide* *on page 135*
- **FS Shampoo**® *see* Fluocinolone* *on page 129*
- **5-FU** *see* Fluorouracil* *on page 130*
- **FUDR** *see* Floxuridine* *on page 128*
- **Fumasorb**® **[OTC]** *see* Ferrous Fumarate *on page 126*
- **Fumerin**® **[OTC]** *see* Ferrous Fumarate *on page 126*
- **Fungizone**® *see* Amphotericin B (Conventional)* *on page 34*
- **Fungoid**® **Solution** *see* Clotrimazole *on page 82*
- **Furadantin**® *see* Nitrofurantoin* *on page 192*
- **Furazosin** *see* Prazosin *on page 217*

Furosemide* (fyoor OH se mide)
Related Information
Drug-Induced Nutrient Depletion Table *on page 498*
U.S. Brand Names Lasix®
Canadian Brand Names Apo®-Furosemide; Furoside®; Novo-Semide; Uritol®
Synonyms Frusemide
Pharmacologic Class Diuretic, Loop
Nutrients Depleted
Calcium *on page 313*
Magnesium *on page 333*
Potassium *on page 340*
Sodium *on page 345*
Vitamin B$_1$ *on page 351*
Vitamin B$_6$ *on page 357*
Vitamin C *on page 360*
Zinc *on page 368*
Scientific Basis Published scientific studies using this pharmacologic agent
Studies & Abstracts 280-311
Additional Information Sodium replacement is not recommended in patients receiving loop diuretics. Potassium replacement should be guided by monitoring of serum concentrations.

- **Furoside**® *see* Furosemide* *on page 135*
- **G-1**® *see* Butalbital Compound and Acetaminophen* *on page 53*

Gabapentin (GA ba pen tin)
U.S. Brand Names Neurontin®
Pharmacologic Class Anticonvulsant, Miscellaneous
Nutrients Depleted
Specific nutrient depletions have not been documented for this agent.

- **Gabitril®** *see* Tiagabine *on page 252*
- **Gamma Benzene Hexachloride** *see* Lindane *on page 166*

Ganciclovir (gan SYE kloe veer)
U.S. Brand Names Cytovene®; Vitrasert®
Synonyms DHPG Sodium; GCV Sodium; Nordeoxyguanosine
Pharmacologic Class Antiviral Agent
Nutrients Depleted
Specific nutrient depletions have not been documented for this agent.

- **Gantanol®** *see* Sulfamethoxazole* *on page 243*
- **Gantrisin®** *see* Sulfisoxazole* *on page 244*
- **Garamycin® Injection** *see* Gentamicin* *on page 138*
- **Garamycin® Ophthalmic** *see* Gentamicin* *on page 138*
- **Garamycin® Topical** *see* Gentamicin* *on page 138*
- **Gas-Ban DS® [OTC]** *see* Aluminum Hydroxide, Magnesium Hydroxide, and Simethicone* *on page 29*
- **Gas Relief®** *see* Simethicone *on page 238*
- **Gastrocrom® Oral** *see* Cromolyn Sodium *on page 87*
- **Gastrosed™** *see* Hyoscyamine *on page 153*
- **Gas-X® [OTC]** *see* Simethicone *on page 238*

Gatifloxacin* (ga ti FLOKS a sin)
U.S. Brand Names Tequin™
Pharmacologic Class Antibiotic, Quinolone
Nutrients Depleted
Bifidobacteria bifidum (bifidus) on page 311
Biotin *on page 311*
Inositol *on page 328*
Lactobacillus acidophilus on page 332
Vitamin B_1 *on page 351*
Vitamin B_2 *on page 353*
Vitamin B_3 *on page 354*
Vitamin B_6 *on page 357*
Vitamin B_{12} *on page 359*
Vitamin K *on page 367*

Scientific Basis Inferred or indirect evidence of depletion based on disruption of physiologic processes
Studies & Abstracts 7-27

- **Gaviscon®-2 Tablet [OTC]** *see* Aluminum Hydroxide and Magnesium Trisilicate* *on page 29*
- **Gaviscon® Liquid [OTC]** *see* Aluminum Hydroxide and Magnesium Carbonate* *on page 28*
- **Gaviscon® Tablet [OTC]** *see* Aluminum Hydroxide and Magnesium Trisilicate* *on page 29*
- **GCV Sodium** *see* Ganciclovir *on page 136*
- **Gee Gee® [OTC]** *see* Guaifenesin *on page 140*
- **Gelusil® [OTC]** *see* Aluminum Hydroxide, Magnesium Hydroxide, and Simethicone* *on page 29*

Gemcitabine* (jem SIT a been)
U.S. Brand Names Gemzar®
Synonyms Gemcitabine Hydrochloride
Pharmacologic Class Antineoplastic Agent, Antimetabolite
Nutrients Depleted
See Nutrient Depletion and Cancer Chemotherapy *on page 515.*
Scientific Basis Inferred or indirect evidence of depletion based on disruption of physiologic processes

♦ **Gemcitabine Hydrochloride** *see Gemcitabine* on page 137*

Gemfibrozil* (jem FI broe zil)
Related Information
Drug-Induced Nutrient Depletion Table *on page 498*
U.S. Brand Names Lopid®
Canadian Brand Names Apo®-Gemfibrozil; Nu-Gemfibrozil
Synonyms CI-719
Pharmacologic Class Antilipemic Agent (Fibric Acid)
Nutrients Depleted
Coenzyme Q_{10} *on page 320*
Vitamin E *on page 365*
Scientific Basis Published scientific studies using this pharmacologic agent
Studies & Abstracts 350

Gemtuzumab Ozogamicin
(gem TUZ yu mab oh zog a MY sin)
U.S. Brand Names Mylotarg™
Pharmacologic Class Antineoplastic Agent, Monoclonal Antibody
Nutrients Depleted
Specific nutrient depletions have not been documented for this agent.

♦ **Gemzar®** *see Gemcitabine* on page 137*
♦ **Genagesic®** *see Guaifenesin and Phenylpropanolamine on page 141*
♦ **Genahist® Oral** *see Diphenhydramine on page 102*
♦ **Genamin® Cold Syrup [OTC]** *see Chlorpheniramine and Phenylpropanolamine on page 73*
♦ **Genamin® Expectorant [OTC]** *see Guaifenesin and Phenylpropanolamine on page 141*
♦ **Genapap® [OTC]** *see Acetaminophen* on page 23*
♦ **Genasoft® Plus [OTC]** *see Docusate and Casanthranol* on page 104*
♦ **Genatap® Elixir [OTC]** *see Brompheniramine and Phenylpropanolamine on page 50*
♦ **Genatuss® [OTC]** *see Guaifenesin on page 140*
♦ **Genatuss DM® [OTC]** *see Guaifenesin and Dextromethorphan on page 141*
♦ **Gen-Glybe** *see Glyburide* on page 139*
♦ **Gen-K®** *see Potassium Chloride (Timed Release)* on page 216*
♦ **Gen-Nifedipine** *see Nifedipine on page 192*

- **Genoptic® Ophthalmic** *see* Gentamicin* *on page 138*
- **Genoptic® S.O.P. Ophthalmic** *see* Gentamicin* *on page 138*
- **Genora® 0.5/35** *see* Ethinyl Estradiol and Norethindrone* *on page 121*
- **Genora® 1/35** *see* Ethinyl Estradiol and Norethindrone* *on page 121*
- **Genpril® [OTC]** *see* Ibuprofen* *on page 153*
- **Gentacidin® Ophthalmic** *see* Gentamicin* *on page 138*
- **Gentak® Ophthalmic** *see* Gentamicin* *on page 138*

Gentamicin* (jen ta MYE sin)

Related Information
Drug-Induced Nutrient Depletion Table *on page 498*

U.S. Brand Names Garamycin® Injection; Garamycin® Ophthalmic; Garamycin® Topical; Genoptic® Ophthalmic; Genoptic® S.O.P. Ophthalmic; Gentacidin® Ophthalmic; Gentak® Ophthalmic; G-myticin® Topical; Jenamicin® Injection

Pharmacologic Class Antibiotic, Aminoglycoside; Antibiotic, Ophthalmic; Antibiotic, Topical

Nutrients Depleted
Bifidobacteria bifidum (bifidus) *on page 311*
Biotin *on page 311*
Calcium *on page 313*
Inositol *on page 328*
Lactobacillus acidophilus *on page 332*
Magnesium *on page 333*
Potassium *on page 340*
Sodium *on page 345*
Vitamin B_1 *on page 351*
Vitamin B_2 *on page 353*
Vitamin B_3 *on page 354*
Vitamin B_6 *on page 357*
Vitamin B_{12} *on page 359*
Vitamin K *on page 367*

Scientific Basis
Published scientific studies of agents from the same pharmacologic class
or
Inferred or indirect evidence of depletion based on disruption of physiologic processes

Studies & Abstracts 7-37

- **Gen-Timolol** *see* Timolol* *on page 254*
- **Gen-Triazolam** *see* Triazolam *on page 261*
- **Gen-XENE®** *see* Clorazepate *on page 81*
- **Geocillin®** *see* Carbenicillin* *on page 57*
- **Geopen®** *see* Carbenicillin* *on page 57*
- **GG** *see* Guaifenesin *on page 140*
- **GG-Cen® [OTC]** *see* Guaifenesin *on page 140*
- **Glibenclamide** *see* Glyburide* *on page 139*

Glimepiride* (GLYE me pye ride)

U.S. Brand Names Amaryl®

Pharmacologic Class Antidiabetic Agent (Sulfonylurea)

Nutrients Depleted

Coenzyme Q_{10} *on page 320*

Scientific Basis Published scientific studies of agents from the same pharmacologic class demonstrate depletion of some nutrients; however, this agent was NOT found to cause a similar depletion

Studies & Abstracts 167

Glipizide* (GLIP i zide)

Related Information

Drug-Induced Nutrient Depletion Table *on page 498*

U.S. Brand Names Glucotrol®; Glucotrol® XL

Synonyms Glydiazinamide

Pharmacologic Class Antidiabetic Agent (Sulfonylurea)

Nutrients Depleted

Coenzyme Q_{10} *on page 320*

Scientific Basis Published scientific studies of agents from the same pharmacologic class demonstrate depletion of some nutrients; however, this agent was NOT found to cause a similar depletion

Studies & Abstracts 167

- ◆ **Glucophage®** *see* Metformin* *on page 175*
- ◆ **Glucotrol®** *see* Glipizide* *on page 139*
- ◆ **Glucotrol® XL** *see* Glipizide* *on page 139*
- ◆ **Glucovance™** *see* Glyburide and Metformin* *on page 139*
- ◆ **Glyate® [OTC]** *see* Guaifenesin *on page 140*
- ◆ **Glybenclamide** *see* Glyburide* *on page 139*
- ◆ **Glybenzcyclamide** *see* Glyburide* *on page 139*

Glyburide* (GLYE byoor ide)

Related Information

Drug-Induced Nutrient Depletion Table *on page 498*

U.S. Brand Names Diaβeta®; Glynase™ PresTab™; Micronase®

Canadian Brand Names Albert® Glyburide; Apo®-Glyburide; Euglucon®; Gen-Glybe; Novo-Glyburide; Nu-Glyburide

Synonyms Glibenclamide; Glybenclamide; Glybenzcyclamide

Pharmacologic Class Antidiabetic Agent (Sulfonylurea)

Nutrients Depleted

Coenzyme Q_{10} *on page 320*

Scientific Basis Published scientific studies using this pharmacologic agent

Studies & Abstracts 167

Glyburide and Metformin*

(GLYE byoor ide & met FOR min)

U.S. Brand Names Glucovance™

Synonyms Glyburide and Metformin Hydrochloride

(Continued)

Glyburide and Metformin* *(Continued)*

Pharmacologic Class Antidiabetic Agent, Oral; Antidiabetic Agent (Sulfonylurea)

Nutrients Depleted
Coenzyme Q_{10} *on page 320*
Folic Acid *on page 325*
Vitamin B_{12} *on page 359*

Scientific Basis
Published scientific studies using these pharmacologic agents
or
Published scientific studies of agents from the same pharmacologic class

Studies & Abstracts 167-176

♦ **Glyburide and Metformin Hydrochloride** *see* Glyburide and Metformin* *on page 139*
♦ **Glycerol Guaiacolate** *see* Guaifenesin *on page 140*
♦ **Glyceryl Trinitrate** *see* Nitroglycerin *on page 192*
♦ **Glycofed®** *see* Guaifenesin and Pseudoephedrine *on page 142*
♦ **Glycotuss® [OTC]** *see* Guaifenesin *on page 140*
♦ **Glycotuss-dM® [OTC]** *see* Guaifenesin and Dextromethorphan *on page 141*
♦ **Glydiazinamide** *see* Glipizide* *on page 139*
♦ **Glynase™ PresTab™** *see* Glyburide* *on page 139*
♦ **Glyset®** *see* Miglitol *on page 181*
♦ **Glytuss® [OTC]** *see* Guaifenesin *on page 140*
♦ **GM-CSF** *see* Sargramostim *on page 236*
♦ **G-myticin® Topical** *see* Gentamicin* *on page 138*
♦ **GP 47680** *see* Oxcarbazepine* *on page 201*
♦ **GR1222311X** *see* Ranitidine Bismuth Citrate* *on page 229*

Granisetron *(gra NI se tron)*

U.S. Brand Names Kytril™
Pharmacologic Class Selective 5-HT_3 Receptor Antagonist
Nutrients Depleted
Specific nutrient depletions have not been documented for this agent.

♦ **Granulocyte-Macrophage Colony Stimulating Factor** *see* Sargramostim *on page 236*
♦ **Guaifed® [OTC]** *see* Guaifenesin and Pseudoephedrine *on page 142*
♦ **Guaifed-PD®** *see* Guaifenesin and Pseudoephedrine *on page 142*

Guaifenesin *(gwye FEN e sin)*

U.S. Brand Names Anti-Tuss® Expectorant [OTC]; Breonesin® [OTC]; Diabetic Tussin® EX [OTC]; Duratuss-G®; Fenesin™; Gee Gee® [OTC]; Genatuss® [OTC]; GG-Cen® [OTC]; Glyate® [OTC]; Glycotuss® [OTC]; Glytuss® [OTC]; Guaifenex® LA; GuiaCough® Expectorant [OTC]; Guiatuss® [OTC]; Halotussin® [OTC]; Humibid® L.A.; Humibid® Sprinkle; Hytuss® [OTC]; Hytuss-2X® [OTC]; Liquibid®; Medi-Tuss®

[OTC]; Monafed®; Muco-Fen-LA®; Mytussin® [OTC]; Naldecon® Senior EX [OTC]; Organidin® NR; Pneumomist®; Respa-GF®; Robitussin® [OTC]; Scot-Tussin® [OTC]; Siltussin® [OTC]; Sinumist®-SR Capsulets®; Touro Ex®; Tusibron® [OTC]; Uni-tussin® [OTC]

Canadian Brand Names Balminil® Expectorant; Calmylin Expectorant

Synonyms GG; Glycerol Guaiacolate

Pharmacologic Class Expectorant

Nutrients Depleted

Specific nutrient depletions have not been documented for this agent.

Guaifenesin and Dextromethorphan

(gwye FEN e sin & deks troe meth OR fan)

U.S. Brand Names Benylin® Expectorant [OTC]; Cheracol® D [OTC]; Clear Tussin® 30; Contac® Cough Formula Liquid [OTC]; Diabetic Tussin DM® [OTC]; Extra Action Cough Syrup [OTC]; Fenesin™ DM; Genatuss DM® [OTC]; Glycotuss-dM® [OTC]; Guaifenex® DM; GuiaCough® [OTC]; Guiatuss-DM® [OTC]; Halotussin® DM [OTC]; Humibid® DM [OTC]; Iobid DM®; Kolephrin® GG/DM [OTC]; Monafed® DM; Muco-Fen-DM®; Mytussin® DM [OTC]; Naldecon® Senior DX [OTC]; Phanatuss® Cough Syrup [OTC]; Phenadex® Senior [OTC]; Respa®-DM; Rhinosyn-DMX® [OTC]; Robafen DM® [OTC]; Robitussin®-DM [OTC]; Safe Tussin® 30 [OTC]; Scot-Tussin® Senior Clear [OTC]; Siltussin DM® [OTC]; Synacol® CF [OTC]; Syracol-CF® [OTC]; Tolu-Sed® DM [OTC]; Tusibron-DM® [OTC]; Tuss-DM® [OTC]; Tussi-Organidin® DM NR; Uni-tussin® DM [OTC]; Vicks® 44E [OTC]; Vicks® Pediatric Formula 44E [OTC]

Synonyms Dextromethorphan and Guaifenesin

Pharmacologic Class Antitussive; Cough Preparation; Expectorant

Nutrients Depleted

Specific nutrient depletions have not been documented for this agent.

Guaifenesin and Phenylephrine

(gwye FEN e sin & fen il EF rin)

U.S. Brand Names Deconsal® Sprinkle®; Endal®; Sinupan®

Synonyms Phenylephrine and Guaifenesin

Pharmacologic Class Decongestant; Expectorant

Nutrients Depleted

Specific nutrient depletions have not been documented for this agent.

Guaifenesin and Phenylpropanolamine

(gwye FEN e sin & fen il proe pa NOLE a meen)

U.S. Brand Names Ami-Tex LA®; Coldlac-LA®; Conex® [OTC]; Contuss® XT; Dura-Vent®; Entex® LA; Genagesic®; Genamin® Expectorant [OTC]; Guaifenex® PPA 75; Guaipax®; Myminic® Expectorant [OTC]; Naldecon-EX® Children's Syrup [OTC]; Nolex® LA; Partuss® LA; Phenylfenesin® L.A.; Profen II®; Profen LA®; Rymed-TR®; Silaminic® Expectorant [OTC]; Sildicon-E® [OTC]; Snaplets-EX® [OTC]; Triaminic® Expectorant [OTC]; Tri-Clear® Expectorant [OTC]; Triphenyl® Expectorant [OTC]; ULR-LA®; Vicks® DayQuil® Sinus Pressure & Congestion Relief [OTC]

(Continued)

Guaifenesin and Phenylpropanolamine
(Continued)

Synonyms Phenylpropanolamine and Guaifenesin

Pharmacologic Class Decongestant; Expectorant

Nutrients Depleted
Specific nutrient depletions have not been documented for this agent.

Guaifenesin and Pseudoephedrine
(gwye FEN e sin & soo doe e FED rin)

U.S. Brand Names Congess® Jr; Congess® Sr; Congestac®; Deconsal® II; Defen-LA®; Entex® PSE; Eudal-SR®; Fedahist® Expectorant [OTC]; Fedahist® Expectorant Pediatric [OTC]; Glycofed®; Guaifed® [OTC]; Guaifed-PD®; Guaifenex® PSE; GuaiMAX-D®; Guaitab®; Guaivent®; Guai-Vent/PSE®; Guiatuss PE® [OTC]; Halotussin® PE [OTC]; Histalet® X; Nasabid™; Respa-1st®; Respaire®-60 SR; Respaire®-120 SR; Robitussin-PE® [OTC]; Robitussin® Severe Congestion Liqui-Gels® [OTC]; Ru-Tuss® DE; Rymed®; Sinufed® Timecelles®; Touro LA®; Tuss-LA®; V-Dec-M®; Versacaps®; Zephrex®; Zephrex LA®

Synonyms Pseudoephedrine and Guaifenesin

Pharmacologic Class Decongestant; Expectorant

Nutrients Depleted
Specific nutrient depletions have not been documented for this agent.

Guaifenesin, Phenylpropanolamine, and Dextromethorphan
(gwye FEN e sin, fen il proe pa NOLE a meen, & deks troe meth OR fan)

U.S. Brand Names Anatuss® [OTC]; Guiatuss CF® [OTC]; Naldecon® DX Adult Liquid [OTC]; Profen II DM®; Robafen® CF [OTC]; Robitussin-CF® [OTC]; Siltussin-CF® [OTC]

Synonyms Dextromethorphan, Guaifenesin, and Phenylpropanolamine; Phenylpropanolamine, Guaifenesin, and Dextromethorphan

Pharmacologic Class Cough Preparation; Decongestant; Expectorant

Nutrients Depleted
Specific nutrient depletions have not been documented for this agent.

Guaifenesin, Phenylpropanolamine, and Phenylephrine
(gwye FEN e sin, fen il proe pa NOLE a meen, & fen il EF rin)

U.S. Brand Names Coldloc®; Contuss®; Dura-Gest®; Enomine®; Entex®; Guaifenex®; Guiatex®

Synonyms Phenylephrine, Guaifenesin, and Phenylpropanolamine; Phenylpropanolamine, Guaifenesin, and Phenylephrine

Pharmacologic Class Decongestant; Expectorant

Nutrients Depleted
Specific nutrient depletions have not been documented for this agent.

Guaifenesin, Pseudoephedrine, and Codeine
(gwye FEN e sin, soo doe e FED rin, & KOE deen)

U.S. Brand Names Codafed® Expectorant; Cycofed® Pediatric; Decohistine® Expectorant; Deproist® Expectorant With Codeine; Dihistine® Expectorant; Guiatuss DAC®; Guiatussin® DAC; Halotussin® DAC; Isoclor® Expectorant; Mytussin® DAC; Nucofed®; Nucofed® Pediatric Expectorant; Nucotuss®; Phenhist® Expectorant; Robitussin®-DAC; Ryna-CX®; Tussar® SF Syrup

Synonyms Codeine, Guaifenesin, and Pseudoephedrine; Pseudoephedrine, Guaifenesin, and Codeine

Pharmacologic Class Antitussive/Decongestant/Expectorant

Nutrients Depleted

Specific nutrient depletions have not been documented for this agent.

Guaifenesin, Pseudoephedrine, and Dextromethorphan
(gwye FEN e sin, soo doe e FED rin, & deks troe meth OR fan)

U.S. Brand Names Anatuss® DM [OTC]; Dimacol® Caplets [OTC]; Rhinosyn-X® Liquid [OTC]; Ru-Tuss® Expectorant [OTC]; Sudafed® Cold & Cough Liquid Caps [OTC]

Synonyms Dextromethorphan, Guaifenesin, and Pseudoephedrine; Pseudoephedrine, Dextromethorphan, and Guaifenesin

Pharmacologic Class Antitussive/Decongestant/Expectorant

Nutrients Depleted

Specific nutrient depletions have not been documented for this agent.

- **Guaifenex®** *see* Guaifenesin, Phenylpropanolamine, and Phenylephrine *on page 142*
- **Guaifenex® DM** *see* Guaifenesin and Dextromethorphan *on page 141*
- **Guaifenex® LA** *see* Guaifenesin *on page 140*
- **Guaifenex® PPA 75** *see* Guaifenesin and Phenylpropanolamine *on page 141*
- **Guaifenex® PSE** *see* Guaifenesin and Pseudoephedrine *on page 142*
- **GuaiMAX-D®** *see* Guaifenesin and Pseudoephedrine *on page 142*
- **Guaipax®** *see* Guaifenesin and Phenylpropanolamine *on page 141*
- **Guaitab®** *see* Guaifenesin and Pseudoephedrine *on page 142*
- **Guaivent®** *see* Guaifenesin and Pseudoephedrine *on page 142*
- **Guai-Vent/PSE®** *see* Guaifenesin and Pseudoephedrine *on page 142*
- **GuiaCough® [OTC]** *see* Guaifenesin and Dextromethorphan *on page 141*
- **GuiaCough® Expectorant [OTC]** *see* Guaifenesin *on page 140*
- **Guiatex®** *see* Guaifenesin, Phenylpropanolamine, and Phenylephrine *on page 142*
- **Guiatuss® [OTC]** *see* Guaifenesin *on page 140*
- **Guiatuss CF® [OTC]** *see* Guaifenesin, Phenylpropanolamine, and Dextromethorphan *on page 142*

- ◆ **Guiatuss DAC**® *see* Guaifenesin, Pseudoephedrine, and Codeine *on page 143*
- ◆ **Guiatuss-DM**® **[OTC]** *see* Guaifenesin and Dextromethorphan *on page 141*
- ◆ **Guiatussin**® **DAC** *see* Guaifenesin, Pseudoephedrine, and Codeine *on page 143*
- ◆ **Guiatuss PE**® **[OTC]** *see* Guaifenesin and Pseudoephedrine *on page 142*
- ◆ **G-well**® *see* Lindane *on page 166*
- ◆ **Gynazole-1**™ *see* Butoconazole *on page 54*
- ◆ **Gynecort**® **[OTC]** *see* Hydrocortisone* *on page 150*
- ◆ **Gyne-Lotrimin**® **[OTC]** *see* Clotrimazole *on page 82*
- ◆ **Gynogen L.A.**® **Injection** *see* Estradiol* *on page 114*
- ◆ **Habitrol**™ **Patch [OTC]** *see* Nicotine *on page 191*

Halazepam (hal AZ e pam)
U.S. Brand Names Paxipam®
Pharmacologic Class Benzodiazepine
Nutrients Depleted
Specific nutrient depletions have not been documented for this agent.

- ◆ **Halcion**® *see* Triazolam *on page 261*
- ◆ **Haldol**® *see* Haloperidol* *on page 145*
- ◆ **Haldol**® **Decanoate** *see* Haloperidol* *on page 145*
- ◆ **Halenol**® **Children's [OTC]** *see* Acetaminophen* *on page 23*
- ◆ **Halfprin**® **81**® **[OTC]** *see* Aspirin* *on page 40*

Halobetasol* (hal oh BAY ta sol)
U.S. Brand Names Ultravate™
Synonyms Halobetasol Propionate
Pharmacologic Class Corticosteroid, Topical
Nutrients Depleted
Calcium *on page 313*
Folic Acid *on page 325*
Magnesium *on page 333*
Potassium *on page 340*
Selenium *on page 343*
Vitamin C *on page 360*
Vitamin D *on page 363*
Zinc *on page 368*
Scientific Basis
Published scientific studies using this pharmacologic agent
or
Published scientific studies of agents from the same pharmacologic class
Studies & Abstracts 182-223
Additional Information Potential for depletion is limited with topical use.

- ◆ **Halobetasol Propionate** *see* Halobetasol* *on page 144*

Haloperidol* (ha loe PER i dole)

Related Information

Drug-Induced Nutrient Depletion Table *on page 498*

U.S. Brand Names Haldol®; Haldol® Decanoate

Synonyms Haloperidol Decanoate; Haloperidol Lactate

Pharmacologic Class Antipsychotic Agent, Butyrophenone

Nutrients Depleted

Coenzyme Q_{10} *on page 320*

Scientific Basis Published scientific studies using this pharmacologic agent

Studies & Abstracts 478

- ◆ **Haloperidol Decanoate** *see Haloperidol* *on page 145*
- ◆ **Haloperidol Lactate** *see Haloperidol* *on page 145*
- ◆ **Halotussin® [OTC]** *see Guaifenesin on page 140*
- ◆ **Halotussin® DAC** *see Guaifenesin, Pseudoephedrine, and Codeine on page 143*
- ◆ **Halotussin® DM [OTC]** *see Guaifenesin and Dextromethorphan on page 141*
- ◆ **Halotussin® PE [OTC]** *see Guaifenesin and Pseudoephedrine on page 142*
- ◆ **Haltran® [OTC]** *see Ibuprofen* *on page 153*
- ◆ **Hayfebrol® Liquid [OTC]** *see Chlorpheniramine and Pseudoephedrine on page 73*
- ◆ **HCTZ** *see Hydrochlorothiazide* *on page 147*
- ◆ **HCTZ and Telmisartan** *see Telmisartan and Hydrochlorothiazide* *on page 248*
- ◆ **Hemocyte® [OTC]** *see Ferrous Fumarate on page 126*
- ◆ **Hemril-HC® Uniserts®** *see Hydrocortisone* *on page 150*
- ◆ **Hexachlorocyclohexane** *see Lindane on page 166*
- ◆ **Hexadrol®** *see Dexamethasone* *on page 95*
- ◆ **Hexadrol® Phosphate** *see Dexamethasone* *on page 95*
- ◆ **Hexit®** *see Lindane on page 166*
- ◆ **Hi-Cor® 1.0** *see Hydrocortisone* *on page 150*
- ◆ **Hi-Cor® 2.5** *see Hydrocortisone* *on page 150*
- ◆ **Histalet® Syrup [OTC]** *see Chlorpheniramine and Pseudoephedrine on page 73*
- ◆ **Histalet® X** *see Guaifenesin and Pseudoephedrine on page 142*
- ◆ **Histatab® Plus Tablet [OTC]** *see Chlorpheniramine and Phenylephrine on page 73*
- ◆ **Histor-D® Syrup** *see Chlorpheniramine and Phenylephrine on page 73*
- ◆ **Hivid®** *see Zalcitabine* *on page 269*
- ◆ **Hold® DM [OTC]** *see Dextromethorphan on page 96*
- ◆ **Honvol®** *see Diethylstilbestrol* *on page 99*
- ◆ **Humalog®** *see Insulin Preparations on page 156*
- ◆ **Humalog® Mix 50/50™** *see Insulin Preparations on page 156*
- ◆ **Humalog® Mix 75/25™** *see Insulin Preparations on page 156*

- **Humibid® DM [OTC]** *see* Guaifenesin and Dextromethorphan *on page 141*
- **Humibid® L.A.** *see* Guaifenesin *on page 140*
- **Humibid® Sprinkle** *see* Guaifenesin *on page 140*
- **Humulin® 50/50** *see* Insulin Preparations *on page 156*
- **Humulin® 70/30** *see* Insulin Preparations *on page 156*
- **Humulin® L** *see* Insulin Preparations *on page 156*
- **Humulin® N** *see* Insulin Preparations *on page 156*
- **Hycamptamine** *see* Topotecan* *on page 257*
- **Hycamtin™** *see* Topotecan* *on page 257*
- **Hycort®** *see* Hydrocortisone* *on page 150*

Hydralazine* (hye DRAL a zeen)
U.S. Brand Names Apresoline®
Canadian Brand Names Apo®-Hydralazine; Novo-Hylazin; Nu-Hydral
Synonyms Hydralazine Hydrochloride
Pharmacologic Class Vasodilator
Nutrients Depleted
  Coenzyme Q_{10} *on page 320*
  Magnesium *on page 333*
  Potassium *on page 340*
  Vitamin B_6 *on page 357*
  Zinc *on page 368*
Scientific Basis Published scientific studies using this pharmacologic agent
Studies & Abstracts 275-279

Hydralazine and Hydrochlorothiazide*
(hye DRAL a zeen & hye droe klor oh THYE a zide)
U.S. Brand Names Apresazide®
Synonyms Hydrochlorothiazide and Hydralazine
Pharmacologic Class Antihypertensive Agent, Combination
Nutrients Depleted
  Coenzyme Q_{10} *on page 320*
  Magnesium *on page 333*
  Phosphorus *on page 339*
  Potassium *on page 340*
  Sodium *on page 345*
  Vitamin B_6 *on page 357*
  Zinc *on page 368*
Scientific Basis Published scientific studies using these pharmacologic agents
Studies & Abstracts 275-279, 320-342
Additional Information Sodium replacement is not recommended.

- **Hydralazine Hydrochloride** *see* Hydralazine* *on page 146*

Hydralazine, Hydrochlorothiazide, and Reserpine*
(hye DRAL a zeen, hye droe klor oh THYE a zide, & re SER peen)

U.S. Brand Names Hydrap-ES®; Marpres®; Ser-Ap-Es®

Synonyms Hydrochlorothiazide, Hydralazine, and Reserpine; Reserpine, Hydralazine, and Hydrochlorothiazide

Pharmacologic Class Antihypertensive Agent, Combination

Nutrients Depleted
Coenzyme Q_{10} *on page 320*
Vitamin B_6 *on page 357*

Scientific Basis Published scientific studies using these pharmacologic agents (hydralazine, hydrochlorothiazide)

Studies & Abstracts 275-279, 320-342

♦ **Hydramyn® Syrup [OTC]** *see* Diphenhydramine *on page 102*

♦ **Hydrap-ES®** *see* Hydralazine, Hydrochlorothiazide, and Reserpine* *on page 147*

♦ **Hydrated Chloral** *see* Chloral Hydrate *on page 72*

♦ **Hydrea®** *see* Hydroxyurea* *on page 152*

♦ **Hydrex®** *see* Benzthiazide* *on page 45*

♦ **Hydrocet®** *see* Hydrocodone and Acetaminophen* *on page 149*

Hydrochlorothiazide* (hye droe klor oh THYE a zide)

Related Information
Drug-Induced Nutrient Depletion Table *on page 498*

U.S. Brand Names Esidrix®; Ezide®; HydroDIURIL®; Hydro-Par®; Microzide™; Oretic®

Canadian Brand Names Apo®-Hydro; Diuchlor®; Neo-Codema®; Novo-Hydrazide; Urozide®

Synonyms HCTZ

Pharmacologic Class Diuretic, Thiazide

Nutrients Depleted
Coenzyme Q_{10} *on page 320*
Magnesium *on page 333*
Phosphorus *on page 339*
Potassium *on page 340*
Sodium *on page 345*
Zinc *on page 368*

Scientific Basis Published scientific studies using this pharmacologic agent

Studies & Abstracts 320-342

Additional Information Although thiazide diuretics deplete sodium, replacement is not recommended, as this may be directly related to the therapeutic effect. Thiazides may deplete potassium, however replacement should be guided by monitoring of serum concentrations and specific instruction by a healthcare provider.

♦ **Hydrochlorothiazide and Amiloride** *see* Amiloride and Hydrochlorothiazide* *on page 31*

- **Hydrochlorothiazide and Enalapril** *see* Enalapril and Hydrochlorothiazide* *on page 110*
- **Hydrochlorothiazide and Hydralazine** *see* Hydralazine and Hydrochlorothiazide* *on page 146*
- **Hydrochlorothiazide and Irbesartan** *see* Irbesartan and Hydrochlorothiazide* *on page 157*
- **Hydrochlorothiazide and Losartan** *see* Losartan and Hydrochlorothiazide* *on page 169*
- **Hydrochlorothiazide and Methyldopa** *see* Methyldopa and Hydrochlorothiazide* *on page 178*
- **Hydrochlorothiazide and Propranolol** *see* Propranolol and Hydrochlorothiazide* *on page 224*

Hydrochlorothiazide and Reserpine*

(hye droe klor oh THYE a zide & re SER peen)

U.S. Brand Names Hydropres®; Hydro-Serp®; Hydroserpine®

Synonyms Reserpine and Hydrochlorothiazide

Pharmacologic Class Antihypertensive Agent, Combination

Nutrients Depleted

Coenzyme Q_{10} *on page 320*
Magnesium *on page 333*
Phosphorus *on page 339*
Potassium *on page 340*
Sodium *on page 345*
Zinc *on page 368*

Scientific Basis Published scientific studies using this pharmacologic agent (hydrochlorothiazide)

Studies & Abstracts 320-342

Additional Information Although thiazide diuretics deplete sodium, replacement is not recommended, as this may be directly related to the therapeutic effect. Thiazides may deplete potassium, however replacement should be guided by monitoring of serum concentrations and specific instruction by a healthcare provider.

Hydrochlorothiazide and Spironolactone*

(hye droe klor oh THYE a zide & speer on oh LAK tone)

U.S. Brand Names Aldactazide®

Canadian Brand Names Apo®-Spirozide; Novo-Spirozine

Synonyms Spironolactone and Hydrochlorothiazide

Pharmacologic Class Antihypertensive Agent, Combination

Nutrients Depleted

Coenzyme Q_{10} *on page 320*
Magnesium *on page 333*
Phosphorus *on page 339*
Potassium *on page 340*
Sodium *on page 345*
Zinc *on page 368*

Scientific Basis Published scientific studies using this pharmacologic agent (hydrochlorothiazide)

Studies & Abstracts 320-342

Additional Information Sodium replacement is not recommended. Although thiazides may deplete potassium, spironolactone counters this action. Potassium replacement should follow adequate serum level monitoring.

♦ **Hydrochlorothiazide and Telmisartan** *see* Telmisartan and Hydrochlorothiazide* *on page 248*

Hydrochlorothiazide and Triamterene*

(hye droe klor oh THYE a zide & trye AM ter een)

Related Information
Drug-Induced Nutrient Depletion Table *on page 498*

U.S. Brand Names Dyazide®; Maxzide®

Canadian Brand Names Apo®-Triazide; Novo-Triamzide; Nu-Triazide

Synonyms Triamterene and Hydrochlorothiazide

Pharmacologic Class Antihypertensive Agent, Combination; Diuretic, Potassium Sparing; Diuretic, Thiazide

Nutrients Depleted
Calcium *on page 313*
Coenzyme Q_{10} *on page 320*
Folic Acid *on page 325*
Magnesium *on page 333*
Potassium *on page 340*
Sodium *on page 345*
Vitamin B_6 *on page 357*
Zinc *on page 368*

Scientific Basis Published scientific studies using these pharmacologic agents

Studies & Abstracts 313-319, 320-342

Additional Information Sodium replacement is not recommended. Although thiazides may deplete potassium, triamterene counters this action. Potassium replacement should follow adequate serum level monitoring.

♦ **Hydrochlorothiazide, Hydralazine, and Reserpine** *see* Hydralazine, Hydrochlorothiazide, and Reserpine* *on page 147*

♦ **Hydrocil® [OTC]** *see* Psyllium *on page 226*

Hydrocodone and Acetaminophen*

(hye droe KOE done & a seet a MIN oh fen)

U.S. Brand Names Anexsia®; Anodynos-DHC®; Bancap HC®; Co-Gesic®; Dolacet®; DuoCet™; Hydrocet®; Hydrogesic®; Hy-Phen®; Lorcet®; Lorcet®-HD; Lorcet® Plus; Lortab®; Margesic® H; Medipain 5®; Norco®; Stagesic®; T-Gesic®; Vicodin®; Vicodin® ES; Vicodin® HP; Zydone®

Canadian Brand Names Vapocet®

Synonyms Acetaminophen and Hydrocodone

Pharmacologic Class Analgesic, Combination (Narcotic)

Nutrients Depleted
Glutathione *on page 327*

Scientific Basis Published scientific studies using this pharmacologic agent (acetaminophen)

(Continued)

Hydrocodone and Acetaminophen* *(Continued)*
Studies & Abstracts 517-518

Hydrocodone and Aspirin*
(hye droe KOE done & AS pir in)
U.S. Brand Names Alor® 5/500; Azdone®; Damason-P®; Lortab® ASA; Panasal® 5/500
Synonyms Aspirin and Hydrocodone
Pharmacologic Class Analgesic, Combination (Narcotic)
Nutrients Depleted
Folic Acid *on page 325*
Iron *on page 331*
Potassium *on page 340*
Sodium *on page 345*
Vitamin C *on page 360*
Scientific Basis Published scientific studies using this pharmacologic agent (aspirin)
Studies & Abstracts 224-236

♦ Hydrocort® *see* Hydrocortisone* *on page 150*

Hydrocortisone* (hye droe KOR ti sone)
Related Information
Drug-Induced Nutrient Depletion Table *on page 498*
U.S. Brand Names Aeroseb-HC®; A-hydroCort®; Ala-Cort®; Ala-Scalp®; Anucort-HC® Suppository; Anuprep HC® Suppository; Anusol® HC 1 [OTC]; Anusol® HC 2.5% [OTC]; Anusol-HC® Suppository; Caldecort®; Caldecort® Anti-Itch Spray; Clocort® Maximum Strength; CortaGel® [OTC]; Cortaid® Maximum Strength [OTC]; Cortaid® With Aloe [OTC]; Cort-Dome®; Cortef®; Cortef® Feminine Itch; Cortenema®; Cortifoam®; Cortizone®-5 [OTC]; Cortizone®-10 [OTC]; Delcort®; Dermacort®; Dermarest Dricort®; DermiCort®; Dermolate® [OTC]; Dermtex® HC With Aloe; Eldecort®; Gynecort® [OTC]; Hemril-HC® Uniserts®; Hi-Cor® 1.0; Hi-Cor® 2.5; Hycort®; Hydrocort®; Hydrocortone® Acetate; Hydrocortone® Phosphate; HydroTex® [OTC]; Hytone®; LactiCare-HC®; Lanacort® [OTC]; Locoid®; Nutracort®; Orabase® HCA; Pandel®; Penecort®; Procort® [OTC]; Proctocort™; Scalpicin®; Solu-Cortef®; S-T Cort®; Synacort®; Tegrin®-HC [OTC]; Westcort®
Synonyms Compound F; Cortisol; Hydrocortisone Acetate; Hydrocortisone Buteprate; Hydrocortisone Butyrate; Hydrocortisone Cypionate; Hydrocortisone Sodium Phosphate; Hydrocortisone Sodium Succinate; Hydrocortisone Valerate
Pharmacologic Class Corticosteroid, Oral; Corticosteroid, Parenteral; Corticosteroid, Rectal; Corticosteroid, Topical
Nutrients Depleted
Calcium *on page 313*
Folic Acid *on page 325*
Magnesium *on page 333*
Potassium *on page 340*
Selenium *on page 343*
Vitamin C *on page 360*

Vitamin D *on page 363*
Zinc *on page 368*

Scientific Basis
Published scientific studies using this pharmacologic agent
or
Published scientific studies of agents from the same pharmacologic class

Studies & Abstracts 182-223

- **Hydrocortisone Acetate** *see* Hydrocortisone* *on page 150*
- **Hydrocortisone Buteprate** *see* Hydrocortisone* *on page 150*
- **Hydrocortisone Butyrate** *see* Hydrocortisone* *on page 150*
- **Hydrocortisone Cypionate** *see* Hydrocortisone* *on page 150*
- **Hydrocortisone Sodium Phosphate** *see* Hydrocortisone* *on page 150*
- **Hydrocortisone Sodium Succinate** *see* Hydrocortisone* *on page 150*
- **Hydrocortisone Valerate** *see* Hydrocortisone* *on page 150*
- **Hydrocortone® Acetate** *see* Hydrocortisone* *on page 150*
- **Hydrocortone® Phosphate** *see* Hydrocortisone* *on page 150*
- **HydroDIURIL®** *see* Hydrochlorothiazide* *on page 147*

Hydroflumethiazide* (hye droe floo meth EYE a zide)
U.S. Brand Names Diucardin®; Saluron®
Pharmacologic Class Diuretic, Thiazide
Nutrients Depleted
Coenzyme Q_{10} *on page 320*
Magnesium *on page 333*
Phosphorus *on page 339*
Potassium *on page 340*
Sodium *on page 345*
Zinc *on page 368*

Scientific Basis Published scientific studies of agents from the same pharmacologic class

Studies & Abstracts 320-342

Additional Information Although thiazide diuretics deplete sodium, replacement is not recommended, as this may be directly related to the therapeutic effect. Thiazides may deplete potassium, however replacement should be guided by monitoring of serum concentrations and specific instruction by a healthcare provider.

- **Hydrogesic®** *see* Hydrocodone and Acetaminophen* *on page 149*
- **Hydromorph Contin®** *see* Hydromorphone *on page 151*

Hydromorphone (hye droe MOR fone)
U.S. Brand Names Dilaudid®; Dilaudid-5®; Dilaudid-HP®; HydroStat IR®
Canadian Brand Names Hydromorph Contin®; PMS-Hydromorphone
Synonyms Dihydromorphinone; Hydromorphone Hydrochloride
Pharmacologic Class Analgesic, Narcotic
Nutrients Depleted
Specific nutrient depletions have not been documented for this agent.

- **Hydromorphone Hydrochloride** *see* Hydromorphone *on page 151*
- **Hydromox**® *see* Quinethazone* *on page 227*
- **Hydro-Par**® *see* Hydrochlorothiazide* *on page 147*
- **Hydropres**® *see* Hydrochlorothiazide and Reserpine* *on page 148*
- **Hydro-Serp**® *see* Hydrochlorothiazide and Reserpine* *on page 148*
- **Hydroserpine**® *see* Hydrochlorothiazide and Reserpine* *on page 148*
- **HydroStat IR**® *see* Hydromorphone *on page 151*
- **HydroTex**® [OTC] *see* Hydrocortisone* *on page 150*
- **Hydroxycarbamide** *see* Hydroxyurea* *on page 152*

Hydroxychloroquine (hye droks ee KLOR oh kwin)
U.S. Brand Names Plaquenil®
Synonyms Hydroxychloroquine Sulfate
Pharmacologic Class Aminoquinoline (Antimalarial)
Nutrients Depleted
  Specific nutrient depletions have not been documented for this agent.

- **Hydroxychloroquine Sulfate** *see* Hydroxychloroquine *on page 152*
- **Hydroxydaunomycin Hydrochloride** *see* Doxorubicin* *on page 106*

Hydroxyurea* (hye droks ee yoor EE a)
U.S. Brand Names Droxia™; Hydrea®
Synonyms Hydroxycarbamide
Pharmacologic Class Antineoplastic Agent, Antimetabolite
Nutrients Depleted
  See Nutrient Depletion and Cancer Chemotherapy *on page 515*.
Scientific Basis Inferred or indirect evidence of depletion based on disruption of physiologic processes

Hydroxyzine (hye DROKS i zeen)
U.S. Brand Names Anxanil®; Atarax®; Hyzine-50®; QYS®; Vistacon®; Vistaquel®; Vistaril®; Vistazine®
Canadian Brand Names Apo®-Hydroxyzine; Multipax®; Novo-Hydroxyzin; PMS-Hydroxyzine
Synonyms Hydroxyzine Hydrochloride; Hydroxyzine Pamoate
Pharmacologic Class Antiemetic; Antihistamine
Nutrients Depleted
  Specific nutrient depletions have not been documented for this agent.

- **Hydroxyzine Hydrochloride** *see* Hydroxyzine *on page 152*
- **Hydroxyzine Pamoate** *see* Hydroxyzine *on page 152*
- **Hygroton**® *see* Chlorthalidone* *on page 74*

Hyoscyamine (hye oh SYE a meen)

U.S. Brand Names Anaspaz®; A-Spas® S/L; Cystospaz®; Cystospaz-M®; Donnamar®; ED-SPAZ®; Gastrosed™; Levbid®; Levsin®; Levsinex®; Levsin/SL®

Synonyms Hyoscyamine Sulfate; *l*-Hyoscyamine Sulfate

Pharmacologic Class Anticholinergic Agent

Nutrients Depleted

Specific nutrient depletions have not been documented for this agent.

♦ **Hyoscyamine Sulfate** *see* Hyoscyamine *on page 153*

♦ **Hy-Phen**® *see* Hydrocodone and Acetaminophen* *on page 149*

♦ **Hyrexin-50**® **Injection** *see* Diphenhydramine *on page 102*

♦ **Hytone**® *see* Hydrocortisone* *on page 150*

♦ **Hytrin**® *see* Terazosin *on page 249*

♦ **Hytuss**® **[OTC]** *see* Guaifenesin *on page 140*

♦ **Hytuss-2X**® **[OTC]** *see* Guaifenesin *on page 140*

♦ **Hyzaar**® *see* Losartan and Hydrochlorothiazide* *on page 169*

♦ **Hyzine-50**® *see* Hydroxyzine *on page 152*

♦ **Iberet-Folic-500**® *see* Ferrous Sulfate, Ascorbic Acid, Vitamin B-Complex, and Folic Acid *on page 127*

♦ **Iberet**®-**Liquid [OTC]** *see* Ferrous Sulfate, Ascorbic Acid, and Vitamin B-Complex *on page 126*

♦ **Ibidomide Hydrochloride** *see* Labetalol* *on page 161*

♦ **IBU**® *see* Ibuprofen* *on page 153*

♦ **Ibuprin**® **[OTC]** *see* Ibuprofen* *on page 153*

Ibuprofen* (eye byoo PROE fen)

Related Information

Drug-Induced Nutrient Depletion Table *on page 498*

U.S. Brand Names Advil® [OTC]; Advil® Migraine Liqui-Gels [OTC]; Bayer® Select® Pain Relief Formula [OTC]; Children's Advil® Oral Suspension [OTC]; Children's Motrin® Oral Suspension [OTC]; Dynafed® IB [OTC]; Genpril® [OTC]; Haltran® [OTC]; IBU®; Ibuprin® [OTC]; Ibuprohm® [OTC]; Junior Strength Motrin® [OTC]; Menadol® [OTC]; Midol® IB [OTC]; Motrin®; Motrin® IB [OTC]; Motrin® Migraine Pain [OTC]; Nuprin® [OTC]; Saleto-200® [OTC]; Saleto-400®; Saleto-600®; Saleto-800®

Canadian Brand Names Actiprofen®; Apo®-Ibuprofen; Novo-Profen®; Nu-Ibuprofen

Synonyms *p*-Isobutylhydratropic Acid

Pharmacologic Class Nonsteroidal Anti-Inflammatory Agent (NSAID)

Nutrients Depleted

Folic Acid *on page 325*

Scientific Basis

Published scientific studies using this pharmacologic agent

or

Published scientific studies of agents from the same pharmacologic class

(Continued)

Ibuprofen* *(Continued)*
Studies & Abstracts 252

Imipramine* (im IP ra meen)
Related Information
  Drug-Induced Nutrient Depletion Table *on page 498*
U.S. Brand Names Janimine®; Tofranil®; Tofranil-PM®
Canadian Brand Names Apo®-Imipramine; Novo-Pramine; PMS-Imipramine
Synonyms Imipramine Hydrochloride; Imipramine Pamoate
Pharmacologic Class Antidepressant, Tricyclic (Tertiary Amine)
Nutrients Depleted
  Coenzyme Q_{10} *on page 320*
  Vitamin B_2 *on page 353*
Scientific Basis Published scientific studies using this pharmacologic agent
Studies & Abstracts 467-472

Indapamide* (in DAP a mide)
Related Information
  Drug-Induced Nutrient Depletion Table *on page 498*
U.S. Brand Names Lozol®
Canadian Brand Names Apo®-Indapadmide; Lozide®
Pharmacologic Class Diuretic, Thiazide
Nutrients Depleted
  Coenzyme Q_{10} *on page 320*
  Magnesium *on page 333*
  Phosphorus *on page 339*
  Potassium *on page 340*
  Sodium *on page 345*
  Zinc *on page 368*
Scientific Basis Published scientific studies of agents with the same mechanism of action
Studies & Abstracts 320-342

Additional Information Sodium replacement is not recommended in patients receiving thiazides or related agents (indapamide). Potassium replacement should be guided by serum level monitoring.

♦ **Inderal**® *see Propranolol* on page 223*

♦ **Inderal**® **LA** *see Propranolol* on page 223*

♦ **Inderide**® *see Propranolol and Hydrochlorothiazide* on page 224*

Indinavir (in DIN a veer)
U.S. Brand Names Crixivan®
Pharmacologic Class Antiretroviral Agent, Reverse Transcriptase Inhibitor (Non-Nucleoside)
Nutrients Depleted
Specific nutrient depletions have not been documented for this agent.

♦ **Indochron E-R**® *see Indomethacin* on page 155*

♦ **Indocid**® *see Indomethacin* on page 155*

♦ **Indocid**® **SR** *see Indomethacin* on page 155*

♦ **Indocin**® *see Indomethacin* on page 155*

♦ **Indocin**® **I.V.** *see Indomethacin* on page 155*

♦ **Indocin**® **SR** *see Indomethacin* on page 155*

♦ **Indometacin** *see Indomethacin* on page 155*

Indomethacin* (in doe METH a sin)
Related Information
Drug-Induced Nutrient Depletion Table *on page 498*
U.S. Brand Names Indochron E-R®; Indocin®; Indocin® I.V.; Indocin® SR
Canadian Brand Names Apo®-Indomethacin; Indocid®; Indocid® SR; Novo-Methacin; Nu-Indo; Pro-Indo®
Synonyms Indometacin; Indomethacin Sodium Trihydrate
Pharmacologic Class Nonsteroidal Anti-Inflammatory Agent (NSAID)
Nutrients Depleted
Folic Acid *on page 325*
Iron *on page 331*
Scientific Basis Published scientific studies using this pharmacologic agent
Studies & Abstracts 246-251

♦ **Indomethacin Sodium Trihydrate** *see Indomethacin* on page 155*

♦ **Infants Feverall**™ **[OTC]** *see Acetaminophen* on page 23*

♦ **Infants' Silapap**® **[OTC]** *see Acetaminophen* on page 23*

♦ **Inflamase**® **Forte Ophthalmic** *see Prednisolone* on page 218*

♦ **Inflamase**® **Mild Ophthalmic** *see Prednisolone* on page 218*

Infliximab (in FLIKS e mab)
U.S. Brand Names Remicade™
Pharmacologic Class Monoclonal Antibody
Nutrients Depleted
Specific nutrient depletions have not been documented for this agent.

- **Infumorph™ Injection** *see* Morphine Sulfate *on page 185*
- **INH** *see* Isoniazid* *on page 158*
- **Innofem®** *see* Estradiol* *on page 114*
- **Innohep®** *see* Tinzaparin *on page 254*

Insulin Preparations (IN su lin prep a RAY shuns)

U.S. Brand Names Humalog®; Humalog® Mix 50/50™; Humalog® Mix 75/25™; Humulin® 50/50; Humulin® 70/30; Humulin® L; Humulin® N; Lantus®; Lente® Iletin® I; Lente® Iletin® II; Lente® Insulin; Lente® L; Novolin® 70/30; Novolin® L; Novolin® N; Novolin® R; NovoLog™; NPH Iletin® I; NPH-N; Pork NPH Iletin® II; Pork Regular Iletin® II; Regular (Concentrated) Iletin® II U-500; Regular Iletin® I; Regular Insulin; Regular Purified Pork Insulin; Velosulin® BR Human (Buffered); Velosulin® Human

Pharmacologic Class Antidiabetic Agent (Insulin); Antidote

Nutrients Depleted

Specific nutrient depletions have not been documented for this agent.

- **Intal® Nebulizer Solution** *see* Cromolyn Sodium *on page 87*
- **Intal® Oral Inhaler** *see* Cromolyn Sodium *on page 87*
- **Integrilin®** *see* Eptifibatide *on page 112*

Interferon Beta-1a (in ter FEER on BAY ta won aye)

U.S. Brand Names Avonex™

Synonyms rIFN-b

Pharmacologic Class Biological Response Modulator

Nutrients Depleted

Specific nutrient depletions have not been documented for this agent.

Interferon Beta-1b (in ter FEER on BAY ta won bee)

U.S. Brand Names Betaseron®

Synonyms rIFN-b

Pharmacologic Class Biological Response Modulator

Nutrients Depleted

Specific nutrient depletions have not been documented for this agent.

- **Intrifiban** *see* Eptifibatide *on page 112*
- **Invirase®** *see* Saquinavir *on page 236*
- **Iobid DM®** *see* Guaifenesin and Dextromethorphan *on page 141*
- **Iofed®** *see* Brompheniramine and Pseudoephedrine *on page 51*
- **Iofed® PD** *see* Brompheniramine and Pseudoephedrine *on page 51*
- **Ionamin®** *see* Phentermine *on page 211*

Ipratropium (i pra TROE pee um)

U.S. Brand Names Atrovent®

Synonyms Ipratropium Bromide

Pharmacologic Class Anticholinergic Agent

Nutrients Depleted

Specific nutrient depletions have not been documented for this agent.

Ipratropium and Albuterol
(i pra TROE pee um & al BYOO ter ole)
U.S. Brand Names Combivent®
Pharmacologic Class Bronchodilator
Nutrients Depleted
Specific nutrient depletions have not been documented for this agent.

♦ **Ipratropium Bromide** *see* Ipratropium *on page 156*

♦ **Iproveratril Hydrochloride** *see* Verapamil *on page 267*

Irbesartan (ir be SAR tan)
U.S. Brand Names Avapro®
Pharmacologic Class Angiotensin II Antagonists
Nutrients Depleted
Specific nutrient depletions have not been documented for this agent.

Irbesartan and Hydrochlorothiazide*
(ir be SAR tan & hye droe klor oh THYE a zide)
U.S. Brand Names Avapro® HCT
Synonyms Hydrochlorothiazide and Irbesartan
Pharmacologic Class Antihypertensive Agent, Combination
Nutrients Depleted
Coenzyme Q_{10} *on page 320*
Magnesium *on page 333*
Phosphorus *on page 339*
Potassium *on page 340*
Sodium *on page 345*
Zinc *on page 368*
Scientific Basis Published scientific studies using this pharmacologic agent (hydrochlorothiazide)
Studies & Abstracts 320-342
Additional Information Sodium replacement is not recommended in patients receiving thiazides. Potassium replacement should be guided by serum level monitoring.

♦ **Ircon® [OTC]** *see* Ferrous Fumarate *on page 126*

Irinotecan* (eye rye no TEE kan)
U.S. Brand Names Camptosar®
Synonyms Camptothecin-11; CPT-11
Pharmacologic Class Antineoplastic Agent, Natural Source (Plant) Derivative
Nutrients Depleted
See Nutrient Depletion and Cancer Chemotherapy *on page 515*.
Scientific Basis Inferred or indirect evidence of depletion based on disruption of physiologic processes

♦ **ISD** *see* Isosorbide Dinitrate *on page 158*

♦ **ISDN** *see* Isosorbide Dinitrate *on page 158*

♦ **ISMN** *see* Isosorbide Mononitrate *on page 158*

♦ **Ismo®** *see* Isosorbide Mononitrate *on page 158*

♦ **Isobamate** *see* Carisoprodol *on page 58*

♦ **Isoclor® Expectorant** *see* Guaifenesin, Pseudoephedrine, and Codeine *on page 143*

♦ **Isollyl® Improved** *see* Butalbital Compound and Aspirin* *on page 54*

Isoniazid* (eye soe NYE a zid)

Related Information
Drug-Induced Nutrient Depletion Table *on page 498*

U.S. Brand Names Laniazid® Oral; Nydrazid® Injection

Canadian Brand Names PMS-Isoniazid

Synonyms INH; Isonicotinic Acid Hydrazide

Pharmacologic Class Antitubercular Agent

Nutrients Depleted
Vitamin B_3 *on page 354*
Vitamin B_6 *on page 357*
Vitamin D *on page 363*

Scientific Basis Published scientific studies using this pharmacologic agent

Studies & Abstracts 39-48

♦ **Isoniazid and Rifampin** *see* Rifampin and Isoniazid* *on page 232*

♦ **Isonicotinic Acid Hydrazide** *see* Isoniazid* *on page 158*

♦ **Isoptin®** *see* Verapamil *on page 267*

♦ **Isoptin® SR** *see* Verapamil *on page 267*

♦ **Isordil®** *see* Isosorbide Dinitrate *on page 158*

Isosorbide Dinitrate (eye soe SOR bide dye NYE trate)

U.S. Brand Names Dilatrate®-SR; Isordil®; Sorbitrate®

Canadian Brand Names Apo®-ISDN; Cedocard®-SR; Coradur®

Synonyms ISD; ISDN

Pharmacologic Class Vasodilator

Nutrients Depleted
Specific nutrient depletions have not been documented for this agent.

Isosorbide Mononitrate
(eye soe SOR bide mon oh NYE trate)

U.S. Brand Names Imdur™; Ismo®; Monoket®

Synonyms ISMN

Pharmacologic Class Vasodilator

Nutrients Depleted
Specific nutrient depletions have not been documented for this agent.

Isradipine (iz RA di peen)

U.S. Brand Names DynaCirc®

Pharmacologic Class Calcium Channel Blocker

Nutrients Depleted
Specific nutrient depletions have not been documented for this agent.

Itraconazole (i tra KOE na zole)
U.S. Brand Names Sporanox®
Pharmacologic Class Antifungal Agent, Oral
Nutrients Depleted
Specific nutrient depletions have not been documented for this agent.

- ♦ **Jaa Amp® Trihydrate** *see* Ampicillin* *on page 35*
- ♦ **Jaa-Prednisone®** *see* Prednisone* *on page 219*
- ♦ **Janimine®** *see* Imipramine* *on page 154*
- ♦ **Jenamicin® Injection** *see* Gentamicin* *on page 138*
- ♦ **Jenest-28™** *see* Ethinyl Estradiol and Norethindrone* *on page 121*
- ♦ **Junior Strength Motrin® [OTC]** *see* Ibuprofen* *on page 153*
- ♦ **Junior Strength Panadol® [OTC]** *see* Acetaminophen* *on page 23*
- ♦ **K+ 10®** *see* Potassium Chloride (Timed Release)* *on page 216*
- ♦ **Kadian™ Capsule** *see* Morphine Sulfate *on page 185*
- ♦ **Kaletra™** *see* Lopinavir and Ritonavir *on page 168*

Kanamycin* (kan a MYE sin)
U.S. Brand Names Kantrex®
Synonyms Kanamycin Sulfate
Pharmacologic Class Antibiotic, Aminoglycoside
Nutrients Depleted
Bifidobacteria bifidum (bifidus) *on page 311*
Biotin *on page 311*
Calcium *on page 313*
Inositol *on page 328*
Lactobacillus acidophilus *on page 332*
Magnesium *on page 333*
Potassium *on page 340*
Vitamin B_1 *on page 351*
Vitamin B_2 *on page 353*
Vitamin B_3 *on page 354*
Vitamin B_6 *on page 357*
Vitamin B_{12} *on page 359*
Vitamin K *on page 367*
Scientific Basis Inferred or indirect evidence of depletion based on disruption of physiologic processes
Studies & Abstracts 7-27, 28-37

- ♦ **Kanamycin Sulfate** *see* Kanamycin* *on page 159*
- ♦ **Kantrex®** *see* Kanamycin* *on page 159*
- ♦ **Kaochlor®** *see* Potassium Chloride (Timed Release)* *on page 216*
- ♦ **Kaochlor® SF** *see* Potassium Chloride (Timed Release)* *on page 216*
- ♦ **Kaodene® [OTC]** *see* Kaolin and Pectin *on page 159*

Kaolin and Pectin (KAY oh lin & PEK tin)
U.S. Brand Names Kaodene® [OTC]; Kao-Spen® [OTC]; Kapectolin® [OTC]
(Continued)

Kaolin and Pectin *(Continued)*

Synonyms Pectin and Kaolin
Pharmacologic Class Antidiarrheal
Nutrients Depleted
Specific nutrient depletions have not been documented for this agent.

Ketoconazole *(kee toe KOE na zole)*

U.S. Brand Names Nizoral®
Pharmacologic Class Antifungal Agent, Oral; Antifungal Agent, Topical
Nutrients Depleted
Specific nutrient depletions have not been documented for this agent.

Ketoprofen* *(kee toe PROE fen)*

Related Information
Drug-Induced Nutrient Depletion Table *on page 498*
U.S. Brand Names Actron® [OTC]; Orudis®; Orudis® KT [OTC]; Oruvail®

Canadian Brand Names Apo®-Keto; Apo®-Keto-E; Novo-Keto-EC; Nu-Ketoprofen; Nu-Ketoprofen-E; Orafen; PMS-Ketoprofen; Rhodis™; Rhodis-EC™

Pharmacologic Class Nonsteroidal Anti-Inflammatory Agent (NSAID)

Nutrients Depleted
Folic Acid *on page 325*

Scientific Basis
Published scientific studies using this pharmacologic agent
  or
Published scientific studies of agents from the same pharmacologic class

Studies & Abstracts 252

Labetalol* (la BET a lole)

Related Information
Drug-Induced Nutrient Depletion Table *on page 498*

U.S. Brand Names Normodyne®; Trandate®

Synonyms Ibidomide Hydrochloride; Labetalol Hydrochloride

Pharmacologic Class Alpha-/Beta- Blocker

Nutrients Depleted
Coenzyme Q_{10} *on page 320*
(Continued)

Labetalol* *(Continued)*
Scientific Basis
Published scientific studies using this pharmacologic agent
or
Published scientific studies of agents from the same pharmacologic class
Studies & Abstracts 348-349

♦ **Labetalol Hydrochloride** *see* Labetalol* *on page 161*
♦ **LactiCare-HC®** *see* Hydrocortisone* *on page 150*
♦ **L-AmB** *see* Amphotericin B (Liposomal)* *on page 35*
♦ **Lamictal®** *see* Lamotrigine *on page 162*
♦ **Lamisil® AT™ Topical** *see* Terbinafine *on page 249*
♦ **Lamisil® Dermgel** *see* Terbinafine *on page 249*
♦ **Lamisil® Topical** *see* Terbinafine *on page 249*

Lamivudine* (la MI vyoo deen)
Related Information
Drug-Induced Nutrient Depletion Table *on page 498*
U.S. Brand Names Epivir®; Epivir® HBV
Synonyms 3TC
Pharmacologic Class Antiretroviral Agent, Nucleoside Reverse Transcriptase Inhibitor (NRTI)
Nutrients Depleted
Carnitine *on page 316*
Copper *on page 322*
Vitamin B_{12} *on page 359*
Zinc *on page 368*
Scientific Basis Published scientific studies of agents from the same pharmacologic class
Studies & Abstracts 260-262

♦ **Lamivudine, Abacavir, and Zidovudine** *see* Abacavir, Lamivudine, and Zidovudine* *on page 22*

Lamotrigine (la MOE tri jeen)
U.S. Brand Names Lamictal®
Synonyms BW-430C; LTG
Pharmacologic Class Anticonvulsant, Miscellaneous
Nutrients Depleted
Specific nutrient depletions have not been documented for this agent.

♦ **Lamprene®** *see* Clofazimine *on page 80*
♦ **Lanacort® [OTC]** *see* Hydrocortisone* *on page 150*
♦ **Laniazid® Oral** *see* Isoniazid* *on page 158*
♦ **Lanophyllin®** *see* Theophylline* *on page 250*
♦ **Lanorinal®** *see* Butalbital Compound and Aspirin* *on page 54*
♦ **Lanoxicaps®** *see* Digoxin* *on page 100*
♦ **Lanoxin®** *see* Digoxin* *on page 100*

Lansoprazole* (lan SOE pra zole)
Related Information
Drug-Induced Nutrient Depletion Table *on page 498*
U.S. Brand Names Prevacid®
Pharmacologic Class Proton Pump Inhibitor
Nutrients Depleted
Vitamin B_{12} *on page 359*
Scientific Basis Published scientific studies of agents from the same pharmacologic class
Studies & Abstracts 511-516

♦ **Lantus®** *see* Insulin Preparations *on page 156*
♦ **Largactil®** *see* Chlorpromazine* *on page 74*
♦ **Larodopa®** *see* Levodopa* *on page 164*
♦ **Lasix®** *see* Furosemide* *on page 135*
♦ **LCR** *see* Vincristine* *on page 268*
♦ **L-Deprenyl** *see* Selegiline *on page 236*
♦ **L-Dopa** *see* Levodopa* *on page 164*
♦ **Lenoltec No 1, 2, 3, 4** *see* Acetaminophen and Codeine* *on page 23*
♦ **Lente® Iletin® I** *see* Insulin Preparations *on page 156*
♦ **Lente® Iletin® II** *see* Insulin Preparations *on page 156*
♦ **Lente® Insulin** *see* Insulin Preparations *on page 156*
♦ **Lente® L** *see* Insulin Preparations *on page 156*
♦ **Lescol®** *see* Fluvastatin* *on page 133*
♦ **Leukeran®** *see* Chlorambucil* *on page 72*
♦ **Leukine™** *see* Sargramostim *on page 236*

Leuprolide Acetate (loo PROE lide AS e tate)
U.S. Brand Names Lupron®; Lupron Depot®; Lupron Depot-3® Month; Lupron Depot-4® Month; Lupron Depot-Ped®
Synonyms Leuprorelin Acetate
Pharmacologic Class Antineoplastic Agent, Miscellaneous; Luteinizing Hormone-Releasing Hormone Analog
Nutrients Depleted
Specific nutrient depletions have not been documented for this agent.

♦ **Leuprorelin Acetate** *see* Leuprolide Acetate *on page 163*
♦ **Leurocristine** *see* Vincristine* *on page 268*
♦ **Leustatin™** *see* Cladribine* *on page 78*

Levalbuterol (leve al BYOO ter ole)
U.S. Brand Names Xopenex™
Synonyms R-albuterol
Pharmacologic Class Beta$_2$ Agonist
Nutrients Depleted
Specific nutrient depletions have not been documented for this agent.

♦ **Levaquin™** *see* Levofloxacin* *on page 164*
♦ **Levate®** *see* Amitriptyline* *on page 32*

♦ **Levbid**® *see* Hyoscyamine *on page 153*

Levetiracetam (lev e tir AS e tam)
U.S. Brand Names Keppra®
Pharmacologic Class Anticonvulsant, Miscellaneous
Nutrients Depleted
Specific nutrient depletions have not been documented for this agent.

♦ **Levlen**® *see* Ethinyl Estradiol and Levonorgestrel* *on page 120*
♦ **Levlite**® *see* Ethinyl Estradiol and Levonorgestrel* *on page 120*

Levodopa* (lee voe DOE pa)
Related Information
Drug-Induced Nutrient Depletion Table *on page 498*
U.S. Brand Names Dopar®; Larodopa®
Synonyms *L*-3-Hydroxytyrosine; *L*-Dopa
Pharmacologic Class Anti-Parkinson's Agent (Dopamine Agonist)
Nutrients Depleted
Potassium *on page 340*
SAMe *on page 341*
Scientific Basis Published scientific studies using this pharmacologic agent
Studies & Abstracts 466-467

Levodopa and Carbidopa*
(lee voe DOE pa & kar bi DOE pa)
U.S. Brand Names Sinemet®; Sinemet® CR
Synonyms Carbidopa and Levodopa
Pharmacologic Class Anti-Parkinson's Agent (Dopamine Agonist)
Nutrients Depleted
Potassium *on page 340*
SAMe *on page 341*
Scientific Basis Published scientific studies using this pharmacologic agent
Studies & Abstracts 466-467

Levofloxacin* (lee voe FLOKS a sin)
U.S. Brand Names Levaquin™; Quixin™ Ophthalmic
Pharmacologic Class Antibiotic, Quinolone
Nutrients Depleted
Bifidobacteria bifidum (bifidus) *on page 311*
Biotin *on page 311*
Inositol *on page 328*
Lactobacillus acidophilus *on page 332*
Vitamin B_1 *on page 351*
Vitamin B_2 *on page 353*
Vitamin B_3 *on page 354*
Vitamin B_6 *on page 357*
Vitamin B_{12} *on page 359*
Vitamin K *on page 367*

Scientific Basis Inferred or indirect evidence of depletion based on disruption of physiologic processes
Studies & Abstracts 7-27

♦ **Levomepromazine** *see* Methotrimeprazine* *on page 176*

Levonorgestrel* (LEE voe nor jes trel)
U.S. Brand Names Norplant® Implant; Plan B™
Pharmacologic Class Contraceptive
Nutrients Depleted
    Folic Acid *on page 325*
    Magnesium *on page 333*
    Vitamin B$_2$ *on page 353*
    Vitamin B$_6$ *on page 357*
    Vitamin B$_{12}$ *on page 359*
    Vitamin C *on page 360*
    Zinc *on page 368*
Scientific Basis Published scientific studies of agents from the same pharmacologic class
Studies & Abstracts 380-436

♦ **Levonorgestrel and Ethinyl Estradiol** *see* Ethinyl Estradiol and Levo-norgestrel* *on page 120*

♦ **Levoprome®** *see* Methotrimeprazine* *on page 176*

♦ **Levora®** *see* Ethinyl Estradiol and Levonorgestrel* *on page 120*

♦ **Levo-T™** *see* Levothyroxine *on page 165*

♦ **Levothroid®** *see* Levothyroxine *on page 165*

Levothyroxine (lee voe thye ROKS een)
U.S. Brand Names Eltroxin®; Levo-T™; Levothroid®; Levoxyl®; Synthroid®; Unithroid™
Canadian Brand Names PMS-Levothyroxine Sodium
Synonyms Levothyroxine Sodium; *L*-Thyroxine Sodium; T$_4$
Pharmacologic Class Thyroid Product
Nutrients Depleted
    Specific nutrient depletions have not been documented for this agent.

♦ **Levothyroxine Sodium** *see* Levothyroxine *on page 165*

♦ **Levoxyl®** *see* Levothyroxine *on page 165*

♦ **Levsin®** *see* Hyoscyamine *on page 153*

♦ **Levsinex®** *see* Hyoscyamine *on page 153*

♦ **Levsin/SL®** *see* Hyoscyamine *on page 153*

♦ **Lexxel™** *see* Enalapril and Felodipine* *on page 110*

♦ *l*-**Hyoscyamine Sulfate** *see* Hyoscyamine *on page 153*

♦ **Libritabs®** *see* Chlordiazepoxide *on page 72*

♦ **Librium®** *see* Chlordiazepoxide *on page 72*

♦ **Lidemol®** *see* Fluocinolone* *on page 129*

♦ **Lidex®** *see* Fluocinonide* *on page 130*

♦ **Lidex-E®** *see* Fluocinonide* *on page 130*

♦ **Linctus Codeine Blac** *see* Codeine *on page 83*

♦ **Linctus With Codeine Phosphate** *see* Codeine *on page 83*

Lindane (LIN dane)
U.S. Brand Names G-well®
Canadian Brand Names Hexit®; Kwellada™; PMS-Lindane
Synonyms Benzene Hexachloride; Gamma Benzene Hexachloride; Hexachlorocyclohexane
Pharmacologic Class Antiparasitic Agent, Topical; Pediculocide; Scabicidal Agent
Nutrients Depleted
Specific nutrient depletions have not been documented for this agent.

Linezolid* (li NE zoh lid)
U.S. Brand Names Zyvox™
Pharmacologic Class Antibiotic, Oxazolidinone
Nutrients Depleted
Bifidobacteria bifidum (bifidus) on page 311
Biotin *on page 311*
Inositol *on page 328*
Lactobacillus acidophilus on page 332
Vitamin B_1 *on page 351*
Vitamin B_2 *on page 353*
Vitamin B_3 *on page 354*
Vitamin B_6 *on page 357*
Vitamin B_{12} *on page 359*
Vitamin K *on page 367*
Scientific Basis Inferred or indirect evidence of depletion based on disruption of physiologic processes
Studies & Abstracts 7-27

- **Lioresal®** *see* Baclofen *on page 44*
- **Lipitor®** *see* Atorvastatin* *on page 42*
- **Liquibid®** *see* Guaifenesin *on page 140*
- **Liquid Pred®** *see* Prednisone* *on page 219*
- **Liquiprin® [OTC]** *see* Acetaminophen* *on page 23*

Lisinopril* (lyse IN oh pril)
Related Information
Drug-Induced Nutrient Depletion Table *on page 498*
U.S. Brand Names Prinivil®; Zestril®
Canadian Brand Names Apo®-Lisinopril
Pharmacologic Class Angiotensin-Converting Enzyme (ACE) Inhibitors
Nutrients Depleted
Zinc *on page 368*
Scientific Basis Published scientific studies of agents from the same pharmacologic class
Studies & Abstracts 269-271

Lithium* (LITH ee um)
Related Information
Drug-Induced Nutrient Depletion Table *on page 498*

U.S. Brand Names Eskalith®; Lithobid®; Lithonate®; Lithotabs®

Synonyms Lithium Carbonate; Lithium Citrate

Pharmacologic Class Lithium

Nutrients Depleted

Inositol *on page 328*

Scientific Basis Published scientific studies using this pharmacologic agent

Studies & Abstracts 479-483

Additional Information Although depletion has been noted, routine replacement of inositol is not recommended due to a possible relationship to lithium's therapeutic effect.

- ◆ **Lithium Carbonate** *see* Lithium* *on page 166*
- ◆ **Lithium Citrate** *see* Lithium* *on page 166*
- ◆ **Lithobid®** *see* Lithium* *on page 166*
- ◆ **Lithonate®** *see* Lithium* *on page 166*
- ◆ **Lithotabs®** *see* Lithium* *on page 166*
- ◆ **Locoid®** *see* Hydrocortisone* *on page 150*
- ◆ **Lodine®** *see* Etodolac* *on page 122*
- ◆ **Lodine® XL** *see* Etodolac* *on page 122*
- ◆ **Loestrin®** *see* Ethinyl Estradiol and Norethindrone* *on page 121*

Lomefloxacin* (loe me FLOKS a sin)

U.S. Brand Names Maxaquin®

Synonyms Lomefloxacin Hydrochloride

Pharmacologic Class Antibiotic, Quinolone

Nutrients Depleted

Bifidobacteria bifidum (bifidus) *on page 311*

Biotin *on page 311*

Inositol *on page 328*

Lactobacillus acidophilus *on page 332*

Vitamin B_1 *on page 351*

Vitamin B_2 *on page 353*

Vitamin B_3 *on page 354*

Vitamin B_6 *on page 357*

Vitamin B_{12} *on page 359*

Vitamin K *on page 367*

Scientific Basis Inferred or indirect evidence of depletion based on disruption of physiologic processes

Studies & Abstracts 7-27

- ◆ **Lomefloxacin Hydrochloride** *see* Lomefloxacin* *on page 167*
- ◆ **Lo/Ovral®** *see* Ethinyl Estradiol and Norgestrel* *on page 122*

Loperamide (loe PER a mide)

U.S. Brand Names Diar-Aid® [OTC]; Imodium®; Imodium® A-D [OTC]; Kaopectate® II [OTC]; Pepto® Diarrhea Control [OTC]

Pharmacologic Class Antidiarrheal

Nutrients Depleted

Specific nutrient depletions have not been documented for this agent.

♦ **Lopid®** *see* Gemfibrozil* *on page 137*
♦ **Lopinavir** *see* Lopinavir and Ritonavir *on page 168*

Lopinavir and Ritonavir (loe PIN a veer & rye TON a veer)
U.S. Brand Names Kaletra™
Synonyms Lopinavir
Pharmacologic Class Antiretroviral Agent, Protease Inhibitor
Nutrients Depleted
Specific nutrient depletions have not been documented for this agent.

♦ **Lopressor®** *see* Metoprolol* *on page 179*
♦ **Lorabid™** *see* Loracarbef* *on page 168*

Loracarbef* (lor a KAR bef)
U.S. Brand Names Lorabid™
Pharmacologic Class Antibiotic, Carbacephem
Nutrients Depleted
Bifidobacteria bifidum (bifidus) *on page 311*
Biotin *on page 311*
Inositol *on page 328*
Lactobacillus acidophilus *on page 332*
Vitamin B_1 *on page 351*
Vitamin B_2 *on page 353*
Vitamin B_3 *on page 354*
Vitamin B_6 *on page 357*
Vitamin B_{12} *on page 359*
Vitamin K *on page 367*
Scientific Basis Inferred or indirect evidence of depletion based on disruption of physiologic processes
Studies & Abstracts 7-27

Loratadine (lor AT a deen)
U.S. Brand Names Claritin® RediTabs®; Claritin® Syrup; Claritin® Tablets
Pharmacologic Class Antihistamine
Nutrients Depleted
Specific nutrient depletions have not been documented for this agent.

Loratadine and Pseudoephedrine
(lor AT a deen & soo doe e FED rin)
U.S. Brand Names Claritin-D® 12-Hour; Claritin-D® 24-Hour
Canadian Brand Names Chlor-Tripolon® N.D.; Claritin® Extra
Synonyms Pseudoephedrine and Loratadine
Pharmacologic Class Antihistamine/Decongestant Combination
Nutrients Depleted
Specific nutrient depletions have not been documented for this agent.

Lorazepam (lor A ze pam)
U.S. Brand Names Ativan®
Canadian Brand Names Apo®-Lorazepam; Novo-Lorazepam; Nu-Loraz; PMS-Lorazepam; Pro-Lorazepam®

Pharmacologic Class Benzodiazepine
Nutrients Depleted
Specific nutrient depletions have not been documented for this agent.

♦ **Lorcet**® *see* Hydrocodone and Acetaminophen* *on page 149*
♦ **Lorcet**®**-HD** *see* Hydrocodone and Acetaminophen* *on page 149*
♦ **Lorcet**® **Plus** *see* Hydrocodone and Acetaminophen* *on page 149*
♦ **Lortab**® *see* Hydrocodone and Acetaminophen* *on page 149*
♦ **Lortab**® **ASA** *see* Hydrocodone and Aspirin* *on page 150*

Losartan (loe SAR tan)
U.S. Brand Names Cozaar®
Synonyms DuP 753; Losartan Potassium; MK594
Pharmacologic Class Angiotensin II Antagonists
Nutrients Depleted
Specific nutrient depletions have not been documented for this agent.

Losartan and Hydrochlorothiazide*
(loe SAR tan & hye droe klor oh THYE a zide)
U.S. Brand Names Hyzaar®
Synonyms Hydrochlorothiazide and Losartan
Pharmacologic Class Antihypertensive Agent, Combination
Nutrients Depleted
Coenzyme Q_{10} *on page 320*
Magnesium *on page 333*
Phosphorus *on page 339*
Potassium *on page 340*
Sodium *on page 345*
Zinc *on page 368*
Scientific Basis Published scientific studies using this pharmacologic agent (hydrochlorothiazide)
Studies & Abstracts 320-342
Additional Information Sodium replacement is not recommended in patients receiving thiazides. Potassium replacement should be guided by serum level monitoring.

♦ **Losartan Potassium** *see* Losartan *on page 169*
♦ **Losec**® *see* Omeprazole* *on page 199*
♦ **Lotensin**® *see* Benazepril* *on page 45*
♦ **Lotrimin**® *see* Clotrimazole *on page 82*
♦ **Lotrimin**® **AF Cream [OTC]** *see* Clotrimazole *on page 82*
♦ **Lotrimin**® **AF Lotion [OTC]** *see* Clotrimazole *on page 82*
♦ **Lotrimin**® **AF Solution [OTC]** *see* Clotrimazole *on page 82*

Lovastatin* (LOE va sta tin)
Related Information
Drug-Induced Nutrient Depletion Table *on page 498*
U.S. Brand Names Mevacor®
Canadian Brand Names Apo®-Lovastatin
Synonyms Mevinolin; Monacolin K
(Continued)

Lovastatin* *(Continued)*

Pharmacologic Class Antilipemic Agent (HMG-CoA Reductase Inhibitor)

Nutrients Depleted
Coenzyme Q_{10} *on page 320*

Scientific Basis Published scientific studies using this pharmacologic agent

Studies & Abstracts 350-361

- **Lovenox® Injection** *see* Enoxaparin *on page 111*
- **Lozide®** *see* Indapamide* *on page 154*
- **Lozol®** *see* Indapamide* *on page 154*
- **LTG** *see* Lamotrigine *on page 162*
- **L-Thyroxine Sodium** *see* Levothyroxine *on page 165*
- **Ludiomil®** *see* Maprotiline *on page 171*
- **Luminal®** *see* Phenobarbital* *on page 210*
- **Lunelle™** *see* Estradiol Cypionate and Medroxyprogesterone Acetate* *on page 115*
- **Lupron®** *see* Leuprolide Acetate *on page 163*
- **Lupron Depot®** *see* Leuprolide Acetate *on page 163*
- **Lupron Depot-3® Month** *see* Leuprolide Acetate *on page 163*
- **Lupron Depot-4® Month** *see* Leuprolide Acetate *on page 163*
- **Lupron Depot-Ped®** *see* Leuprolide Acetate *on page 163*
- **Luvox®** *see* Fluvoxamine *on page 133*
- **Lyderm** *see* Fluocinonide* *on page 130*
- **Lydonide** *see* Fluocinonide* *on page 130*
- **Lyphocin®** *see* Vancomycin *on page 266*
- **Maalox® [OTC]** *see* Aluminum Hydroxide and Magnesium Hydroxide* *on page 29*
- **Maalox® Anti-Gas [OTC]** *see* Simethicone *on page 238*
- **Maalox® Plus [OTC]** *see* Aluminum Hydroxide, Magnesium Hydroxide, and Simethicone* *on page 29*
- **Maalox® Therapeutic Concentrate [OTC]** *see* Aluminum Hydroxide and Magnesium Hydroxide* *on page 29*
- **Macrobid®** *see* Nitrofurantoin* *on page 192*
- **Macrodantin®** *see* Nitrofurantoin* *on page 192*
- **Magalox Plus® [OTC]** *see* Aluminum Hydroxide, Magnesium Hydroxide, and Simethicone* *on page 29*
- **Magnesia Magma** *see* Magnesium Hydroxide* *on page 170*

Magnesium Hydroxide* (mag NEE zhum hye DROKS ide)

Related Information
Drug-Induced Nutrient Depletion Table *on page 498*

U.S. Brand Names Phillips'® Milk of Magnesia [OTC]

Synonyms Magnesia Magma; Milk of Magnesia; MOM

Pharmacologic Class Antacid; Laxative, Saline; Magnesium Salt

Nutrients Depleted
Calcium *on page 313*

Phosphorus *on page 339*
Vitamin D *on page 363*
Scientific Basis Published scientific studies of agents from the same pharmacologic class
Studies & Abstracts 1-5

♦ **Magnesium Hydroxide and Aluminum Hydroxide** *see* Aluminum Hydroxide and Magnesium Hydroxide* *on page 29*

Magnesium Oxide* (mag NEE zhum OKS ide)
Related Information
Drug-Induced Nutrient Depletion Table *on page 498*
U.S. Brand Names Maox®
Pharmacologic Class Antacid; Electrolyte Supplement, Oral; Laxative, Saline; Magnesium Salt
Nutrients Depleted
Calcium *on page 313*
Phosphorus *on page 339*
Scientific Basis Published scientific studies of agents from the same pharmacologic class
Studies & Abstracts 1-5

Magnesium Sulfate* (mag NEE zhum SUL fate)
Related Information
Drug-Induced Nutrient Depletion Table *on page 498*
Synonyms Epsom Salts
Pharmacologic Class Antacid; Anticonvulsant, Miscellaneous; Electrolyte Supplement, Parenteral; Laxative, Saline; Magnesium Salt
Nutrients Depleted
Calcium *on page 313*
Phosphorus *on page 339*
Scientific Basis Published scientific studies of agents from the same pharmacologic class
Studies & Abstracts 1-5

♦ **Malarone™** *see* Atovaquone and Proguanil *on page 42*
♦ **Mandol®** *see* Cefamandole* *on page 61*
♦ **Maox®** *see* Magnesium Oxide* *on page 171*
♦ **Mapap® [OTC]** *see* Acetaminophen* *on page 23*

Maprotiline (ma PROE ti leen)
U.S. Brand Names Ludiomil®
Synonyms Maprotiline Hydrochloride
Pharmacologic Class Antidepressant, Tetracyclic
Nutrients Depleted
Specific nutrient depletions have not been documented for this agent.

♦ **Maprotiline Hydrochloride** *see* Maprotiline *on page 171*
♦ **Maranox® [OTC]** *see* Acetaminophen* *on page 23*
♦ **Marazide®** *see* Benzthiazide* *on page 45*
♦ **Marcillin®** *see* Ampicillin* *on page 35*

- **Marezine®** [OTC] *see* Cyclizine *on page 88*
- **Margesic® H** *see* Hydrocodone and Acetaminophen* *on page 149*
- **Marpres®** *see* Hydralazine, Hydrochlorothiazide, and Reserpine* *on page 147*
- **Marthritic®** *see* Salsalate* *on page 235*
- **Matulane®** *see* Procarbazine* *on page 221*
- **Mavik®** *see* Trandolapril* *on page 258*
- **Maxair™ Inhalation Aerosol** *see* Pirbuterol *on page 214*
- **Maxaquin®** *see* Lomefloxacin* *on page 167*
- **Maxeran®** *see* Metoclopramide *on page 179*
- **Maxidex®** *see* Dexamethasone* *on page 95*
- **Maxiflor®** *see* Diflorasone* *on page 99*
- **Maximum Strength Dex-A-Diet®** [OTC] *see* Phenylpropanolamine *on page 211*
- **Maximum Strength Dexatrim®** [OTC] *see* Phenylpropanolamine *on page 211*
- **Maximum Strength Nytol®** [OTC] *see* Diphenhydramine *on page 102*
- **Maxipime®** *see* Cefepime* *on page 62*
- **Maxivate®** *see* Betamethasone* *on page 46*
- **Maxolon®** *see* Metoclopramide *on page 179*
- **Maxzide®** *see* Hydrochlorothiazide and Triamterene* *on page 149*
- **Mazepine®** *see* Carbamazepine* *on page 57*

Mebendazole (me BEN da zole)
U.S. Brand Names Vermox®
Pharmacologic Class Anthelmintic
Nutrients Depleted
   Specific nutrient depletions have not been documented for this agent.

- **Meclan® Topical** *see* Meclocycline* *on page 172*

Meclizine (MEK li zeen)
U.S. Brand Names Antivert®; Antrizine®; Bonine® [OTC]; Dizmiss® [OTC]; Dramamine® II [OTC]; Meni-D®; Ru-Vert-M®; Vergon® [OTC]
Synonyms Meclizine Hydrochloride; Meclozine Hydrochloride
Pharmacologic Class Antihistamine
Nutrients Depleted
   Specific nutrient depletions have not been documented for this agent.

- **Meclizine Hydrochloride** *see* Meclizine *on page 172*

Meclocycline* (me kloe SYE kleen)
U.S. Brand Names Meclan® Topical
Synonyms Meclocycline Sulfosalicylate
Pharmacologic Class Antibiotic, Topical;   Topical Skin Product, Acne
Nutrients Depleted
   Bifidobacteria bifidum (bifidus) on page 311

Biotin *on page 311*
Calcium *on page 313*
Inositol *on page 328*
Iron *on page 331*
Lactobacillus acidophilus on page 332
Magnesium *on page 333*
Vitamin B_1 *on page 351*
Vitamin B_2 *on page 353*
Vitamin B_3 *on page 354*
Vitamin B_6 *on page 357*
Vitamin B_{12} *on page 359*
Vitamin K *on page 367*

Scientific Basis
Published scientific studies using this pharmacologic agent
> or

Inferred or indirect evidence of depletion based on disruption of physiologic processes

Studies & Abstracts 7-27, 62-68

- **Meclocycline Sulfosalicylate** *see* Meclocycline* *on page 172*
- **Meclozine Hydrochloride** *see* Meclizine *on page 172*
- **Medigesic**® *see* Butalbital Compound and Acetaminophen* *on page 53*
- **Medilium**® *see* Chlordiazepoxide *on page 72*
- **Medimet**® *see* Methyldopa* *on page 177*
- **Medipain 5**® *see* Hydrocodone and Acetaminophen* *on page 149*
- **Medi-Tuss**® **[OTC]** *see* Guaifenesin *on page 140*
- **Medralone**® **Injection** *see* Methylprednisolone* *on page 178*
- **Medrol**® **Oral** *see* Methylprednisolone* *on page 178*

Medroxyprogesterone Acetate
(me DROKS ee proe JES te rone AS e tate)

U.S. Brand Names Amen® Oral; Curretab® Oral; Cycrin® Oral; Depo-Provera® Injection; Provera® Oral

Canadian Brand Names Novo-Medrone

Synonyms Acetoxymethylprogesterone; Methylacetoxyprogesterone

Pharmacologic Class Contraceptive; Progestin

Nutrients Depleted
Specific nutrient depletions have not been documented for this agent.

- **Medroxyprogesterone Acetate and Estradiol Cypionate** *see* Estradiol Cypionate and Medroxyprogesterone Acetate* *on page 115*
- **Medroxyprogesterone and Estrogens** *see* Estrogen and Medroxyprogesterone* *on page 116*
- **Mefoxin**® *see* Cefoxitin* *on page 65*
- **Megace**® *see* Megestrol Acetate *on page 174*
- **Megacillin**® **Susp** *see* Penicillin G Benzathine* *on page 205*

Megestrol Acetate (me JES trole AS e tate)
U.S. Brand Names Megace®
Pharmacologic Class Antineoplastic Agent, Miscellaneous; Progestin
Nutrients Depleted
Specific nutrient depletions have not been documented for this agent.

♦ **Mellaril**® see Thioridazine* on page 251
♦ **Mellaril-S**® see Thioridazine* on page 251

Meloxicam* (mel OX ee cam)
U.S. Brand Names Mobic®
Pharmacologic Class Nonsteroidal Anti-Inflammatory Agent (NSAID)
Nutrients Depleted
Folic Acid on page 325
Scientific Basis
Published scientific studies using this pharmacologic agent
or
Published scientific studies of agents from the same pharmacologic class
Studies & Abstracts 252

♦ **Menadol**® [OTC] see Ibuprofen* on page 153
♦ **Menest**® see Estrogens (Esterified)* on page 118
♦ **Meni-D**® see Meclizine on page 172
♦ **Meridia**™ see Sibutramine on page 237

Mesalamine* (me SAL a meen)
Related Information
Drug-Induced Nutrient Depletion Table on page 498
U.S. Brand Names Asacol® Oral; Pentasa® Oral; Rowasa® Rectal
Synonyms 5-Aminosalicylic Acid; 5-ASA; Fisalamine; Mesalazine
Pharmacologic Class 5-Aminosalicylic Acid Derivative
Nutrients Depleted
Folic Acid on page 325
Scientific Basis Published scientific studies of agents with the same mechanism of action
Studies & Abstracts 237-245

♦ **Mesalazine** see Mesalamine* on page 174
♦ **M-Eslon**® see Morphine Sulfate on page 185

Mesoridazine* (mez oh RID a zeen)
U.S. Brand Names Serentil®
Synonyms Mesoridazine Besylate
Pharmacologic Class Antipsychotic Agent, Phenothiazine, Piperidine
Nutrients Depleted
Coenzyme Q_{10} on page 320

Vitamin B₂ *on page 353*

Scientific Basis Published scientific studies of agents from the same pharmacologic class

Studies & Abstracts 474-477

- ♦ **Mesoridazine Besylate** *see Mesoridazine* on page 174*
- ♦ **Metacortandralone** *see Prednisolone* on page 218*
- ♦ **Metadate ER®** *see Methylphenidate on page 178*
- ♦ **Metahydrin®** *see Trichlormethiazide* on page 261*
- ♦ **Metamucil® [OTC]** *see Psyllium on page 226*
- ♦ **Metamucil® Instant Mix [OTC]** *see Psyllium on page 226*

Metformin* (met FOR min)

Related Information

Drug-Induced Nutrient Depletion Table *on page 498*

U.S. Brand Names Glucophage®

Canadian Brand Names Novo-Metformin

Synonyms Metformin Hydrochloride

Pharmacologic Class Antidiabetic Agent (Biguanide)

Nutrients Depleted

Folic Acid *on page 325*

Vitamin B₁₂ *on page 359*

Scientific Basis

Published scientific studies using this pharmacologic agent

or

Published scientific studies of agents from the same pharmacologic class

Studies & Abstracts 168-176

Additional Information Diarrhea/loose stools often accompany initial titration and may lead to nutrient loss.

- ♦ **Metformin Hydrochloride** *see Metformin* on page 175*
- ♦ **Methaminodiazepoxide Hydrochloride** *see Chlordiazepoxide on page 72*

Methdilazine* (meth DIL a zeen)

U.S. Brand Names Tacaryl®

Pharmacologic Class Antihistamine; Phenothiazine Derivative

Nutrients Depleted

Coenzyme Q₁₀ *on page 320*

Vitamin B₂ *on page 353*

Scientific Basis Published scientific studies of agents from the same pharmacologic class

Studies & Abstracts 474-477

Methimazole (meth IM a zole)

U.S. Brand Names Tapazole®

Synonyms Thiamazole

Pharmacologic Class Antithyroid Agent

Nutrients Depleted

Specific nutrient depletions have not been documented for this agent.

Methocarbamol (meth oh KAR ba mole)
U.S. Brand Names Robaxin®
Pharmacologic Class Skeletal Muscle Relaxant
Nutrients Depleted
Specific nutrient depletions have not been documented for this agent.

Methocarbamol and Aspirin*
(meth oh KAR ba mole & AS pir in)
U.S. Brand Names Robaxisal®
Pharmacologic Class Skeletal Muscle Relaxant
Nutrients Depleted
Folic Acid *on page 325*
Iron *on page 331*
Potassium *on page 340*
Sodium *on page 345*
Vitamin C *on page 360*
Scientific Basis Published scientific studies using this pharmacologic agent (aspirin)
Studies & Abstracts 224-236

Methotrexate* (meth oh TREKS ate)
Related Information
Drug-Induced Nutrient Depletion Table *on page 498*
U.S. Brand Names Folex® PFS; Rheumatrex®
Synonyms Amethopterin; Methotrexate Sodium; MTX
Pharmacologic Class Antineoplastic Agent, Antimetabolite
Nutrients Depleted
Folic Acid *on page 325*
Scientific Basis Published scientific studies using this pharmacologic agent
Studies & Abstracts 519-522

♦ **Methotrexate Sodium** *see* Methotrexate* *on page 176*

Methotrimeprazine* (meth oh trye MEP ra zeen)
U.S. Brand Names Levoprome®
Canadian Brand Names Nozinan®
Synonyms Levomepromazine; Methotrimeprazine Hydrochloride
Pharmacologic Class Analgesic, Non-narcotic; Phenothiazine Derivative; Sedative
Nutrients Depleted
Coenzyme Q_{10} *on page 320*
Vitamin B_2 *on page 353*
Scientific Basis Published scientific studies of agents from the same pharmacologic class
Studies & Abstracts 474-477

♦ **Methotrimeprazine Hydrochloride** *see* Methotrimeprazine* *on page 176*

Methsuximide* (meth SUKS i mide)
U.S. Brand Names Celontin®
Canadian Brand Names Celontin®
Pharmacologic Class Anticonvulsant, Succinimide
Nutrients Depleted
Calcium *on page 313*
Folic Acid *on page 325*
Vitamin D *on page 363*
Vitamin K *on page 367*
Scientific Basis Published scientific studies of agents with the same mechanism of action
Studies & Abstracts 73-92

Methyclothiazide* (meth i kloe THYE a zide)
Related Information
Drug-Induced Nutrient Depletion Table *on page 498*
U.S. Brand Names Aquatensen®; Enduron®
Pharmacologic Class Diuretic, Thiazide
Nutrients Depleted
Coenzyme Q_{10} *on page 320*
Magnesium *on page 333*
Phosphorus *on page 339*
Potassium *on page 340*
Sodium *on page 345*
Zinc *on page 368*
Scientific Basis Published scientific studies of agents from the same pharmacologic class
Studies & Abstracts 320-342
Additional Information Although thiazide diuretics deplete sodium, replacement is not recommended, as this may be directly related to the therapeutic effect. Thiazides may deplete potassium, however replacement should be guided by monitoring of serum concentrations and specific instruction by a healthcare provider.

♦ **Methylacetoxyprogesterone** *see* Medroxyprogesterone Acetate *on page 173*

Methyldopa* (meth il DOE pa)
Related Information
Drug-Induced Nutrient Depletion Table *on page 498*
U.S. Brand Names Aldomet®
Canadian Brand Names Apo®-Methyldopa; Dopamet®; Medimet®; Novo-Medopa®; Nu-Medopa
Synonyms Methyldopate Hydrochloride
Pharmacologic Class False Neurotransmitter
Nutrients Depleted
Coenzyme Q_{10} *on page 320*
Scientific Basis Published scientific studies using this pharmacologic agent
Studies & Abstracts 312

Methyldopa and Hydrochlorothiazide*

(meth il DOE pa & hye droe klor oh THYE a zide)

U.S. Brand Names Aldoril®

Canadian Brand Names Aldoril®-15; Aldoril®-25; Apo®-Methazide; Novo-Doparil; PMS-Dopazide

Synonyms Hydrochlorothiazide and Methyldopa

Pharmacologic Class Antihypertensive Agent, Combination

Nutrients Depleted

Coenzyme Q_{10} on page 320

Magnesium on page 333

Phosphorus on page 339

Potassium on page 340

Sodium on page 345

Vitamin B_6 on page 357

Zinc on page 368

Scientific Basis Published scientific studies using these pharmacologic agents

Studies & Abstracts 312, 320-342

Additional Information Sodium replacement is not recommended in patients receiving thiazides. Potassium replacement should be guided by serum level monitoring.

♦ **Methyldopate Hydrochloride** see Methyldopa* on page 177

♦ **Methylin™ ER** see Methylphenidate on page 178

♦ **Methylmorphine** see Codeine on page 83

Methylphenidate (meth il FEN i date)

U.S. Brand Names Concerta™; Metadate ER®; Methylin™ ER; Ritalin®; Ritalin-SR®

Canadian Brand Names PMS-Methylphenidate; Riphenidate

Synonyms Methylphenidate Hydrochloride

Pharmacologic Class Stimulant

Nutrients Depleted

Specific nutrient depletions have not been documented for this agent.

♦ **Methylphenidate Hydrochloride** see Methylphenidate on page 178

Methylprednisolone* (meth il pred NIS oh lone)

Related Information

Drug-Induced Nutrient Depletion Table on page 498

U.S. Brand Names Adlone® Injection; A-methaPred® Injection; depMedalone® Injection; Depoject® Injection; Depo-Medrol® Injection; Depopred® Injection; D-Med® Injection; Duralone® Injection; Medralone® Injection; Medrol® Oral; M-Prednisol® Injection; Solu-Medrol® Injection

Synonyms 6-α-Methylprednisolone; Methylprednisolone Acetate; Methylprednisolone Sodium Succinate

Pharmacologic Class Corticosteroid, Parenteral

Nutrients Depleted

Calcium on page 313

Folic Acid *on page 325*
Magnesium *on page 333*
Potassium *on page 340*
Selenium *on page 343*
Vitamin C *on page 360*
Vitamin D *on page 363*
Zinc *on page 368*

Scientific Basis
Published scientific studies using this pharmacologic agent
or
Published scientific studies of agents from the same pharmacologic class

Studies & Abstracts 182-223

♦ **6-α-Methylprednisolone** *see* Methylprednisolone* *on page 178*
♦ **Methylprednisolone Acetate** *see* Methylprednisolone* *on page 178*
♦ **Methylprednisolone Sodium Succinate** *see* Methylprednisolone* *on page 178*
♦ **4-Methylpyrazole** *see* Fomepizole *on page 133*
♦ **Meticorten®** *see* Prednisone* *on page 219*

Metoclopramide (met oh kloe PRA mide)
U.S. Brand Names Maxolon®; Octamide® PFS; Reglan®
Canadian Brand Names Apo®-Metoclop; Maxeran®
Pharmacologic Class Gastrointestinal Agent, Prokinetic
Nutrients Depleted
Specific nutrient depletions have not been documented for this agent.

Metolazone* (me TOLE a zone)
Related Information
Drug-Induced Nutrient Depletion Table *on page 498*
U.S. Brand Names Mykrox®; Zaroxolyn®
Pharmacologic Class Diuretic, Miscellaneous
Nutrients Depleted
Coenzyme Q_{10} *on page 320*
Magnesium *on page 333*
Phosphorus *on page 339*
Potassium *on page 340*
Sodium *on page 345*
Zinc *on page 368*

Scientific Basis Published scientific studies of agents with the same mechanism of action

Studies & Abstracts 320-342

Additional Information Sodium replacement is not recommended in patients receiving thiazides (and related agents such as metolazone). Potassium replacement should be guided by serum level monitoring.

Metoprolol* (me toe PROE lole)
Related Information
Drug-Induced Nutrient Depletion Table *on page 498*
(Continued)

Metoprolol* *(Continued)*

U.S. Brand Names Lopressor®; Toprol XL®
Canadian Brand Names Apo®-Metoprolol (Type L); Betaloc®; Betaloc® Durules®; Novo-Metoprolol; Nu-Metop
Synonyms Metoprolol Tartrate
Pharmacologic Class Beta Blocker, Beta₁ Selective
Nutrients Depleted
 Coenzyme Q₁₀ *on page 320*
Scientific Basis
 Published scientific studies using this pharmacologic agent
  or
 Published scientific studies of agents from the same pharmacologic class
Studies & Abstracts 348-349

♦ **Metoprolol Tartrate** *see* Metoprolol* *on page 179*
♦ **MetroCream™** *see* Metronidazole* *on page 180*
♦ **MetroGel® Topical** *see* Metronidazole* *on page 180*
♦ **MetroGel®-Vaginal** *see* Metronidazole* *on page 180*
♦ **Metro I.V.® Injection** *see* Metronidazole* *on page 180*
♦ **MetroLotion®** *see* Metronidazole* *on page 180*

Metronidazole* (me troe NI da zole)

U.S. Brand Names Flagyl®; Flagyl ER®; MetroCream™; MetroGel® Topical; MetroGel®-Vaginal; Metro I.V.® Injection; MetroLotion®; Noritate® Cream; Protostat® Oral
Canadian Brand Names Apo®-Metronidazole; Novo-Nidazol
Synonyms Metronidazole Hydrochloride
Pharmacologic Class Amebicide; Antibiotic, Topical; Antibiotic, Miscellaneous; Antiprotozoal
Nutrients Depleted
 Bifidobacteria bifidum (bifidus) on page 311
 Lactobacillus acidophilus on page 332
Scientific Basis Published scientific studies of agents with the same mechanism of action
Studies & Abstracts 7-27

♦ **Metronidazole Hydrochloride** *see* Metronidazole* *on page 180*
♦ **Mevacor®** *see* Lovastatin* *on page 169*
♦ **Meval®** *see* Diazepam *on page 97*
♦ **Mevinolin** *see* Lovastatin* *on page 169*

Mexiletine (MEKS i le teen)

U.S. Brand Names Mexitil®
Pharmacologic Class Antiarrhythmic Agent, Class I-B
Nutrients Depleted
 Specific nutrient depletions have not been documented for this agent.

♦ **Mexitil®** *see* Mexiletine *on page 180*
♦ **Miacalcin® Injection** *see* Calcitonin *on page 55*

- **Miacalcin**® **Nasal Spray** *see* Calcitonin *on page 55*
- **Micardis**® *see* Telmisartan *on page 248*
- **Micardis**® **HCT** *see* Telmisartan and Hydrochlorothiazide* *on page 248*
- **Micro-K**® **10** *see* Potassium Chloride (Timed Release)* *on page 216*
- **Micro-K**® **Extencaps**® *see* Potassium Chloride (Timed Release)* *on page 216*
- **Micro-K**® **LS**® *see* Potassium Chloride (Timed Release)* *on page 216*
- **Micronase**® *see* Glyburide* *on page 139*
- **Micronor**® *see* Norethindrone* *on page 193*
- **Microsulfon**® *see* Sulfadiazine* *on page 243*
- **Microzide**™ *see* Hydrochlorothiazide* *on page 147*
- **Midamor**® *see* Amiloride* *on page 31*

Midodrine (MI doe dreen)
U.S. Brand Names ProAmatine
Synonyms Midodrine Hydrochloride
Pharmacologic Class Alpha₁ Agonist
Nutrients Depleted
Specific nutrient depletions have not been documented for this agent.

- **Midodrine Hydrochloride** *see* Midodrine *on page 181*
- **Midol**® **IB [OTC]** *see* Ibuprofen* *on page 153*
- **Mifeprex**™ *see* Mifepristone *on page 181*

Mifepristone (mi fe PRIS tone)
U.S. Brand Names Mifeprex™
Synonyms RU-486; RU-38486
Pharmacologic Class Abortifacient; Antineoplastic Agent, Hormone Antagonist; Antiprogestin
Nutrients Depleted
Specific nutrient depletions have not been documented for this agent.

Miglitol (MIG li tol)
U.S. Brand Names Glyset®
Pharmacologic Class Antidiabetic Agent (Miscellaneous)
Nutrients Depleted
Specific nutrient depletions have not been documented for this agent.

- **Miles Nervine**® **Caplets [OTC]** *see* Diphenhydramine *on page 102*
- **Milkinol**® **[OTC]** *see* Mineral Oil* *on page 181*
- **Milk of Magnesia** *see* Magnesium Hydroxide* *on page 170*
- **Milophene**® *see* Clomiphene *on page 80*

Mineral Oil* (MIN er al oyl)
Related Information
Drug-Induced Nutrient Depletion Table *on page 498*
U.S. Brand Names Agoral® Plain [OTC]; Fleet® Mineral Oil Enema [OTC]; Kondremul® [OTC]; Milkinol® [OTC]; Neo-Cultol® [OTC]; Zymenol® [OTC]
(Continued)

Mineral Oil* *(Continued)*

Pharmacologic Class Laxative, Lubricant

Nutrients Depleted

Beta-Carotene *on page 310*

Calcium *on page 313*

Phosphorus *on page 339*

Vitamin A *on page 349*

Vitamin D *on page 363*

Vitamin E *on page 365*

Vitamin K *on page 367*

Scientific Basis Published scientific studies using this pharmacologic agent

Studies & Abstracts 455-456

♦ **Minipress**® *see* Prazosin *on page 217*

♦ **Minitran**™ **Patch** *see* Nitroglycerin *on page 192*

♦ **Minizide**® *see* Prazosin and Polythiazide* *on page 217*

♦ **Minocin**® **IV Injection** *see* Minocycline* *on page 182*

♦ **Minocin**® **Oral** *see* Minocycline* *on page 182*

Minocycline* (mi noe SYE kleen)

Related Information

Drug-Induced Nutrient Depletion Table *on page 498*

U.S. Brand Names Dynacin® Oral; Minocin® IV Injection; Minocin® Oral

Canadian Brand Names Apo®-Minocycline; Syn-Minocycline

Synonyms Minocycline Hydrochloride

Pharmacologic Class Antibiotic, Tetracycline Derivative

Nutrients Depleted

Bifidobacteria bifidum (bifidus) on page 311

Biotin *on page 311*

Calcium *on page 313*

Inositol *on page 328*

Iron *on page 331*

Lactobacillus acidophilus on page 332

Magnesium *on page 333*

Vitamin B₁ *on page 351*

Vitamin B₂ *on page 353*

Vitamin B₃ *on page 354*

Vitamin B₆ *on page 357*

Vitamin B₁₂ *on page 359*

Vitamin K *on page 367*

Scientific Basis Published scientific studies of agents from the same pharmacologic class

Studies & Abstracts 7-27, 62-68

Additional Information Calcium, iron, and magnesium depletion may be minimal during brief treatments. Replacement should not be attempted unless the time of administration is separated from the dosing of the tetracycline.

♦ **Minocycline Hydrochloride** *see* Minocycline* *on page 182*

♦ **Mirapex**® *see* Pramipexole *on page 217*

♦ **Mircette**™ *see* Ethinyl Estradiol and Desogestrel* *on page 119*

Misoprostol (mye soe PROST ole)
U.S. Brand Names Cytotec®
Pharmacologic Class Prostaglandin
Nutrients Depleted
Specific nutrient depletions have not been documented for this agent.

♦ **Misoprostol and Diclofenac** *see* Diclofenac and Misoprostol* *on page 98*

♦ **Mithracin**® *see* Plicamycin* *on page 215*

Mitoxantrone* (mye toe ZAN trone)
U.S. Brand Names Novantrone®
Synonyms DHAD; Mitoxantrone Hydrochloride
Pharmacologic Class Antineoplastic Agent, Antibiotic
Nutrients Depleted
See Nutrient Depletion and Cancer Chemotherapy *on page 515*.
Scientific Basis Inferred or indirect evidence of depletion based on disruption of physiologic processes

♦ **Mitoxantrone Hydrochloride** *see* Mitoxantrone* *on page 183*

♦ **Mitran**® **Oral** *see* Chlordiazepoxide *on page 72*

♦ **MK 383** *see* Tirofiban *on page 255*

♦ **MK594** *see* Losartan *on page 169*

♦ **Mobenol**® *see* Tolbutamide* *on page 256*

♦ **Mobic**® *see* Meloxicam* *on page 174*

Modafinil (moe DAF i nil)
U.S. Brand Names Provigil®
Pharmacologic Class Stimulant
Nutrients Depleted
Specific nutrient depletions have not been documented for this agent.

♦ **Modane**® **Bulk [OTC]** *see* Psyllium *on page 226*

♦ **Modane**® **Soft [OTC]** *see* Docusate *on page 104*

♦ **Modecate**® *see* Fluphenazine* *on page 131*

♦ **Modecate**® **Enanthate** *see* Fluphenazine* *on page 131*

♦ **Modicon**™ *see* Ethinyl Estradiol and Norethindrone* *on page 121*

♦ **Moditen**® **Hydrochloride** *see* Fluphenazine* *on page 131*

♦ **Moduret**® *see* Amiloride and Hydrochlorothiazide* *on page 31*

♦ **Moduretic**® *see* Amiloride and Hydrochlorothiazide* *on page 31*

Moexipril* (mo EKS i pril)
Related Information
Drug-Induced Nutrient Depletion Table *on page 498*
U.S. Brand Names Univasc®
Synonyms Moexipril Hydrochloride
Pharmacologic Class Angiotensin-Converting Enzyme (ACE) Inhibitors
(Continued)

Moexipril* *(Continued)*
Nutrients Depleted
Zinc *on page 368*
Scientific Basis Published scientific studies of agents from the same pharmacologic class
Studies & Abstracts 269-271

Moexipril and Hydrochlorothiazide*
(mo EKS i pril & hye droe klor oh THYE a zide)
U.S. Brand Names Uniretic™
Pharmacologic Class Antihypertensive Agent, Combination
Nutrients Depleted
Coenzyme Q_{10} *on page 320*
Magnesium *on page 333*
Phosphorus *on page 339*
Potassium *on page 340*
Sodium *on page 345*
Zinc *on page 368*
Scientific Basis Published scientific studies using these pharmacologic agents
Studies & Abstracts 320-342
Additional Information Although thiazide diuretics deplete sodium, replacement is not recommended, as this may be directly related to the therapeutic effect. Thiazides may deplete potassium, however ACE-inhibitors may increase this ion. Replacement should be guided by monitoring of serum concentrations and specific instruction by a healthcare provider.

♦ **Moexipril Hydrochloride** *see* Moexipril* *on page 183*
♦ **Mol-Iron® [OTC]** *see* Ferrous Sulfate *on page 126*
♦ **MOM** *see* Magnesium Hydroxide* *on page 170*

Mometasone Furoate* (moe MET a sone FYOOR oh ate)
Related Information
Drug-Induced Nutrient Depletion Table *on page 498*
U.S. Brand Names Elocon®; Nasonex®
Canadian Brand Names Elocom
Pharmacologic Class Corticosteroid, Topical
Nutrients Depleted
Calcium *on page 313*
Folic Acid *on page 325*
Magnesium *on page 333*
Potassium *on page 340*
Selenium *on page 343*
Vitamin C *on page 360*
Vitamin D *on page 363*
Zinc *on page 368*
Scientific Basis
Published scientific studies using this pharmacologic agent
or
Published scientific studies of agents from the same pharmacologic class

Studies & Abstracts 182-223

Additional Information Nutrient depletion with topical administration is limited.

- ◆ **Monacolin K** *see* Lovastatin* *on page 169*
- ◆ **Monafed®** *see* Guaifenesin *on page 140*
- ◆ **Monafed® DM** *see* Guaifenesin and Dextromethorphan *on page 141*
- ◆ **Monitan®** *see* Acebutolol* *on page 22*
- ◆ **Monocid®** *see* Cefonicid* *on page 63*
- ◆ **Mono-Gesic®** *see* Salsalate* *on page 235*
- ◆ **Monoket®** *see* Isosorbide Mononitrate *on page 158*
- ◆ **Monopril®** *see* Fosinopril* *on page 134*

Montelukast (mon te LOO kast)

U.S. Brand Names Singulair®
Synonyms Montelukast Sodium
Pharmacologic Class Leukotriene Receptor Antagonist
Nutrients Depleted
Specific nutrient depletions have not been documented for this agent.

- ◆ **Montelukast Sodium** *see* Montelukast *on page 185*
- ◆ **Morning After Pill** *see* Ethinyl Estradiol and Norgestrel* *on page 122*
- ◆ **Morphine-HP®** *see* Morphine Sulfate *on page 185*

Morphine Sulfate (MOR feen SUL fate)

U.S. Brand Names Astramorph™ PF Injection; Duramorph® Injection; Infumorph™ Injection; Kadian™ Capsule; MS Contin® Oral; MSIR® Oral; MS/L®; MS/S®; OMS® Oral; Oramorph SR™ Oral; RMS® Rectal; Roxanol™ Oral; Roxanol Rescudose®; Roxanol SR™ Oral
Canadian Brand Names Epimorph®; M-Eslon®; Morphine-HP®; MS-IR®; MST Continus; Statex®
Synonyms MS
Pharmacologic Class Analgesic, Narcotic
Nutrients Depleted
Specific nutrient depletions have not been documented for this agent.

- ◆ **Motrin®** *see* Ibuprofen* *on page 153*
- ◆ **Motrin® IB [OTC]** *see* Ibuprofen* *on page 153*
- ◆ **Motrin® IB Sinus [OTC]** *see* Pseudoephedrine and Ibuprofen* *on page 226*
- ◆ **Motrin® Migraine Pain [OTC]** *see* Ibuprofen* *on page 153*

Moxifloxacin* (mox i FLOKS a sin)

U.S. Brand Names Avelox™
Synonyms Moxifloxacin Hydrochloride
Pharmacologic Class Antibiotic, Quinolone
Nutrients Depleted
Bifidobacteria bifidum (bifidus) on page 311
(Continued)

Moxifloxacin* *(Continued)*

Biotin *on page 311*
Inositol *on page 328*
Lactobacillus acidophilus on page 332
Vitamin B$_1$ *on page 351*
Vitamin B$_2$ *on page 353*
Vitamin B$_3$ *on page 354*
Vitamin B$_6$ *on page 357*
Vitamin B$_{12}$ *on page 359*
Vitamin K *on page 367*

Scientific Basis Inferred or indirect evidence of depletion based on disruption of physiologic processes

Studies & Abstracts 7-27

- **Moxifloxacin Hydrochloride** *see* Moxifloxacin* *on page 185*
- **4-MP** *see* Fomepizole *on page 133*
- **M-Prednisol® Injection** *see* Methylprednisolone* *on page 178*
- **MS** *see* Morphine Sulfate *on page 185*
- **MS Contin® Oral** *see* Morphine Sulfate *on page 185*
- **MSD® Enteric Coated ASA** *see* Aspirin* *on page 40*
- **MS-IR®** *see* Morphine Sulfate *on page 185*
- **MSIR® Oral** *see* Morphine Sulfate *on page 185*
- **MS/L®** *see* Morphine Sulfate *on page 185*
- **MS/S®** *see* Morphine Sulfate *on page 185*
- **MST Continus** *see* Morphine Sulfate *on page 185*
- **MTX** *see* Methotrexate* *on page 176*
- **Muco-Fen-DM®** *see* Guaifenesin and Dextromethorphan *on page 141*
- **Muco-Fen-LA®** *see* Guaifenesin *on page 140*
- **Multipax®** *see* Hydroxyzine *on page 152*
- **Muse® Pellet** *see* Alprostadil *on page 28*
- **Myambutol®** *see* Ethambutol* *on page 119*
- **Mycelex®** *see* Clotrimazole *on page 82*
- **Mycelex®-7** *see* Clotrimazole *on page 82*
- **Mycelex®-G** *see* Clotrimazole *on page 82*
- **Mycifradin® Sulfate Oral** *see* Neomycin* *on page 190*
- **Mycifradin® Sulfate Topical** *see* Neomycin* *on page 190*
- **Mycobutin®** *see* Rifabutin* *on page 231*
- **Mykrox®** *see* Metolazone* *on page 179*
- **Mylanta® [OTC]** *see* Aluminum Hydroxide, Magnesium Hydroxide, and Simethicone* *on page 29*
- **Mylanta® Gas [OTC]** *see* Simethicone *on page 238*
- **Mylanta®-II [OTC]** *see* Aluminum Hydroxide, Magnesium Hydroxide, and Simethicone* *on page 29*
- **Myleran®** *see* Busulfan* *on page 53*
- **Mylicon® [OTC]** *see* Simethicone *on page 238*
- **Mylotarg™** *see* Gemtuzumab Ozogamicin *on page 137*

- ◆ **Myminic® Expectorant [OTC]** *see* Guaifenesin and Phenylpropanolamine *on page 141*
- ◆ **Myotonachol™** *see* Bethanechol *on page 47*
- ◆ **Myphetane DC®** *see* Brompheniramine, Phenylpropanolamine, and Codeine *on page 51*
- ◆ **Mysoline®** *see* Primidone* *on page 220*
- ◆ **Mytussin® [OTC]** *see* Guaifenesin *on page 140*
- ◆ **Mytussin® DAC** *see* Guaifenesin, Pseudoephedrine, and Codeine *on page 143*
- ◆ **Mytussin® DM [OTC]** *see* Guaifenesin and Dextromethorphan *on page 141*
- ◆ **N-Acetyl-P-Aminophenol** *see* Acetaminophen* *on page 23*

Nadolol* (nay DOE lole)
Related Information
  Drug-Induced Nutrient Depletion Table *on page 498*
U.S. Brand Names Corgard®
Canadian Brand Names Apo®-Nadol; Syn-Nadolol
Pharmacologic Class Beta Blocker, Nonselective
Nutrients Depleted
  Coenzyme Q_{10} *on page 320*
Scientific Basis Published scientific studies of agents from the same pharmacologic class
Studies & Abstracts 348-349

- ◆ **Nadopen-V®** *see* Penicillin V Potassium* *on page 207*
- ◆ **Nafcil™ Injection** *see* Nafcillin* *on page 187*

Nafcillin* (naf SIL in)
Related Information
  Drug-Induced Nutrient Depletion Table *on page 498*
U.S. Brand Names Nafcil™ Injection; Nallpen® Injection; Unipen® Injection; Unipen® Oral
Synonyms Ethoxynaphthamido Penicillin Sodium; Nafcillin Sodium; Sodium Nafcillin
Pharmacologic Class Antibiotic, Penicillin
Nutrients Depleted
  Bifidobacteria bifidum (bifidus) *on page 311*
  Biotin *on page 311*
  Inositol *on page 328*
  Lactobacillus acidophilus *on page 332*
  Potassium *on page 340*
  Vitamin B_1 *on page 351*
  Vitamin B_2 *on page 353*
  Vitamin B_3 *on page 354*
  Vitamin B_6 *on page 357*
  Vitamin B_{12} *on page 359*
  Vitamin K *on page 367*
Scientific Basis Inferred or indirect evidence of depletion based on disruption of physiologic processes
Studies & Abstracts 7-27, 49-57

- **Nafcillin Sodium** *see* Nafcillin* *on page 187*
- **NaHCO₃** *see* Sodium Bicarbonate* *on page 239*
- **Naldecon® DX Adult Liquid [OTC]** *see* Guaifenesin, Phenylpropanolamine, and Dextromethorphan *on page 142*
- **Naldecon-EX® Children's Syrup [OTC]** *see* Guaifenesin and Phenylpropanolamine *on page 141*
- **Naldecon® Senior DX [OTC]** *see* Guaifenesin and Dextromethorphan *on page 141*
- **Naldecon® Senior EX [OTC]** *see* Guaifenesin *on page 140*
- **Nalfon®** *see* Fenoprofen* *on page 125*

Nalidixic Acid* (nal i DIKS ik AS id)
U.S. Brand Names NegGram®
Synonyms Nalidixinic Acid
Pharmacologic Class Antibiotic, Quinolone
Nutrients Depleted
  Bifidobacteria bifidum (bifidus) on page 311
  Biotin *on page 311*
  Inositol *on page 328*
  Lactobacillus acidophilus on page 332
  Vitamin B₁ *on page 351*
  Vitamin B₂ *on page 353*
  Vitamin B₃ *on page 354*
  Vitamin B₆ *on page 357*
  Vitamin B₁₂ *on page 359*
  Vitamin K *on page 367*
Scientific Basis Inferred or indirect evidence of depletion based on disruption of physiologic processes
Studies & Abstracts 7-27

- **Nalidixinic Acid** *see* Nalidixic Acid* *on page 188*
- **Nallpen® Injection** *see* Nafcillin* *on page 187*

Nalmefene (NAL me feen)
U.S. Brand Names Revex®
Synonyms Nalmefene Hydrochloride
Pharmacologic Class Antidote
Nutrients Depleted
  Specific nutrient depletions have not been documented for this agent.

- **Nalmefene Hydrochloride** *see* Nalmefene *on page 188*

Naltrexone (nal TREKS one)
U.S. Brand Names Depade®; ReVia®
Synonyms Naltrexone Hydrochloride
Pharmacologic Class Antidote
Nutrients Depleted
  Specific nutrient depletions have not been documented for this agent.

- **Naltrexone Hydrochloride** *see* Naltrexone *on page 188*
- **Naprelan®** *see* Naproxen* *on page 189*
- **Naprosyn®** *see* Naproxen* *on page 189*

Naproxen* (na PROKS en)

Related Information
Drug-Induced Nutrient Depletion Table *on page 498*

U.S. Brand Names Aleve® [OTC]; Anaprox®; EC-Naprosyn®; Naprelan®; Naprosyn®

Canadian Brand Names Apo®-Naproxen; Naxen®; Novo-Naprox; Nu-Naprox

Synonyms Naproxen Sodium

Pharmacologic Class Nonsteroidal Anti-Inflammatory Agent (NSAID)

Nutrients Depleted
Folic Acid *on page 325*

Scientific Basis
Published scientific studies using this pharmacologic agent
or
Published scientific studies of agents from the same pharmacologic class

Studies & Abstracts 252

- **Naproxen Sodium** *see* Naproxen* *on page 189*
- **Naqua®** *see* Trichlormethiazide* *on page 261*

Naratriptan (NAR a trip tan)

U.S. Brand Names Amerge®

Synonyms Naratriptan Hydrochloride

Pharmacologic Class Serotonin 5-HT$_{1D}$ Receptor Agonist

Nutrients Depleted
Specific nutrient depletions have not been documented for this agent.

- **Naratriptan Hydrochloride** *see* Naratriptan *on page 189*
- **Nasabid™** *see* Guaifenesin and Pseudoephedrine *on page 142*
- **Nasacort®** *see* Triamcinolone* *on page 259*
- **Nasacort® AQ** *see* Triamcinolone* *on page 259*
- **Nasahist B®** *see* Brompheniramine *on page 50*
- **Nasalcrom® Nasal Solution [OTC]** *see* Cromolyn Sodium *on page 87*
- **Nasalide® Nasal Aerosol** *see* Flunisolide* *on page 129*
- **Nasarel® Nasal Spray** *see* Flunisolide* *on page 129*
- **Nasonex®** *see* Mometasone Furoate* *on page 184*
- **Navane®** *see* Thiothixene *on page 252*
- **Navelbine®** *see* Vinorelbine* *on page 268*
- **Naxen®** *see* Naproxen* *on page 189*
- **ND-Stat®** *see* Brompheniramine *on page 50*
- **Nebcin® Injection** *see* Tobramycin* *on page 255*
- **NebuPent™ Inhalation** *see* Pentamidine* *on page 208*
- **N.E.E.® 1/35** *see* Ethinyl Estradiol and Norethindrone* *on page 121*

Nefazodone (nef AY zoe done)

U.S. Brand Names Serzone®

Synonyms Nefazodone Hydrochloride
(Continued)

Nefazodone *(Continued)*

Pharmacologic Class Antidepressant, Serotonin Reuptake Inhibitor/ Antagonist

Nutrients Depleted
Specific nutrient depletions have not been documented for this agent.

♦ **Nefazodone Hydrochloride** *see* Nefazodone *on page 189*
♦ **NegGram®** *see* Nalidixic Acid* *on page 188*

Nelfinavir (nel FIN a veer)

U.S. Brand Names Viracept®

Pharmacologic Class Antiretroviral Agent, Reverse Transcriptase Inhibitor (Non-Nucleoside)

Nutrients Depleted
Specific nutrient depletions have not been documented for this agent.

♦ **Nelova™ 0.5/35E** *see* Ethinyl Estradiol and Norethindrone* *on page 121*
♦ **Nelova™ 10/11** *see* Ethinyl Estradiol and Norethindrone* *on page 121*
♦ **Neo-Codema®** *see* Hydrochlorothiazide* *on page 147*
♦ **Neo-Cultol® [OTC]** *see* Mineral Oil* *on page 181*
♦ **Neo-Estrone®** *see* Estrogens (Esterified)* *on page 118*
♦ **Neo-fradin® Oral** *see* Neomycin* *on page 190*

Neomycin* (nee oh MYE sin)

Related Information
Drug-Induced Nutrient Depletion Table *on page 498*

U.S. Brand Names Mycifradin® Sulfate Oral; Mycifradin® Sulfate Topical; Neo-fradin® Oral; Neo-Tabs® Oral

Synonyms Neomycin Sulfate

Pharmacologic Class Ammonium Detoxicant; Antibiotic, Topical

Nutrients Depleted
Beta-Carotene *on page 310*
Bifidobacteria bifidum (bifidus) *on page 311*
Calcium *on page 313*
Iron *on page 331*
Lactobacillus acidophilus *on page 332*
Magnesium *on page 333*
Potassium *on page 340*
Vitamin A *on page 349*
Vitamin B_{12} *on page 359*

Scientific Basis Published scientific studies using this pharmacologic agent

Studies & Abstracts 7-27, 28-37

♦ **Neomycin Sulfate** *see* Neomycin* *on page 190*
♦ **Neopap® [OTC]** *see* Acetaminophen* *on page 23*
♦ **Neoral® Oral** *see* Cyclosporine* *on page 88*
♦ **Neosar® Injection** *see* Cyclophosphamide* *on page 88*
♦ **Neo-Tabs® Oral** *see* Neomycin* *on page 190*

- **Nephro-Fer™ [OTC]** *see* Ferrous Fumarate *on page 126*
- **Nephronex®** *see* Nitrofurantoin* *on page 192*
- **Nephrox Suspension [OTC]** *see* Aluminum Hydroxide* *on page 28*
- **Neurontin®** *see* Gabapentin *on page 135*
- **Neut® Injection** *see* Sodium Bicarbonate* *on page 239*

Nevirapine* (ne VYE ra peen)
Related Information
Drug-Induced Nutrient Depletion Table *on page 498*
U.S. Brand Names Viramune®
Pharmacologic Class Antiretroviral Agent, Protease Inhibitor
Nutrients Depleted
Carnitine *on page 316*
Copper *on page 322*
Vitamin B$_{12}$ *on page 359*
Zinc *on page 368*
Scientific Basis Published scientific studies of agents from the same pharmacologic class
Studies & Abstracts 260-262

Nicardipine (nye KAR de peen)
U.S. Brand Names Cardene®; Cardene® SR
Canadian Brand Names Ridene
Synonyms Nicardipine Hydrochloride
Pharmacologic Class Calcium Channel Blocker
Nutrients Depleted
Specific nutrient depletions have not been documented for this agent.

- **Nicardipine Hydrochloride** *see* Nicardipine *on page 191*
- **Nicoderm® Patch [OTC]** *see* Nicotine *on page 191*
- **Nicorette®** *see* Nicotine *on page 191*
- **Nicorette® DS Gum [OTC]** *see* Nicotine *on page 191*
- **Nicorette® Gum** *see* Nicotine *on page 191*
- **Nicorette® Plus** *see* Nicotine *on page 191*

Nicotine (nik oh TEEN)
U.S. Brand Names Habitrol™ Patch [OTC]; Nicoderm® Patch [OTC]; Nicorette® DS Gum [OTC]; Nicorette® Gum; Nicotrol® Inhaler; Nicotrol® NS Nasal Spray; Nicotrol® Patch; ProStep® Patch
Canadian Brand Names Nicorette®; Nicorette® Plus
Pharmacologic Class Smoking Cessation Aid
Nutrients Depleted
Specific nutrient depletions have not been documented for this agent.

- **Nicotrol® Inhaler** *see* Nicotine *on page 191*
- **Nicotrol® NS Nasal Spray** *see* Nicotine *on page 191*
- **Nicotrol® Patch** *see* Nicotine *on page 191*

Nifedipine (nye FED i peen)
U.S. Brand Names Adalat®; Adalat® CC; Procardia®; Procardia XL®
Canadian Brand Names Adalat PA®; Apo®-Nifed; Gen-Nifedipine; Novo-Nifedin; Nu-Nifedin
Pharmacologic Class Calcium Channel Blocker
Nutrients Depleted
Specific nutrient depletions have not been documented for this agent.

Nimodipine (nye MOE di peen)
U.S. Brand Names Nimotop®
Pharmacologic Class Calcium Channel Blocker
Nutrients Depleted
Specific nutrient depletions have not been documented for this agent.

♦ **Nimotop®** *see* Nimodipine *on page 192*

Nisoldipine (NYE sole di peen)
U.S. Brand Names Sular®
Pharmacologic Class Calcium Channel Blocker
Nutrients Depleted
Specific nutrient depletions have not been documented for this agent.

♦ **Nitalapram** *see* Citalopram *on page 78*
♦ **Nitrek® Patch** *see* Nitroglycerin *on page 192*
♦ **Nitro-Bid® I.V. Injection** *see* Nitroglycerin *on page 192*
♦ **Nitro-Bid® Ointment** *see* Nitroglycerin *on page 192*
♦ **Nitrodisc® Patch** *see* Nitroglycerin *on page 192*
♦ **Nitro-Dur® Patch** *see* Nitroglycerin *on page 192*

Nitrofurantoin* (nye troe fyoor AN toyn)
U.S. Brand Names Furadantin®; Macrobid®; Macrodantin®
Canadian Brand Names Apo®-Nitrofurantoin; Nephronex®; Novo-Furan
Pharmacologic Class Antibiotic, Miscellaneous
Nutrients Depleted
Bifidobacteria bifidum (bifidus) on page 311
Lactobacillus acidophilus on page 332
Scientific Basis Published scientific studies using this pharmacologic agent
Studies & Abstracts 7-27

♦ **Nitrogard® Buccal** *see* Nitroglycerin *on page 192*

Nitroglycerin (nye troe GLI ser in)
U.S. Brand Names Deponit® Patch; Minitran™ Patch; Nitrek® Patch; Nitro-Bid® I.V. Injection; Nitro-Bid® Ointment; Nitrodisc® Patch; Nitro-Dur® Patch; Nitrogard® Buccal; Nitroglyn® Oral; Nitrolingual® Trans-lingual Spray; Nitrol® Ointment; Nitrong® Oral Tablet; Nitrostat® Sublin-gual; Transdermal-NTG® Patch; Transderm-Nitro® Patch; Tridil® Injection
Synonyms Glyceryl Trinitrate; Nitroglycerol; NTG

Pharmacologic Class Vasodilator
Nutrients Depleted
  Specific nutrient depletions have not been documented for this agent.

♦ **Nitroglycerol** *see* Nitroglycerin *on page 192*
♦ **Nitroglyn® Oral** *see* Nitroglycerin *on page 192*
♦ **Nitrolingual® Translingual Spray** *see* Nitroglycerin *on page 192*
♦ **Nitrol® Ointment** *see* Nitroglycerin *on page 192*
♦ **Nitrong® Oral Tablet** *see* Nitroglycerin *on page 192*
♦ **Nitrostat® Sublingual** *see* Nitroglycerin *on page 192*

Nizatidine* (ni ZA ti deen)
Related Information
  Drug-Induced Nutrient Depletion Table *on page 498*
U.S. Brand Names Axid®; Axid® AR [OTC]
Canadian Brand Names Apo®-Nizatidine
Pharmacologic Class Histamine H_2 Antagonist
Nutrients Depleted
  Calcium *on page 313*
  Folic Acid *on page 325*
  Iron *on page 331*
  Vitamin B_{12} *on page 359*
  Vitamin D *on page 363*
  Zinc *on page 368*
Scientific Basis Published scientific studies of agents from the same pharmacologic class
Studies & Abstracts 484-510

♦ **Nizoral®** *see* Ketoconazole *on page 160*
♦ **N-Methylhydrazine** *see* Procarbazine* *on page 221*
♦ **Nobesine®** *see* Diethylpropion *on page 99*
♦ **Nolex® LA** *see* Guaifenesin and Phenylpropanolamine *on page 141*
♦ **Nolvadex®** *see* Tamoxifen *on page 247*
♦ **Norco®** *see* Hydrocodone and Acetaminophen* *on page 149*
♦ **Nordeoxyguanosine** *see* Ganciclovir *on page 136*
♦ **Nordette®** *see* Ethinyl Estradiol and Levonorgestrel* *on page 120*
♦ **Norethin™ 1/35E** *see* Ethinyl Estradiol and Norethindrone* *on page 121*

Norethindrone* (nor eth IN drone)
U.S. Brand Names Aygestin®; Micronor®; NOR-QD®
Synonyms Norethindrone Acetate; Norethisterone
Pharmacologic Class Contraceptive; Progestin
Nutrients Depleted
  Folic Acid *on page 325*
  Magnesium *on page 333*
  Vitamin B_2 *on page 353*
  Vitamin B_6 *on page 357*
  Vitamin B_{12} *on page 359*
  Vitamin C *on page 360*
  (Continued)

Norethindrone* *(Continued)*

Zinc *on page 368*
Scientific Basis
Published scientific studies using this pharmacologic agent
or
Published scientific studies of agents from the same pharmacologic class
Studies & Abstracts 380-436

♦ **Norethindrone Acetate** *see* Norethindrone* *on page 193*
♦ **Norethindrone Acetate and Ethinyl Estradiol** *see* Ethinyl Estradiol and Norethindrone* *on page 121*
♦ **Norethisterone** *see* Norethindrone* *on page 193*

Norfloxacin* *(nor FLOKS a sin)*
U.S. Brand Names Chibroxin™ Ophthalmic; Noroxin® Oral
Pharmacologic Class Antibiotic, Quinolone
Nutrients Depleted
Bifidobacteria bifidum (bifidus) on page 311
Biotin *on page 311*
Inositol *on page 328*
Lactobacillus acidophilus on page 332
Vitamin B_1 *on page 351*
Vitamin B_2 *on page 353*
Vitamin B_3 *on page 354*
Vitamin B_6 *on page 357*
Vitamin B_{12} *on page 359*
Vitamin K *on page 367*
Scientific Basis Inferred or indirect evidence of depletion based on disruption of physiologic processes
Studies & Abstracts 7-27

♦ **Norgestimate and Ethinyl Estradiol** *see* Ethinyl Estradiol and Norgestimate* *on page 121*
♦ **Norgestrel and Ethinyl Estradiol** *see* Ethinyl Estradiol and Norgestrel* *on page 122*
♦ **Norinyl®** 1+35 *see* Ethinyl Estradiol and Norethindrone* *on page 121*
♦ **Noritate® Cream** *see* Metronidazole* *on page 180*
♦ **Normodyne®** *see* Labetalol* *on page 161*
♦ **Noroxin® Oral** *see* Norfloxacin* *on page 194*
♦ **Norpace®** *see* Disopyramide *on page 103*
♦ **Norplant® Implant** *see* Levonorgestrel* *on page 165*
♦ **Norpramin®** *see* Desipramine* *on page 94*
♦ **NOR-QD®** *see* Norethindrone* *on page 193*

Nortriptyline* *(nor TRIP ti leen)*
Related Information
Drug-Induced Nutrient Depletion Table *on page 498*
U.S. Brand Names Aventyl® Hydrochloride; Pamelor®
Canadian Brand Names Apo®-Nortriptyline

Synonyms Nortriptyline Hydrochloride
Pharmacologic Class Antidepressant, Tricyclic (Secondary Amine)
Nutrients Depleted
   Coenzyme Q_{10} *on page 320*
   Vitamin B_2 *on page 353*
Scientific Basis Published scientific studies of agents from the same pharmacologic class
   Studies & Abstracts 467-472

♦ **Nortriptyline Hydrochloride** *see* Nortriptyline* *on page 194*
♦ **Norvasc**® *see* Amlodipine *on page 32*
♦ **Norvir**® *see* Ritonavir *on page 233*
♦ **Norzine**® *see* Thiethylperazine* *on page 251*
♦ **Novamilor** *see* Amiloride and Hydrochlorothiazide* *on page 31*
♦ **Novamoxin**® *see* Amoxicillin* *on page 33*
♦ **Novantrone**® *see* Mitoxantrone* *on page 183*
♦ **Novasen** *see* Aspirin* *on page 40*
♦ **Novo-Alprazol** *see* Alprazolam *on page 28*
♦ **Novo-Atenol** *see* Atenolol* *on page 41*
♦ **Novo-AZT** *see* Zidovudine* *on page 270*
♦ **Novo-Butamide** *see* Tolbutamide* *on page 256*
♦ **Novo-Captopril** *see* Captopril* *on page 57*
♦ **Novo-Carbamaz** *see* Carbamazepine* *on page 57*
♦ **Novo-Chlorhydrate** *see* Chloral Hydrate *on page 72*
♦ **Novo-Chlorpromazine** *see* Chlorpromazine* *on page 74*
♦ **Novo-Cimetine** *see* Cimetidine* *on page 76*
♦ **Novo-Clonidine** *see* Clonidine* *on page 81*
♦ **Novo-Clopate** *see* Clorazepate *on page 81*
♦ **Novo-Cromolyn** *see* Cromolyn Sodium *on page 87*
♦ **Novo-Cycloprine** *see* Cyclobenzaprine *on page 88*
♦ **Novo-Difenac**® *see* Diclofenac* *on page 97*
♦ **Novo-Difenac**®-**SR** *see* Diclofenac* *on page 97*
♦ **Novo-Diflunisal** *see* Diflunisal *on page 100*
♦ **Novo-Digoxin** *see* Digoxin* *on page 100*
♦ **Novo-Diltazem** *see* Diltiazem *on page 101*
♦ **Novo-Dipam** *see* Diazepam *on page 97*
♦ **Novo-Dipiradol** *see* Dipyridamole *on page 103*
♦ **Novo-Doparil** *see* Methyldopa and Hydrochlorothiazide* *on page 178*
♦ **Novo-Doxepin** *see* Doxepin* *on page 106*
♦ **Novo-Doxylin** *see* Doxycycline* *on page 106*
♦ **Novo-Famotidine** *see* Famotidine* *on page 123*
♦ **Novo-Fibrate** *see* Clofibrate *on page 80*
♦ **Novo-Flupam** *see* Flurazepam *on page 131*
♦ **Novo-Flurprofen** *see* Flurbiprofen* *on page 131*
♦ **Novo-Flutamide** *see* Flutamide *on page 132*
♦ **Novo-Furan** *see* Nitrofurantoin* *on page 192*

- **Novo-Gesic-C8** *see* Acetaminophen and Codeine* *on page 23*
- **Novo-Gesic-C15** *see* Acetaminophen and Codeine* *on page 23*
- **Novo-Gesic-C30** *see* Acetaminophen and Codeine* *on page 23*
- **Novo-Glyburide** *see* Glyburide* *on page 139*
- **Novo-Hydrazide** *see* Hydrochlorothiazide* *on page 147*
- **Novo-Hydroxyzin** *see* Hydroxyzine *on page 152*
- **Novo-Hylazin** *see* Hydralazine* *on page 146*
- **Novo-Keto-EC** *see* Ketoprofen* *on page 160*
- **Novo-Lexin** *see* Cephalexin* *on page 69*
- **Novolin® 70/30** *see* Insulin Preparations *on page 156*
- **Novolin® L** *see* Insulin Preparations *on page 156*
- **Novolin® N** *see* Insulin Preparations *on page 156*
- **Novolin® R** *see* Insulin Preparations *on page 156*
- **NovoLog™** *see* Insulin Preparations *on page 156*
- **Novo-Lorazepam** *see* Lorazepam *on page 168*
- **Novo-Medopa®** *see* Methyldopa* *on page 177*
- **Novo-Medrone** *see* Medroxyprogesterone Acetate *on page 173*
- **Novo-Metformin** *see* Metformin* *on page 175*
- **Novo-Methacin** *see* Indomethacin* *on page 155*
- **Novo-Metoprolol** *see* Metoprolol* *on page 179*
- **Novo-Mucilax** *see* Psyllium *on page 226*
- **Novo-Naprox** *see* Naproxen *on page 189*
- **Novo-Nidazol** *see* Metronidazole* *on page 180*
- **Novo-Nifedin** *see* Nifedipine *on page 192*
- **Novo-Oxazepam** *see* Oxazepam *on page 201*
- **Novo-Pen-VK®** *see* Penicillin V Potassium* *on page 207*
- **Novo-Piroxicam** *see* Piroxicam* *on page 214*
- **Novo-Poxide** *see* Chlordiazepoxide *on page 72*
- **Novo-Pramine** *see* Imipramine* *on page 154*
- **Novo-Prazin** *see* Prazosin *on page 217*
- **Novo-Prednisolone** *see* Prednisolone* *on page 218*
- **Novo-Prednisone** *see* Prednisone* *on page 219*
- **Novo-Profen®** *see* Ibuprofen* *on page 153*
- **Novo-Propamide** *see* Chlorpropamide *on page 74*
- **Novo-Propoxyn** *see* Propoxyphene *on page 223*
- **Novo-Purol** *see* Allopurinol *on page 27*
- **Novo-Ranidine** *see* Ranitidine Hydrochloride* *on page 229*
- **Novo-Ridazine** *see* Thioridazine* *on page 251*
- **Novo-Rythro Encap** *see* Erythromycin (Systemic)* *on page 113*
- **Novo-Salmol** *see* Albuterol *on page 26*
- **Novo-Selegiline** *see* Selegiline *on page 236*
- **Novo-Semide** *see* Furosemide* *on page 135*
- **Novo-Spiroton** *see* Spironolactone *on page 241*
- **Novo-Spirozine** *see* Hydrochlorothiazide and Spironolactone* *on page 148*
- **Novo-Sucralate** *see* Sucralfate* *on page 242*

- **Novo-Sundac** *see* Sulindac* *on page 245*
- **Novo-Tamoxifen** *see* Tamoxifen *on page 247*
- **Novo-Tetra** *see* Tetracycline* *on page 249*
- **Novo-Thalidone** *see* Chlorthalidone* *on page 74*
- **Novo-Timol** *see* Timolol* *on page 254*
- **Novo-Tolmetin** *see* Tolmetin* *on page 256*
- **Novo-Triamzide** *see* Hydrochlorothiazide and Triamterene* *on page 149*
- **Novo-Trimel** *see* Co-Trimoxazole* *on page 86*
- **Novo-Triolam** *see* Triazolam *on page 261*
- **Novo-Tripramine** *see* Trimipramine* *on page 262*
- **Novo-Tryptin** *see* Amitriptyline* *on page 32*
- **Novo-Veramil** *see* Verapamil *on page 267*
- **Novo-Zolamide** *see* Acetazolamide* *on page 24*
- **Nozinan®** *see* Methotrimeprazine* *on page 176*
- **NPH Iletin® I** *see* Insulin Preparations *on page 156*
- **NPH-N** *see* Insulin Preparations *on page 156*
- **NSC 26271** *see* Cyclophosphamide* *on page 88*
- **NSC-106977** *see* Erwinia Asparaginase* *on page 112*
- **NSC 125066** *see* Bleomycin* *on page 49*
- **NTG** *see* Nitroglycerin *on page 192*
- **Nu-Alprax** *see* Alprazolam *on page 28*
- **Nu-Amilzide** *see* Amiloride and Hydrochlorothiazide* *on page 31*
- **Nu-Amoxi** *see* Amoxicillin* *on page 33*
- **Nu-Ampi Trihydrate** *see* Ampicillin* *on page 35*
- **Nu-Atenol** *see* Atenolol* *on page 41*
- **Nu-Capto** *see* Captopril* *on page 57*
- **Nu-Carbamazepine** *see* Carbamazepine* *on page 57*
- **Nu-Cephalex** *see* Cephalexin* *on page 69*
- **Nu-Cimet** *see* Cimetidine* *on page 76*
- **Nu-Clonidine** *see* Clonidine* *on page 81*
- **Nucofed®** *see* Guaifenesin, Pseudoephedrine, and Codeine *on page 143*
- **Nucofed® Pediatric Expectorant** *see* Guaifenesin, Pseudoephedrine, and Codeine *on page 143*
- **Nu-Cotrimox** *see* Co-Trimoxazole* *on page 86*
- **Nucotuss®** *see* Guaifenesin, Pseudoephedrine, and Codeine *on page 143*
- **Nu-Diclo** *see* Diclofenac* *on page 97*
- **Nu-Diflunisal** *see* Diflunisal* *on page 100*
- **Nu-Diltiaz** *see* Diltiazem *on page 101*
- **Nu-Doxycycline** *see* Doxycycline* *on page 106*
- **Nu-Famotidine** *see* Famotidine* *on page 123*
- **Nu-Flurprofen** *see* Flurbiprofen* *on page 131*
- **Nu-Gemfibrozil** *see* Gemfibrozil* *on page 137*
- **Nu-Glyburide** *see* Glyburide* *on page 139*
- **Nu-Hydral** *see* Hydralazine* *on page 146*

- **Nu-Ibuprofen** *see* Ibuprofen* *on page 153*
- **Nu-Indo** *see* Indomethacin* *on page 155*
- **Nu-Ketoprofen** *see* Ketoprofen* *on page 160*
- **Nu-Ketoprofen-E** *see* Ketoprofen* *on page 160*
- **Nu-Loraz** *see* Lorazepam *on page 168*
- **Nu-Medopa** *see* Methyldopa* *on page 177*
- **Nu-Metop** *see* Metoprolol* *on page 179*
- **Nu-Naprox** *see* Naproxen* *on page 189*
- **Nu-Nifedin** *see* Nifedipine *on page 192*
- **Nu-Pen-VK** *see* Penicillin V Potassium* *on page 207*
- **Nu-Pirox** *see* Piroxicam* *on page 214*
- **Nu-Prazo** *see* Prazosin *on page 217*
- **Nuprin® [OTC]** *see* Ibuprofen* *on page 153*
- **Nu-Prochlor** *see* Prochlorperazine* *on page 221*
- **Nu-Propranolol** *see* Propranolol* *on page 223*
- **Nu-Ranit** *see* Ranitidine Hydrochloride* *on page 229*
- **Nu-Tetra** *see* Tetracycline* *on page 249*
- **Nu-Timolol** *see* Timolol* *on page 254*
- **Nutracort®** *see* Hydrocortisone* *on page 150*
- **Nu-Triazide** *see* Hydrochlorothiazide and Triamterene* *on page 149*
- **Nu-Triazo** *see* Triazolam *on page 261*
- **Nu-Trimipramine** *see* Trimipramine* *on page 262*
- **Nu-Verap** *see* Verapamil *on page 267*
- **Nydrazid® Injection** *see* Isoniazid* *on page 158*
- **Nytol® Extra Strength** *see* Diphenhydramine *on page 102*
- **Nytol® Oral [OTC]** *see* Diphenhydramine *on page 102*
- **Occlucort®** *see* Betamethasone* *on page 46*
- **Octamide® PFS** *see* Metoclopramide *on page 179*

Octreotide Acetate (ok TREE oh tide AS e tate)
U.S. Brand Names Sandostatin®; Sandostatin LAR®
Pharmacologic Class Antidiarrheal; Antisecretory Agent; Somatostatin Analog
Nutrients Depleted
Specific nutrient depletions have not been documented for this agent.

- **Ocufen® Ophthalmic** *see* Flurbiprofen* *on page 131*
- **Ocuflox™ Ophthalmic** *see* Ofloxacin* *on page 198*
- **Ocupress® Ophthalmic** *see* Carteolol* *on page 59*

Ofloxacin* (oh FLOKS a sin)
U.S. Brand Names Floxin®; Ocuflox™ Ophthalmic
Pharmacologic Class Antibiotic, Quinolone
Nutrients Depleted
Bifidobacteria bifidum (bifidus) *on page 311*
Biotin *on page 311*
Inositol *on page 328*
Lactobacillus acidophilus *on page 332*

Vitamin B$_1$ *on page 351*
Vitamin B$_2$ *on page 353*
Vitamin B$_3$ *on page 354*
Vitamin B$_6$ *on page 357*
Vitamin B$_{12}$ *on page 359*
Vitamin K *on page 367*
Scientific Basis Inferred or indirect evidence of depletion based on disruption of physiologic processes
Studies & Abstracts 7-27

♦ **Ogen® Oral** *see* Estropipate* *on page 118*
♦ **Ogen® Vaginal** *see* Estropipate* *on page 118*

Olopatadine (oh LOP ah tah deen)
U.S. Brand Names Patanol®
Pharmacologic Class Antihistamine; Ophthalmic Agent, Miscellaneous
Nutrients Depleted
Specific nutrient depletions have not been documented for this agent.

Olsalazine* (ole SAL a zeen)
Related Information
Drug-Induced Nutrient Depletion Table *on page 498*
U.S. Brand Names Dipentum®
Synonyms Olsalazine Sodium
Pharmacologic Class 5-Aminosalicylic Acid Derivative
Nutrients Depleted
Folic Acid *on page 325*
Scientific Basis Published scientific studies using this pharmacologic agent
Studies & Abstracts 237-245

♦ **Olsalazine Sodium** *see* Olsalazine* *on page 199*

Omeprazole* (oh ME pray zol)
Related Information
Drug-Induced Nutrient Depletion Table *on page 498*
U.S. Brand Names Prilosec™
Canadian Brand Names Losec®
Pharmacologic Class Proton Pump Inhibitor
Nutrients Depleted
Vitamin B$_{12}$ *on page 359*
Scientific Basis Published scientific studies using this pharmacologic agent
Studies & Abstracts 511-516

♦ **Omnicef®** *see* Cefdinir* *on page 62*
♦ **Omnipen®** *see* Ampicillin* *on page 35*
♦ **Omnipen®-N** *see* Ampicillin* *on page 35*
♦ **OMS® Oral** *see* Morphine Sulfate *on page 185*
♦ **Oncovin® Injection** *see* Vincristine* *on page 268*

Ondansetron (on DAN se tron)
U.S. Brand Names Zofran®
Synonyms Ondansetron Hydrochloride
Pharmacologic Class Selective 5-HT₃ Receptor Antagonist
Nutrients Depleted
Specific nutrient depletions have not been documented for this agent.

- **Ondansetron Hydrochloride** *see* Ondansetron *on page 200*
- **Opticrom®** *see* Cromolyn Sodium *on page 87*
- **Orabase® HCA** *see* Hydrocortisone* *on page 150*
- **Orafen** *see* Ketoprofen* *on page 160*
- **Oramorph SR™ Oral** *see* Morphine Sulfate *on page 185*
- **Orap™** *see* Pimozide *on page 213*
- **Orasone®** *see* Prednisone* *on page 219*
- **Oretic®** *see* Hydrochlorothiazide* *on page 147*
- **Organidin® NR** *see* Guaifenesin *on page 140*
- **Orgaran®** *see* Danaparoid *on page 91*
- **Orinase® Diagnostic Injection** *see* Tolbutamide* *on page 256*
- **Orinase® Oral** *see* Tolbutamide* *on page 256*

Orlistat* (OR li stat)
Related Information
Drug-Induced Nutrient Depletion Table *on page 498*
U.S. Brand Names Xenical®
Pharmacologic Class Lipase Inhibitor
Nutrients Depleted
Beta-Carotene *on page 310*
Vitamin D *on page 363*
Vitamin E *on page 365*
Scientific Basis Published scientific studies using this pharmacologic agent
Studies & Abstracts 525-528

- **Ormazine** *see* Chlorpromazine* *on page 74*
- **Ornidyl® Injection** *see* Eflornithine *on page 109*
- **Ortho-Cept®** *see* Ethinyl Estradiol and Desogestrel* *on page 119*
- **Ortho-Cyclen®** *see* Ethinyl Estradiol and Norgestimate* *on page 121*
- **Ortho-Est® Oral** *see* Estropipate* *on page 118*
- **Ortho-Novum® 1/35** *see* Ethinyl Estradiol and Norethindrone* *on page 121*
- **Ortho-Novum® 7/7/7** *see* Ethinyl Estradiol and Norethindrone* *on page 121*
- **Ortho-Novum® 10/11** *see* Ethinyl Estradiol and Norethindrone* *on page 121*
- **Ortho-Prefest®** *see* Ethinyl Estradiol and Norgestimate* *on page 121*
- **Ortho Tri-Cyclen®** *see* Ethinyl Estradiol and Norgestimate* *on page 121*
- **Or-Tyl® Injection** *see* Dicyclomine *on page 98*

- **Orudis®** *see Ketoprofen* on page 160*
- **Orudis® KT [OTC]** *see Ketoprofen* on page 160*
- **Oruvail®** *see Ketoprofen* on page 160*

Oseltamivir (o sel TAM e veer)
U.S. Brand Names Tamiflu™
Pharmacologic Class Neuraminidase Inhibitor
Nutrients Depleted
Specific nutrient depletions have not been documented for this agent.

- **Osteocalcin® Injection** *see Calcitonin on page 55*
- **Ovcon® 35** *see Ethinyl Estradiol and Norethindrone* on page 121*
- **Ovcon® 50** *see Ethinyl Estradiol and Norethindrone* on page 121*
- **Ovral®** *see Ethinyl Estradiol and Norgestrel* on page 122*

Oxaprozin* (oks a PROE zin)
U.S. Brand Names Daypro™
Pharmacologic Class Nonsteroidal Anti-Inflammatory Agent (NSAID)
Nutrients Depleted
Folic Acid *on page 325*
Scientific Basis Published scientific studies of agents from the same pharmacologic class
Studies & Abstracts 252

Oxazepam (oks A ze pam)
U.S. Brand Names Serax®
Canadian Brand Names Apo®-Oxazepam; Novo-Oxazepam; Oxpam®; PMS-Oxazepam; Zapex®
Pharmacologic Class Benzodiazepine
Nutrients Depleted
Specific nutrient depletions have not been documented for this agent.

Oxcarbazepine* (ox car BAZ e peen)
U.S. Brand Names Trileptal®
Synonyms GP 47680
Pharmacologic Class Anticonvulsant, Miscellaneous
Nutrients Depleted
Biotin *on page 311*
Calcium *on page 313*
Folic Acid *on page 325*
Vitamin D *on page 363*
Scientific Basis Published scientific studies of agents from the same pharmacologic class
Studies & Abstracts 93-111

- **Oxpam®** *see Oxazepam on page 201*
- **Oxpentifylline** *see Pentoxifylline on page 209*
- **Oxycocet** *see Oxycodone and Acetaminophen* on page 202*
- **Oxycodan** *see Oxycodone and Aspirin* on page 202*

Oxycodone (oks i KOE done)
U.S. Brand Names OxyContin®; OxyIR™; Percolone®; Roxicodone™
Canadian Brand Names Supeudol®
Synonyms Dihydrohydroxycodeinone; Oxycodone Hydrochloride
Pharmacologic Class Analgesic, Narcotic
Nutrients Depleted
  Specific nutrient depletions have not been documented for this agent.

Oxycodone and Acetaminophen*
(oks i KOE done & a seet a MIN oh fen)
U.S. Brand Names Endocet®; Percocet® 2.5/325; Percocet® 5/325;
  Percocet® 7.5/500; Percocet® 10/650; Roxicet® 5/500; Roxilox™;
  Tylox®
Canadian Brand Names Endocet®; Oxycocet; Percocet®-Demi
Synonyms Acetaminophen and Oxycodone
Pharmacologic Class Analgesic, Narcotic
Nutrients Depleted
  Glutathione *on page 327*
Scientific Basis Published scientific studies using this pharmacologic
  agent (acetaminophen)
Studies & Abstracts 517-518

Oxycodone and Aspirin* (oks i KOE done & AS pir in)
U.S. Brand Names Codoxy®; Percodan®; Percodan®-Demi; Roxiprin®
Canadian Brand Names Endodan®; Oxycodan
Synonyms Aspirin and Oxycodone
Pharmacologic Class Analgesic, Narcotic
Nutrients Depleted
  Folic Acid *on page 325*
  Iron *on page 331*
  Potassium *on page 340*
  Sodium *on page 345*
  Vitamin C *on page 360*
Scientific Basis Published scientific studies using this pharmacologic
  agent (aspirin)
Studies & Abstracts 224-236

♦ **Oxycodone Hydrochloride** *see* Oxycodone *on page 202*
♦ **OxyContin®** *see* Oxycodone *on page 202*
♦ **OxyIR™** *see* Oxycodone *on page 202*

Oxytetracycline* (oks i tet ra SYE kleen)
Related Information
  Drug-Induced Nutrient Depletion Table *on page 498*
U.S. Brand Names Terramycin® I.M. Injection; Terramycin® Oral; Uri-
  Tet® Oral
Synonyms Oxytetracycline Hydrochloride
Pharmacologic Class Antibiotic, Tetracycline Derivative
Nutrients Depleted
  Bifidobacteria bifidum (bifidus) on page 311

Biotin *on page 311*
Calcium *on page 313*
Inositol *on page 328*
Iron *on page 331*
Lactobacillus acidophilus on page 332
Magnesium *on page 333*
Vitamin B$_1$ *on page 351*
Vitamin B$_2$ *on page 353*
Vitamin B$_3$ *on page 354*
Vitamin B$_6$ *on page 357*
Vitamin B$_{12}$ *on page 359*
Vitamin K *on page 367*

Scientific Basis Published scientific studies of agents from the same pharmacologic class

Studies & Abstracts 7-27, 62-68

Additional Information Calcium, iron, and magnesium depletion may be minimal during brief treatments. Replacement should not be attempted unless the time of administration is separated from the dosing of the tetracycline.

♦ **Oxytetracycline Hydrochloride** *see* Oxytetracycline* *on page 202*

♦ **P-071** *see* Cetirizine *on page 71*

♦ **Pacerone**® *see* Amiodarone *on page 32*

Paclitaxel* (PAK li taks el)

U.S. Brand Names Paxene®; Taxol®

Pharmacologic Class Antineoplastic Agent, Natural Source (Plant) Derivative

Nutrients Depleted

See Nutrient Depletion and Cancer Chemotherapy *on page 515*.

Scientific Basis Inferred or indirect evidence of depletion based on disruption of physiologic processes

♦ **Pamelor**® *see* Nortriptyline* *on page 194*

Pamidronate (pa mi DROE nate)

U.S. Brand Names Aredia™

Synonyms Pamidronate Disodium

Pharmacologic Class Antidote; Bisphosphonate Derivative

Nutrients Depleted

Specific nutrient depletions have not been documented for this agent.

Additional Information Bisphosphonates have been (rarely) associated with hypocalcemia, as a natural extension of their therapeutic action. Correction of hypocalcemia is recommended prior to alendronate treatment. Calcium administration should be separated from alendronate by at least 30 minutes.

♦ **Pamidronate Disodium** *see* Pamidronate *on page 203*

♦ **Panadol**® **[OTC]** *see* Acetaminophen* *on page 23*

♦ **Panasal**® **5/500** *see* Hydrocodone and Aspirin* *on page 150*

♦ **Pandel**® *see* Hydrocortisone* *on page 150*

Pantoprazole* (pan TOE pra zole)
U.S. Brand Names Protonix®
Pharmacologic Class Proton Pump Inhibitor
Nutrients Depleted
Vitamin B_{12} *on page 359*
Scientific Basis Published scientific studies of agents from the same pharmacologic class
Studies & Abstracts 511-516

- **Parabromdylamine** *see* Brompheniramine *on page 50*
- **Paracetamol** *see* Acetaminophen* *on page 23*
- **Paraflex®** *see* Chlorzoxazone *on page 75*
- **Parafon Forte™ DSC** *see* Chlorzoxazone *on page 75*
- **Paraplatin®** *see* Carboplatin* *on page 58*
- **Pariprazole** *see* Rabeprazole* *on page 228*
- **Parlodel®** *see* Bromocriptine *on page 50*

Paroxetine (pa ROKS e teen)
U.S. Brand Names Paxil™; Paxil® CR™
Pharmacologic Class Antidepressant, Selective Serotonin Reuptake Inhibitor
Nutrients Depleted
Specific nutrient depletions have not been documented for this agent.
Additional Information Selective serotonin reuptake inhibitors have been associated with rare, potentially severe hyponatremia. However, this is generally associated with fluid excess (SIADH), rather than a sodium deficiency. Treatment must be guided by a qualified healthcare provider.

- **Partuss® LA** *see* Guaifenesin and Phenylpropanolamine *on page 141*
- **Patanol®** *see* Olopatadine *on page 199*
- **Pathocil®** *see* Dicloxacillin* *on page 98*
- **Paveral Stanley Syrup With Codeine Phosphate** *see* Codeine *on page 83*
- **Paxene®** *see* Paclitaxel* *on page 203*
- **Paxil™** *see* Paroxetine *on page 204*
- **Paxil® CR™** *see* Paroxetine *on page 204*
- **Paxipam®** *see* Halazepam *on page 144*
- **PCA** *see* Procainamide *on page 220*
- **PCE® Oral** *see* Erythromycin (Systemic)* *on page 113*
- **Pectin and Kaolin** *see* Kaolin and Pectin *on page 159*
- **Pedia Care® Oral** *see* Pseudoephedrine *on page 225*
- **Pediapred® Oral** *see* Prednisolone* *on page 218*
- **Pediatrix** *see* Acetaminophen* *on page 23*

Pemoline (PEM oh leen)
U.S. Brand Names Cylert®
Synonyms Phenylisohydantoin; PIO

Pharmacologic Class Stimulant
Nutrients Depleted
Specific nutrient depletions have not been documented for this agent.

Penciclovir (pen SYE kloe veer)
U.S. Brand Names Denavir™
Pharmacologic Class Antiviral Agent
Nutrients Depleted
Specific nutrient depletions have not been documented for this agent.

♦ **Penecort®** *see Hydrocortisone* on page 150*
♦ **Penetrex™** *see Enoxacin* on page 111*

Penicillamine* (pen i SIL a meen)
Related Information
Drug-Induced Nutrient Depletion Table *on page 498*
U.S. Brand Names Cuprimine®; Depen®
Synonyms D-3-Mercaptovaline; β,β-Dimethylcysteine; D-Penicillamine
Pharmacologic Class Chelating Agent
Nutrients Depleted
Copper *on page 322*
Magnesium *on page 333*
Vitamin B$_6$ *on page 357*
Zinc *on page 368*
Scientific Basis Published scientific studies using this pharmacologic agent
Studies & Abstracts 529-536

Penicillin G Benzathine* (pen i SIL in jee BENZ a theen)
U.S. Brand Names Bicillin® L-A; Permapen®
Canadian Brand Names Megacillin® Susp
Synonyms Benzathine Benzylpenicillin; Benzathine Penicillin G; Benzylpenicillin Benzathine
Pharmacologic Class Antibiotic, Penicillin
Nutrients Depleted
Bifidobacteria bifidum (bifidus) on page 311
Biotin *on page 311*
Inositol *on page 328*
Lactobacillus acidophilus on page 332
Potassium *on page 340*
Vitamin B$_1$ *on page 351*
Vitamin B$_2$ *on page 353*
Vitamin B$_3$ *on page 354*
Vitamin B$_6$ *on page 357*
Vitamin B$_{12}$ *on page 359*
Vitamin K *on page 367*
Scientific Basis Inferred or indirect evidence of depletion based on disruption of physiologic processes
Studies & Abstracts 7-27, 49-57
(Continued)

Penicillin G Benzathine* *(Continued)*

Additional Information Potassium depletion has been documented primarily with high dose, parenteral penicillins, primarily from the ureidopenicillin group.

Penicillin G Benzathine and Procaine Combined*

(pen i SIL in jee BENZ a theen & PROE kane KOM bined)

Related Information

Drug-Induced Nutrient Depletion Table *on page 498*

U.S. Brand Names Bicillin® C-R 900/300 Injection; Bicillin® C-R Injection

Synonyms Penicillin G Procaine and Benzathine Combined

Pharmacologic Class Antibiotic, Penicillin

Nutrients Depleted

Bifidobacteria bifidum (bifidus) on page 311

Biotin *on page 311*

Inositol *on page 328*

Lactobacillus acidophilus on page 332

Potassium *on page 340*

Vitamin B$_1$ *on page 351*

Vitamin B$_2$ *on page 353*

Vitamin B$_3$ *on page 354*

Vitamin B$_6$ *on page 357*

Vitamin B$_{12}$ *on page 359*

Vitamin K *on page 367*

Scientific Basis Inferred or indirect evidence of depletion based on disruption of physiologic processes

Studies & Abstracts 7-27, 49-57

Additional Information Potassium depletion has been documented primarily with high dose, parenteral penicillins, primarily from the ureidopenicillin group.

Penicillin G (Parenteral/Aqueous)*

(pen i SIL in jee, pa REN ter al, AYE kwee us)

U.S. Brand Names Pfizerpen®

Synonyms Benzylpenicillin Potassium; Benzylpenicillin Sodium; Crystalline Penicillin; Penicillin G Potassium; Penicillin G Sodium

Pharmacologic Class Antibiotic, Penicillin

Nutrients Depleted

Bifidobacteria bifidum (bifidus) on page 311

Biotin *on page 311*

Inositol *on page 328*

Lactobacillus acidophilus on page 332

Potassium *on page 340*

Vitamin B$_1$ *on page 351*

Vitamin B$_2$ *on page 353*

Vitamin B$_3$ *on page 354*

Vitamin B$_6$ *on page 357*

Vitamin B$_{12}$ *on page 359*

Vitamin K *on page 367*

Scientific Basis Inferred or indirect evidence of depletion based on disruption of physiologic processes

Studies & Abstracts 7-27, 49-57

Additional Information Potassium depletion has been documented primarily with high dose, parenteral penicillins, primarily from the ureidopenicillin group.

♦ **Penicillin G Potassium** *see* Penicillin G (Parenteral/Aqueous)* *on page 206*

Penicillin G Procaine* (pen i SIL in jee PROE kane)
Related Information

Drug-Induced Nutrient Depletion Table *on page 498*

U.S. Brand Names Crysticillin® A.S.; Wycillin®

Canadian Brand Names Ayercillin®

Synonyms APPG; Aqueous Procaine Penicillin G; Procaine Benzyl-penicillin; Procaine Penicillin G

Pharmacologic Class Antibiotic, Penicillin

Nutrients Depleted

Bifidobacteria bifidum (bifidus) on page 311
Biotin *on page 311*
Inositol *on page 328*
Lactobacillus acidophilus on page 332
Potassium *on page 340*
Vitamin B_1 *on page 351*
Vitamin B_2 *on page 353*
Vitamin B_3 *on page 354*
Vitamin B_6 *on page 357*
Vitamin B_{12} *on page 359*
Vitamin K *on page 367*

Scientific Basis Inferred or indirect evidence of depletion based on disruption of physiologic processes

Studies & Abstracts 7-27, 49-57

Additional Information Potassium depletion has been documented primarily with high dose, parenteral penicillins, primarily from the ureidopenicillin group.

♦ **Penicillin G Procaine and Benzathine Combined** *see* Penicillin G Benzathine and Procaine Combined* *on page 206*

♦ **Penicillin G Sodium** *see* Penicillin G (Parenteral/Aqueous)* *on page 206*

Penicillin V Potassium* (pen i SIL in vee poe TASS ee um)
Related Information

Drug-Induced Nutrient Depletion Table *on page 498*

U.S. Brand Names Beepen-VK®; Betapen®-VK; Pen.Vee® K; Robi-cillin® VK; Veetids®

Canadian Brand Names Apo®-Pen VK; Nadopen-V®; Novo-Pen-VK®; Nu-Pen-VK; PVF® K

Synonyms Pen VK; Phenoxymethyl Penicillin

Pharmacologic Class Antibiotic, Penicillin

(Continued)

Penicillin V Potassium* *(Continued)*
Nutrients Depleted
Bifidobacteria bifidum (bifidus) on page 311
Biotin *on page 311*
Inositol *on page 328*
Lactobacillus acidophilus on page 332
Potassium *on page 340*
Vitamin B_1 *on page 351*
Vitamin B_2 *on page 353*
Vitamin B_3 *on page 354*
Vitamin B_6 *on page 357*
Vitamin B_{12} *on page 359*
Vitamin K *on page 367*
Scientific Basis
Inferred or indirect evidence of depletion based on disruption of physiologic processes
Studies & Abstracts
7-27, 49-57
Additional Information
Potassium depletion has been documented primarily with high dose, parenteral penicillins, primarily from the ureidopenicillin group.

♦ **Pentacarinat® Injection** *see* Pentamidine* *on page 208*
♦ **Pentam-300® Injection** *see* Pentamidine* *on page 208*

Pentamidine* (pen TAM i deen)
Related Information
Drug-Induced Nutrient Depletion Table *on page 498*
U.S. Brand Names
NebuPent™ Inhalation; Pentacarinat® Injection; Pentam-300® Injection
Pharmacologic Class
Antibiotic, Miscellaneous
Nutrients Depleted
Magnesium *on page 333*
Scientific Basis
Published scientific studies using this pharmacologic agent
Studies & Abstracts
7-27, 58

♦ **Pentasa® Oral** *see* Mesalamine* *on page 174*

Pentazocine (pen TAZ oh seen)
U.S. Brand Names
Talwin®; Talwin® NX
Synonyms
Pentazocine Hydrochloride; Pentazocine Lactate
Pharmacologic Class
Analgesic, Narcotic
Nutrients Depleted
Specific nutrient depletions have not been documented for this agent.

Pentazocine Compound (pen TAZ oh seen KOM pownd)
U.S. Brand Names
Talacen®; Talwin® Compound
Pharmacologic Class
Analgesic, Combination (Narcotic)
Nutrients Depleted
Specific nutrient depletions have not been documented for this agent.

♦ **Pentazocine Hydrochloride** *see* Pentazocine *on page 208*
♦ **Pentazocine Lactate** *see* Pentazocine *on page 208*

Pentoxifylline (pen toks I fi leen)
U.S. Brand Names Trental®
Canadian Brand Names Albert® Pentoxifylline; Apo®-Pentoxifylline SR
Synonyms Oxpentifylline
Pharmacologic Class Blood Viscosity Reducer Agent
Nutrients Depleted
Specific nutrient depletions have not been documented for this agent.

♦ **Pen.Vee® K** *see* Penicillin V Potassium* *on page 207*
♦ **Pen VK** *see* Penicillin V Potassium* *on page 207*
♦ **Pepcid®** *see* Famotidine* *on page 123*
♦ **Pepcid® AC Acid Controller [OTC]** *see* Famotidine* *on page 123*
♦ **Pepto® Diarrhea Control [OTC]** *see* Loperamide *on page 167*
♦ **Peptol®** *see* Cimetidine* *on page 76*
♦ **Percocet® 2.5/325** *see* Oxycodone and Acetaminophen* *on page 202*
♦ **Percocet® 5/325** *see* Oxycodone and Acetaminophen* *on page 202*
♦ **Percocet® 7.5/500** *see* Oxycodone and Acetaminophen* *on page 202*
♦ **Percocet® 10/650** *see* Oxycodone and Acetaminophen* *on page 202*
♦ **Percocet®-Demi** *see* Oxycodone and Acetaminophen* *on page 202*
♦ **Percodan®** *see* Oxycodone and Aspirin* *on page 202*
♦ **Percodan®-Demi** *see* Oxycodone and Aspirin* *on page 202*
♦ **Percolone®** *see* Oxycodone *on page 202*
♦ **Perdiem® Plain [OTC]** *see* Psyllium *on page 226*

Pergolide (PER go lide)
U.S. Brand Names Permax®
Synonyms Pergolide Mesylate
Pharmacologic Class Anti-Parkinson's Agent (Dopamine Agonist); Ergot Derivative
Nutrients Depleted
Specific nutrient depletions have not been documented for this agent.

♦ **Pergolide Mesylate** *see* Pergolide *on page 209*
♦ **Periactin®** *see* Cyproheptadine *on page 89*
♦ **Peri-Colace® [OTC]** *see* Docusate and Casanthranol* *on page 104*

Perindopril Erbumine* (per IN doe pril er BYOO meen)
Related Information
Drug-Induced Nutrient Depletion Table *on page 498*
U.S. Brand Names Aceon®
Pharmacologic Class Angiotensin-Converting Enzyme (ACE) Inhibitors
Nutrients Depleted
Zinc *on page 368*
Scientific Basis Published scientific studies of agents from the same pharmacologic class
(Continued)

Perindopril Erbumine* *(Continued)*
Studies & Abstracts 269-271

- ◆ **Periostat**® *see* Doxycycline* *on page 106*
- ◆ **Permapen**® *see* Penicillin G Benzathine* *on page 205*
- ◆ **Permax**® *see* Pergolide *on page 209*
- ◆ **Permitil**® **Oral** *see* Fluphenazine* *on page 131*

Perphenazine* *(per FEN a zeen)*
U.S. Brand Names Trilafon®
Canadian Brand Names Apo®-Perphenazine; PMS-Perphenazine
Pharmacologic Class Antipsychotic Agent, Phenothazine, Piperazine
Nutrients Depleted
Coenzyme Q₁₀ *on page 320*
Vitamin B₂ *on page 353*
Scientific Basis Published scientific studies of agents from the same pharmacologic class
Studies & Abstracts 474-477

- ◆ **Persantine**® *see* Dipyridamole *on page 103*
- ◆ **Pertussin**® **CS [OTC]** *see* Dextromethorphan *on page 96*
- ◆ **Pertussin**® **ES [OTC]** *see* Dextromethorphan *on page 96*
- ◆ **PFA** *see* Foscarnet* *on page 134*
- ◆ **Pfizerpen**® *see* Penicillin G (Parenteral/Aqueous)* *on page 206*
- ◆ **PGE₁** *see* Alprostadil *on page 28*
- ◆ **Phanatuss**® **Cough Syrup [OTC]** *see* Guaifenesin and Dextromethorphan *on page 141*
- ◆ **Phazyme**® **[OTC]** *see* Simethicone *on page 238*
- ◆ **Phenadex**® **Senior [OTC]** *see* Guaifenesin and Dextromethorphan *on page 141*
- ◆ **Phenaphen**® **With Codeine** *see* Acetaminophen and Codeine* *on page 23*
- ◆ **Phenazine**® *see* Promethazine* *on page 222*
- ◆ **Phenazopyridine and Sulfisoxazole** *see* Sulfisoxazole and Phenazopyridine* *on page 244*
- ◆ **Phendry**® **Oral [OTC]** *see* Diphenhydramine *on page 102*
- ◆ **Phenergan**® *see* Promethazine* *on page 222*
- ◆ **Phenhist**® **Expectorant** *see* Guaifenesin, Pseudoephedrine, and Codeine *on page 143*

Phenobarbital* *(fee noe BAR bi tal)*
U.S. Brand Names Barbita®; Luminal®; Solfoton®
Canadian Brand Names Barbilixir®
Synonyms Phenobarbital Sodium; Phenobarbitone; Phenylethylmalonylurea
Pharmacologic Class Anticonvulsant, Miscellaneous; Barbiturate
Nutrients Depleted
Biotin *on page 311*

Calcium *on page 313*
Folic Acid *on page 325*
Vitamin D *on page 363*
Vitamin K *on page 367*

Scientific Basis Published scientific studies using this pharmacologic agent

Studies & Abstracts 73-92

- **Phenobarbital Sodium** *see Phenobarbital* on page 210*
- **Phenobarbitone** *see Phenobarbital* on page 210*
- **Phenoxine® [OTC]** *see Phenylpropanolamine on page 211*
- **Phenoxymethyl Penicillin** *see Penicillin V Potassium* on page 207*

Phentermine (FEN ter meen)
U.S. Brand Names Adipex-P®; Fastin®; Ionamin®; Zantryl®
Synonyms Phentermine Hydrochloride
Pharmacologic Class Anorexiant
Nutrients Depleted
Specific nutrient depletions have not been documented for this agent.

- **Phentermine Hydrochloride** *see Phentermine on page 211*
- **Phenyldrine® [OTC]** *see Phenylpropanolamine on page 211*
- **Phenylephrine and Chlorpheniramine** *see Chlorpheniramine and Phenylephrine on page 73*
- **Phenylephrine and Guaifenesin** *see Guaifenesin and Phenylephrine on page 141*
- **Phenylephrine, Guaifenesin, and Phenylpropanolamine** *see Guaifenesin, Phenylpropanolamine, and Phenylephrine on page 142*
- **Phenylethylmalonylurea** *see Phenobarbital* on page 210*
- **Phenylfenesin® L.A.** *see Guaifenesin and Phenylpropanolamine on page 141*
- **Phenylisohydantoin** *see Pemoline on page 204*

Phenylpropanolamine (fen il proe pa NOLE a meen)
U.S. Brand Names Acutrim® 16 Hours [OTC]; Acutrim® II, Maximum Strength [OTC]; Acutrim® Late Day [OTC]; Control® [OTC]; Dexatrim® Pre-Meal [OTC]; Maximum Strength Dex-A-Diet® [OTC]; Maximum Strength Dexatrim® [OTC]; Phenoxine® [OTC]; Phenyldrine® [OTC]; Propagest® [OTC]; Unitrol® [OTC]
Synonyms *dl*-Norephedrine Hydrochloride; Phenylpropanolamine Hydrochloride; PPA
Pharmacologic Class Alpha/Beta Agonist
Nutrients Depleted
Specific nutrient depletions have not been documented for this agent.

- **Phenylpropanolamine and Brompheniramine** *see Brompheniramine and Phenylpropanolamine on page 50*
- **Phenylpropanolamine and Chlorpheniramine** *see Chlorpheniramine and Phenylpropanolamine on page 73*
- **Phenylpropanolamine and Guaifenesin** *see Guaifenesin and Phenylpropanolamine on page 141*

- ♦ **Phenylpropanolamine, Brompheniramine, and Codeine** *see* Brompheniramine, Phenylpropanolamine, and Codeine *on page 51*
- ♦ **Phenylpropanolamine, Guaifenesin, and Dextromethorphan** *see* Guaifenesin, Phenylpropanolamine, and Dextromethorphan *on page 142*
- ♦ **Phenylpropanolamine, Guaifenesin, and Phenylephrine** *see* Guaifenesin, Phenylpropanolamine, and Phenylephrine *on page 142*
- ♦ **Phenylpropanolamine Hydrochloride** *see* Phenylpropanolamine *on page 211*

Phenytoin* (FEN i toyn)

Related Information
Drug-Induced Nutrient Depletion Table *on page 498*

U.S. Brand Names Dilantin®; Diphenylan Sodium®

Canadian Brand Names Tremytoine®

Synonyms Diphenylhydantoin; DPH; Phenytoin Sodium; Phenytoin Sodium, Extended; Phenytoin Sodium, Prompt

Pharmacologic Class Antiarrhythmic Agent, Class I-B; Anticonvulsant, Hydantoin

Nutrients Depleted
Biotin *on page 311*
Calcium *on page 313*
Folic Acid *on page 325*
Vitamin B_1 *on page 351*
Vitamin B_{12} *on page 359*
Vitamin D *on page 363*
Vitamin K *on page 367*

Scientific Basis Published scientific studies using this pharmacologic agent

Studies & Abstracts 112-150

Additional Information The addition of folic acid to patients on a stable dose of phenytoin may alter serum concentrations and/or result in breakthrough seizures. Consultation with the prescriber and careful monitoring should be instituted prior to beginning supplementation.

- ♦ **Phenytoin Sodium** *see* Phenytoin* *on page 212*
- ♦ **Phenytoin Sodium, Extended** *see* Phenytoin* *on page 212*
- ♦ **Phenytoin Sodium, Prompt** *see* Phenytoin* *on page 212*
- ♦ **Phillips'® Milk of Magnesia [OTC]** *see* Magnesium Hydroxide* *on page 170*
- ♦ **PhosLo®** *see* Calcium Acetate *on page 55*
- ♦ **Phosphonoformate** *see* Foscarnet* *on page 134*
- ♦ **Phosphonoformic Acid** *see* Foscarnet* *on page 134*
- ♦ **Phrenilin®** *see* Butalbital Compound and Acetaminophen* *on page 53*
- ♦ **Phrenilin® Forte** *see* Butalbital Compound and Acetaminophen* *on page 53*
- ♦ **p-Hydroxyampicillin** *see* Amoxicillin* *on page 33*
- ♦ **Phyllocontin®** *see* Theophylline* *on page 250*

Pimozide (PI moe zide)
U.S. Brand Names Orap™
Pharmacologic Class Antipsychotic Agent, Diphenylbutylperidine
Nutrients Depleted
Specific nutrient depletions have not been documented for this agent.

Pindolol* (PIN doe lole)
Related Information
Drug-Induced Nutrient Depletion Table *on page 498*
U.S. Brand Names Visken®
Pharmacologic Class Beta Blocker (with Intrinsic Sympathomimetic Activity)
Nutrients Depleted
Coenzyme Q_{10} *on page 320*
Scientific Basis Published scientific studies using this pharmacologic agent
Studies & Abstracts 348-349

♦ **PIO** *see* Pemoline *on page 204*

Pioglitazone (pye oh GLI ta zone)
U.S. Brand Names Actos™
Pharmacologic Class Antidiabetic Agent (Thiazolidinedione)
Nutrients Depleted
Specific nutrient depletions have not been documented for this agent.

Piperacillin* (pi PER a sil in)
Related Information
Drug-Induced Nutrient Depletion Table *on page 498*
U.S. Brand Names Pipracil®
Synonyms Piperacillin Sodium
Pharmacologic Class Antibiotic, Penicillin
Nutrients Depleted
Bifidobacteria bifidum (bifidus) *on page 311*
Biotin *on page 311*
Inositol *on page 328*
Lactobacillus acidophilus *on page 332*
Potassium *on page 340*
Vitamin B_1 *on page 351*
Vitamin B_2 *on page 353*
Vitamin B_3 *on page 354*
Vitamin B_6 *on page 357*
Vitamin B_{12} *on page 359*
Vitamin K *on page 367*
Scientific Basis Inferred or indirect evidence of depletion based on disruption of physiologic processes
Studies & Abstracts 7-27, 49-57

Piperacillin and Tazobactam Sodium*
(pi PER a sil in & ta zoe BAK tam SOW dee um)
Related Information
Drug-Induced Nutrient Depletion Table *on page 498*
U.S. Brand Names Zosyn™
Synonyms Piperacillin Sodium and Tazobactam Sodium
Pharmacologic Class Antibiotic, Penicillin
Nutrients Depleted
Bifidobacteria bifidum (bifidus) on page 311
Biotin *on page 311*
Inositol *on page 328*
Lactobacillus acidophilus on page 332
Potassium *on page 340*
Vitamin B_1 *on page 351*
Vitamin B_2 *on page 353*
Vitamin B_3 *on page 354*
Vitamin B_6 *on page 357*
Vitamin B_{12} *on page 359*
Vitamin K *on page 367*
Scientific Basis Inferred or indirect evidence of depletion based on disruption of physiologic processes
Studies & Abstracts 7-27, 49-57

♦ **Piperacillin Sodium** *see* Piperacillin* *on page 213*
♦ **Piperacillin Sodium and Tazobactam Sodium** *see* Piperacillin and Tazobactam Sodium* *on page 214*
♦ **Piperazine Estrone Sulfate** *see* Estropipate* *on page 118*
♦ **Pipracil®** *see* Piperacillin* *on page 213*

Pirbuterol (peer BYOO ter ole)
U.S. Brand Names Maxair™ Inhalation Aerosol
Pharmacologic Class Beta$_2$ Agonist
Nutrients Depleted
Specific nutrient depletions have not been documented for this agent.

Piroxicam* (peer OKS i kam)
Related Information
Drug-Induced Nutrient Depletion Table *on page 498*
U.S. Brand Names Feldene®
Canadian Brand Names Apo®-Piroxicam; Novo-Piroxicam; Nu-Pirox; Pro-Piroxicam®
Pharmacologic Class Nonsteroidal Anti-Inflammatory Agent (NSAID)
Nutrients Depleted
Folic Acid *on page 325*
Scientific Basis
Published scientific studies using this pharmacologic agent
   or
Published scientific studies of agents from the same pharmacologic class

Studies & Abstracts 252

♦ **p-Isobutylhydratropic Acid** *see* Ibuprofen* *on page 153*
♦ **Plan B™** *see* Levonorgestrel* *on page 165*
♦ **Plantago Seed** *see* Psyllium *on page 226*
♦ **Plantain Seed** *see* Psyllium *on page 226*
♦ **Plaquenil®** *see* Hydroxychloroquine *on page 152*
♦ **Platinol®** *see* Cisplatin* *on page 78*
♦ **Platinol®-AQ** *see* Cisplatin* *on page 78*
♦ **Plavix®** *see* Clopidogrel *on page 81*
♦ **Plendil®** *see* Felodipine *on page 124*

Plicamycin* (plye kay MYE sin)
Related Information
  Drug-Induced Nutrient Depletion Table *on page 498*
U.S. Brand Names Mithracin®
Pharmacologic Class Antidote; Antineoplastic Agent, Antibiotic
Nutrients Depleted
  Calcium *on page 313*
Scientific Basis Published scientific studies using this pharmacologic agent
Studies & Abstracts 523-524

♦ **PMS-Amantadine** *see* Amantadine *on page 30*
♦ **PMS-Baclofen** *see* Baclofen *on page 44*
♦ **PMS-Benztropine** *see* Benztropine *on page 46*
♦ **PMS-Bethanechol Chloride** *see* Bethanechol *on page 47*
♦ **PMS-Carbamazepine** *see* Carbamazepine* *on page 57*
♦ **PMS-Chloral Hydrate** *see* Chloral Hydrate *on page 72*
♦ **PMS-Cholestyramine** *see* Cholestyramine Resin* *on page 75*
♦ **PMS-Clonazepam** *see* Clonazepam *on page 81*
♦ **PMS-Cyproheptadine** *see* Cyproheptadine *on page 89*
♦ **PMS-Desipramine** *see* Desipramine* *on page 94*
♦ **PMS-Diazepam** *see* Diazepam *on page 97*
♦ **PMS-Docusate Calcium** *see* Docusate *on page 104*
♦ **PMS-Dopazide** *see* Methyldopa and Hydrochlorothiazide* *on page 178*
♦ **PMS-Erythromycin** *see* Erythromycin (Systemic)* *on page 113*
♦ **PMS-Flupam** *see* Flurazepam *on page 131*
♦ **PMS-Fluphenazine** *see* Fluphenazine* *on page 131*
♦ **PMS-Hydromorphone** *see* Hydromorphone *on page 151*
♦ **PMS-Hydroxyzine** *see* Hydroxyzine *on page 152*
♦ **PMS-Imipramine** *see* Imipramine* *on page 154*
♦ **PMS-Isoniazid** *see* Isoniazid* *on page 158*
♦ **PMS-Ketoprofen** *see* Ketoprofen* *on page 160*
♦ **PMS-Levothyroxine Sodium** *see* Levothyroxine *on page 165*
♦ **PMS-Lindane** *see* Lindane *on page 166*
♦ **PMS-Lorazepam** *see* Lorazepam *on page 168*

- **PMS-Methylphenidate** *see* Methylphenidate *on page 178*
- **PMS-Oxazepam** *see* Oxazepam *on page 201*
- **PMS-Perphenazine** *see* Perphenazine* *on page 210*
- **PMS-Prochlorperazine** *see* Prochlorperazine* *on page 221*
- **PMS-Progesterone** *see* Progesterone *on page 221*
- **PMS-Pseudoephedrine** *see* Pseudoephedrine *on page 225*
- **PMS-Sodium Cromoglycate** *see* Cromolyn Sodium *on page 87*
- **PMS-Sulfasalazine** *see* Sulfasalazine* *on page 244*
- **PMS-Thioridazine** *see* Thioridazine* *on page 251*
- **Pneumomist®** *see* Guaifenesin *on page 140*
- **Poladex®** *see* Dexchlorpheniramine *on page 95*
- **Polaramine®** *see* Dexchlorpheniramine *on page 95*
- **Polycillin-N®** *see* Ampicillin* *on page 35*
- **Poly-Histine CS®** *see* Brompheniramine, Phenylpropanolamine, and Codeine *on page 51*

Polythiazide* (pol i THYE a zide)

U.S. Brand Names Renese®

Pharmacologic Class Diuretic, Thiazide

Nutrients Depleted

Coenzyme Q_{10} *on page 320*
Magnesium *on page 333*
Phosphorus *on page 339*
Potassium *on page 340*
Sodium *on page 345*
Zinc *on page 368*

Scientific Basis Published scientific studies of agents from the same pharmacologic class

Studies & Abstracts 320-342

Additional Information Although thiazide diuretics deplete sodium, replacement is not recommended, as this may be directly related to the therapeutic effect. Thiazides may deplete potassium, however replacement should be guided by monitoring of serum concentrations and specific instruction by a healthcare provider.

- **Pork NPH Iletin® II** *see* Insulin Preparations *on page 156*
- **Pork Regular Iletin® II** *see* Insulin Preparations *on page 156*
- **Porton Asparaginase** *see* Erwinia Asparaginase* *on page 112*
- **Potasalan®** *see* Potassium Chloride (Timed Release)* *on page 216*

Potassium Chloride (Timed Release)*

(poe TASS ee um KLOR ide)

Related Information

Drug-Induced Nutrient Depletion Table *on page 498*

U.S. Brand Names Cena-K®; Gen-K®; K+ 10®; Kaochlor®; Kaochlor® SF; Kaon-Cl®; Kaon Cl-10®; Kay Ciel®; K+ Care®; K-Dur® 10; K-Dur® 20; K-Lease®; K-Lor™; Klor-Con®; Klor-Con® 8; Klor-Con® 10; Klor-Con/25®; Klorvess®; Klotrix®; K-Lyte/Cl®; K-Norm®; K-Tab®; Micro-K® 10; Micro-K® Extencaps®; Micro-K® LS®; Potasalan®; Rum-K®; Slow-K®; Ten-K®

Synonyms KCl
Pharmacologic Class Electrolyte Supplement, Oral; Electrolyte Supplement, Parenteral; Potassium Salt
Nutrients Depleted
Vitamin B_{12} *on page 359*
Scientific Basis Published scientific studies using this pharmacologic agent
Studies & Abstracts 376-377

♦ **PPA** *see* Phenylpropanolamine *on page 211*

Pramipexole (pra mi PEX ole)
U.S. Brand Names Mirapex®
Pharmacologic Class Anti-Parkinson's Agent (Dopamine Agonist)
Nutrients Depleted
Specific nutrient depletions have not been documented for this agent.

♦ **Prandin™** *see* Repaglinide* *on page 230*
♦ **Pravachol®** *see* Pravastatin* *on page 217*

Pravastatin* (PRA va stat in)
Related Information
Drug-Induced Nutrient Depletion Table *on page 498*
U.S. Brand Names Pravachol®
Synonyms Pravastatin Sodium
Pharmacologic Class Antilipemic Agent (HMG-CoA Reductase Inhibitor)
Nutrients Depleted
Coenzyme Q_{10} *on page 320*
Scientific Basis Published scientific studies using this pharmacologic agent
Studies & Abstracts 350-361

♦ **Pravastatin Sodium** *see* Pravastatin* *on page 217*

Prazosin (PRA zoe sin)
U.S. Brand Names Minipress®
Canadian Brand Names Apo®-Prazo; Novo-Prazin; Nu-Prazo
Synonyms Furazosin; Prazosin Hydrochloride
Pharmacologic Class Alpha$_1$ Blockers
Nutrients Depleted
Specific nutrient depletions have not been documented for this agent.

Prazosin and Polythiazide*
(PRA zoe sin & pol i THYE a zide)
U.S. Brand Names Minizide®
Pharmacologic Class Antihypertensive Agent, Combination
Nutrients Depleted
Coenzyme Q_{10} *on page 320*
Magnesium *on page 333*
Phosphorus *on page 339*
Potassium *on page 340*
(Continued)

Prazosin and Polythiazide* *(Continued)*

Sodium *on page 345*
Zinc *on page 368*

Scientific Basis Published scientific studies of agents from the same pharmacologic class

Studies & Abstracts 320-342

Additional Information Sodium replacement is not recommended in patients receiving thiazides. Potassium replacement should be guided by serum level monitoring.

♦ **Prazosin Hydrochloride** *see* Prazosin *on page 217*

♦ **Precose®** *see* Acarbose *on page 22*

♦ **Predcor-TBA® Injection** *see* Prednisolone* *on page 218*

♦ **Pred Forte® Ophthalmic** *see* Prednisolone* *on page 218*

♦ **Pred Mild® Ophthalmic** *see* Prednisolone* *on page 218*

♦ **Prednicen-M®** *see* Prednisone* *on page 219*

Prednisolone* (pred NIS oh lone)

Related Information

Drug-Induced Nutrient Depletion Table *on page 498*

U.S. Brand Names AK-Pred® Ophthalmic; Articulose-50® Injection; Delta-Cortef® Oral; Econopred® Ophthalmic; Econopred® Plus Ophthalmic; Inflamase® Forte Ophthalmic; Inflamase® Mild Ophthalmic; Key-Pred® Injection; Key-Pred-SP® Injection; Pediapred® Oral; Predcor-TBA® Injection; Pred Forte® Ophthalmic; Pred Mild® Ophthalmic; Prednisol® TBA Injection; Prelone® Oral

Canadian Brand Names Novo-Prednisolone

Synonyms Deltahydrocortisone; Metacortandralone; Prednisolone Acetate; Prednisolone Acetate, Ophthalmic; Prednisolone Sodium Phosphate; Prednisolone Sodium Phosphate, Ophthalmic; Prednisolone Tebutate

Pharmacologic Class Corticosteroid, Ophthalmic; Corticosteroid, Parenteral

Nutrients Depleted

Calcium *on page 313*
Folic Acid *on page 325*
Magnesium *on page 333*
Potassium *on page 340*
Selenium *on page 343*
Vitamin C *on page 360*
Vitamin D *on page 363*
Zinc *on page 368*

Scientific Basis

Published scientific studies using this pharmacologic agent
or
Published scientific studies of agents from the same pharmacologic class

Studies & Abstracts 182-223

Additional Information Nutrient depletion with topical administration is limited.

- **Prednisolone Acetate** *see* Prednisolone* *on page 218*
- **Prednisolone Acetate, Ophthalmic** *see* Prednisolone* *on page 218*
- **Prednisolone Sodium Phosphate** *see* Prednisolone* *on page 218*
- **Prednisolone Sodium Phosphate, Ophthalmic** *see* Prednisolone* *on page 218*
- **Prednisolone Tebutate** *see* Prednisolone* *on page 218*
- **Prednisol® TBA Injection** *see* Prednisolone* *on page 218*

Prednisone* (PRED ni sone)

Related Information
Drug-Induced Nutrient Depletion Table *on page 498*

U.S. Brand Names Deltasone®; Liquid Pred®; Meticorten®; Orasone®; Prednicen-M®

Canadian Brand Names Apo®-Prednisone; Jaa-Prednisone®; Novo-Prednisone; Wimpred

Synonyms Deltacortisone; Deltadehydrocortisone

Pharmacologic Class Corticosteroid, Oral

Nutrients Depleted
Calcium *on page 313*
Folic Acid *on page 325*
Magnesium *on page 333*
Potassium *on page 340*
Selenium *on page 343*
Vitamin C *on page 360*
Vitamin D *on page 363*
Zinc *on page 368*

Scientific Basis
Published scientific studies using this pharmacologic agent
  or
Published scientific studies of agents from the same pharmacologic class

Studies & Abstracts 182-223

- **Pregnenedione** *see* Progesterone *on page 221*
- **Prelone® Oral** *see* Prednisolone* *on page 218*
- **Premarin®** *see* Estrogens (Conjugated)* *on page 117*
- **Premarin® With Methyltestosterone** *see* Estrogens and Methyltestosterone* *on page 117*
- **Premphase™** *see* Estrogen and Medroxyprogesterone* *on page 116*
- **Prempro™** *see* Estrogen and Medroxyprogesterone* *on page 116*
- **Prevacid®** *see* Lansoprazole* *on page 163*
- **Prevalite®** *see* Cholestyramine Resin* *on page 75*
- **PREVEN™** *see* Ethinyl Estradiol and Levonorgestrel* *on page 120*
- **Priftin®** *see* Rifapentine* *on page 232*
- **Prilosec™** *see* Omeprazole* *on page 199*
- **Primaclone** *see* Primidone* *on page 220*

Primidone* (PRI mi done)
Related Information
  Drug-Induced Nutrient Depletion Table *on page 498*
U.S. Brand Names Mysoline®
Canadian Brand Names Apo®-Primidone; Sertan®
Synonyms Desoxyphenobarbital; Primaclone
Pharmacologic Class Anticonvulsant, Miscellaneous
Nutrients Depleted
  Biotin *on page 311*
  Calcium *on page 313*
  Folic Acid *on page 325*
  Vitamin D *on page 363*
  Vitamin K *on page 367*
Scientific Basis Published scientific studies using this pharmacologic agent and related agents
Studies & Abstracts 151-156

- **Primsol**® *see* Trimethoprim* *on page 262*
- **Principen**® *see* Ampicillin* *on page 35*
- **Prinivil**® *see* Lisinopril* *on page 166*
- **ProAmatine** *see* Midodrine *on page 181*
- **Pro-Amox**® *see* Amoxicillin* *on page 33*
- **Pro-Ampi**® **Trihydrate** *see* Ampicillin* *on page 35*
- **Proaqua**® *see* Benzthiazide* *on page 45*

Probenecid (proe BEN e sid)
Canadian Brand Names Benuryl™
Pharmacologic Class Uricosuric Agent
Nutrients Depleted
  Specific nutrient depletions have not been documented for this agent.

- **Probenecid and Colchicine** *see* Colchicine and Probenecid* *on page 84*

Procainamide (proe kane A mide)
U.S. Brand Names Procanbid®; Pronestyl®
Canadian Brand Names Apo®-Procainamide
Synonyms PCA; Procainamide Hydrochloride; Procaine Amide Hydrochloride
Pharmacologic Class Antiarrhythmic Agent, Class I-A
Nutrients Depleted
  Specific nutrient depletions have not been documented for this agent.

- **Procainamide Hydrochloride** *see* Procainamide *on page 220*
- **Procaine Amide Hydrochloride** *see* Procainamide *on page 220*
- **Procaine Benzylpenicillin** *see* Penicillin G Procaine* *on page 207*
- **Procaine Penicillin G** *see* Penicillin G Procaine* *on page 207*
- **Pro-Cal-Sof**® **[OTC]** *see* Docusate *on page 104*
- **Procanbid**® *see* Procainamide *on page 220*

Procarbazine* (proe KAR ba zeen)
U.S. Brand Names Matulane®
Synonyms Benzmethyzin; N-Methylhydrazine; Procarbazine Hydrochloride
Pharmacologic Class Antineoplastic Agent, Alkylating Agent
Nutrients Depleted
See Nutrient Depletion and Cancer Chemotherapy *on page 515.*
Scientific Basis Inferred or indirect evidence of depletion based on disruption of physiologic processes

♦ **Procarbazine Hydrochloride** *see* Procarbazine* *on page 221*

♦ **Procardia**® *see* Nifedipine *on page 192*

♦ **Procardia XL**® *see* Nifedipine *on page 192*

♦ **Procetofene** *see* Fenofibrate* *on page 124*

Prochlorperazine* (proe klor PER a zeen)
U.S. Brand Names Compazine®
Canadian Brand Names Nu-Prochlor; PMS-Prochlorperazine; Prorazin®; Stemetil®
Synonyms Prochlorperazine Edisylate; Prochlorperazine Maleate
Pharmacologic Class Antipsychotic Agent, Phenothazine, Piperazine
Nutrients Depleted
Coenzyme Q_{10} *on page 320*
Vitamin B_2 *on page 353*
Scientific Basis Published scientific studies of agents from the same pharmacologic class
Studies & Abstracts 474-477

♦ **Prochlorperazine Edisylate** *see* Prochlorperazine* *on page 221*

♦ **Prochlorperazine Maleate** *see* Prochlorperazine* *on page 221*

♦ **Procort**® **[OTC]** *see* Hydrocortisone* *on page 150*

♦ **Proctocort**™ *see* Hydrocortisone* *on page 150*

♦ **Proctofene** *see* Fenofibrate* *on page 124*

♦ **Procytox**® *see* Cyclophosphamide* *on page 88*

♦ **Prodiem**® **Plain** *see* Psyllium *on page 226*

♦ **Profenal**® **Ophthalmic** *see* Suprofen* *on page 245*

♦ **Profen II**® *see* Guaifenesin and Phenylpropanolamine *on page 141*

♦ **Profen II DM**® *see* Guaifenesin, Phenylpropanolamine, and Dextromethorphan *on page 142*

♦ **Profen LA**® *see* Guaifenesin and Phenylpropanolamine *on page 141*

♦ **Progestasert**® *see* Progesterone *on page 221*

Progesterone (proe JES ter one)
U.S. Brand Names Crinone™; Progestasert®; Prometrium®
Canadian Brand Names PMS-Progesterone; Progesterone Oil
Synonyms Pregnenedione; Progestin
Pharmacologic Class Progestin
Nutrients Depleted
Specific nutrient depletions have not been documented for this agent.

- **Progesterone Oil** see Progesterone *on page 221*
- **Progestin** see Progesterone *on page 221*
- **Prograf®** see Tacrolimus* *on page 246*
- **Pro-Indo®** see Indomethacin* *on page 155*
- **Prolixin Decanoate® Injection** see Fluphenazine* *on page 131*
- **Prolixin Enanthate® Injection** see Fluphenazine* *on page 131*
- **Prolixin® Injection** see Fluphenazine* *on page 131*
- **Prolixin® Oral** see Fluphenazine* *on page 131*
- **Proloprim®** see Trimethoprim* *on page 262*
- **Pro-Lorazepam®** see Lorazepam *on page 168*

Promazine* (PROE ma zeen)
U.S. Brand Names Sparine®
Synonyms Promazine Hydrochloride
Pharmacologic Class Antipsychotic Agent, Phenothiazine, Aliphatic
Nutrients Depleted
Coenzyme Q_{10} *on page 320*
Vitamin B_2 *on page 353*
Scientific Basis Published scientific studies of agents from the same pharmacologic class
Studies & Abstracts 474-477

- **Promazine Hydrochloride** see Promazine* *on page 222*

Promethazine* (proe METH a zeen)
U.S. Brand Names Anergan®; Phenazine®; Phenergan®; Prorex®
Synonyms Promethazine Hydrochloride
Pharmacologic Class Antiemetic
Nutrients Depleted
Coenzyme Q_{10} *on page 320*
Vitamin B_2 *on page 353*
Scientific Basis Published scientific studies of agents from the same pharmacologic class
Studies & Abstracts 474-477

- **Promethazine Hydrochloride** see Promethazine* *on page 222*
- **Prometrium®** see Progesterone *on page 221*
- **Pronestyl®** see Procainamide *on page 220*
- **Propacet®** see Propoxyphene and Acetaminophen* *on page 223*

Propafenone* (proe pa FEEN one)
U.S. Brand Names Rythmol®
Synonyms Propafenone Hydrochloride
Pharmacologic Class Antiarrhythmic Agent, Class I-C
Nutrients Depleted
Coenzyme Q_{10} *on page 320*
Scientific Basis Published scientific studies of agents with the same mechanism of action (specifically, beta-blocking activity)
Studies & Abstracts 348-349

- **Propafenone Hydrochloride** see Propafenone* *on page 222*

- **Propagest**® [OTC] *see* Phenylpropanolamine *on page 211*
- **Pro-Piroxicam**® *see* Piroxicam* *on page 214*

Propoxyphene (proe POKS i feen)

U.S. Brand Names Darvon®; Darvon-N®; Dolene®

Canadian Brand Names Novo-Propoxyn; 624® Tablets

Synonyms Dextropropoxyphene; Propoxyphene Hydrochloride; Propoxyphene Napsylate

Pharmacologic Class Analgesic, Narcotic

Nutrients Depleted

Specific nutrient depletions have not been documented for this agent.

Propoxyphene and Acetaminophen*

(proe POKS i feen & a seet a MIN oh fen)

U.S. Brand Names Darvocet-N®; Darvocet-N® 100; Propacet®; Wygesic®

Synonyms Propoxyphene Hydrochloride and Acetaminophen; Propoxyphene Napsylate and Acetaminophen

Pharmacologic Class Analgesic, Combination (Narcotic)

Nutrients Depleted

Glutathione *on page 327*

Scientific Basis Published scientific studies using this pharmacologic agent (acetaminophen)

Studies & Abstracts 517-518

- **Propoxyphene Hydrochloride** *see* Propoxyphene *on page 223*
- **Propoxyphene Hydrochloride and Acetaminophen** *see* Propoxyphene and Acetaminophen* *on page 223*
- **Propoxyphene Napsylate** *see* Propoxyphene *on page 223*
- **Propoxyphene Napsylate and Acetaminophen** *see* Propoxyphene and Acetaminophen* *on page 223*

Propranolol* (proe PRAN oh lole)

Related Information

Drug-Induced Nutrient Depletion Table *on page 498*

U.S. Brand Names Betachron E-R® Capsule; Inderal®; Inderal® LA

Canadian Brand Names Apo®-Propranolol; Detensol®; Nu-Propranolol

Synonyms Propranolol Hydrochloride

Pharmacologic Class Antiarrhythmic Agent, Class II; Beta Blocker, Nonselective

Nutrients Depleted

Coenzyme Q_{10} *on page 320*

Scientific Basis

Published scientific studies using this pharmacologic agent

or

Published scientific studies of agents from the same pharmacologic class

Studies & Abstracts 348-349

Propranolol and Hydrochlorothiazide*
(proe PRAN oh lole & hye droe klor oh THYE a zide)

U.S. Brand Names Inderide®

Synonyms Hydrochlorothiazide and Propranolol

Pharmacologic Class Antihypertensive Agent, Combination

Nutrients Depleted

Coenzyme Q_{10} *on page 320*

Magnesium *on page 333*

Phosphorus *on page 339*

Potassium *on page 340*

Sodium *on page 345*

Zinc *on page 368*

Scientific Basis

Published scientific studies using these pharmacologic agents

or

Published scientific studies of agents from the same pharmacologic class

Studies & Abstracts 320-342, 348-349

Additional Information Although thiazide diuretics deplete sodium, replacement is not recommended, as this may be directly related to the therapeutic effect. Thiazides may deplete potassium, however replacement should be guided by monitoring of serum concentrations and specific instruction by a healthcare provider.

- ◆ **Propranolol Hydrochloride** *see* Propranolol* *on page 223*
- ◆ **2-Propylpentanoic Acid** *see* Valproic Acid and Derivatives* *on page 265*

Propylthiouracil (proe pil thye oh YOOR a sil)
Canadian Brand Names Propyl-Thyracil®

Synonyms PTU

Pharmacologic Class Antithyroid Agent

Nutrients Depleted

Specific nutrient depletions have not been documented for this agent.

- ◆ **Propyl-Thyracil®** *see* Propylthiouracil *on page 224*
- ◆ **2-Propylvaleric Acid** *see* Valproic Acid and Derivatives* *on page 265*
- ◆ **Prorazin®** *see* Prochlorperazine* *on page 221*
- ◆ **Prorex®** *see* Promethazine* *on page 222*
- ◆ **Proscar®** *see* Finasteride *on page 127*
- ◆ **Pro-Sof® Plus [OTC]** *see* Docusate and Casanthranol* *on page 104*
- ◆ **ProSom™** *see* Estazolam *on page 113*
- ◆ **Prostaglandin E_1** *see* Alprostadil *on page 28*
- ◆ **ProStep® Patch** *see* Nicotine *on page 191*
- ◆ **Prostin VR Pediatric® Injection** *see* Alprostadil *on page 28*
- ◆ **Protonix®** *see* Pantoprazole* *on page 204*
- ◆ **Protostat® Oral** *see* Metronidazole* *on page 180*
- ◆ **Pro-Trin®** *see* Co-Trimoxazole* *on page 86*

Protriptyline* (proe TRIP ti leen)
U.S. Brand Names Vivactil®

Canadian Brand Names Triptil®

Synonyms Protriptyline Hydrochloride

Pharmacologic Class Antidepressant, Tricyclic (Secondary Amine)

Nutrients Depleted

Coenzyme Q$_{10}$ on page 320

Vitamin B$_2$ on page 353

Scientific Basis Published scientific studies of agents from the same pharmacologic class

Studies & Abstracts 467-472

♦ **Protriptyline Hydrochloride** see Protriptyline* on page 225

♦ **Proventil®** see Albuterol on page 26

♦ **Proventil® HFA** see Albuterol on page 26

♦ **Provera® Oral** see Medroxyprogesterone Acetate on page 173

♦ **Provigil®** see Modafinil on page 183

♦ **Prozac®** see Fluoxetine on page 130

Pseudoephedrine (soo doe e FED rin)
U.S. Brand Names Actifed® Allergy Tablet (Day) [OTC]; Afrin® Tablet [OTC]; Cenafed® [OTC]; Children's Silfedrine® [OTC]; Decofed® Syrup [OTC]; Drixoral® Non-Drowsy [OTC]; Efidac/24® [OTC]; Pedia Care® Oral; Sudafed® [OTC]; Sudafed® 12 Hour [OTC]; Triaminic® AM Decongestant Formula [OTC]

Canadian Brand Names Balminil® Decongestant; Eltor®; PMS-Pseudoephedrine; Robidrine®

Synonyms d-Isoephedrine Hydrochloride; Pseudoephedrine Hydrochloride; Pseudoephedrine Sulfate

Pharmacologic Class Alpha/Beta Agonist

Nutrients Depleted

Specific nutrient depletions have not been documented for this agent.

♦ **Pseudoephedrine and Chlorpheniramine** see Chlorpheniramine and Pseudoephedrine on page 73

Pseudoephedrine and Dextromethorphan
(soo doe e FED rin & deks troe meth OR fan)

U.S. Brand Names Drixoral® Cough & Congestion Liquid Caps [OTC]; Vicks® 44D Cough & Head Congestion; Vicks® 44 Non-Drowsy Cold & Cough Liqui-Caps [OTC]

Pharmacologic Class Antitussive/Decongestant

Nutrients Depleted

Specific nutrient depletions have not been documented for this agent.

♦ **Pseudoephedrine and Guaifenesin** see Guaifenesin and Pseudoephedrine on page 142

Pseudoephedrine and Ibuprofen*
(soo doe e FED rin & eye byoo PROE fen)

U.S. Brand Names Advil® Cold & Sinus Caplets [OTC]; Dimetapp® Sinus Caplets [OTC]; Dristan® Sinus Caplets [OTC]; Motrin® IB Sinus [OTC]; Sine-Aid® IB [OTC]

Pharmacologic Class Decongestant/Analgesic

Nutrients Depleted

Folic Acid *on page 325*

Scientific Basis

Published scientific studies using this pharmacologic agent (ibuprofen)

or

Published scientific studies of agents from the same pharmacologic class

Studies & Abstracts 252

- ♦ **Pseudoephedrine and Loratadine** *see* Loratadine and Pseudoephedrine *on page 168*
- ♦ **Pseudoephedrine, Dextromethorphan, and Guaifenesin** *see* Guaifenesin, Pseudoephedrine, and Dextromethorphan *on page 143*
- ♦ **Pseudoephedrine, Guaifenesin, and Codeine** *see* Guaifenesin, Pseudoephedrine, and Codeine *on page 143*
- ♦ **Pseudoephedrine Hydrochloride** *see* Pseudoephedrine *on page 225*
- ♦ **Pseudoephedrine Sulfate** *see* Pseudoephedrine *on page 225*
- ♦ **Pseudo-Gest Plus® Tablet [OTC]** *see* Chlorpheniramine and Pseudoephedrine *on page 73*
- ♦ **Psorcon™** *see* Diflorasone* *on page 99*

Psyllium (SIL i yum)

U.S. Brand Names Effer-Syllium® [OTC]; Fiberall® Powder [OTC]; Fiberall® Wafer [OTC]; Hydrocil® [OTC]; Konsyl® [OTC]; Konsyl-D® [OTC]; Metamucil® [OTC]; Metamucil® Instant Mix [OTC]; Modane® Bulk [OTC]; Perdiem® Plain [OTC]; Reguloid® [OTC]; Serutan® [OTC]; Syllact® [OTC]; V-Lax® [OTC]

Canadian Brand Names Fibrepur®; Novo-Mucilax; Prodiem® Plain

Synonyms Plantago Seed; Plantain Seed; Psyllium Hydrophilic Mucilloid

Pharmacologic Class Laxative, Bulk-Producing

Nutrients Depleted

Specific nutrient depletions have not been documented for this agent.

- ♦ **Psyllium Hydrophilic Mucilloid** *see* Psyllium *on page 226*
- ♦ **PTU** *see* Propylthiouracil *on page 224*
- ♦ **Pulmicort®** *see* Budesonide* *on page 51*
- ♦ **Pulmicort® Turbuhaler®** *see* Budesonide* *on page 51*
- ♦ **Pulmophylline** *see* Theophylline* *on page 250*
- ♦ **Purinol®** *see* Allopurinol *on page 27*
- ♦ **PVF® K** *see* Penicillin V Potassium* *on page 207*

Quazepam (KWAY ze pam)
U.S. Brand Names Doral®
Pharmacologic Class Benzodiazepine
Nutrients Depleted
Specific nutrient depletions have not been documented for this agent.

♦ **Questran®** *see* Cholestyramine Resin* *on page 75*
♦ **Questran® Light** *see* Cholestyramine Resin* *on page 75*

Quetiapine (kwe TYE a peen)
U.S. Brand Names Seroquel®
Synonyms Quetiapine Fumarate
Pharmacologic Class Antipsychotic Agent, Dibenzothiazepine
Nutrients Depleted
Specific nutrient depletions have not been documented for this agent.

♦ **Quetiapine Fumarate** *see* Quetiapine *on page 227*
♦ **Quibron®-T** *see* Theophylline* *on page 250*
♦ **Quibron®-T/SR** *see* Theophylline* *on page 250*

Quinapril* (KWIN a pril)
Related Information
Drug-Induced Nutrient Depletion Table *on page 498*
U.S. Brand Names Accupril®
Synonyms Quinapril Hydrochloride
Pharmacologic Class Angiotensin-Converting Enzyme (ACE) Inhibitors
Nutrients Depleted
Zinc *on page 368*
Scientific Basis Published scientific studies of agents from the same pharmacologic class
Studies & Abstracts 269-271

♦ **Quinapril Hydrochloride** *see* Quinapril* *on page 227*

Quinestrol* (kwin ES trole)
U.S. Brand Names Estrovis®
Pharmacologic Class Estrogen Derivative
Nutrients Depleted
Magnesium *on page 333*
Vitamin B_6 *on page 357*
Scientific Basis Published scientific studies of agents from the same pharmacologic class
Studies & Abstracts 378-379

Quinethazone* (kwin ETH a zone)
U.S. Brand Names Hydromox®
Pharmacologic Class Diuretic, Thiazide
Nutrients Depleted
Coenzyme Q_{10} *on page 320*
(Continued)

Quinethazone* *(Continued)*

Magnesium *on page 333*
Potassium *on page 340*
Zinc *on page 368*

Scientific Basis Published scientific studies of agents from the same pharmacologic class

Studies & Abstracts 320-342

♦ **Quixin™ Ophthalmic** *see* Levofloxacin* *on page 164*

♦ **QYS®** *see* Hydroxyzine *on page 152*

Rabeprazole* (ra BE pray zole)

U.S. Brand Names Aciphex™

Synonyms Pariprazole

Pharmacologic Class Gastric Acid Secretion Inhibitor

Nutrients Depleted

Vitamin B_{12} *on page 359*

Scientific Basis Published scientific studies of agents from the same pharmacologic class

Studies & Abstracts 511-516

♦ **Racemic Amphetamine Sulfate** *see* Amphetamine *on page 33*

♦ **R-albuterol** *see* Levalbuterol *on page 163*

Raloxifene* (ral OX i feen)

Related Information

Drug-Induced Nutrient Depletion Table *on page 498*

U.S. Brand Names Evista®

Synonyms Keoxifene Hydrochloride; Raloxifene Hydrochloride

Pharmacologic Class Selective Estrogen Receptor Modulator (SERM)

Nutrients Depleted

Magnesium *on page 333*
Vitamin B_6 *on page 357*

Scientific Basis Published scientific studies of agents with the same mechanism of action

Studies & Abstracts 378-379

♦ **Raloxifene Hydrochloride** *see* Raloxifene* *on page 228*

Ramipril* (ra MI pril)

Related Information

Drug-Induced Nutrient Depletion Table *on page 498*

U.S. Brand Names Altace™

Pharmacologic Class Angiotensin-Converting Enzyme (ACE) Inhibitors

Nutrients Depleted

Zinc *on page 368*

Scientific Basis Published scientific studies of agents from the same pharmacologic class

Studies & Abstracts 269-271

Ranitidine Bismuth Citrate*

(ra NI ti deen BIZ muth SIT rate)

U.S. Brand Names Tritec®

Synonyms GR1222311X; RBC

Pharmacologic Class Histamine H_2 Antagonist

Nutrients Depleted

Calcium *on page 313*

Folic Acid *on page 325*

Iron *on page 331*

Vitamin B_{12} *on page 359*

Vitamin D *on page 363*

Zinc *on page 368*

Scientific Basis Published scientific studies using this pharmacologic agent

Studies & Abstracts 484-510

Ranitidine Hydrochloride*

(ra NI ti deen hye droe KLOR ide)

Related Information

Drug-Induced Nutrient Depletion Table *on page 498*

U.S. Brand Names Zantac®; Zantac® 75 [OTC]

Canadian Brand Names Apo®-Ranitidine; Novo-Ranidine; Nu-Ranit

Pharmacologic Class Histamine H_2 Antagonist

Nutrients Depleted

Calcium *on page 313*

Folic Acid *on page 325*

Iron *on page 331*

Vitamin B_{12} *on page 359*

Vitamin D *on page 363*

Zinc *on page 368*

Scientific Basis Published scientific studies using this pharmacologic agent

Studies & Abstracts 484-510

- **Rapamune®** *see Sirolimus* on page 238*
- **RBC** *see Ranitidine Bismuth Citrate* on page 229*
- **Redutemp® [OTC]** *see Acetaminophen* on page 23*
- **Reglan®** *see Metoclopramide on page 179*
- **Regulace® [OTC]** *see Docusate and Casanthranol* on page 104*
- **Regular (Concentrated) Iletin® II U-500** *see Insulin Preparations on page 156*
- **Regular Iletin® I** *see Insulin Preparations on page 156*
- **Regular Insulin** *see Insulin Preparations on page 156*
- **Regular Purified Pork Insulin** *see Insulin Preparations on page 156*
- **Regular Strength Bayer® Enteric 500 Aspirin [OTC]** *see Aspirin* on page 40*
- **Regulax SS® [OTC]** *see Docusate on page 104*
- **Regulex®** *see Docusate on page 104*
- **Reguloid® [OTC]** *see Psyllium on page 226*

- **Relenza**® *see* Zanamivir *on page 270*
- **Remicade**™ *see* Infliximab *on page 155*
- **Renedil**® *see* Felodipine *on page 124*
- **Renese**® *see* Polythiazide* *on page 216*
- **Renormax**® *see* Spirapril* *on page 241*
- **Renova**® *see* Tretinoin (Topical) *on page 259*

Repaglinide* (re PAG li nide)
Related Information
Drug-Induced Nutrient Depletion Table *on page 498*
U.S. Brand Names Prandin™
Pharmacologic Class Antidiabetic Agent (Miscellaneous)
Nutrients Depleted
Coenzyme Q_{10} *on page 320*
Scientific Basis Published scientific studies of agents with the same mechanism of action
Studies & Abstracts 167

- **Repan**® *see* Butalbital Compound and Acetaminophen* *on page 53*
- **Reposans-10**® **Oral** *see* Chlordiazepoxide *on page 72*
- **Resaid**® *see* Chlorpheniramine and Phenylpropanolamine *on page 73*
- **Rescon Liquid [OTC]** *see* Chlorpheniramine and Phenylpropanolamine *on page 73*
- **Rescriptor**® *see* Delavirdine* *on page 92*
- **Reserpine and Hydrochlorothiazide** *see* Hydrochlorothiazide and Reserpine* *on page 148*
- **Reserpine, Hydralazine, and Hydrochlorothiazide** *see* Hydralazine, Hydrochlorothiazide, and Reserpine* *on page 147*
- **Respa-1st**® *see* Guaifenesin and Pseudoephedrine *on page 142*
- **Respa**®**-DM** *see* Guaifenesin and Dextromethorphan *on page 141*
- **Respa-GF**® *see* Guaifenesin *on page 140*
- **Respaire**®**-60 SR** *see* Guaifenesin and Pseudoephedrine *on page 142*
- **Respaire**®**-120 SR** *see* Guaifenesin and Pseudoephedrine *on page 142*
- **Respbid**® *see* Theophylline* *on page 250*
- **Restoril**® *see* Temazepam *on page 248*
- **Retin-A**® **Micro Topical** *see* Tretinoin (Topical) *on page 259*
- **Retin-A**® **Topical** *see* Tretinoin (Topical) *on page 259*
- **Retinoic Acid** *see* Tretinoin (Topical) *on page 259*
- **Retisol-A**® *see* Tretinoin (Topical) *on page 259*
- **Retrovir**® *see* Zidovudine* *on page 270*
- **Revex**® *see* Nalmefene *on page 188*
- **ReVia**® *see* Naltrexone *on page 188*
- **rGM-CSF** *see* Sargramostim *on page 236*
- **Rheumatrex**® *see* Methotrexate* *on page 176*
- **Rhinalar**® *see* Flunisolide* *on page 129*
- **Rhinaris**®**-F** *see* Flunisolide* *on page 129*

- **Rhinocort**® *see* Budesonide* *on page 51*
- **Rhinocort**® **Aqua**™ *see* Budesonide* *on page 51*
- **Rhinosyn-DMX**® **[OTC]** *see* Guaifenesin and Dextromethorphan *on page 141*
- **Rhinosyn**® **Liquid [OTC]** *see* Chlorpheniramine and Pseudoephedrine *on page 73*
- **Rhinosyn-PD**® **Liquid [OTC]** *see* Chlorpheniramine and Pseudoephedrine *on page 73*
- **Rhinosyn-X**® **Liquid [OTC]** *see* Guaifenesin, Pseudoephedrine, and Dextromethorphan *on page 143*
- **Rhodis**™ *see* Ketoprofen* *on page 160*
- **Rhodis-EC**™ *see* Ketoprofen* *on page 160*
- **Rhoprolene** *see* Betamethasone* *on page 46*
- **Rhoprosone** *see* Betamethasone* *on page 46*
- **Rhotral** *see* Acebutolol* *on page 22*
- **Rhotrimine**® *see* Trimipramine* *on page 262*
- **Ridene** *see* Nicardipine *on page 191*
- **Ridenol**® **[OTC]** *see* Acetaminophen* *on page 23*

Rifabutin* (rif a BYOO tin)
U.S. Brand Names Mycobutin®
Synonyms Ansamycin
Pharmacologic Class Antibiotic, Miscellaneous; Antitubercular Agent
Nutrients Depleted
 Vitamin D *on page 363*
Scientific Basis Published scientific studies of agents from the same pharmacologic class
Studies & Abstracts 59-61

- **Rifadin**® *see* Rifampin* *on page 231*
- **Rifadin**® **Injection** *see* Rifampin* *on page 231*
- **Rifadin**® **Oral** *see* Rifampin* *on page 231*
- **Rifamate**® *see* Rifampin and Isoniazid* *on page 232*
- **Rifampicin** *see* Rifampin* *on page 231*

Rifampin* (RIF am pin)
Related Information
 Drug-Induced Nutrient Depletion Table *on page 498*
U.S. Brand Names Rifadin® Injection; Rifadin® Oral; Rimactane® Oral
Canadian Brand Names Rifadin®; Rimactane®; Rofact™
Synonyms Rifampicin
Pharmacologic Class Antibiotic, Miscellaneous; Antitubercular Agent
Nutrients Depleted
 Vitamin D *on page 363*
Scientific Basis Published scientific studies using this pharmacologic agent
Studies & Abstracts 59-61

Rifampin and Isoniazid* (RIF am pin & eye soe NYE a zid)
U.S. Brand Names Rifamate®
Synonyms Isoniazid and Rifampin
Pharmacologic Class Antibiotic, Miscellaneous
Nutrients Depleted
  Vitamin B_3 *on page 354*
  Vitamin B_6 *on page 357*
  Vitamin D *on page 363*
Scientific Basis Published scientific studies using these pharmacologic agents
Studies & Abstracts 39-48, 59-61

Rifapentine* (RIF a pen teen)
U.S. Brand Names Priftin®
Pharmacologic Class Antitubercular Agent
Nutrients Depleted
  Vitamin D *on page 363*
Scientific Basis Published scientific studies of agents from the same pharmacologic class
Studies & Abstracts 59-61

♦ **rIFN-b** *see* Interferon Beta-1a *on page 156*
♦ **Rilutek®** *see* Riluzole *on page 232*

Riluzole (RIL yoo zole)
U.S. Brand Names Rilutek®
Synonyms 2-Amino-6-Trifluoromethoxy-benzothiazole; RP54274
Pharmacologic Class Glutamate Inhibitor
Nutrients Depleted
  Specific nutrient depletions have not been documented for this agent.

♦ **Rimactane®** *see* Rifampin* *on page 231*
♦ **Rimactane® Oral** *see* Rifampin* *on page 231*

Rimantadine (ri MAN ta deen)
U.S. Brand Names Flumadine®
Synonyms Rimantadine Hydrochloride
Pharmacologic Class Antiviral Agent
Nutrients Depleted
  Specific nutrient depletions have not been documented for this agent.

♦ **Rimantadine Hydrochloride** *see* Rimantadine *on page 232*
♦ **Riphenidate** *see* Methylphenidate *on page 178*

Risedronate (ris ED roe nate)
U.S. Brand Names Actonel™
Synonyms Risedronate Sodium
Pharmacologic Class Bisphosphonate Derivative
Nutrients Depleted
  Specific nutrient depletions have not been documented for this agent.

Additional Information Bisphosphonates have been (rarely) associated with hypocalcemia, as a natural extension of their therapeutic action. Correction of hypocalcemia is recommended prior to treatment. When used for Paget's disease, adequate vitamin D and calcium intake should be ensured to provide for enhanced needs. Calcium administration should be separated from risedronate by at least 30 minutes.

♦ **Risedronate Sodium** *see* Risedronate *on page 232*
♦ **Risperdal®** *see* Risperidone *on page 233*

Risperidone (ris PER i done)
U.S. Brand Names Risperdal®
Pharmacologic Class Antipsychotic Agent, Benzisoxazole
Nutrients Depleted
Specific nutrient depletions have not been documented for this agent.

♦ **Ritalin®** *see* Methylphenidate *on page 178*
♦ **Ritalin-SR®** *see* Methylphenidate *on page 178*

Ritonavir (rye TON a veer)
U.S. Brand Names Norvir®
Pharmacologic Class Antiretroviral Agent, Reverse Transcriptase Inhibitor (Non-Nucleoside)
Nutrients Depleted
Specific nutrient depletions have not been documented for this agent.

Rivastigmine (ri va STIG meen)
U.S. Brand Names Exelon®
Pharmacologic Class Acetylcholinesterase Inhibitor (Central)
Nutrients Depleted
Specific nutrient depletions have not been documented for this agent.

♦ **Rivotril®** *see* Clonazepam *on page 81*
♦ **rIFN-b** *see* Interferon Beta-1b *on page 156*
♦ **RMS® Rectal** *see* Morphine Sulfate *on page 185*
♦ **Robafen® CF [OTC]** *see* Guaifenesin, Phenylpropanolamine, and Dextromethorphan *on page 142*
♦ **Robafen DM® [OTC]** *see* Guaifenesin and Dextromethorphan *on page 141*
♦ **Robaxin®** *see* Methocarbamol *on page 176*
♦ **Robaxisal®** *see* Methocarbamol and Aspirin* *on page 176*
♦ **Robicillin® VK** *see* Penicillin V Potassium* *on page 207*
♦ **Robidrine®** *see* Pseudoephedrine *on page 225*
♦ **Robitussin® [OTC]** *see* Guaifenesin *on page 140*
♦ **Robitussin-CF® [OTC]** *see* Guaifenesin, Phenylpropanolamine, and Dextromethorphan *on page 142*
♦ **Robitussin® Cough Calmers [OTC]** *see* Dextromethorphan *on page 96*
♦ **Robitussin®-DAC** *see* Guaifenesin, Pseudoephedrine, and Codeine *on page 143*

- **Robitussin®-DM [OTC]** *see* Guaifenesin and Dextromethorphan *on page 141*
- **Robitussin-PE® [OTC]** *see* Guaifenesin and Pseudoephedrine *on page 142*
- **Robitussin® Pediatric [OTC]** *see* Dextromethorphan *on page 96*
- **Robitussin® Severe Congestion Liqui-Gels® [OTC]** *see* Guaifenesin and Pseudoephedrine *on page 142*
- **Rocephin®** *see* Ceftriaxone* *on page 67*
- **Rofact™** *see* Rifampin* *on page 231*

Rofecoxib* (roe fe COX ib)
U.S. Brand Names Vioxx®
Pharmacologic Class Nonsteroidal Anti-inflammatory Drug (NSAID), COX-2 Selective
Nutrients Depleted
Folic Acid *on page 325*
Scientific Basis Inferred or indirect evidence of depletion based on disruption of physiologic processes
Studies & Abstracts 252
Additional Information Selective COX-2 inhibitors may not share potential depletions of nonselective agents

- **Rolatuss® Plain Liquid** *see* Chlorpheniramine and Phenylephrine *on page 73*

Rosiglitazone (ROSE i gli ta zone)
U.S. Brand Names Avandia®
Pharmacologic Class Antidiabetic Agent (Thiazolidinedione)
Nutrients Depleted
Specific nutrient depletions have not been documented for this agent.

- **Roubac®** *see* Co-Trimoxazole* *on page 86*
- **Rowasa® Rectal** *see* Mesalamine* *on page 174*
- **Roxanol™ Oral** *see* Morphine Sulfate *on page 185*
- **Roxanol Rescudose®** *see* Morphine Sulfate *on page 185*
- **Roxanol SR™ Oral** *see* Morphine Sulfate *on page 185*
- **Roxicet® 5/500** *see* Oxycodone and Acetaminophen* *on page 202*
- **Roxicodone™** *see* Oxycodone *on page 202*
- **Roxilox™** *see* Oxycodone and Acetaminophen* *on page 202*
- **Roxiprin®** *see* Oxycodone and Aspirin* *on page 202*
- **RP54274** *see* Riluzole *on page 232*
- **RU-486** *see* Mifepristone *on page 181*
- **RU-38486** *see* Mifepristone *on page 181*
- **Rubex®** *see* Doxorubicin* *on page 106*
- **Rum-K®** *see* Potassium Chloride (Timed Release)* *on page 216*
- **Ru-Tuss® DE** *see* Guaifenesin and Pseudoephedrine *on page 142*
- **Ru-Tuss® Expectorant [OTC]** *see* Guaifenesin, Pseudoephedrine, and Dextromethorphan *on page 143*
- **Ru-Tuss® Liquid** *see* Chlorpheniramine and Phenylephrine *on page 73*

- **Ru-Vert-M**® *see* Meclizine *on page 172*
- **Rymed**® *see* Guaifenesin and Pseudoephedrine *on page 142*
- **Rymed-TR**® *see* Guaifenesin and Phenylpropanolamine *on page 141*
- **Rynacrom**® *see* Cromolyn Sodium *on page 87*
- **Ryna-CX**® *see* Guaifenesin, Pseudoephedrine, and Codeine *on page 143*
- **Ryna**® **Liquid [OTC]** *see* Chlorpheniramine and Pseudoephedrine *on page 73*
- **Rythmol**® *see* Propafenone* *on page 222*
- **Sabulin** *see* Albuterol *on page 26*
- **Safe Tussin**® **30 [OTC]** *see* Guaifenesin and Dextromethorphan *on page 141*
- **Salazopyrin**® *see* Sulfasalazine* *on page 244*
- **Salazopyrin EN-Tabs**® *see* Sulfasalazine* *on page 244*
- **Salbutamol** *see* Albuterol *on page 26*
- **Saleto-200**® **[OTC]** *see* Ibuprofen* *on page 153*
- **Saleto-400**® *see* Ibuprofen* *on page 153*
- **Saleto-600**® *see* Ibuprofen* *on page 153*
- **Saleto-800**® *see* Ibuprofen* *on page 153*
- **Salflex**® *see* Salsalate* *on page 235*
- **Salgesic**® *see* Salsalate* *on page 235*
- **Salicylazosulfapyridine** *see* Sulfasalazine* *on page 244*
- **Salicylsalicylic Acid** *see* Salsalate* *on page 235*

Salmeterol (sal ME te role)
U.S. Brand Names Serevent®
Synonyms Salmeterol Xinafoate
Pharmacologic Class Beta₂ Agonist
Nutrients Depleted
  Specific nutrient depletions have not been documented for this agent.

- **Salmeterol and Fluticasone** *see* Fluticasone and Salmeterol* *on page 132*
- **Salmeterol Xinafoate** *see* Salmeterol *on page 235*
- **Salmonine**® **Injection** *see* Calcitonin *on page 55*

Salsalate* (SAL sa late)
Related Information
  Drug-Induced Nutrient Depletion Table *on page 498*
U.S. Brand Names Argesic®-SA; Artha-G®; Disalcid®; Marthritic®; Mono-Gesic®; Salflex®; Salgesic®; Salsitab®
Synonyms Disalicylic Acid; Salicylsalicylic Acid
Pharmacologic Class Salicylate
Nutrients Depleted
  Folic Acid *on page 325*
Scientific Basis Published scientific studies of agents with the same mechanism of action
Studies & Abstracts 252

- **Salsitab**® *see* Salsalate* *on page 235*

• **Saluron**® *see* Hydroflumethiazide* *on page 151*
• **Sandimmune**® **Injection** *see* Cyclosporine* *on page 88*
• **Sandimmune**® **Oral** *see* Cyclosporine* *on page 88*
• **Sandostatin**® *see* Octreotide Acetate *on page 198*
• **Sandostatin LAR**® *see* Octreotide Acetate *on page 198*

Saquinavir (sa KWIN a veer)
U.S. Brand Names Fortovase®; Invirase®
Synonyms Saquinavir Mesylate
Pharmacologic Class Antiretroviral Agent, Reverse Transcriptase Inhibitor (Non-Nucleoside)
Nutrients Depleted
  Specific nutrient depletions have not been documented for this agent.

• **Saquinavir Mesylate** *see* Saquinavir *on page 236*
• **Sarafem**™ *see* Fluoxetine *on page 130*

Sargramostim (sar GRAM oh stim)
U.S. Brand Names Leukine™
Synonyms GM-CSF; Granulocyte-Macrophage Colony Stimulating Factor; rGM-CSF
Pharmacologic Class Colony Stimulating Factor
Nutrients Depleted
  Specific nutrient depletions have not been documented for this agent.

• **S.A.S**™ *see* Sulfasalazine* *on page 244*
• **Scalpicin**® *see* Hydrocortisone* *on page 150*
• **Scot-Tussin**® **[OTC]** *see* Guaifenesin *on page 140*
• **Scot-Tussin DM**® **Cough Chasers [OTC]** *see* Dextromethorphan *on page 96*
• **Scot-Tussin**® **Senior Clear [OTC]** *see* Guaifenesin and Dextromethorphan *on page 141*
• **Sectral**® *see* Acebutolol* *on page 22*
• **Sedapap-10**® *see* Butalbital Compound and Acetaminophen* *on page 53*
• **Selax**® *see* Docusate *on page 104*

Selegiline (seh LEDGE ah leen)
U.S. Brand Names Eldepryl®
Canadian Brand Names Apo®-Selegiline; Novo-Selegiline
Synonyms Deprenyl; L-Deprenyl; Selegiline Hydrochloride
Pharmacologic Class Antidepressant, Monoamine Oxidase Inhibitor; Anti-Parkinson's Agent (Monoamine Oxidase Inhibitor)
Nutrients Depleted
  Specific nutrient depletions have not been documented for this agent.

• **Selegiline Hydrochloride** *see* Selegiline *on page 236*
• **Septra**® *see* Co-Trimoxazole* *on page 86*
• **Septra**® **DS** *see* Co-Trimoxazole* *on page 86*
• **Ser-Ap-Es**® *see* Hydralazine, Hydrochlorothiazide, and Reserpine* *on page 147*

+ **Serax**® *see* Oxazepam *on page 201*
+ **Serentil**® *see* Mesoridazine* *on page 174*
+ **Serevent**® *see* Salmeterol *on page 235*
+ **Seromycin**® **Pulvules**® *see* Cycloserine *on page 88*
+ **Serophene**® *see* Clomiphene *on page 80*
+ **Seroquel**® *see* Quetiapine *on page 227*
+ **Sertan**® *see* Primidone* *on page 220*

Sertraline (SER tra leen)
U.S. Brand Names Zoloft®
Synonyms Sertraline Hydrochloride
Pharmacologic Class Antidepressant, Selective Serotonin Reuptake Inhibitor
Nutrients Depleted
Specific nutrient depletions have not been documented for this agent.
Additional Information Selective serotonin reuptake inhibitors have been associated with rare, potentially severe hyponatremia. However, this is generally associated with fluid excess (SIADH), rather than a sodium deficiency. Treatment must be guided by a qualified healthcare provider.

+ **Sertraline Hydrochloride** *see* Sertraline *on page 237*
+ **Serutan**® **[OTC]** *see* Psyllium *on page 226*
+ **Serzone**® *see* Nefazodone *on page 189*

Sibutramine (si BYOO tra meen)
U.S. Brand Names Meridia™
Synonyms Sibutramine Hydrochloride Monohydrate
Pharmacologic Class Anorexiant
Nutrients Depleted
Specific nutrient depletions have not been documented for this agent.

+ **Sibutramine Hydrochloride Monohydrate** *see* Sibutramine *on page 237*
+ **Silace-C**® **[OTC]** *see* Docusate and Casanthranol* *on page 104*
+ **Siladryl**® **Oral [OTC]** *see* Diphenhydramine *on page 102*
+ **Silaminic**® **Cold Syrup [OTC]** *see* Chlorpheniramine and Phenylpropanolamine *on page 73*
+ **Silaminic**® **Expectorant [OTC]** *see* Guaifenesin and Phenylpropanolamine *on page 141*

Sildenafil (sil DEN a fil)
U.S. Brand Names Viagra®
Synonyms UK 92480
Pharmacologic Class Phosphodiesterase Enzyme Inhibitor
Nutrients Depleted
Specific nutrient depletions have not been documented for this agent.

+ **Sildicon-E**® **[OTC]** *see* Guaifenesin and Phenylpropanolamine *on page 141*
+ **Silphen**® **Cough [OTC]** *see* Diphenhydramine *on page 102*

- **Silphen DM® [OTC]** *see* Dextromethorphan *on page 96*
- **Siltussin® [OTC]** *see* Guaifenesin *on page 140*
- **Siltussin-CF® [OTC]** *see* Guaifenesin, Phenylpropanolamine, and Dextromethorphan *on page 142*
- **Siltussin DM® [OTC]** *see* Guaifenesin and Dextromethorphan *on page 141*

Simethicone (sye METH i kone)
U.S. Brand Names Degas® [OTC]; Flatulex® [OTC]; Gas Relief®; Gas-X® [OTC]; Maalox® Anti-Gas [OTC]; Mylanta® Gas [OTC]; Mylicon® [OTC]; Phazyme® [OTC]

Synonyms Activated Dimethicone; Activated Methylpolysiloxane

Pharmacologic Class Antiflatulent

Nutrients Depleted
Specific nutrient depletions have not been documented for this agent.

- **Simron® [OTC]** *see* Ferrous Gluconate *on page 126*

Simvastatin* (SIM va stat in)
Related Information
Drug-Induced Nutrient Depletion Table *on page 498*

U.S. Brand Names Zocor®

Pharmacologic Class Antilipemic Agent (HMG-CoA Reductase Inhibitor)

Nutrients Depleted
Coenzyme Q_{10} *on page 320*

Scientific Basis Published scientific studies using this pharmacologic agent

Studies & Abstracts 351-362

- **Sine-Aid® IB [OTC]** *see* Pseudoephedrine and Ibuprofen* *on page 226*
- **Sinemet®** *see* Levodopa and Carbidopa* *on page 164*
- **Sinemet® CR** *see* Levodopa and Carbidopa* *on page 164*
- **Sinequan® Oral** *see* Doxepin* *on page 106*
- **Singulair®** *see* Montelukast *on page 185*
- **Sinufed® Timecelles®** *see* Guaifenesin and Pseudoephedrine *on page 142*
- **Sinumist®-SR Capsulets®** *see* Guaifenesin *on page 140*
- **Sinupan®** *see* Guaifenesin and Phenylephrine *on page 141*
- **Sirdalud®** *see* Tizanidine *on page 255*

Sirolimus* (sir OH li mus)
U.S. Brand Names Rapamune®

Pharmacologic Class Immunosuppressant Agent

Nutrients Depleted
Potassium *on page 340*

Scientific Basis Published scientific studies of agents from the same pharmacologic class

Studies & Abstracts 449-450

Additional Information Electrolyte monitoring must be evaluated and replacement directed by prescriber due to the nature of the drug effect and the impact on transplant organ function.

♦ **SK and F 104864** *see* Topotecan* *on page 257*

♦ **Skelid®** *see* Tiludronate *on page 253*

♦ **SKF 104864** *see* Topotecan* *on page 257*

♦ **SKF 104864-A** *see* Topotecan* *on page 257*

♦ **Sleep-eze 3® Oral [OTC]** *see* Diphenhydramine *on page 102*

♦ **Sleepinal® [OTC]** *see* Diphenhydramine *on page 102*

♦ **Sleepwell 2-nite® [OTC]** *see* Diphenhydramine *on page 102*

♦ **Slo-bid™** *see* Theophylline* *on page 250*

♦ **Slo-Phyllin®** *see* Theophylline* *on page 250*

♦ **Slow FE® [OTC]** *see* Ferrous Sulfate *on page 126*

♦ **Slow-K®** *see* Potassium Chloride (Timed Release)* *on page 216*

♦ **SMZ-TMP** *see* Co-Trimoxazole* *on page 86*

♦ **Snaplets-EX® [OTC]** *see* Guaifenesin and Phenylpropanolamine *on page 141*

♦ **Snooze Fast® [OTC]** *see* Diphenhydramine *on page 102*

♦ **Sodium Acid Carbonate** *see* Sodium Bicarbonate* *on page 239*

Sodium Bicarbonate* (SOW dee um bye KAR bun ate)
Related Information
Drug-Induced Nutrient Depletion Table *on page 498*
U.S. Brand Names Neut® Injection
Synonyms Baking Soda; NaHCO₃; Sodium Acid Carbonate; Sodium Hydrogen Carbonate
Pharmacologic Class Alkalinizing Agent; Antacid; Electrolyte Supplement, Oral; Electrolyte Supplement, Parenteral
Nutrients Depleted
Potassium *on page 340*
Scientific Basis Published scientific studies using this pharmacologic agent
Studies & Abstracts 6

♦ **Sodium Ferric Gluconate** *see* Ferric Gluconate *on page 125*

♦ **Sodium Hydrogen Carbonate** *see* Sodium Bicarbonate* *on page 239*

♦ **Sodium Nafcillin** *see* Nafcillin* *on page 187*

Sodium Phosphates* (SOW dee um FOS fates)
Related Information
Drug-Induced Nutrient Depletion Table *on page 498*
U.S. Brand Names Fleet® Enema [OTC]; Fleet® Phospho®-Soda [OTC]
Pharmacologic Class Electrolyte Supplement, Oral; Laxative
Nutrients Depleted
Calcium *on page 313*
Magnesium *on page 333*
Potassium *on page 340*
(Continued)

Sodium Phosphates* *(Continued)*

Sodium *on page 345*

Scientific Basis Published scientific studies using this pharmacologic agent.

Studies & Abstracts 459-465

Sodium Polystyrene Sulfonate

(SOW dee um pol ee STYE reen SUL fon ate)

U.S. Brand Names Kayexalate®; SPS®

Pharmacologic Class Antidote

Nutrients Depleted

Specific nutrient depletions have not been documented for this agent.

♦ **SoFlax™** *see* Docusate *on page 104*

♦ **Solfoton®** *see* Phenobarbital* *on page 210*

♦ **Solium®** *see* Chlordiazepoxide *on page 72*

♦ **Solu-Cortef®** *see* Hydrocortisone* *on page 150*

♦ **Solu-Medrol® Injection** *see* Methylprednisolone* *on page 178*

♦ **Solurex®** *see* Dexamethasone* *on page 95*

♦ **Solurex L.A.®** *see* Dexamethasone* *on page 95*

♦ **Soma®** *see* Carisoprodol *on page 58*

♦ **Soma® Compound** *see* Carisoprodol and Aspirin* *on page 58*

♦ **Soma® Compound w/Codeine** *see* Carisoprodol, Aspirin, and Codeine* *on page 59*

♦ **Sominex® Oral [OTC]** *see* Diphenhydramine *on page 102*

♦ **Somnol®** *see* Flurazepam *on page 131*

♦ **Som Pam®** *see* Flurazepam *on page 131*

♦ **Sorbitrate®** *see* Isosorbide Dinitrate *on page 158*

♦ **Sotacor®** *see* Sotalol* *on page 240*

Sotalol* (SOE ta lole)

Related Information

Drug-Induced Nutrient Depletion Table *on page 498*

U.S. Brand Names Betapace®; Betapace AF®

Canadian Brand Names Sotacor®

Synonyms Sotalol Hydrochloride

Pharmacologic Class Antiarrhythmic Agent, Class II; Antiarrhythmic Agent, Class III; Beta Blocker, Beta₁ Selective

Nutrients Depleted

Coenzyme Q_{10} *on page 320*

Scientific Basis

Published scientific studies using this pharmacologic agent
   or
Published scientific studies of agents from the same pharmacologic class

Studies & Abstracts 348-349

♦ **Sotalol Hydrochloride** *see* Sotalol* *on page 240*

♦ **Span-FF® [OTC]** *see* Ferrous Fumarate *on page 126*

Sparfloxacin* (spar FLOKS a sin)
U.S. Brand Names Zagam®
Pharmacologic Class Antibiotic, Quinolone
Nutrients Depleted
  Bifidobacteria bifidum (bifidus) on page 311
  Biotin *on page 311*
  Inositol *on page 328*
  Lactobacillus acidophilus on page 332
  Vitamin B_1 *on page 351*
  Vitamin B_2 *on page 353*
  Vitamin B_3 *on page 354*
  Vitamin B_6 *on page 357*
  Vitamin B_{12} *on page 359*
  Vitamin K *on page 367*
Scientific Basis Inferred or indirect evidence of depletion based on disruption of physiologic processes
Studies & Abstracts 7-27

♦ **Sparine**® *see* Promazine* *on page 222*
♦ **Spectrobid**® *see* Bacampicillin* *on page 43*

Spirapril* (SPYE ra pril)
U.S. Brand Names Renormax®
Pharmacologic Class Angiotensin-Converting Enzyme (ACE) Inhibitors
Nutrients Depleted
  Zinc *on page 368*
Scientific Basis Published scientific studies of agents from the same pharmacologic class
Studies & Abstracts 269-271

Spironolactone (speer on oh LAK tone)
U.S. Brand Names Aldactone®
Canadian Brand Names Novo-Spiroton
Pharmacologic Class Diuretic, Potassium Sparing
Nutrients Depleted
  Specific nutrient depletions have not been documented for this agent.

♦ **Spironolactone and Hydrochlorothiazide** *see* Hydrochlorothiazide and Spironolactone* *on page 148*
♦ **Sporanox**® *see* Itraconazole *on page 159*
♦ **SPS**® *see* Sodium Polystyrene Sulfonate *on page 240*
♦ **S-P-T** *see* Thyroid *on page 252*
♦ **Stadol**® *see* Butorphanol *on page 55*
♦ **Stadol**® **NS** *see* Butorphanol *on page 55*
♦ **Stagesic**® *see* Hydrocodone and Acetaminophen* *on page 149*
♦ **Statex**® *see* Morphine Sulfate *on page 185*

Stavudine* (STAV yoo deen)
Related Information
  Drug-Induced Nutrient Depletion Table *on page 498*
  (Continued)

Stavudine* *(Continued)*
U.S. Brand Names Zerit®
Synonyms d4T
Pharmacologic Class Antiretroviral Agent, Reverse Transcriptase Inhibitor (Nucleoside)
Nutrients Depleted
Carnitine *on page 316*
Copper *on page 322*
Vitamin B$_{12}$ *on page 359*
Zinc *on page 368*
Scientific Basis Published scientific studies of agents from the same pharmacologic class
Studies & Abstracts 260-262

- ♦ **S-T Cort®** *see* Hydrocortisone* *on page 150*
- ♦ **Stelazine®** *see* Trifluoperazine* *on page 261*
- ♦ **Stemetil®** *see* Prochlorperazine* *on page 221*
- ♦ **Stieva-A®** *see* Tretinoin (Topical) *on page 259*
- ♦ **Stieva-A® Forte** *see* Tretinoin (Topical) *on page 259*
- ♦ **Stilbestrol** *see* Diethylstilbestrol* *on page 99*
- ♦ **Stilphostrol®** *see* Diethylstilbestrol* *on page 99*
- ♦ **St Joseph® Adult Chewable Aspirin [OTC]** *see* Aspirin* *on page 40*
- ♦ **St. Joseph® Cough Suppressant [OTC]** *see* Dextromethorphan *on page 96*
- ♦ **Sublimaze® Injection** *see* Fentanyl *on page 125*

Sucralfate* *(soo KRAL fate)*
U.S. Brand Names Carafate®
Canadian Brand Names Novo-Sucralate; Sulcrate®; Sulcrate® Suspension Plus
Synonyms Aluminum Sucrose Sulfate, Basic
Pharmacologic Class Gastrointestinal Agent, Miscellaneous
Nutrients Depleted
Calcium *on page 313*
Phosphorus *on page 339*
Scientific Basis Inferred or indirect evidence of depletion based on disruption of physiologic processes
Studies & Abstracts 484-490
Additional Information Aluminum salts (including sucralfate) may be used to prevent hyperphophatemia.

- ♦ **Sucrets® Cough Calmers [OTC]** *see* Dextromethorphan *on page 96*
- ♦ **Sudafed® [OTC]** *see* Pseudoephedrine *on page 225*
- ♦ **Sudafed® 12 Hour [OTC]** *see* Pseudoephedrine *on page 225*
- ♦ **Sudafed® Cold & Cough Liquid Caps [OTC]** *see* Guaifenesin, Pseudoephedrine, and Dextromethorphan *on page 143*
- ♦ **Sudafed® Plus Tablet [OTC]** *see* Chlorpheniramine and Pseudoephedrine *on page 73*

♦ **Sular**® *see* Nisoldipine *on page 192*

♦ **Sulcrate**® *see* Sucralfate* *on page 242*

♦ **Sulcrate**® **Suspension Plus** *see* Sucralfate* *on page 242*

Sulfadiazine* (sul fa DYE a zeen)
U.S. Brand Names Microsulfon®
Canadian Brand Names Coptin®
Pharmacologic Class Antibiotic, Sulfonamide Derivative
Nutrients Depleted
    Bifidobacteria bifidum (bifidus) on page 311
    Biotin *on page 311*
    Inositol *on page 328*
    Lactobacillus acidophilus on page 332
    Vitamin B_1 *on page 351*
    Vitamin B_2 *on page 353*
    Vitamin B_3 *on page 354*
    Vitamin B_6 *on page 357*
    Vitamin B_{12} *on page 359*
    Vitamin K *on page 367*
Scientific Basis
    Published scientific studies of agents from the same pharmacologic
      class
      or
    Inferred or indirect evidence of depletion based on disruption of physi-
      ologic processes
Studies & Abstracts 7-27

♦ **Sulfalax**® **[OTC]** *see* Docusate *on page 104*

Sulfamethoxazole* (sul fa meth OKS a zole)
U.S. Brand Names Gantanol®; Urobak®
Canadian Brand Names Apo®-Sulfamethoxazole
Pharmacologic Class Antibiotic, Sulfonamide Derivative
Nutrients Depleted
    Bifidobacteria bifidum (bifidus) on page 311
    Biotin *on page 311*
    Inositol *on page 328*
    Lactobacillus acidophilus on page 332
    Vitamin B_1 *on page 351*
    Vitamin B_2 *on page 353*
    Vitamin B_3 *on page 354*
    Vitamin B_6 *on page 357*
    Vitamin B_{12} *on page 359*
    Vitamin K *on page 367*
Scientific Basis
    Published scientific studies of agents from the same pharmacologic
      class
      or
    Inferred or indirect evidence of depletion based on disruption of physi-
      ologic processes
Studies & Abstracts 7-27

♦ **Sulfamethoxazole and Trimethoprim** *see* Co-Trimoxazole* *on page 86*

Sulfasalazine* (sul fa SAL a zeen)
Related Information
Drug-Induced Nutrient Depletion Table *on page 498*
U.S. Brand Names Azulfidine®; Azulfidine® EN-tabs®
Canadian Brand Names Apo®-Sulfasalazine; PMS-Sulfasalazine; Salazopyrin®; Salazopyrin EN-Tabs®; S.A.S™
Synonyms Salicylazosulfapyridine
Pharmacologic Class 5-Aminosalicylic Acid Derivative
Nutrients Depleted
Folic Acid *on page 325*
Scientific Basis Published scientific studies using this pharmacologic agent
Studies & Abstracts 237-245

♦ **Sulfatrim®** *see* Co-Trimoxazole* *on page 86*

Sulfisoxazole* (sul fi SOKS a zole)
U.S. Brand Names Gantrisin®
Pharmacologic Class Antibiotic, Sulfonamide Derivative
Nutrients Depleted
Bifidobacteria bifidum (bifidus) on page 311
Biotin *on page 311*
Inositol *on page 328*
Lactobacillus acidophilus on page 332
Vitamin B_1 *on page 351*
Vitamin B_2 *on page 353*
Vitamin B_3 *on page 354*
Vitamin B_6 *on page 357*
Vitamin B_{12} *on page 359*
Vitamin K *on page 367*
Scientific Basis
Published scientific studies of agents from the same pharmacologic class
or
Inferred or indirect evidence of depletion based on disruption of physiologic processes
Studies & Abstracts 7-27

Sulfisoxazole and Phenazopyridine*
(sul fi SOKS a zole & fen az oh PEER i deen)
U.S. Brand Names Azo-Sulfisoxazole
Synonyms Phenazopyridine and Sulfisoxazole
Pharmacologic Class Antibiotic, Sulfonamide Derivative; Local Anesthetic
Nutrients Depleted
Bifidobacteria bifidum (bifidus) on page 311
Biotin *on page 311*
Inositol *on page 328*

Lactobacillus acidophilus on page 332
Vitamin B_1 *on page 351*
Vitamin B_2 *on page 353*
Vitamin B_3 *on page 354*
Vitamin B_6 *on page 357*
Vitamin B_{12} *on page 359*
Vitamin K *on page 367*

Scientific Basis
Published scientific studies of agents from the same pharmacologic class
    or
Inferred or indirect evidence of depletion based on disruption of physiologic processes
Studies & Abstracts 7-27

Sulindac* (sul IN dak)
Related Information
Drug-Induced Nutrient Depletion Table *on page 498*
U.S. Brand Names Clinoril®
Canadian Brand Names Apo®-Sulin; Novo-Sundac
Pharmacologic Class Nonsteroidal Anti-Inflammatory Agent (NSAID)
Nutrients Depleted
Folic Acid *on page 325*
Scientific Basis Published scientific studies of agents from the same pharmacologic class
Studies & Abstracts 252

Sumatriptan Succinate (SOO ma trip tan SUKS i nate)
U.S. Brand Names Imitrex®
Pharmacologic Class Serotonin 5-HT_{1D} Receptor Agonist
Nutrients Depleted
Specific nutrient depletions have not been documented for this agent.

♦ **Sumycin® Oral** *see* Tetracycline* *on page 249*
♦ **Supeudol®** *see* Oxycodone *on page 202*
♦ **Suppress® [OTC]** *see* Dextromethorphan *on page 96*
♦ **Suprax®** *see* Cefixime* *on page 62*

Suprofen* (soo PROE fen)
U.S. Brand Names Profenal® Ophthalmic
Pharmacologic Class Nonsteroidal Anti-Inflammatory Agent (NSAID)
Nutrients Depleted
Folic Acid *on page 325*
Scientific Basis Published scientific studies of agents from the same pharmacologic class
Studies & Abstracts 252

♦ **Surfak® [OTC]** *see* Docusate *on page 104*
♦ **Surmontil®** *see* Trimipramine* *on page 262*

Tacrine (TAK reen)

U.S. Brand Names Cognex®
Synonyms Tacrine Hydrochloride; Tetrahydroaminoacrine; THA
Pharmacologic Class Acetylcholinesterase Inhibitor (Central)
Nutrients Depleted
Specific nutrient depletions have not been documented for this agent.

Tacrolimus* (ta KROE li mus)

U.S. Brand Names Prograf®
Synonyms FK506
Pharmacologic Class Immunosuppressant Agent
Nutrients Depleted
Magnesium *on page 333*
Potassium *on page 340*
Scientific Basis
Published scientific studies of agents with the same mechanism of action
or
Published scientific studies using this pharmacologic agent
Studies & Abstracts 449-450
Additional Information Electrolyte changes may be extremely complex during immunosuppressive therapy. In particular, tacrolimus may be associated with either a decrease **OR** increase in potassium

serum concentrations. Excessive levels of electrolytes may be dangerous. Potassium replacement and/or magnesium supplementation MUST be guided by a qualified healthcare practitioner based on serum level monitoring.

◆ **Tagamet**® *see* Cimetidine* *on page 76*

◆ **Tagamet**® **HB [OTC]** *see* Cimetidine* *on page 76*

◆ **Talacen**® *see* Pentazocine Compound *on page 208*

◆ **Talwin**® *see* Pentazocine *on page 208*

◆ **Talwin**® **Compound** *see* Pentazocine Compound *on page 208*

◆ **Talwin**® **NX** *see* Pentazocine *on page 208*

◆ **Tamiflu**™ *see* Oseltamivir *on page 201*

◆ **Tamine**® **[OTC]** *see* Brompheniramine and Phenylpropanolamine *on page 50*

◆ **Tamofen**® *see* Tamoxifen *on page 247*

◆ **Tamone**® *see* Tamoxifen *on page 247*

Tamoxifen (ta MOKS i fen)

U.S. Brand Names Nolvadex®
Canadian Brand Names Alpha-Tamoxifen®; Apo®-Tamox; Novo-Tamoxifen; Tamofen®; Tamone®
Synonyms Tamoxifen Citrate
Pharmacologic Class Antineoplastic Agent, Miscellaneous
Nutrients Depleted
  Specific nutrient depletions have not been documented for this agent.

◆ **Tamoxifen Citrate** *see* Tamoxifen *on page 247*

◆ **Tantaphen**® *see* Acetaminophen* *on page 23*

◆ **Tapazole**® *see* Methimazole *on page 175*

◆ **Tarka**® *see* Trandolapril and Verapamil* *on page 258*

◆ **Taro-Ampicillin**® **Trihydrate** *see* Ampicillin* *on page 35*

◆ **Taro-Atenol**® *see* Atenolol* *on page 41*

◆ **Taro-Sone** *see* Betamethasone* *on page 46*

◆ **Tasmar**® *see* Tolcapone *on page 256*

◆ **Tavist**® *see* Clemastine *on page 79*

◆ **Tavist**®**-1 [OTC]** *see* Clemastine *on page 79*

◆ **Tavist-D**® *see* Clemastine and Phenylpropanolamine *on page 79*

◆ **Taxol**® *see* Paclitaxel* *on page 203*

◆ **Taxotere**® *see* Docetaxel* *on page 104*

◆ **Tazicef**® *see* Ceftazidime* *on page 66*

◆ **Tazidime**® *see* Ceftazidime* *on page 66*

◆ **3TC** *see* Lamivudine* *on page 162*

◆ **3TC, Abacavir, and Zidovudine** *see* Abacavir, Lamivudine, and Zidovudine* *on page 22*

◆ **TCN** *see* Tetracycline* *on page 249*

◆ **Tecnal** *see* Butalbital Compound and Aspirin* *on page 54*

◆ **Tecnal C¹/₄, C¹/₂** *see* Butalbital Compound and Codeine* *on page 54*

◆ **Teczem**® *see* Enalapril and Diltiazem* *on page 110*

- **Teejel®** *see* Choline Salicylate* *on page 76*
- **Tegopen®** *see* Cloxacillin* *on page 82*
- **Tegretol®** *see* Carbamazepine* *on page 57*
- **Tegretol®-XR** *see* Carbamazepine* *on page 57*
- **Tegrin®-HC [OTC]** *see* Hydrocortisone* *on page 150*
- **Telachlor®** *see* Chlorpheniramine *on page 73*
- **Teladar®** *see* Betamethasone* *on page 46*
- **Teldrin® [OTC]** *see* Chlorpheniramine *on page 73*

Telmisartan (tel mi SAR tan)
U.S. Brand Names Micardis®
Pharmacologic Class Angiotensin II Antagonists
Nutrients Depleted
  Specific nutrient depletions have not been documented for this agent.

- **Telmisartan and HCTZ** *see* Telmisartan and Hydrochlorothiazide* *on page 248*

Telmisartan and Hydrochlorothiazide*
(tel mi SAR tan & hye droe klor oh THYE a zide)
U.S. Brand Names Micardis® HCT
Synonyms HCTZ and Telmisartan; Hydrochlorothiazide and Telmisartan; Telmisartan and HCTZ
Pharmacologic Class Angiotensin II Antagonist Combination; Antihypertensive Agent, Combination
Nutrients Depleted
  Coenzyme Q_{10} *on page 320*
  Magnesium *on page 333*
  Phosphorus *on page 339*
  Potassium *on page 340*
  Sodium *on page 345*
  Zinc *on page 368*
Scientific Basis Published scientific studies using this pharmacologic agent (hydrochlorothiazide)
Studies & Abstracts 320-342
Additional Information Although thiazide diuretics deplete sodium, replacement is not recommended, as this may be directly related to the therapeutic effect. Thiazides may deplete potassium, however replacement should be guided by monitoring of serum concentrations and specific instruction by a healthcare provider.

Temazepam (te MAZ e pam)
U.S. Brand Names Restoril®
Canadian Brand Names Apo®-Temazepam
Pharmacologic Class Benzodiazepine
Nutrients Depleted
  Specific nutrient depletions have not been documented for this agent.

- **Temazin® Cold Syrup [OTC]** *see* Chlorpheniramine and Phenylpropanolamine *on page 73*
- **Temodar®** *see* Temozolomide* *on page 249*

Temozolomide* (te mo ZOLE oh mide)
U.S. Brand Names Temodar®
Pharmacologic Class Antineoplastic Agent, Alkylating Agent
Nutrients Depleted
See Nutrient Depletion and Cancer Chemotherapy *on page 515.*
Scientific Basis Inferred or indirect evidence of depletion based on disruption of physiologic processes

♦ **Tempra® [OTC]** *see* Acetaminophen* *on page 23*
♦ **Ten-K®** *see* Potassium Chloride (Timed Release)* *on page 216*
♦ **Tenoretic®** *see* Atenolol and Chlorthalidone* *on page 41*
♦ **Tenormin®** *see* Atenolol* *on page 41*
♦ **Tenuate®** *see* Diethylpropion *on page 99*
♦ **Tenuate® Dospan®** *see* Diethylpropion *on page 99*
♦ **Tequin™** *see* Gatifloxacin* *on page 136*

Terazosin (ter AY zoe sin)
U.S. Brand Names Hytrin®
Pharmacologic Class Alpha$_1$ Blockers
Nutrients Depleted
Specific nutrient depletions have not been documented for this agent.

Terbinafine (TER bin a feen)
U.S. Brand Names Lamisil® AT™ Topical; Lamisil® Dermgel; Lamisil® Topical
Synonyms Terbinafine Hydrochloride
Pharmacologic Class Antifungal Agent, Oral; Antifungal Agent, Topical
Nutrients Depleted
Specific nutrient depletions have not been documented for this agent.

♦ **Terbinafine Hydrochloride** *see* Terbinafine *on page 249*
♦ **Terramycin® I.M. Injection** *see* Oxytetracycline *on page 202*
♦ **Terramycin® Oral** *see* Oxytetracycline* *on page 202*
♦ **Tessalon® Perles** *see* Benzonatate *on page 45*
♦ **Testosterone and Estradiol** *see* Estradiol and Testosterone* *on page 115*

Tetracycline* (tet ra SYE kleen)
Related Information
Drug-Induced Nutrient Depletion Table *on page 498*
U.S. Brand Names Achromycin® Ophthalmic; Achromycin® Topical; Sumycin® Oral; Topicycline® Topical
Canadian Brand Names Apo®-Tetra; Novo-Tetra; Nu-Tetra
Synonyms TCN; Tetracycline Hydrochloride
Pharmacologic Class Antibiotic, Ophthalmic; Antibiotic, Tetracycline Derivative; Antibiotic, Topical
Nutrients Depleted
Bifidobacteria bifidum (bifidus) on page 311
(Continued)

Tetracycline* *(Continued)*

Biotin *on page 311*
Calcium *on page 313*
Inositol *on page 328*
Iron *on page 331*
Lactobacillus acidophilus on page 332
Magnesium *on page 333*
Vitamin B_1 *on page 351*
Vitamin B_2 *on page 353*
Vitamin B_3 *on page 354*
Vitamin B_6 *on page 357*
Vitamin B_{12} *on page 359*
Vitamin K *on page 367*

Scientific Basis

Published scientific studies using this pharmacologic agent
  or
Inferred or indirect evidence of depletion based on disruption of physiologic processes

Studies & Abstracts 7-27, 62-68

- **Tetracycline Hydrochloride** *see* Tetracycline* *on page 249*
- **Tetrahydroaminoacrine** *see* Tacrine *on page 246*
- **Teveten®** *see* Eprosartan *on page 112*
- **T-Gesic®** *see* Hydrocodone and Acetaminophen* *on page 149*
- **THA** *see* Tacrine *on page 246*

Thalidomide *(tha LI doe mide)*

U.S. Brand Names Contergan®; Distaval®; Kevadon®; Thalomid®
Pharmacologic Class Immunosuppressant Agent
Nutrients Depleted
Specific nutrient depletions have not been documented for this agent.

- **Thalitone®** *see* Chlorthalidone* *on page 74*
- **Thalomid®** *see* Thalidomide *on page 250*
- **Theo-24®** *see* Theophylline* *on page 250*
- **Theobid®** *see* Theophylline* *on page 250*
- **Theochron®** *see* Theophylline* *on page 250*
- **Theoclear-80®** *see* Theophylline* *on page 250*
- **Theoclear® L.A.** *see* Theophylline* *on page 250*
- **Theo-Dur®** *see* Theophylline* *on page 250*
- **Theolair™** *see* Theophylline* *on page 250*

Theophylline* *(thee OF i lin)*

Related Information

Drug-Induced Nutrient Depletion Table *on page 498*
U.S. Brand Names Aerolate III®; Aerolate JR®; Aerolate SR®; Aquaphyllin®; Asmalix®; Bronkodyl®; Elixomin®; Elixophyllin®; Lanophyllin®; Quibron®-T; Quibron®-T/SR; Respbid®; Slo-bid™; Slo-Phyllin®;

Sustaire®; Theo-24®; Theobid®; Theochron®; Theoclear-80®; Theo-clear® L.A.; Theo-Dur®; Theolair™; Theo-Sav®; Theospan®-SR; Theo-stat-80®; Theovent®; Theo-X®; T-Phyl®; Uni-Dur®; Uniphyl®

Canadian Brand Names Apo®-Theo LA; Phyllocontin®; Pulmophyl-line

Synonyms Theophylline Anhydrous

Pharmacologic Class Theophylline Derivative

Nutrients Depleted

Vitamin B₁ *on page 351*

Vitamin B₆ *on page 357*

Scientific Basis Published scientific studies using this pharmacologic agent

Studies & Abstracts 263-268

♦ **Theophylline Anhydrous** *see Theophylline* on page 250*

♦ **Theo-Sav®** *see Theophylline* on page 250*

♦ **Theospan®-SR** *see Theophylline* on page 250*

♦ **Theostat-80®** *see Theophylline* on page 250*

♦ **Theovent®** *see Theophylline* on page 250*

♦ **Theo-X®** *see Theophylline* on page 250*

♦ **Thera-Hist® Syrup [OTC]** *see Chlorpheniramine and Phenylpropanola-mine on page 73*

♦ **Thiamazole** *see Methimazole on page 175*

Thiethylperazine* (thye eth il PER a zeen)

U.S. Brand Names Norzine®; Torecan®

Synonyms Thiethylperazine Maleate

Pharmacologic Class Antiemetic

Nutrients Depleted

Coenzyme Q₁₀ *on page 320*

Vitamin B₂ *on page 353*

Scientific Basis Published scientific studies of agents from the same pharmacologic class

Studies & Abstracts 474-477

♦ **Thiethylperazine Maleate** *see Thiethylperazine* on page 251*

Thioridazine* (thye oh RID a zeen)

Related Information

Drug-Induced Nutrient Depletion Table *on page 498*

U.S. Brand Names Mellaril®; Mellaril-S®

Canadian Brand Names Apo®-Thioridazine; Novo-Ridazine; PMS-Thioridazine

Synonyms Thioridazine Hydrochloride

Pharmacologic Class Antipsychotic Agent, Phenothazine, Piperidine

Nutrients Depleted

Coenzyme Q₁₀ *on page 320*

Vitamin B₂ *on page 353*

Scientific Basis Published scientific studies of agents from the same pharmacologic class

Studies & Abstracts 474-477

♦ **Thioridazine Hydrochloride** *see* Thioridazine* *on page 251*

Thiothixene (thye oh THIKS een)
U.S. Brand Names Navane®
Synonyms Tiotixene
Pharmacologic Class Antipsychotic Agent, Thioxanthene Derivative
Nutrients Depleted
Specific nutrient depletions have not been documented for this agent.

♦ **Thorazine®** *see* Chlorpromazine* *on page 74*
♦ **Thyrar®** *see* Thyroid *on page 252*

Thyroid (THYE royd)
U.S. Brand Names Armour® Thyroid; S-P-T; Thyrar®; Thyroid Strong®
Synonyms Desiccated Thyroid; Thyroid Extract; Thyroid USP
Pharmacologic Class Thyroid Product
Nutrients Depleted
Specific nutrient depletions have not been documented for this agent.

♦ **Thyroid Extract** *see* Thyroid *on page 252*
♦ **Thyroid Strong®** *see* Thyroid *on page 252*
♦ **Thyroid USP** *see* Thyroid *on page 252*

Tiagabine (tye AG a bene)
U.S. Brand Names Gabitril®
Synonyms Tiagabine Hydrochloride
Pharmacologic Class Anticonvulsant, Miscellaneous
Nutrients Depleted
Specific nutrient depletions have not been documented for this agent.

♦ **Tiagabine Hydrochloride** *see* Tiagabine *on page 252*
♦ **Tiamate®** *see* Diltiazem *on page 101*
♦ **Tiamol®** *see* Fluocinonide* *on page 130*
♦ **Tiazac™** *see* Diltiazem *on page 101*
♦ **Ticar®** *see* Ticarcillin* *on page 252*

Ticarcillin* (tye kar SIL in)
U.S. Brand Names Ticar®
Synonyms Ticarcillin Disodium
Pharmacologic Class Antibiotic, Penicillin
Nutrients Depleted
Bifidobacteria bifidum (bifidus) *on page 311*
Biotin *on page 311*
Inositol *on page 328*
Lactobacillus acidophilus *on page 332*
Potassium *on page 340*
Vitamin B_1 *on page 351*
Vitamin B_2 *on page 353*
Vitamin B_3 *on page 354*
Vitamin B_6 *on page 357*
Vitamin B_{12} *on page 359*
Vitamin K *on page 367*

Scientific Basis Inferred or indirect evidence of depletion based on disruption of physiologic processes

Studies & Abstracts 7-27, 49-57

Additional Information Potassium depletion has been documented primarily with high dose, parenteral penicillins, primarily from the ureidopenicillin group.

Ticarcillin and Clavulanate Potassium*

(tye kar SIL in & klav yoo LAN ate poe TASS ee um)

U.S. Brand Names Timentin®

Synonyms Ticarcillin and Clavulanic Acid

Pharmacologic Class Antibiotic, Penicillin

Nutrients Depleted

Bifidobacteria bifidum (bifidus) on page 311

Biotin *on page 311*

Inositol *on page 328*

Lactobacillus acidophilus on page 332

Potassium *on page 340*

Vitamin B$_1$ *on page 351*

Vitamin B$_2$ *on page 353*

Vitamin B$_3$ *on page 354*

Vitamin B$_6$ *on page 357*

Vitamin B$_{12}$ *on page 359*

Vitamin K *on page 367*

Scientific Basis Inferred or indirect evidence of depletion based on disruption of physiologic processes

Studies & Abstracts 7-27, 49-57

Additional Information Potassium depletion has been documented primarily with high dose, parenteral penicillins, primarily from the ureidopenicillin group.

♦ **Ticarcillin and Clavulanic Acid** *see* Ticarcillin and Clavulanate Potassium* *on page 253*

♦ **Ticarcillin Disodium** *see* Ticarcillin* *on page 252*

♦ **Ticlid®** *see* Ticlopidine *on page 253*

Ticlopidine (tye KLOE pi deen)

U.S. Brand Names Ticlid®

Synonyms Ticlopidine Hydrochloride

Pharmacologic Class Antiplatelet Agent

Nutrients Depleted

Specific nutrient depletions have not been documented for this agent.

♦ **Ticlopidine Hydrochloride** *see* Ticlopidine *on page 253*

♦ **Tikosyn™** *see* Dofetilide *on page 105*

Tiludronate (tye LOO droe nate)

U.S. Brand Names Skelid®

Synonyms Tiludronate Disodium

Pharmacologic Class Bisphosphonate Derivative

Nutrients Depleted

Specific nutrient depletions have not been documented for this agent.
(Continued)

Tiludronate *(Continued)*

Additional Information Bisphosphonates have been (rarely) associated with hypocalcemia, as a natural extension of their therapeutic action. Correction of hypocalcemia is recommended prior to tiludronate treatment. When used in Paget's disease, adequate vitamin D and calcium intake should be ensured to provide for enhanced needs. Calcium administration should be separated from tiludronate by at least 30 minutes.

♦ **Tiludronate Disodium** *see* Tiludronate *on page 253*
♦ **Timentin®** *see* Ticarcillin and Clavulanate Potassium* *on page 253*

Timolol* *(TYE moe lole)*
Related Information
Drug-Induced Nutrient Depletion Table *on page 498*
U.S. Brand Names Betimol® Ophthalmic; Blocadren® Oral; Timoptic® Ophthalmic; Timoptic® Ophthalmic in OcuDose®; Timoptic-XE® Ophthalmic
Canadian Brand Names Apo®-Timol; Apo®-Timop; Gen-Timolol; Novo-Timol; Nu-Timolol
Synonyms Timolol Hemihydrate; Timolol Maleate
Pharmacologic Class Beta Blocker, Nonselective; Ophthalmic Agent, Antiglaucoma
Nutrients Depleted
Coenzyme Q_{10} *on page 320*
Scientific Basis
Published scientific studies using this pharmacologic agent
or
Published scientific studies of agents from the same pharmacologic class
Studies & Abstracts 348-349

♦ **Timolol Hemihydrate** *see* Timolol* *on page 254*
♦ **Timolol Maleate** *see* Timolol* *on page 254*
♦ **Timoptic® Ophthalmic** *see* Timolol* *on page 254*
♦ **Timoptic® Ophthalmic in OcuDose®** *see* Timolol* *on page 254*
♦ **Timoptic-XE® Ophthalmic** *see* Timolol* *on page 254*
♦ **Tindal®** *see* Acetophenazine* *on page 24*

Tinzaparin *(tin ZA pa rin)*
U.S. Brand Names Innohep®
Synonyms Tinzaparin Sodium
Pharmacologic Class Low Molecular Weight Heparin
Nutrients Depleted
Specific nutrient depletions have not been documented for this agent.

♦ **Tinzaparin Sodium** *see* Tinzaparin *on page 254*
♦ **Tiotixene** *see* Thiothixene *on page 252*

Tirofiban (tye roe FYE ban)
U.S. Brand Names Aggrastat®
Synonyms MK 383; Tirofiban Hydrochloride
Pharmacologic Class Antiplatelet Agent
Nutrients Depleted
  Specific nutrient depletions have not been documented for this agent.

♦ **Tirofiban Hydrochloride** see Tirofiban on page 255

Tizanidine (tye ZAN i deen)
U.S. Brand Names Zanaflex®
Synonyms Sirdalud®
Pharmacologic Class Alpha$_2$ Agonist
Nutrients Depleted
  Specific nutrient depletions have not been documented for this agent.

♦ **TMP** see Trimethoprim* on page 262
♦ **TMP-SMZ** see Co-Trimoxazole* on page 86

Tobramycin* (toe bra MYE sin)
Related Information
  Drug-Induced Nutrient Depletion Table on page 498
U.S. Brand Names AKTob® Ophthalmic; Nebcin® Injection; Tobrex® Ophthalmic
Synonyms Tobramycin Sulfate
Pharmacologic Class Antibiotic, Aminoglycoside;   Antibiotic, Ophthalmic
Nutrients Depleted
  Bifidobacteria bifidum (bifidus) on page 311
  Biotin on page 311
  Calcium on page 313
  Inositol on page 328
  Lactobacillus acidophilus on page 332
  Magnesium on page 333
  Potassium on page 340
  Sodium on page 345
  Vitamin B$_1$ on page 351
  Vitamin B$_2$ on page 353
  Vitamin B$_3$ on page 354
  Vitamin B$_6$ on page 357
  Vitamin B$_{12}$ on page 359
  Vitamin K on page 367
Scientific Basis
  Published scientific studies of agents from the same pharmacologic class
    or
  Inferred or indirect evidence of depletion based on disruption of physiologic processes
Studies & Abstracts 7-37

♦ **Tobramycin Sulfate** see Tobramycin* on page 255
♦ **Tobrex® Ophthalmic** see Tobramycin* on page 255

♦ **Tofranil**® *see* Imipramine* *on page 154*

♦ **Tofranil-PM**® *see* Imipramine* *on page 154*

Tolazamide* (tole AZ a mide)
Related Information
  Drug-Induced Nutrient Depletion Table *on page 498*
U.S. Brand Names Tolinase®
Pharmacologic Class Antidiabetic Agent (Sulfonylurea)
Nutrients Depleted
  Coenzyme Q_{10} *on page 320*
Scientific Basis Published scientific studies using this pharmacologic agent
Studies & Abstracts 167

Tolbutamide* (tole BYOO ta mide)
U.S. Brand Names Orinase® Diagnostic Injection; Orinase® Oral
Canadian Brand Names Apo®-Tolbutamide; Mobenol®; Novo-Butamide
Synonyms Tolbutamide Sodium
Pharmacologic Class Antidiabetic Agent (Sulfonylurea)
Nutrients Depleted
  Coenzyme Q_{10} *on page 320*
Scientific Basis Published scientific studies of agents from the same pharmacologic class demonstrate depletion of some nutrients; however, this agent was NOT found to cause a similar depletion
Studies & Abstracts 167

♦ **Tolbutamide Sodium** *see* Tolbutamide* *on page 256*

Tolcapone (TOLE ka pone)
U.S. Brand Names Tasmar®
Pharmacologic Class Anti-Parkinson's Agent (COMT Inhibitor)
Nutrients Depleted
  Specific nutrient depletions have not been documented for this agent.

♦ **Tolectin**® *see* Tolmetin* *on page 256*

♦ **Tolectin**® **DS** *see* Tolmetin* *on page 256*

♦ **Tolinase**® *see* Tolazamide* *on page 256*

Tolmetin* (TOLE met in)
Related Information
  Drug-Induced Nutrient Depletion Table *on page 498*
U.S. Brand Names Tolectin®; Tolectin® DS
Canadian Brand Names Novo-Tolmetin
Synonyms Tolmetin Sodium
Pharmacologic Class Nonsteroidal Anti-Inflammatory Agent (NSAID)
Nutrients Depleted
  Folic Acid *on page 325*

Scientific Basis
Published scientific studies using this pharmacologic agent
or
Published scientific studies of agents from the same pharmacologic class
Studies & Abstracts 252

♦ **Tolmetin Sodium** *see* Tolmetin* *on page 256*

Tolterodine (tole TER oh dine)
U.S. Brand Names Detrol™
Pharmacologic Class Anticholinergic Agent
Nutrients Depleted
Specific nutrient depletions have not been documented for this agent.

♦ **Tolu-Sed® DM [OTC]** *see* Guaifenesin and Dextromethorphan *on page 141*

♦ **Topactin®** *see* Fluocinonide* *on page 130*

♦ **Topamax®** *see* Topiramate *on page 257*

♦ **Topicycline® Topical** *see* Tetracycline* *on page 249*

♦ **Topilene** *see* Betamethasone* *on page 46*

Topiramate (toe PYE ra mate)
U.S. Brand Names Topamax®
Pharmacologic Class Anticonvulsant, Miscellaneous
Nutrients Depleted
Specific nutrient depletions have not been documented for this agent.

♦ **Topisone** *see* Betamethasone* *on page 46*

♦ **TOPO** *see* Topotecan* *on page 257*

♦ **Toposar® Injection** *see* Etoposide* *on page 123*

Topotecan* (toe poe TEE kan)
U.S. Brand Names Hycamtin™
Synonyms Hycamptamine; SK and F 104864; SKF 104864; SKF 104864-A; TOPO; Topotecan Hydrochloride; TPT
Pharmacologic Class Antineoplastic Agent, Natural Source (Plant) Derivative
Nutrients Depleted
See Nutrient Depletion and Cancer Chemotherapy *on page 515.*
Scientific Basis Inferred or indirect evidence of depletion based on disruption of physiologic processes

♦ **Topotecan Hydrochloride** *see* Topotecan* *on page 257*

♦ **Toprol XL®** *see* Metoprolol* *on page 179*

♦ **Topsyn®** *see* Fluocinonide* *on page 130*

♦ **Torecan®** *see* Thiethylperazine* *on page 251*

Torsemide* (TOR se mide)
U.S. Brand Names Demadex®
Pharmacologic Class Diuretic, Loop
Nutrients Depleted
Calcium *on page 313*
(Continued)

Torsemide* *(Continued)*

    Magnesium *on page 333*
    Potassium *on page 340*
    Sodium *on page 345*
    Vitamin B₁ *on page 351*
    Vitamin B₆ *on page 357*
    Vitamin C *on page 360*
    Zinc *on page 368*
  Scientific Basis Published scientific studies of agents from the same
    pharmacologic class
  Studies & Abstracts 280-311
  Additional Information Sodium replacement is not routinely recom-
    mended in patients receiving loop diuretics. Potassium replacement
    should be guided by serum level monitoring.

♦ **Touro Ex®** *see* Guaifenesin *on page 140*
♦ **Touro LA®** *see* Guaifenesin and Pseudoephedrine *on page 142*
♦ **T-Phyl®** *see* Theophylline* *on page 250*
♦ **TPT** *see* Topotecan* *on page 257*

Tramadol (TRA ma dole)
  U.S. Brand Names Ultram®
  Synonyms Tramadol Hydrochloride
  Pharmacologic Class Analgesic, Non-narcotic
  Nutrients Depleted
    Specific nutrient depletions have not been documented for this agent.

♦ **Tramadol Hydrochloride** *see* Tramadol *on page 258*
♦ **Trandate®** *see* Labetalol* *on page 161*

Trandolapril* (tran DOE la pril)
  Related Information
    Drug-Induced Nutrient Depletion Table *on page 498*
  U.S. Brand Names Mavik®
  Pharmacologic Class Angiotensin-Converting Enzyme (ACE) Inhibi-
    tors
  Nutrients Depleted
    Zinc *on page 368*
  Scientific Basis Published scientific studies of agents from the same
    pharmacologic class
  Studies & Abstracts 269-271

Trandolapril and Verapamil*
    (tran DOE la pril & ver AP a mil)
  U.S. Brand Names Tarka®
  Pharmacologic Class Antihypertensive Agent, Combination
  Nutrients Depleted
    Zinc *on page 368*
  Scientific Basis Published scientific studies of agents from the same
    pharmacologic class
  Studies & Abstracts 269-271

- ◆ **Transdermal-NTG® Patch** *see* Nitroglycerin *on page 192*
- ◆ **Transderm-Nitro® Patch** *see* Nitroglycerin *on page 192*
- ◆ ***trans*-Retinoic Acid** *see* Tretinoin (Topical) *on page 259*
- ◆ **Tranxene®** *see* Clorazepate *on page 81*

Trazodone (TRAZ oh done)
U.S. Brand Names Desyrel®
Synonyms Trazodone Hydrochloride
Pharmacologic Class Antidepressant, Serotonin Reuptake Inhibitor/ Antagonist
Nutrients Depleted
Specific nutrient depletions have not been documented for this agent.

- ◆ **Trazodone Hydrochloride** *see* Trazodone *on page 259*
- ◆ **Tremytoine®** *see* Phenytoin* *on page 212*
- ◆ **Trental®** *see* Pentoxifylline *on page 209*

Tretinoin (Topical) (TRET i noyn, TOP i kal)
U.S. Brand Names Avita®; Renova®; Retin-A® Micro Topical; Retin-A® Topical
Canadian Brand Names Retisol-A®; Stieva-A®; Stieva-A® Forte
Synonyms Retinoic Acid; *trans*-Retinoic Acid; Vitamin A Acid
Pharmacologic Class Retinoic Acid Derivative
Nutrients Depleted
Specific nutrient depletions have not been documented for this agent.

- ◆ **Triacet™** *see* Triamcinolone* *on page 259*
- ◆ **Triadapin®** *see* Doxepin* *on page 106*
- ◆ **Triam-A®** *see* Triamcinolone* *on page 259*

Triamcinolone* (trye am SIN oh lone)
Related Information
Drug-Induced Nutrient Depletion Table *on page 498*
U.S. Brand Names Amcort®; Aristocort®; Aristocort® A; Aristocort® Forte; Aristocort® Intralesional; Aristospan® Intra-Articular; Aristospan® Intralesional; Atolone®; Azmacort™; Delta-Tritex®; Flutex®; Kenacort®; Kenaject-40®; Kenalog®; Kenalog-10®; Kenalog-40®; Kenalog® H; Kenalog® in Orabase®; Kenonel®; Nasacort®; Nasacort® AQ; Tac™-3; Tac™-40; Triacet™; Triam-A®; Triam Forte®; Triderm®; Tri-Kort®; Trilog®; Trilone®; Tri-Nasal® Spray; Tristoject®
Synonyms Triamcinolone Acetonide, Aerosol; Triamcinolone Acetonide, Parenteral; Triamcinolone Diacetate, Oral; Triamcinolone Diacetate, Parenteral; Triamcinolone Hexacetonide; Triamcinolone, Oral
Pharmacologic Class Corticosteroid, Adrenal; Corticosteroid, Oral Inhaler; Corticosteroid, Nasal; Corticosteroid, Parenteral; Corticosteroid, Topical
Nutrients Depleted
Calcium *on page 313*
Folic Acid *on page 325*
Magnesium *on page 333*
Potassium *on page 340*
(Continued)

Triamcinolone* *(Continued)*

Selenium *on page 343*
Vitamin C *on page 360*
Vitamin D *on page 363*
Zinc *on page 368*

Scientific Basis

Published scientific studies using this pharmacologic agent
or
Published scientific studies of agents from the same pharmacologic
class

Studies & Abstracts 182-223

- **Triamcinolone Acetonide, Aerosol** *see* Triamcinolone* *on page 259*
- **Triamcinolone Acetonide, Parenteral** *see* Triamcinolone* *on page 259*
- **Triamcinolone Diacetate, Oral** *see* Triamcinolone* *on page 259*
- **Triamcinolone Diacetate, Parenteral** *see* Triamcinolone* *on page 259*
- **Triamcinolone Hexacetonide** *see* Triamcinolone* *on page 259*
- **Triamcinolone, Oral** *see* Triamcinolone* *on page 259*
- **Triam Forte®** *see* Triamcinolone* *on page 259*
- **Triaminic® Allergy Tablet [OTC]** *see* Chlorpheniramine and Phenylpropanolamine *on page 73*
- **Triaminic® AM Decongestant Formula [OTC]** *see* Pseudoephedrine *on page 225*
- **Triaminic® Cold Tablet [OTC]** *see* Chlorpheniramine and Phenylpropanolamine *on page 73*
- **Triaminic® Expectorant [OTC]** *see* Guaifenesin and Phenylpropanolamine *on page 141*
- **Triaminic® Syrup [OTC]** *see* Chlorpheniramine and Phenylpropanolamine *on page 73*

Triamterene* (trye AM ter een)

Related Information

Drug-Induced Nutrient Depletion Table *on page 498*

U.S. Brand Names Dyrenium®

Pharmacologic Class Diuretic, Potassium Sparing

Nutrients Depleted

Calcium *on page 313*
Folic Acid *on page 325*
Zinc *on page 368*

Scientific Basis Published scientific studies using this pharmacologic agent

Studies & Abstracts 313-319

- **Triamterene and Hydrochlorothiazide** *see* Hydrochlorothiazide and Triamterene* *on page 149*
- **Triapin®** *see* Butalbital Compound and Acetaminophen* *on page 53*

Triazolam (trye AY zoe lam)
U.S. Brand Names Halcion®
Canadian Brand Names Apo®-Triazo; Gen-Triazolam; Novo-Triolam; Nu-Triazo
Pharmacologic Class Benzodiazepine
Nutrients Depleted
Specific nutrient depletions have not been documented for this agent.

Trichlormethiazide* (trye klor meth EYE a zide)
U.S. Brand Names Metahydrin®; Naqua®
Pharmacologic Class Diuretic, Thiazide
Nutrients Depleted
Coenzyme Q_{10} *on page 320*
Magnesium *on page 333*
Phosphorus *on page 339*
Potassium *on page 340*
Sodium *on page 345*
Zinc *on page 368*
Scientific Basis Published scientific studies of agents from the same pharmacologic class
Studies & Abstracts 320-342
Additional Information Although thiazide diuretics deplete sodium, replacement is not recommended, as this may be directly related to the therapeutic effect. Thiazides may deplete potassium, however replacement should be guided by monitoring of serum concentrations and specific instruction by a healthcare provider.

♦ **Trichloroacetaldehyde Monohydrate** *see* Chloral Hydrate *on page 72*
♦ **Tri-Clear® Expectorant [OTC]** *see* Guaifenesin and Phenylpropanolamine *on page 141*
♦ **TriCor™** *see* Fenofibrate* *on page 124*
♦ **Tricosal®** *see* Choline Magnesium Trisalicylate* *on page 76*
♦ **Tri-Cyclen®** *see* Ethinyl Estradiol and Norgestimate* *on page 121*
♦ **Triderm®** *see* Triamcinolone* *on page 259*
♦ **Tridil® Injection** *see* Nitroglycerin *on page 192*

Trifluoperazine* (trye floo oh PER a zeen)
U.S. Brand Names Stelazine®
Synonyms Trifluoperazine Hydrochloride
Pharmacologic Class Antipsychotic Agent, Phenothiazine, Piperazine
Nutrients Depleted
Coenzyme Q_{10} *on page 320*
Vitamin B_2 *on page 353*
Scientific Basis Published scientific studies of agents from the same pharmacologic class
Studies & Abstracts 474-477

♦ **Trifluoperazine Hydrochloride** *see* Trifluoperazine* *on page 261*
♦ **Tri-Kort®** *see* Triamcinolone* *on page 259*

- **Trilafon**® *see* Perphenazine* *on page 210*
- **Trileptal**® *see* Oxcarbazepine* *on page 201*
- **Tri-Levlen**® *see* Ethinyl Estradiol and Levonorgestrel* *on page 120*
- **Trilisate**® *see* Choline Magnesium Trisalicylate* *on page 76*
- **Trilog**® *see* Triamcinolone* *on page 259*
- **Trilone**® *see* Triamcinolone* *on page 259*

Trimethoprim* (trye METH oh prim)
U.S. Brand Names Primsol®; Proloprim®; Trimpex®
Synonyms TMP
Pharmacologic Class Antibiotic, Miscellaneous
Nutrients Depleted
  Bifidobacteria bifidum (bifidus) on page 311
  Biotin *on page 311*
  Folic Acid *on page 325*
  Inositol *on page 328*
  Lactobacillus acidophilus on page 332
  Vitamin B_1 *on page 351*
  Vitamin B_2 *on page 353*
  Vitamin B_3 *on page 354*
  Vitamin B_6 *on page 357*
  Vitamin B_{12} *on page 359*
  Vitamin K *on page 367*
Scientific Basis
  Published scientific studies using this pharmacologic agent
    or
  Inferred or indirect evidence of depletion based on disruption of physiologic processes
Studies & Abstracts 7-27, 69-71

- **Trimethoprim and Sulfamethoxazole** *see* Co-Trimoxazole* *on page 86*

Trimipramine* (trye MI pra meen)
U.S. Brand Names Surmontil®
Canadian Brand Names Apo®-Trimip; Novo-Tripramine; Nu-Trimipramine; Rhotrimine®
Synonyms Trimipramine Maleate
Pharmacologic Class Antidepressant, Tricyclic (Tertiary Amine)
Nutrients Depleted
  Coenzyme Q_{10} *on page 320*
  Vitamin B_2 *on page 353*
Scientific Basis Published scientific studies of agents from the same pharmacologic class
Studies & Abstracts 467-472

- **Trimipramine Maleate** *see* Trimipramine* *on page 262*
- **Trimox**® *see* Amoxicillin* *on page 33*
- **Trimpex**® *see* Trimethoprim* *on page 262*
- **Tri-Nasal**® **Spray** *see* Triamcinolone* *on page 259*

- **Tri-Nefrin® Extra Strength Tablet [OTC]** *see* Chlorpheniramine and Phenylpropanolamine *on page 73*
- **Tri-Norinyl®** *see* Ethinyl Estradiol and Norethindrone* *on page 121*
- **Triphasil®** *see* Ethinyl Estradiol and Levonorgestrel* *on page 120*
- **Triphenyl® Expectorant [OTC]** *see* Guaifenesin and Phenylpropanolamine *on page 141*
- **Triphenyl® Syrup [OTC]** *see* Chlorpheniramine and Phenylpropanolamine *on page 73*
- **Triptil®** *see* Protriptyline* *on page 225*
- **Trisenox™** *see* Arsenic Trioxide *on page 39*
- **Tristoject®** *see* Triamcinolone* *on page 259*
- **Trisulfa®** *see* Co-Trimoxazole* *on page 86*
- **Trisulfa-S®** *see* Co-Trimoxazole* *on page 86*
- **Tritec®** *see* Ranitidine Bismuth Citrate* *on page 229*
- **Trivagizole 3™ [OTC]** *see* Clotrimazole *on page 82*
- **Trizivir™** *see* Abacavir, Lamivudine, and Zidovudine* *on page 22*
- **Trocal® [OTC]** *see* Dextromethorphan *on page 96*

Trovafloxacin* (TROE va flox a sin)

U.S. Brand Names Trovan®
Synonyms Alatrofloxacin Mesylate; CP-99,219-27
Pharmacologic Class Antibiotic, Quinolone
Nutrients Depleted
Bifidobacteria bifidum (bifidus) *on page 311*
Biotin *on page 311*
Inositol *on page 328*
Lactobacillus acidophilus *on page 332*
Vitamin B_1 *on page 351*
Vitamin B_2 *on page 353*
Vitamin B_3 *on page 354*
Vitamin B_6 *on page 357*
Vitamin B_{12} *on page 359*
Vitamin K *on page 367*
Scientific Basis Inferred or indirect evidence of depletion based on disruption of physiologic processes
Studies & Abstracts 7-27

- **Trovan®** *see* Trovafloxacin* *on page 263*
- **Tusibron® [OTC]** *see* Guaifenesin *on page 140*
- **Tusibron-DM® [OTC]** *see* Guaifenesin and Dextromethorphan *on page 141*
- **Tussar® SF Syrup** *see* Guaifenesin, Pseudoephedrine, and Codeine *on page 143*
- **Tuss-DM® [OTC]** *see* Guaifenesin and Dextromethorphan *on page 141*
- **Tussi-Organidin® DM NR** *see* Guaifenesin and Dextromethorphan *on page 141*
- **Tuss-LA®** *see* Guaifenesin and Pseudoephedrine *on page 142*
- **Tusstat® Syrup** *see* Diphenhydramine *on page 102*
- **Twilite® Oral [OTC]** *see* Diphenhydramine *on page 102*

- **Two-Dyne®** *see* Butalbital Compound and Acetaminophen* *on page 53*
- **Tylenol® [OTC]** *see* Acetaminophen* *on page 23*
- **Tylenol® Extended Relief [OTC]** *see* Acetaminophen* *on page 23*
- **Tylenol® With Codeine** *see* Acetaminophen and Codeine* *on page 23*
- **Tylox®** *see* Oxycodone and Acetaminophen* *on page 202*
- **U-90152S** *see* Delavirdine* *on page 92*
- **UCB-P071** *see* Cetirizine *on page 71*
- **UK 92480** *see* Sildenafil *on page 237*
- **ULR-LA®** *see* Guaifenesin and Phenylpropanolamine *on page 141*
- **Ultram®** *see* Tramadol *on page 258*
- **Ultravate™** *see* Halobetasol* *on page 144*
- **Uni-Ace® [OTC]** *see* Acetaminophen* *on page 23*
- **Uni-Bent® Cough Syrup** *see* Diphenhydramine *on page 102*
- **Uni-Dur®** *see* Theophylline* *on page 250*
- **Unipen® Injection** *see* Nafcillin* *on page 187*
- **Unipen® Oral** *see* Nafcillin* *on page 187*
- **Uniphyl®** *see* Theophylline* *on page 250*
- **Uniretic™** *see* Moexipril and Hydrochlorothiazide* *on page 184*
- **Unithroid™** *see* Levothyroxine *on page 165*
- **Unitrol® [OTC]** *see* Phenylpropanolamine *on page 211*
- **Uni-tussin® [OTC]** *see* Guaifenesin *on page 140*
- **Uni-tussin® DM [OTC]** *see* Guaifenesin and Dextromethorphan *on page 141*
- **Univasc®** *see* Moexipril* *on page 183*

Uracil Mustard* (YOOR a sil MUS tard)

Pharmacologic Class Antineoplastic Agent, Alkylating Agent
Nutrients Depleted
    See Nutrient Depletion and Cancer Chemotherapy *on page 515.*
Scientific Basis Inferred or indirect evidence of depletion based on disruption of physiologic processes

- **Urecholine®** *see* Bethanechol *on page 47*
- **Uridon®** *see* Chlorthalidone* *on page 74*
- **Uri-Tet® Oral** *see* Oxytetracycline* *on page 202*
- **Uritol®** *see* Furosemide* *on page 135*
- **Urobak®** *see* Sulfamethoxazole* *on page 243*
- **Urozide®** *see* Hydrochlorothiazide* *on page 147*
- **Vagifem®** *see* Estradiol* *on page 114*

Valacyclovir (val ay SYE kloe veer)

U.S. Brand Names Valtrex®
Pharmacologic Class Antiviral Agent, Ophthalmic
Nutrients Depleted
    Specific nutrient depletions have not been documented for this agent.

- **Valertest No.1® Injection** *see* Estradiol and Testosterone* *on page 115*
- **Valium® Injection** *see* Diazepam *on page 97*
- **Valium® Oral** *see* Diazepam *on page 97*
- **Valproate Semisodium** *see* Valproic Acid and Derivatives* *on page 265*
- **Valproate Sodium** *see* Valproic Acid and Derivatives* *on page 265*
- **Valproic Acid** *see* Valproic Acid and Derivatives* *on page 265*

Valproic Acid and Derivatives*
(val PROE ik AS id & dah RIV ah tives)
Related Information
Drug-Induced Nutrient Depletion Table *on page 498*
U.S. Brand Names Depacon™; Depakene®; Depakote® Delayed Release; Depakote® ER
Canadian Brand Names Deproic
Synonyms Dipropylacetic Acid; Divalproex Sodium; DPA; 2-Propylpentanoic Acid; 2-Propylvaleric Acid; Valproate Semisodium; Valproate Sodium; Valproic Acid
Pharmacologic Class Anticonvulsant, Miscellaneous
Nutrients Depleted
Carnitine *on page 316*
Folic Acid *on page 325*
Scientific Basis Published scientific studies using this pharmacologic agent
Studies & Abstracts 157-166

Valrubicin* (val ru BYE cin)
U.S. Brand Names Valstar™
Pharmacologic Class Antineoplastic Agent, Anthracycline
Nutrients Depleted
See Nutrient Depletion and Cancer Chemotherapy *on page 515*.
Scientific Basis Inferred or indirect evidence of depletion based on disruption of physiologic processes

Valsartan (val SAR tan)
U.S. Brand Names Diovan™
Pharmacologic Class Angiotensin II Antagonists
Nutrients Depleted
Specific nutrient depletions have not been documented for this agent.

Valsartan and Hydrochlorothiazide*
(val SAR tan & hye droe klor oh THYE a zide)
U.S. Brand Names Diovan HCTZ®
Pharmacologic Class Antihypertensive Agent, Combination
Nutrients Depleted
Coenzyme Q_{10} *on page 320*
Magnesium *on page 333*
Phosphorus *on page 339*
Potassium *on page 340*
(Continued)

Valsartan and Hydrochlorothiazide* *(Continued)*

Sodium *on page 345*

Zinc *on page 368*

Scientific Basis Published scientific studies using this pharmacologic agent (hydrochlorothiazide)

Studies & Abstracts 320-342

Additional Information Sodium replacement is not recommended in patients receiving thiazides. Potassium replacement should be guided by serum level monitoring.

♦ **Valstar™** *see* Valrubicin* *on page 265*

♦ **Valtrex®** *see* Valacyclovir *on page 264*

♦ **Vancocin®** *see* Vancomycin *on page 266*

♦ **Vancocin® CP** *see* Vancomycin *on page 266*

♦ **Vancoled®** *see* Vancomycin *on page 266*

Vancomycin (van koe MYE sin)

U.S. Brand Names Lyphocin®; Vancocin®; Vancoled®

Canadian Brand Names Vancocin® CP

Synonyms Vancomycin Hydrochloride

Pharmacologic Class Antibiotic, Miscellaneous

Nutrients Depleted

Specific nutrient depletions have not been documented for this agent.

♦ **Vancomycin Hydrochloride** *see* Vancomycin *on page 266*

♦ **Vaniqa™ Cream** *see* Eflornithine *on page 109*

♦ **Vantin®** *see* Cefpodoxime* *on page 65*

♦ **Vapocet®** *see* Hydrocodone and Acetaminophen* *on page 149*

♦ **Vaseretic®** *see* Enalapril and Hydrochlorothiazide* *on page 110*

♦ **Vaseretic® 10-25** *see* Enalapril and Hydrochlorothiazide* *on page 110*

♦ **Vasotec®** *see* Enalapril* *on page 110*

♦ **Vasotec® I.V.** *see* Enalapril* *on page 110*

♦ **VCR** *see* Vincristine* *on page 268*

♦ **V-Dec-M®** *see* Guaifenesin and Pseudoephedrine *on page 142*

♦ **Veetids®** *see* Penicillin V Potassium* *on page 207*

♦ **Velban®** *see* Vinblastine* *on page 267*

♦ **Velosef®** *see* Cephradine* *on page 70*

♦ **Velosulin® BR Human (Buffered)** *see* Insulin Preparations *on page 156*

♦ **Velosulin® Human** *see* Insulin Preparations *on page 156*

Venlafaxine (VEN la faks een)

U.S. Brand Names Effexor®; Effexor-XR®

Pharmacologic Class Antidepressant, Serotonin/Norepinephrine Reuptake Inhibitor

Nutrients Depleted

Specific nutrient depletions have not been documented for this agent.

- **Ventolin**® *see* Albuterol *on page 26*
- **Ventolin**® **Rotocaps**® *see* Albuterol *on page 26*
- **VePesid**® **Injection** *see* Etoposide* *on page 123*
- **VePesid**® **Oral** *see* Etoposide* *on page 123*

Verapamil (ver AP a mil)

U.S. Brand Names Calan®; Calan® SR; Covera-HS®; Isoptin®; Isoptin® SR; Verelan®
Canadian Brand Names Apo®-Verap; Novo-Veramil; Nu-Verap
Synonyms Iproveratril Hydrochloride; Verapamil Hydrochloride
Pharmacologic Class Antiarrhythmic Agent, Class IV; Calcium Channel Blocker
Nutrients Depleted
Specific nutrient depletions have not been documented for this agent.

- **Verapamil Hydrochloride** *see* Verapamil *on page 267*
- **Verelan**® *see* Verapamil *on page 267*
- **Vergon**® [OTC] *see* Meclizine *on page 172*
- **Vermox**® *see* Mebendazole *on page 172*
- **Versacaps**® *see* Guaifenesin and Pseudoephedrine *on page 142*
- **Viagra**® *see* Sildenafil *on page 237*
- **Vibramycin**® *see* Doxycycline* *on page 106*
- **Vibramycin**® **IV** *see* Doxycycline* *on page 106*
- **Vibra-Tabs**® *see* Doxycycline* *on page 106*
- **Vicks**® **44D Cough & Head Congestion** *see* Pseudoephedrine and Dextromethorphan *on page 225*
- **Vicks**® **44E [OTC]** *see* Guaifenesin and Dextromethorphan *on page 141*
- **Vicks**® **44 Non-Drowsy Cold & Cough Liqui-Caps [OTC]** *see* Pseudoephedrine and Dextromethorphan *on page 225*
- **Vicks**® **DayQuil**® **Allergy Relief 4 Hour Tablet [OTC]** *see* Brompheniramine and Phenylpropanolamine *on page 50*
- **Vicks**® **DayQuil**® **Sinus Pressure & Congestion Relief [OTC]** *see* Guaifenesin and Phenylpropanolamine *on page 141*
- **Vicks Formula 44**® **[OTC]** *see* Dextromethorphan *on page 96*
- **Vicks Formula 44**® **Pediatric Formula [OTC]** *see* Dextromethorphan *on page 96*
- **Vicks**® **Pediatric Formula 44E [OTC]** *see* Guaifenesin and Dextromethorphan *on page 141*
- **Vicodin**® *see* Hydrocodone and Acetaminophen* *on page 149*
- **Vicodin**® **ES** *see* Hydrocodone and Acetaminophen* *on page 149*
- **Vicodin**® **HP** *see* Hydrocodone and Acetaminophen* *on page 149*
- **Videx**® *see* Didanosine* *on page 99*

Vinblastine* (vin BLAS teen)

U.S. Brand Names Alkaban-AQ®; Velban®
Synonyms Vinblastine Sulfate; Vincaleukoblastine; VLB
Pharmacologic Class Antineoplastic Agent, Natural Source (Plant) Derivative
(Continued)

Vinblastine* *(Continued)*

Nutrients Depleted
See Nutrient Depletion and Cancer Chemotherapy *on page 515.*

Scientific Basis Inferred or indirect evidence of depletion based on disruption of physiologic processes

- **Vinblastine Sulfate** *see* Vinblastine* *on page 267*
- **Vincaleukoblastine** *see* Vinblastine* *on page 267*
- **Vincasar® PFS™ Injection** *see* Vincristine* *on page 268*

Vincristine* (vin KRIS teen)
U.S. Brand Names Oncovin® Injection; Vincasar® PFS™ Injection
Synonyms LCR; Leurocristine; VCR; Vincristine Sulfate
Pharmacologic Class Antineoplastic Agent, Natural Source (Plant) Derivative

Nutrients Depleted
See Nutrient Depletion and Cancer Chemotherapy *on page 515.*

Scientific Basis Inferred or indirect evidence of depletion based on disruption of physiologic processes

- **Vincristine Sulfate** *see* Vincristine* *on page 268*

Vinorelbine* (vi NOR el been)
U.S. Brand Names Navelbine®
Synonyms Vinorelbine Tartrate
Pharmacologic Class Antineoplastic Agent, Natural Source (Plant) Derivative

Nutrients Depleted
See Nutrient Depletion and Cancer Chemotherapy *on page 515.*

Scientific Basis Inferred or indirect evidence of depletion based on disruption of physiologic processes

- **Vinorelbine Tartrate** *see* Vinorelbine* *on page 268*
- **Vioxx®** *see* Rofecoxib* *on page 234*
- **Viracept®** *see* Nelfinavir *on page 190*
- **Viramune®** *see* Nevirapine* *on page 191*
- **Visken®** *see* Pindolol* *on page 213*
- **Vistacon®** *see* Hydroxyzine *on page 152*
- **Vistaquel®** *see* Hydroxyzine *on page 152*
- **Vistaril®** *see* Hydroxyzine *on page 152*
- **Vistazine®** *see* Hydroxyzine *on page 152*
- **Vistide®** *see* Cidofovir *on page 76*
- **Vitamin A Acid** *see* Tretinoin (Topical) *on page 259*
- **Vitrasert®** *see* Ganciclovir *on page 136*
- **Vivactil®** *see* Protriptyline* *on page 225*
- **Vivelle® Transdermal** *see* Estradiol* *on page 114*
- **Vivol®** *see* Diazepam *on page 97*
- **V-Lax® [OTC]** *see* Psyllium *on page 226*
- **VLB** *see* Vinblastine* *on page 267*
- **Volmax®** *see* Albuterol *on page 26*

- ◆ **Voltaren**® **Ophthalmic** *see* Diclofenac* *on page 97*
- ◆ **Voltaren**® **Oral** *see* Diclofenac* *on page 97*
- ◆ **Voltaren Rapide**® *see* Diclofenac* *on page 97*
- ◆ **Voltaren**®**-XR Oral** *see* Diclofenac* *on page 97*
- ◆ **VP-16** *see* Etoposide* *on page 123*
- ◆ **VP-16-213** *see* Etoposide* *on page 123*

Warfarin (WAR far in)
U.S. Brand Names Coumadin®
Canadian Brand Names Warfilone®
Synonyms Warfarin Sodium
Pharmacologic Class Anticoagulant, Coumarin Derivative
Nutrients Depleted
  Specific nutrient depletions have not been documented for this agent.
Additional Information Warfarin blocks the action of vitamin K. However, supplementation of vitamin K is **NOT** recommended.

- ◆ **Warfarin Sodium** *see* Warfarin *on page 269*
- ◆ **Warfilone**® *see* Warfarin *on page 269*
- ◆ **Welchol**™ *see* Colesevelam* *on page 84*
- ◆ **Wellbutrin**® *see* Bupropion *on page 52*
- ◆ **Wellbutrin**® **SR** *see* Bupropion *on page 52*
- ◆ **Westcort**® *see* Hydrocortisone* *on page 150*
- ◆ **Wimpred** *see* Prednisone* *on page 219*
- ◆ **40 Winks**® **[OTC]** *see* Diphenhydramine *on page 102*
- ◆ **Wycillin**® *see* Penicillin G Procaine* *on page 207*
- ◆ **Wygesic**® *see* Propoxyphene and Acetaminophen* *on page 223*
- ◆ **Wymox**® *see* Amoxicillin* *on page 33*
- ◆ **Xanax**® *see* Alprazolam *on page 28*
- ◆ **Xeloda**® *see* Capecitabine* *on page 56*
- ◆ **Xenical**® *see* Orlistat* *on page 200*
- ◆ **Xopenex**™ *see* Levalbuterol *on page 163*

Zafirlukast (za FIR loo kast)
U.S. Brand Names Accolate®
Synonyms ICI 204, 219
Pharmacologic Class Leukotriene Receptor Antagonist
Nutrients Depleted
  Specific nutrient depletions have not been documented for this agent.

- ◆ **Zagam**® *see* Sparfloxacin* *on page 241*

Zalcitabine* (zal SITE a been)
Related Information
  Drug-Induced Nutrient Depletion Table *on page 498*
U.S. Brand Names Hivid®
Synonyms ddC; Dideoxycytidine
Pharmacologic Class Antiretroviral Agent, Reverse Transcriptase Inhibitor (Nucleoside)
(Continued)

Zalcitabine* *(Continued)*
Nutrients Depleted
Carnitine *on page 316*
Copper *on page 322*
Vitamin B$_{12}$ *on page 359*
Zinc *on page 368*
Scientific Basis Published scientific studies of agents from the same pharmacologic class
Studies & Abstracts 260-262

Zaleplon (ZAL e plon)
Pharmacologic Class Hypnotic, Nonbenzodiazepine
Nutrients Depleted
Specific nutrient depletions have not been documented for this agent.

♦ **Zanaflex®** *see* Tizanidine *on page 255*

Zanamivir (za NA mi veer)
U.S. Brand Names Relenza®
Pharmacologic Class Antiviral Agent
Nutrients Depleted
Specific nutrient depletions have not been documented for this agent.

♦ **Zantac®** *see* Ranitidine Hydrochloride* *on page 229*
♦ **Zantac® 75 [OTC]** *see* Ranitidine Hydrochloride* *on page 229*
♦ **Zantryl®** *see* Phentermine *on page 211*
♦ **Zapex®** *see* Oxazepam *on page 201*
♦ **Zarontin®** *see* Ethosuximide* *on page 122*
♦ **Zaroxolyn®** *see* Metolazone* *on page 179*
♦ **ZDV, Abacavir, and Lamivudine** *see* Abacavir, Lamivudine, and Zidovudine* *on page 22*
♦ **Zebeta®** *see* Bisoprolol* *on page 48*
♦ **Zefazone®** *see* Cefmetazole* *on page 63*
♦ **Zephrex®** *see* Guaifenesin and Pseudoephedrine *on page 142*
♦ **Zephrex LA®** *see* Guaifenesin and Pseudoephedrine *on page 142*
♦ **Zerit®** *see* Stavudine* *on page 241*
♦ **Zestril®** *see* Lisinopril* *on page 166*
♦ **Ziagen®** *see* Abacavir *on page 22*

Zidovudine* (zye DOE vyoo deen)
Related Information
Drug-Induced Nutrient Depletion Table *on page 498*
U.S. Brand Names Retrovir®
Canadian Brand Names Apo®-Zidovudine; Novo-AZT
Synonyms Azidothymidine; AZT; Compound S
Pharmacologic Class Antiretroviral Agent, Reverse Transcriptase Inhibitor (Nucleoside)
Nutrients Depleted
Carnitine *on page 316*
Copper *on page 322*
Vitamin B$_{12}$ *on page 359*

Zinc *on page 368*

Scientific Basis Published scientific studies using this pharmacologic agent

Studies & Abstracts 260-262

♦ **Zidovudine, Abacavir, and Lamivudine** *see* Abacavir, Lamivudine, and Zidovudine* *on page 22*

Zidovudine and Lamivudine*

(zye DOE vyoo deen & la MI vyoo deen)

U.S. Brand Names Combivir®

Synonyms AZT + 3TC

Pharmacologic Class Antiretroviral Agent, Protease Inhibitor; Antiretroviral Agent, Reverse Transcriptase Inhibitor (Nucleoside)

Nutrients Depleted

Carnitine *on page 316*

Copper *on page 322*

Vitamin B_{12} *on page 359*

Zinc *on page 368*

Scientific Basis Published scientific studies using these pharmacologic agents

Studies & Abstracts 260-262

Zileuton (zye LOO ton)

U.S. Brand Names Zyflo™

Pharmacologic Class 5-Lipoxygenase Inhibitor

Nutrients Depleted

Specific nutrient depletions have not been documented for this agent.

♦ **Zinacef® Injection** *see* Cefuroxime* *on page 68*

♦ **Zithromax™** *see* Azithromycin* *on page 43*

♦ **Zocor®** *see* Simvastatin* *on page 238*

♦ **Zofran®** *see* Ondansetron *on page 200*

♦ **Zolicef®** *see* Cefazolin* *on page 61*

Zolmitriptan (zohl mi TRIP tan)

U.S. Brand Names Zomig®

Synonyms 311C90

Pharmacologic Class Serotonin 5-HT_{1D} Receptor Agonist

Nutrients Depleted

Specific nutrient depletions have not been documented for this agent.

♦ **Zoloft®** *see* Sertraline *on page 237*

Zolpidem (zole PI dem)

U.S. Brand Names Ambien™

Synonyms Zolpidem Tartrate

Pharmacologic Class Hypnotic, Nonbenzodiazepine

Nutrients Depleted

Specific nutrient depletions have not been documented for this agent.

♦ **Zolpidem Tartrate** *see* Zolpidem *on page 271*

♦ **Zomig**® *see* Zolmitriptan *on page 271*

♦ **Zonalon**® **Topical Cream** *see* Doxepin* *on page 106*

♦ **Zonegran**™ *see* Zonisamide* *on page 272*

Zonisamide* (zoe NIS a mide)

Related Information
Drug-Induced Nutrient Depletion Table *on page 498*

U.S. Brand Names Zonegran™

Pharmacologic Class Anticonvulsant, Miscellaneous

Nutrients Depleted

Biotin *on page 311*

Calcium *on page 313*

Folic Acid *on page 325*

Inositol *on page 328*

Vitamin B_1 *on page 351*

Scientific Basis Inferred or indirect evidence of depletion based on disruption of physiologic processes

♦ **ZORprin**® *see* Aspirin* *on page 40*

♦ **Zosyn**™ *see* Piperacillin and Tazobactam Sodium* *on page 214*

♦ **Zovia**® *see* Estradiol and Ethynodiol Diacetate* *on page 114*

♦ **Zovirax**® *see* Acyclovir *on page 25*

♦ **Zyban**™ *see* Bupropion *on page 52*

♦ **Zydone**® *see* Hydrocodone and Acetaminophen* *on page 149*

♦ **Zyflo**™ *see* Zileuton *on page 271*

♦ **Zyloprim**® *see* Allopurinol *on page 27*

♦ **Zymenol**® **[OTC]** *see* Mineral Oil* *on page 181*

♦ **Zyrtec**® *see* Cetirizine *on page 71*

♦ **Zyvox**™ *see* Linezolid* *on page 166*

ALPHABETICAL LISTING OF NUTRIENTS AND THE DRUGS THAT DEPLETE

Beta-Carotene

Bifidobacteria bifidum (Bifidus)

Biotin

(Continued)

Biotin *(Continued)*

Calcium

(Continued)

Calcium *(Continued)*

Carnitine

Coenzyme Q$_{10}$

(Continued)

Coenzyme Q$_{10}$ *(Continued)*

Copper

Folic Acid

(Continued)

Folic Acid *(Continued)*

Glutathione

Inositol

Inositol *(Continued)*

Iron

Lactobacillus acidophilus

(Continued)

Lactobacillus acidophilus (Continued)

Magnesium

(Continued)

Magnesium *(Continued)*

Phosphorus

Potassium

(Continued)

Potassium *(Continued)*

SAMe

Selenium

Sodium

Sodium *(Continued)*

Tyrosine

Vitamin A

Vitamin B$_1$

(Continued)

Vitamin B₁ *(Continued)*

Vitamin B₂

(Continued)

Vitamin B₂ *(Continued)*

Vitamin B₃

Vitamin B$_6$

(Continued)

Vitamin B$_6$ *(Continued)*

Vitamin B₆ *(Continued)*

Vitamin B₁₂

Vitamin B$_{12}$ *(Continued)*

Vitamin C

Vitamin D

(Continued)

Vitamin D *(Continued)*

Vitamin E

Vitamin K

Zinc

(Continued)

Zinc *(Continued)*

ALPHABETICAL LISTING OF
NUTRIENT MONOGRAPHS

- ♦ **Acidulated Phosphate Fluoride** *see* Fluoride *on page 323*
- ♦ **Alpha Tocopherol** *see* Vitamin E *on page 365*
- ♦ **Ascorbic Acid** *see* Vitamin C *on page 360*

Beta-Carotene

Drugs That Deplete

See the Alphabetical Listing of Nutrients and the Drugs That Deplete *on page 273* for a complete listing.

Effects of Depletion Since beta-carotene is the dietary precursor of vitamin A, deficiencies of this nutrient are associated with the symptoms of vitamin A deficiency.

Low dietary intake of beta-carotene is associated with a weaker immune system, which is probably due to increased amounts of free radical damage. The incidence of numerous types of cancer is also associated with low dietary intake of beta-carotene.

Although several drugs are capable of reducing blood levels, the primary cause for a deficiency of beta-carotene is not eating enough colored fruits and vegetables.

Overview Beta-carotene belongs to a group of plant compounds called carotenoids. To date, over 500 carotenoids have been found to occur in nature. Carotenoids are the pigments that provide the yellow, orange, and red coloration in fruits and vegetables. Beta-carotene is the most abundant carotenoid in human foods and is generally thought to be the most important carotenoid for humans.

Beta-carotene, which is also known as pro-vitamin A, consists of two molecules of vitamin A linked head to head (A-A). Enzymes in the epithelial lining of the intestinal tract split beta-carotene into two molecules of vitamin A whenever the body needs it. This makes beta-carotene the most abundant precursor of vitamin A in fruits and vegetables.

Biological Function & Effect

- **Antioxidant:** Beta-carotene functions as a chain-breaking antioxidant. This means it does not prevent the initiation of lipid peroxidation, but rather, it stops the chain reaction by trapping free radicals, which halts the progression of free radical activity. Beta-carotene is the most effective natural agent capable of quenching single oxygen free radicals in humans.

Side Effects & Toxicity There are no known toxicities associated with beta-carotene. However, ingestion of large doses of beta-carotene can result in a harmless side effect called carotenosis, which is characterized by the appearance of an orange coloring in the skin. This coloration is most noticeable on the palms of the hands and the soles of the feet. The discoloration subsides when the dosage is lowered or stopped.

RDA No RDA has been established for beta-carotene; the most common supplemental dose of beta-carotene is 25,000 international units (IU) daily.

Dosage Range 5000-30,000 international units (IU)/day

Dietary Sources Beta-carotene occurs exclusively in plant (fruit and vegetable) foods. Foods containing high amounts of beta-carotene are green leafy vegetables, carrots, sweet potatoes, squash, spinach, apricots, peaches, cantaloupe, and green, yellow, and red peppers.

Forms Capsule: 15 mg, 30 mg

Bifidobacteria bifidum (bifidus)

Drugs That Deplete

See the Alphabetical Listing of Nutrients and the Drugs That Deplete *on page 273* for a complete listing.

Effects of Depletion

- Gas and bloating
- Diarrhea or constipation
- Bad breath
- Chronic vaginal yeast infections

Overview *Bifidobacteria bifidum* or *bifidus* is primary strain of beneficial bacteria that inhabits the large intestine. If the balance between the beneficial and pathological bacteria gets upset a condition known as dysbiosis develops. The use of antibiotics is a frequent cause of dysbiosis. When antibiotics are taken, most of the bifidobacteria are killed in addition to the pathological bacteria that are destroyed. Products containing beneficial bacteria are frequently referred to as probiotics.

Biological Function & Effect Bifidobacteria produce short chain fatty acids (SCFAs) in the colon which create a slight acidic environment that is unfavorable for the growth of pathological bacteria, yeasts, and molds. The short chain fatty acids produced by bifidobacteria are the main source of energy for the colonocytes, which are the cells that form the inner surface of the colon.

Side Effects & Toxicity There is no toxicity associated with probiotics and they do not interfere with other medications.

RDA No RDA has been set. Dosages for probiotics are measures in terms of cfu (colony forming units) which denote the number of live organisms per dose. Many probiotic products contain a combination of acidophilus and bifidobacteria.

- Dosage range for prevention: Healthy people can take a probiotic containing 1-2 billion cfu/day
- Patients with dysbiosis or after antibiotics: 10-15 billion cfu twice daily with a probiotic containing both bifidobacteria and acidophilus

Dosage Range 1-20 billion units

Dietary Sources Substantial amounts of bifidobacteria do not occur in foods. They are best obtained by purchasing commercial probiotic products that contain bifidobacteria.

Forms Capsules; Powder

Biotin

Synonyms Coenzyme R; Vitamin Bw; Vitamin H

Drugs That Deplete

See the Alphabetical Listing of Nutrients and the Drugs That Deplete *on page 273* for a complete listing.

Effects of Depletion Biotin deficiency in humans is very rare. Some diabetics may have an abnormality in the biotin-dependent enzyme (Continued)

Biotin *(Continued)*

pyruvate carboxylase, which can lead to dysfunctions of the nervous system. Deficiency symptoms include progressive hair loss, loss of hair color, depression, scaly dermatitis, lesions on the nose and mouth, anorexia, nausea, numbness and tingling of the extremities, muscle pain, and cardiac irregularities.

Overview Biotin is one of the more recently discovered water-soluble B vitamins. It was first isolated in 1936, the structure finally identified in 1942, and synthesized in 1943. Biotin is essential for the activity of many enzyme systems. Orally ingested biotin from plant and animal sources is protein bound. It is liberated by enzymatic action in the proximal small intestine where it is absorbed. Biotin is also absorbed from the distal small intestine where it is biosynthesized by the "friendly" intestinal bacteria.

Biological Function & Effect Biotin-containing enzymes play a vital role in the production of energy from the metabolism of carbohydrates and fats. Biotin-containing enzymes are also involved in the manufacture of fats and the excretion of byproducts from protein metabolism. Biotin-containing enzymes participate in a) carboxylation reactions (adding CO_2 to acceptor molecules), b) decarboxylation reactions where CO_2 groups are removed, and c) deamination reactions where NH_2 groups are removed from certain amino acids.

- **Healthy hair:** Biotin is known as the vitamin that produces healthy hair and helps prevent graying and baldness. Supplementation in cases of severe deficiency will help, but since biotin deficiency is very rare, these claims are suspect. However, biotin does help with "uncombable hair syndrome," a condition in children with multiple cowlicks where hair sticks up in all directions and will not lie down.
- **Fingernails:** In many cases, biotin helps people with dry, splitting fingernails.

Side Effects & Toxicity There are no known toxic effects from biotin. Excess is easily eliminated via urination.

RDA The RDA for biotin is 0.3 mg/day. Pharmacologic doses in the scientific literature range from 0.3 mg up to 3 mg. Since biotin is seldom deficient in humans, excessive intake of this vitamin is unwarranted.

Dosage Range 30-5000 mcg/day

Dietary Sources Biotin is found abundantly in many plant and animal foods. A considerable amount of biotin is also synthesized by the "friendly" intestinal bacteria.

Best food sources include liver, milk, brewer's yeast, bananas, grapefruit, watermelon, strawberries, and peanuts.

Forms Capsule; Liquid; Tablet

Boron

Available Compounds Boron Citrate; Boron Aspartate; Boron Glycinate

Drugs That Deplete
No medications were identified that deplete this nutrient.

Effects of Depletion
- Increased urinary loss of calcium and magnesium.
- Increased rate of bone demineralization, which probably influences the development of osteoporosis in postmenopausal women.

Overview Boron is a trace mineral. It is most prevalent in nature as borax, which is a mixture of boron, sodium and oxygen. Boron has been recognized as an essential nutrient for plants for almost 100 years, but its essentiality in humans was not discovered until the mid-1980s. Since boron is a relatively newly discovered essential nutrient for humans, some of the information about its metabolic activity and function is still somewhat speculative. Research in the past decade however, is strongly implicating that boron plays critical roles in metabolism and bone health.

Biological Function & Effect Boron has a powerful effect on the metabolism of calcium. When given to boron-deficient women, it caused a 44% reduction in urinary excretion of calcium. Boron also plays an important role in the metabolism of magnesium. In addition, boron has a regulatory effect on the production of estrogens and testosterone.

Biochemically, boron facilitates hydroxylation reactions, which is the addition of OH groups in chemical processes. The synthesis of estrogens and testosterone both require hydroxylation steps, so there is a strong indication that boron influences the production of these hormones.

- **Osteoporosis:** Boron may play a factor in the prevention of osteoporosis in postmenopausal women since it has been shown that boron substantially reduces urinary calcium loss.
- **Prevention of bone loss:** Boron may influence the synthesis of vitamin D, which plays a role in the prevention of bone loss.
- **Arthritis:** Individuals living in geographic areas with low soil boron levels have an increased incidence of osteoarthritis.

Side Effects & Toxicity Excessive intake of boron can cause nausea, vomiting, diarrhea, skin rashes, and fatigue. No health or medical problems have been reported in areas of the world where the daily diet supplies up to 41 mg/day of boron.

RDA No RDA has been set for boron. Based on animal studies, the human requirement for boron is estimated to be from 1-2 mg/day. Pharmacologic doses in the scientific literature range from 1-9 mg/day.

Dosage Range 1-9 mg/day

Dietary Sources Boron is readily available and easily absorbable from fruits and vegetables.

Forms Capsule; Liquid; Tablet

♦ **Calciferol** *see* Vitamin D *on page 363*

Calcium

Available Compounds Calcium Citrate; Aspartate; Ascorbate; Lactate; Phosphate; Carbonate; Glycinate; Maleate; Amino Acid Chelate; Microcrystalline Hydroxyapatite Compound (MCHC) (Continued)

Calcium *(Continued)*

Drugs That Deplete

See the Alphabetical Listing of Nutrients and the Drugs That Deplete *on page 273* for a complete listing.

Effects of Depletion Rickets is the classic calcium deficiency disease. It occurs most frequently in children and causes a variety of bone deformities. A lack of vitamin D and/or a lack of sunshine can cause the calcium deficiency that leads to rickets. Symptoms of calcium deficiency include muscle cramps, heart palpitations, high blood pressure, brittle or soft bones, tooth decay, back and leg pains, insomnia, nervous disorders, rickets, osteoporosis, and osteomalacia.

Osteoporosis and osteomalacia are the two main adult conditions caused by calcium deficiency. Bone deformities and fractures are the result.

Magnesium deficiency causes various abnormalities in calcium metabolism. Ingestion of foods high in phosphorus (soft drinks and animal protein) promote the urinary loss of calcium. Other significant factors that can negatively influence calcium levels include caffeine, excess dietary fat and fiber, and lack of exercise. Intestinal inflammatory conditions will decrease calcium absorption.

Overview Calcium is the most abundant mineral in the human body, and the fifth most common substance behind carbon, hydrogen, oxygen and nitrogen. Average healthy male bodies contain about 2.5-3 pounds of calcium while female bodies contain about 2 pounds. Approximately 99% of our calcium is present in the bones and teeth, which leaves only about 1% in cells and body fluids.

Although only a small amount of calcium is in the blood, the body goes to great lengths to maintain blood-calcium levels within a relatively narrow range. Three regulatory mechanisms control blood-calcium. If levels drop too low intestinal calcium absorption increases, bones increase calcium release, and the kidneys reduce calcium excretion.

Phosphorus displaces calcium. Ingesting large amounts of phosphorus-containing foods will cause increased urinary excretion of calcium, which can cause the body to leach calcium from the bones and thus contribute to osteoporosis. The main sources of dietary phosphorus are soft drinks and animal protein.

In bones and teeth, calcium exists primarily as hydroxyapatite, which is a calcium carbonate/calcium phosphate crystalline compound that provides rigidity and strength to these tissues.

There is some question about the appropriateness of cow's milk as a source of calcium. First, milk is a frequent cause of food allergies due to the ingestion of foreign (cow) proteins. Second, many people suffer digestive problems caused by lactose intolerance. Third, an enzyme from cow's milk, called xanthine oxidase, is capable of causing damage to arterial membranes, and antibodies to bovine xanthine oxidase have been found in the blood of individuals with atherosclerosis.

Biological Function & Effect

- **Bones & teeth:** Calcium's most important, documented function is in the development and maintenance of healthy bones and teeth. Need is greatest during periods of rapid growth including childhood, pregnancy and lactation.

- **Osteoporosis:** Calcium supplements are only minimally effective when taken alone. In one study, a nutritional supplement containing a broad range of micronutrients increased bone density 2-3 times more effectively than calcium alone.

- **High blood pressure:** Low levels of calcium are associated with high blood pressure, and many studies have shown that calcium supplementation provides hypertensive patients with a slight lowering of blood pressure. However, the gains are so small that calcium cannot be suggested as a treatment.

- **Cancer:** Several studies report that men with low levels of calcium intake have higher rates of colorectal cancer. Calcium supplementation in high risk individuals also decreased the rate of abnormal cell division in the colon.

- **Muscle contraction:** Ionized serum calcium helps to initiate muscle contractions. As such, it plays a vital role in the contraction-relaxation cycle that regulates a normal heart beat.

- **Blood clotting:** Calcium is involved in several steps of the blood clotting mechanism.

- **Cell wall permeability:** Ionized calcium regulates the passage of fluids across cellular membranes by affecting cell wall permeability.

- **Enzyme function:** Calcium activates various enzyme systems responsible for muscle contraction, fat digestion, and protein metabolism.

Side Effects & Toxicity Large doses of calcium are efficiently excreted by the body and do not usually produce toxic effects. Regularly taking large doses of calcium may interfere with the absorption of zinc, iron, and magnesium.

Recommended Dietary Allowance (RDA) for Calcium

Age/Condition	Amount of Calcium (elemental calcium/day)
0-6 months	400 mg
6-12 months	600 mg
1-5 years	800 mg
6-10 years	800-1200 mg
11-24 years	1200 mg
Males 25-65 years	1000 mg
Females 25-50 years	1000 mg
Pregnancy	1200-1500 mg
Females 51-65 years taking estrogen	1000 mg
Females 51-65 years NOT taking estrogen	1500 mg
>65 years	1500 mg

(Continued)

Calcium *(Continued)*

RDA Pharmacologic doses in the scientific literature range from 1000-2000 mg/day. See table on previous page for RDA information.

Dosage Range 800-2000 mg

Dietary Sources Milk and dairy products are the major source of dietary calcium for most people. Other good sources are dark green leafy vegetables, broccoli, legumes, nuts, and whole grains.

Forms Capsule; Liquid; Powder; Spray, liposomal; Tablet; Tablet, chewable

Carnitine

Drugs That Deplete

See the Alphabetical Listing of Nutrients and the Drugs That Deplete *on page 273* for a complete listing.

Effects of Depletion Carnitine deficiencies are rare because the body produces carnitine relatively easily. Symptoms include elevated blood lipids, abnormal liver function, muscle weakness, reduced energy, and impaired glucose control.

Overview Although carnitine is a nonessential amino acid, it also exhibits vitamin-like properties. It can be synthesized from the essential amino acids lysine and methionine. The highest concentrations of carnitine are found in the heart, muscles, liver, and kidney.

Biological Function & Effect

- **Cardiac function:** Carnitine's primary role seems to be the regulation of heart function because it regulates the production of energy in muscle tissue.
- **Fat metabolism:** Carnitine regulates fat metabolism by facilitating the transport of fats across cell membranes into the mitochondria for energy production.
- **Energy production:** Carnitine helps the body oxidize amino acids to produce energy when necessary.
- **Ketone metabolism:** Carnitine also helps to metabolize ketones.
- **Athletic performance:** Although it has not been well researched, many athletes take carnitine supplements to increase their energy and endurance.
- **Weight loss:** Carnitine's ability to increase the oxidation of fats suggests that it may be useful in weight-loss diets.

Side Effects & Toxicity Carnitine is quite safe with no significant side effects reported, even at high doses.

RDA No RDA has been set; dosage range: 1500-4000 mg/day in divided doses

Dosage Range 50 mg to 2 g

Dietary Sources Mostly found in foods of animal origin, and to a lesser extent, in foods of plant origin.

Forms Capsule; Powder; Tablet

Chloride

Drugs That Deplete

No medications were identified that deplete this nutrient.

Effects of Depletion Chloride deficiency is quite rare due to the widespread availability and use of salt (sodium chloride). A chloride deficiency creates a condition called metabolic alkalosis, which can cause diarrhea, vomiting, and sweating. Other symptoms of chloride deficiency include weakness, poor digestion, loss of appetite, and hair loss.

Chloride deficiency can be caused by extensive diarrhea, frequent vomiting, adrenal insufficiency, long-term use of diuretics, and systemic acidosis. Increased sweating can also cause chloride depletion.

Overview Chloride is one of the body's three major electrolytes (the other two being sodium and potassium). They exist as fully dissociated ions and are the main particles responsible for osmotic pressure in body fluids. The osmotic pressure is very rigidly controlled, primarily by regulatory mechanisms that determine the rate of resorption of ions and water through the kidney. These substances are called electrolytes because they carry an electronic charge in the dissociated (ionic) state. Their ionic strength enables them to influence the solubility of proteins and other substances throughout the body.

Hormonal control of chloride, sodium, and potassium is mediated through the hormones of the adrenal cortex and the anterior pituitary gland. Chloride and the other electrolytes are readily absorbed through the intestinal tract and are primarily excreted in the urine and sweat. Under normal conditions, chloride represents about 3% of the total mineral content of the body.

Biological Function & Effect Chloride is the primary anion functioning in the extracellular fluids throughout the body, which includes the blood, lymph, and the fluid in the spaces between the cells. Approximately 85% of the chloride ions reside in extracellular fluids and 15% in the intracellular fluids. Chloride, along with sodium and potassium helps to maintain normal osmotic equilibrium by controlling the distribution and balance of water throughout the body.

Chloride ions participate in the chloride-bicarbonate shift by having the ability to move in and out of red blood cells and blood plasma. This action permits the plasma transport of tissue CO_2 as bicarbonate to the lungs for excretion.

The electrolytes, in conjunction with calcium and magnesium, function in the maintenance of nerve transmission and normal muscle activity (contraction and relaxation).

- **pH**: Chloride, along with phosphate and sulfate ions, help to maintain the acid/alkaline pH balance throughout the body.
- **Digestion:** As part of gastric hydrochloric acid, chloride is necessary to maintain the normal acidity of the stomach for the processes of digestion.

Side Effects & Toxicity Excess chloride is efficiently excreted through the kidneys and, therefore, chloride toxicity is virtually impossible in humans. Due to efficient excretion of excess chloride, side effects are also a nonissue.
(Continued)

Chloride *(Continued)*

RDA No RDA has been set for chloride because it is so readily available; estimated safe and adequate intake of chloride for adults is from 1.5-5 g/day.

Dosage Range No dosage range has been established. Replenishment in amounts greater than the estimated safe and adequate intake should be done under a healthcare provider's supervision.

Dietary Sources The primary dietary source of chloride is table salt (sodium chloride). Chloride also occurs abundantly in vegetables and animal foods.

Forms As an anion, paired with a cation (such as sodium or potassium): Capsule; Powder; Tablet

Choline

Available Compounds Choline Bitartrate; Choline Citrate; Choline Chloride; CDP-Choline; Phosphatidyl Choline (Lecithin)

Drugs That Deplete
No medications were identified that deplete this nutrient.

Effects of Depletion Clear cases of deficiency in humans have not been reported.

Overview Choline is a member of the water-soluble B-complex vitamin group. Classifying choline as a vitamin is questionable since humans synthesize it. However, because the rate of synthesis is normally insufficient to meet human metabolic needs, choline has been included as an essential vitamin nutrient.

Biological Function & Effect Choline is the precursor to and a component of the neurotransmitter acetylcholine. As such, choline is intimately involved in a wide range of neurological activities, including the functions of movement, coordination, and the stimulation of muscle contraction. It also plays a critical role in the higher level cerebrocortical functions of thoughts, memory, and intellect.

Choline is a lipotropic (fat emulsifying) agent. Structurally, it contains three methyl groups which enable it to serve as a methyl donor in many important biochemical pathways.

Choline is also a part of phosphatidylcholine, a phospholipid that is a major structural component of cell walls and cellular membranes throughout the body. As part of phosphatidylcholine, choline functions in the metabolism of fat and in the transport of fat from the liver.

Choline is converted to betaine and then functions in transmethylation reactions (methyl donor) in the synthesis of amino acids and proteins.

- **Alzheimer's disease:** One of the main characteristics of Alzheimer's disease is a deficiency of acetylcholine. Some patients with mild to moderate Alzheimer's disease experience improvement in memory and cognitive function with high-dose phosphatidylcholine.
- **Tardive dyskinesia**: Choline is useful in reducing the tremors associated with tardive dyskinesia and other diseases of the nervous system.

Side Effects & Toxicity The toxicity of choline is very low. Oral ingestion of high doses of choline salts such as choline chloride can easily produce nausea, diarrhea, and dizziness Oral ingestion of choline also produces an unpleasant "fishy" odor. This is due to gut bacteria metabolizing the choline and releasing the odorous substance trimethylamine.

RDA No RDA has been set for choline. Pharmacologic doses in the scientific literature range from 2-10 g in divided doses. Larger doses are not practical because they cause diarrhea and the unpleasant "fishy" smell.

Dosage Range 150 mg to 10 g

Dietary Sources The richest source of dietary choline is egg yolk. Other good sources include organ meats, brewer's yeast, wheat germ, soy beans, peanuts, and legumes

Forms Capsule, gelatin; Liquid; Powder; Tablet

Chromium

Available Compounds Chromium Picolinate; Chromium Polynicotinate; Chromium Chloride; Chromium-Enriched Yeast (grown in a growth medium with added chromium)

Drugs That Deplete
No medications were identified that deplete this nutrient.

Effects of Depletion Poor dietary intake is the main cause of chromium deficiency. It is claimed to be one of the major nutritional deficiencies in the United States. High sugar consumption is a major contributing cause of chromium deficiency because sugar raises serum chromium levels, increasing its urinary excretion and accelerating chromium deficiency.

Chromium deficiency symptoms parallel those of diabetes. They include elevated blood sugar, numbness and tingling in the extremities, nerve disorders in the limbs, and glucose intolerance. Disturbances in protein and lipid metabolism have also been reported in conjunction with chromium deficiency.

Low levels of chromium are associated with cardiovascular disease.

Overview Chromium is an essential trace mineral that is very commonly deficient in American diets. One survey reported that the diets of 90% of Americans contained less than sufficient amounts of chromium. The body of an average healthy individual only contains several milligrams. However, this small amount plays important roles in the enhancement of insulin's effectiveness, regulation of blood sugar levels, and the activation of various enzymes for energy production.

Chromium is only biologically active in the trivalent state in which it forms complexes with organic compounds. One such complex is glucose tolerance factor (GTF) which has been identified as chromium (III) dinicotinic acid-glutathione complex. The components of the GTF complex include trivalent chromium, niacin, glycine, glutamic acid, and cysteine. In addition to potentiating the effect of insulin, GTF also seems to help lower elevated serum cholesterol and triglycerides.

Biological Function & Effect
- **Blood sugar and diabetes:** Chromium, as a component of glucose tolerance factor, enhances the blood sugar-lowering effects of insulin

(Continued)

319

Chromium *(Continued)*

by facilitating the uptake of glucose into cells. Chromium has been shown to increase insulin activity, possibly resulting in lower amounts of exogenous insulin necessary for blood sugar control. Studies suggest chromium is helpful in the prevention of Type 2 diabetes. This appears to be a significant finding for many elderly individuals.

- **Cholesterol:** Numerous studies indicate that chromium decreases total cholesterol, LDL cholesterol and triglycerides while increasing levels of HDL cholesterol. However, some studies have not shown these benefits.
- **Hypoglycemia:** Chromium may also be helpful for hypoglycemia.
- **Body mass:** Some studies have shown that supplemental chromium increases lean body mass.

Side Effects & Toxicity The occurrence of side effects and toxicity with supplemental chromium is virtually nonexistent in humans.

RDA There is no RDA for chromium. However, in 1989, the National Research Council recommended the Safe and Adequate Range for adults to be from 50-200 mcg/day. Pharmacologic doses in the scientific literature are frequently in the 200-400 mcg/day range.

Dosage Range 50-400 mcg/day

Dietary Sources Good chromium food sources include whole grain breads and cereals, lean meats, cheeses, and some condiments, such as black pepper and thyme.

In nutritional supplements, chromium is available in nutritional brewer's yeast, which is grown on a chromium-enriched growth medium; chromium picolinate; and chromium polynicotinate. All forms are fairly well absorbed.

Forms Capsule; Powder; Spray; Tablet

♦ **Cobalamin** *see* Vitamin B₁₂ *on page 359*

Coenzyme Q₁₀
Drugs That Deplete

See the Alphabetical Listing of Nutrients and the Drugs That Deplete *on page 273* for a complete listing.

Effects of Depletion Although we get a limited amount of coenzyme Q₁₀ (CoQ₁₀) from dietary sources, the majority of CoQ₁₀ in humans is manufactured by our own cells. The biosynthesis of coenzyme Q₁₀ is a 17-step process that requires the following nutrients: riboflavin (132), niacinamide (133), pantothenic acid (B₅), pyridoxine (136), cobalamin (B₁₂), folic acid, vitamin C, and numerous other trace elements. Consequently, there are many ways the complex synthesis of coenzyme Q₁₀ can be interrupted. It is probable that many people with health problems are suffering from a coenzyme Q₁₀ deficiency due to inadequate dietary intake of the necessary nutrients and/or ingestion of one or more drugs that interrupt the synthesis of coenzyme Q₁₀.

Symptoms of coenzyme Q₁₀ deficiency include congestive heart failure, high blood pressure, angina, mitral valve prolapse, stroke, cardiac arrhythmias, cardiomyopathy, lack of energy, gingivitis, and generalized weakening of the immune system.

Since coenzyme Q$_{10}$ is intimately involved in the production of energy, a deficiency of CoQ$_{10}$ first affects the heart and cardiovascular system because the heart is the most energy demanding muscle in the human body. The results of some studies suggest that congestive heart failure is primarily a coenzyme Q$_{10}$ deficiency disease.

Overview Coenzyme Q$_{10}$ is one of the most important nutrients in the human body. It is a fat-soluble vitamin-like compound that is also known as ubiquinone, from the word ubiquitous, meaning "everywhere." Coenzyme Q or ubiquinone compounds are synthesized in the cells of all living organisms including plants, animals and man. There are ten coenzyme Q compounds that occur throughout nature, but only coenzyme Q$_{10}$ is synthesized in humans.

In 1958, Professor Karl Folkers elucidated the chemical structure of coenzyme Q$_{10}$ while working at Merck, Inc. Working with minute quantities, Folkers was able to determine that CoQ$_{10}$ had great promise in the treatment of cardiovascular disease. However, Professor Folkers was not able to convince his superiors to pursue the development of CoQ$_{10}$ because Merck had recently launched their new blockbuster drug in the cardiovascular arena called Diuril®. Consequently, the formula and patent rights for coenzyme Q$_{10}$ were sold to a Japanese company. The Japanese quickly developed new methods of synthesizing large quantities, and coenzyme Q$_{10}$ has become the best selling natural product for cardiovascular disease in Japan. The story of the miracle nutrient, coenzyme Q$_{10}$, is just beginning to be recognized in the United States.

Biological Function & Effect

- **Energy:** Coenzyme Q$_{10}$ plays critical roles in the production of energy within the mitochondria. It is a coenzyme for numerous enzymes that are involved in the production of adenosine triphosphate (ATP), which is the high-energy fuel for all living cells.
- **Antioxidant:** Coenzyme Q$_{10}$ is also an important antioxidant. Because it is fat-soluble, it is able to reside in the mitochondrial cell membranes where it provides protection against free radical damage.
- **Cardiovascular disease:** CoQ$_{10}$ is reportedly useful in all kinds of cardiovascular disease. CoQ$_{10}$ has been found to be effective for periodontal disease.
- **Protective:** Coenzyme Q$_{10}$ also helps to protect against the toxic side effects of drugs such as Adriamycin®, beta-blockers, and drugs used for psychiatric disorders.

Side Effects & Toxicity Coenzyme Q$_{10}$ appears to be very safe. No studies have reported toxicity or adverse side effects.

RDA No RDA has been set for coenzyme Q$_{10}$. Normal supplement dosage range is 30-100 mg. There have been some reports of benefits for certain health conditions (eg, severe cardiovascular disease and advanced breast cancer) with dosages of 300-360 mg/day. Utilization of high dosages for severe health problems should only be done under the supervision of a physician.

(Continued)

Coenzyme Q₁₀ *(Continued)*

Dosage Range 30-100 mg

Dietary Sources Coenzyme Q compounds exist in the cells of all plants and animals. However, the level of coenzyme Q_{10} that we obtain from the diet is believed to be inadequate to meet the needs for optimal health and wellness.

Forms Capsule, powder-filled; Capsule, softgel; Spray, liposomal; Tablet, powder-based

♦ **Coenzyme R** *see* Biotin *on page 311*

Copper

Available Compounds Copper Gluconate; Copper Amino Acid Chelates; Copper Glycinate; Copper Lysinate; Copper Citrate; Copper Sulfate; Copper Sebacate

Drugs That Deplete

See the Alphabetical Listing of Nutrients and the Drugs That Deplete *on page 273* for a complete listing.

Effects of Depletion Severe copper deficiency is rare, but marginal copper deficiency is common since the diet of most Americans only supplies about 50% of the RDA. Symptoms of copper deficiency include loss of color in the hair and skin (due to decreased synthesis of melanin), anemia, fatigue, kinky hair, low body temperature, breakdown of connective tissue, various cardiovascular problems, nervous system disorders, and reduced resistance to infection.

Zinc interferes with copper absorption. High intake of zinc supplements can lead to copper deficiency.

Menkes' disease, also called kinky or steely hair syndrome, is a genetic defect in copper absorption characterized by stunted growth, abnormalities in cardiovascular and skeletal development, progressive cognitive decline, and premature death.

Some researchers have shown that copper deficiency is associated with elevated cholesterol and triglycerides, and the development of atherosclerosis. Thus, copper deficiency may play a role in the risk of cardiovascular disease. Copper deficiency has also been associated with emphysema.

Overview Copper is an essential trace mineral that is a cofactor in many cuproenzyme systems throughout the body. Copper is absorbed in the small intestine and carried on transcuprein and albumin to the liver where it is incorporated into liver enzymes and secreted into the blood on ceruloplasmin. Ceruloplasmin is a copper-carrying protein that is an important blood-based antioxidant. The results of some dietary surveys suggest that the diet of most Americans provides about 50% of the RDA for copper.

Biological Function & Effect

• **Oxygen transport:** Copper is required for the synthesis and function of hemoglobin, and therefore it plays a central role in the transport of oxygen throughout the body. Copper also stimulates the absorption of iron.

- **Collagen production:** Collagen synthesis, which determines the integrity of bone, cartilage, skin, and tendons, is copper dependent.
- **Elastin production:** Copper is involved in the production of elastin, which is the protein that provides the structural elasticity to tissues in the lungs, blood vessels, and skin.
- **Antioxidant component:** Copper is a component of many important enzymes such as copper-zinc superoxide dismutase (SOD), which is one of the body's most important antioxidant enzymes, and dopamine beta-hydroxylase, which oxidizes ascorbic acid and synthesizes norepinephrine.
- **Arthritis:** Copper chelates have anti-inflammatory activity and are effective in some forms of arthritis. A double-blind study has shown that wearing copper bracelets helps some arthritic individuals.
- **Cardiovascular disease:** Copper's role remains controversial. Studies show that both high and low copper levels can increase cardiovascular abnormalities.
- **Osteoporosis/Diabetes:** There is some indication that copper may also play a role in osteoporosis and diabetes.

Side Effects & Toxicity Copper toxicity is rare. Tissue elevations usually occur only when intake is 300-500 times above normal. Symptoms include GI disturbances, salivation, a metallic taste in the mouth, headache, dizziness, and weakness. Severe cases cause hypertension, liver damage, kidney failure, and death. In cases of elevated copper, the problems that develop may not be due to copper toxicity, but rather its interference with the absorption and distribution of other metal ions such as iron and zinc.

Wilson's disease is a genetic disorder that causes a toxic accumulation of copper in the liver, kidney, cornea of the eye, and central nervous system. Treatment involves a low copper diet and use of penicillamine which facilitates copper excretion.

Occasional copper toxicity has been reported in individuals who live in houses with copper water pipes where copper leaches into the drinking water.

RDA The RDA for copper is 2 mg/day. Pharmacologic doses of copper in scientific studies usually range from 2-4 mg/day.

Dosage Range 0.2-4 mg/day

Dietary Sources Copper-containing foods include oysters, organ meats, whole grain breads and cereals, shellfish, dark green leafy vegetables, dried legumes, nuts, and chocolate.

Forms Capsule; Tablet

♦ **Drug-Induced Nutrient Depletion Table** *see page 498*

Fluoride

Synonyms Acidulated Phosphate Fluoride; Sodium Fluoride; Stannous Fluoride

Drugs That Deplete

No medications were identified that deplete this nutrient.

Effects of Depletion The primary symptom of fluoride deficiency is an increase in the incidence of dental caries occurring in areas where natural levels are low and municipal water supplies are not fluoridated. (Continued)

Fluoride *(Continued)*

Overview Fluoride is a very controversial nutrient. Fluoridation of community water supplies is the main issue. Proponents claim that fluoridation reduces the incidence of dental caries and strengthens bone. However, the opponents of fluoridation claim that it does more harm than good. This issue is far from being resolved. Hotly contested, emotionally charged debates still occur in U.S. cities considering fluoridation, in other countries, and in scientific journals.

It is generally accepted that fluoride prevents cavities and has an effect on bone metabolism. Fluoride hardens tooth enamel and increases the stability of the bone mineral matrix. Health benefits include teeth that are less prone to developing cavities and possibly creating bones that are less susceptible to osteoporosis.

On the other hand, critics of fluoridation cite studies showing that children in fluoridated cities have about the same incidence of dental caries as those in nonfluoridated cities. They also cite studies reporting higher rates of osteoporotic bone fractures in fluoridated communities. Cancer is another concern. In 1977, results of a study presented at a Congressional hearing revealed that people living in the 10 largest fluoridated U.S. cities had a 15% higher incidence of cancer than those living in the 10 largest nonfluoridated cities.

Whether or not municipal water supplies should be fluoridated is a medical, social, and political issue, and is far from being resolved. Individuals on both sides of the argument agree that fluoride produces some beneficial effects on teeth. In 1989, the American Dental Association reduced its long standing official estimate of 60% benefit, and now states that fluoride provides a 25% reduction in tooth decay.

There are two points in the fluoride debate that are beyond argument. First, ingestion of too much fluoride can produce a number of undesirable side effects. Second, there is a relatively narrow dosage range between benefits and side effects, and there are big differences in an individual's sensitivity to fluoride.

Biological Function & Effect

- **Teeth:** Fluoride's primary function is related to the prevention of dental caries. In children, fluoride creates stronger teeth because it gets incorporated into dental structure during tooth formation. Its effects are greatest when given during early childhood when teeth are still forming. After eruption, topical fluoride gets deposited into the enamel creating a stronger protective surface.
- **Function:** Fluoride replaces the hydroxy portion of hydroxyapatite in bone crystalline structure, producing a less water-soluble, more stable substance called fluorapatite.
- **Osteoporosis:** Some reports suggest that fluoride protects against osteoporosis and is also useful for osteoporosis. Fluoride works in conjunction with calcium to stimulate new bone growth, and it is also incorporated into the bone crystalline matrix making bone stronger.

Side Effects & Toxicity Fluorosis is the main side effect from excess fluoride. This is a mottling discoloration of the teeth that occurs in children if they ingest too much fluoride during tooth development.

There are studies that report that in sensitive individuals, fluoride does damage to immune and nervous systems, possibly setting the stage for multiple chemical sensitivities. Fluoride may also interfere with various enzyme systems, harm a developing fetus, and play a role in arthritis, gastric ulcers, atherosclerosis, kidney disorders, and migraine headaches.

It is relatively easy to get too much fluoride since it is found in soils, plants, animal tissues, water supplies, dental products, and fluoride vitamin supplements, as well as foods and beverages processed with fluoridated water. Moderate fluorosis occurs in 1% to 2% of children exposed to 1 ppm fluoride and in approximately 10% of children exposed to 2 ppm. Moderate to severe fluorosis occurs in varying percentages up to as high as 33% of children exposed to 2.4-4.1 ppm. Groups that are potentially at higher risk for fluoride-associated problems include formula-fed infants, heavy exercisers, individuals with high consumption of water-based beverages, people with malfunctioning kidneys, and the elderly.

RDA No RDA has been established for fluoride. The U.S. Environmental Protection Agency's limit for fluoride in municipal water supply is 0.7-1.2 ppm. The maximal acceptable limit is 4 ppm.

Dosage Range 0.25-1 mg daily of the fluoride ion (1 mg of fluoride ion = 2.2 mg of sodium fluoride). Supplemental fluoride should only be given under the supervision of a healthcare provider.

Dietary Sources Fluoride content varies widely in soil, water, plants, and animals in different areas of the United States. Many cities have fluoridated water supplies. However, more and more people believe that municipal water supplies contain unacceptable levels of toxins and opt for bottled or filtered water. Fluoride is also available in toothpaste, mouthwash, topical dental applications, and fluoride vitamin supplements.

Forms Drops, oral; Gel; Lozenge; Rinse, topical; Solution, oral; Tablet; Tablet, chewable

Note: With the exception of the topical products, the above forms are available only by prescription in the United States.

♦ **Folacin** see Folic Acid on page 325

Folic Acid

Synonyms Folacin

Available Compounds Folate; Folinic Acid

Drugs That Deplete

See the Alphabetical Listing of Nutrients and the Drugs That Deplete on page 273 for a complete listing.

Effects of Depletion Folic acid deficiency harms DNA metabolism, which causes abnormal cellular development, especially in cells with the most rapid rates of turnover (ie, red blood cells, leukocytes, and epithelial cells of the stomach, intestine, vagina and uterine cervix). Folic acid needs are greater during pregnancy. Folic acid is one of the most common vitamin deficiencies. It is easily destroyed by heat, light, and oxygen. Substantial losses occur in cooking and storage. (Continued)

Folic Acid *(Continued)*

Symptoms of folic acid deficiency include megaloblastic anemia, birth defects, cervical dysplasia, elevated homocysteine, headache, fatigue, hair loss, anorexia, insomnia, diarrhea, nausea, and increased infections.

Folic acid is necessary for the production of red blood cells (erythrocytes) which carry oxygen from the lungs to the tissues and carbon dioxide from tissues to the lungs. Folic acid deficiency results in anemia and reduced tissue oxygenation. This results in a condition known as megaloblastic anemia, which is a condition characterized by enlarged nucleated abnormal red blood cells. This condition can produce symptoms of tiredness, weakness, diarrhea, and weight loss.

Folic acid helps regulate neural development and the transfer of genetic material to new cells. Numerous drugs have been shown to deplete folic acid. During pregnancy, the rapidly growing fetus substantially increases a woman's need for folic acid. Folic acid deficiency during pregnancy dramatically increases the risk of birth defects such as spina bifida and cleft palate. The link between folic acid deficiency and birth defects is so strong, the authors recommend that all women have their folic acid status checked before trying to become pregnant. If this practice were followed, thousands of birth defects would probably be prevented each year. A laboratory test called the Neutrophilic Hypersegmentation Index (NHI) has been developed that can identify the earliest stages of folate insufficiency.

Cervical dysplasia is a term that refers to the development of abnormal cells in the uterus. It is a precancerous condition that is usually discovered when a woman has her annual PAP exam. This condition may contribute to an increased number of hysterectomies. Over 800,000 women have hysterectomies every year in the United States. Some professionals believe that the folic acid depletion caused by oral contraceptives is linked to this high incidence of cervical dysplasia and hysterectomies.

Elevated homocysteine is now recognized as one of the most critical independent risk factors to cardiovascular disease. Homocysteine is a toxic intermediate metabolite in the metabolism of the amino acid methionine. It is capable of directly damaging the vascular system and initiating the process of atherosclerosis. Folic acid is one of the nutrients that is required to metabolize homocysteine so that it does not build up in the blood and begin to damage the lining of the blood vessels.

Overview Folic acid is a member of the B vitamin group. Isolated in 1946 from spinach leaves, its name comes from folium, the Latin word for leaf. In the body, folic acid is converted to its biologically active form tetrahydrofolic acid (THFA). Niacin and vitamin C are necessary for this conversion. Structurally, folic acid consists of a pteridine (containing two rings) nucleus, conjugated with para-aminobenzoic acid, and glutamic acid. Hence, its chemical name is pteroylmonoglutamate.

Biological Function & Effect

- **Cell division:** Like vitamin B_{12}, folic acid is intimately involved in the synthesis of both DNA and RNA. Hence, it is essential for proper cellular division and the transmission of our genetic code to all newly formed cells.
- **Cancer:** Folic acid may protect against certain types of cancers including precancerous cervical dysplasia in women (especially those taking oral contraceptives), bronchial squamous metaplasia in long-time heavy cigarette smokers, and dysplasia associated with ulcerative colitis and colon cancer.
- **Birth defects:** Folic acid prevents birth abnormalities such as neural tube defects, cleft palate, and cleft lip and is essential for the healthy maturation of both red and white blood cells.
- **Cervical dysplasia:** Folic acid supplementation has been shown to prevent and reverse cervical dysplasia, which is recognized as a precancerous condition.
- **Atherosclerosis:** Folic acid is required for the conversion of homocysteine to methionine. High blood levels of homocysteine are associated with the development of atherosclerosis.

Side Effects & Toxicity Folic acid is essentially nontoxic, even at very high doses. Large doses of folic acid can mask an underlying vitamin B_{12} deficiency, which if gone undetected, could result in irreversible nerve damage. Consequently, folic acid is limited to 800 mcg in OTC nutritional supplements.

RDA The RDA for folic acid is 200 mcg/day. Pregnant and lactating women require dosages higher than the RDA. Pharmacologic dosages in the scientific literature range from 400-4000 mcg.

Dosage Range 200-800 mcg/day; however, physicians occasionally need to administer doses to severely deficient patients ranging from 5000-10,000 mcg/day. Supplementation in patients receiving phenytoin and/or co-trimoxazole should not be initiated without consultation with the prescriber. For additional information, see phenytoin *on page 212* and co-trimoxazole *on page 86.*

Dietary Sources Folic acid occurs in a wide variety of foods. Best sources include dark green leafy vegetables, brewer's yeast, liver, and eggs. Other good sources are beets, broccoli, brussel sprouts, orange juice, cabbage, cauliflower, cantaloupe, kidney and lima beans, wheat germ, whole grain cereals and breads. Folic acid is also synthesized by the "friendly" intestinal bacteria.

Forms Capsule; Liquid; Spray, liposomal; Tablet; Tablet, effervescent

♦ **Food-Drug Interactions, Key Summary** *see page 519*

Glutathione

Available Compounds L-glutathione

Drugs That Deplete

See the Alphabetical Listing of Nutrients and the Drugs That Deplete *on page 273* for a complete listing.

Effects of Depletion Decreased capacity for hepatic detoxification. Decreased immunity and suppression of macrophage activity. A lack of glutathione may lead to increased free radical damage throughout (Continued)

Glutathione *(Continued)*

the body, especially in the membranes of red blood cells and mitochondria. Glutathione deficiency could result in hair loss and baldness.

Overview Glutathione is a part of critical detoxifying and antioxidant enzyme systems. Supplementation may aid in protecting the liver from toxic damage, strengthen the immune system, and protect against oxidative damage to tissues.

Special note: Glutathione must be in its reduced form to be active. Some manufacturers do not indicate if their product is reduced. In general, the unreduced form is cheaper, but it is not metabolically active.

Biological Function & Effect Glutathione is a sulfur-containing tripeptide that is composed of cysteine, glycine, and glutamic acid.

- **Detoxification:** Glutathione participates in the hepatic detoxification of many compounds via glutathione S-transferase. This enzyme participates in the detoxification of compounds from cigarette smoke, ethanol, and overdoses of aspirin or acetaminophen.
- **Antioxidant:** Glutathione is part of the antioxidant enzyme systems, including glutathione peroxidase. It reduces oxidative damage, particularly in mitochondria and red blood cells, and appears to reduce free radical damage due to radiation.
- **Fatty acid synthesis:** Glutathione is involved in cellular transmembrane amino acid transport systems and is involved in fatty acid synthesis.
- **Immune function:** It facilitates the development and function of a variety of immune cells, including macrophages and lymphoctyes.

Side Effects & Toxicity There are no known toxicities or serious side effects.

RDA Nutritional guidelines have not been established.

Dosage Range 500-3000 mg/day in divided doses

Dietary Sources Asparagus, avocado, walnuts, fresh fruit, raw vegetables, fish, meat

♦ **Herb/Nutrient Depletions** *see page 512*

Inositol

Available Compounds Inositol Monophosphate

Drugs That Deplete

See the Alphabetical Listing of Nutrients and the Drugs That Deplete *on page 273* for a complete listing.

Effects of Depletion No inositol deficiency has been identified in humans, and a deficiency is not likely because of its widespread occurrence in foods.

Overview Inositol is a compound that has been known for a long time, but in 1940 scientists first realized that it was a vitamin. It is a sugar-like, water-soluble substance and is part of the B vitamin complex. It is found in the liver, kidney, skeletal and heart muscle, and in the leaves and seeds of most plants. In animal tissues, inositol occurs as a component of phospholipids and in plants, it usually occurs as phytic acid, which is the hexaphosphate ester of inositol. In humans, inositol is synthesized in the intestinal tract by the normal or "friendly" bacteria.

Biological Function & Effect

- **Phospholipids:** Inositol is an essential component of phospholipids in cellular membranes of animals and humans. The metabolically active form of myo-inositol is phosphatidylinositol. As part of phospholipids in cellular membranes, phosphatidylinositol helps to mediate cellular responses to external stimuli. Phosphatidylinositol also facilitates the production of arachidonic acid.
- **Diabetic neuropathy:** Myo-inositol may be helpful in diabetic neuropathy.
- **Psychiatric:** Several studies have shown that inositol can offer benefit for depression, panic, and obsessive-compulsive disorders.

Side Effects & Toxicity No toxicity has been reported or observed.

RDA No RDA has been set for inositol. Pharmacologic doses in the scientific literature range from 100-1000 mg.

Dosage Range 100-1000 mg/day

Dietary Sources Myo-inositol occurs in foods in three different forms: free myo-inositol, phytic acid, and inositol-containing phospholipids. The richest sources of myo-inositol are the seeds of plants such as beans, grains, and nuts. The richest animal sources are organ meats. Free myo-inositol predominates in brain and kidney, whereas phospholipid-inositol is concentrated in skeletal muscle, heart, liver, and pancreas.

Forms Capsule; Powder; Tablet

Iodine

Drugs That Deplete

No medications were identified that deplete this nutrient.

Effects of Depletion Hypothyroidism: A lack of iodine decreases thyroid hormone synthesis. Low thyroid activity reduces the rate of energy production and can cause fatigue and weight gain.

Goiter: A deficiency of iodine can result in enlargement of the thyroid gland. When this becomes visible it is called a simple goiter. This condition can be prevented and frequently cured by administration of iodine.

Cretinism: Iodine deficiency during pregnancy can cause cretinism. This condition imparts serious injury to the developing fetus, resulting in both mental and physical retardation.

Myxedema: Iodine deficiency is one cause of this condition. The resulting hypofunction of the thyroid gland causes decreased metabolic rate, anemia, enlarged tongue, slow speech, puffiness of the hands and face, problems with skin and hair, drowsiness, and mental apathy.

Goitrogens are naturally-occurring substances in some foods that can inhibit the synthesis and secretion of thyroid hormones. Some common foods containing goitrogens are raw cabbage, turnips, cauliflower, soybeans, and peanuts. Problems are unlikely unless an
(Continued)

Iodine *(Continued)*

iodine-deficient individual engages in prolonged consumption of these foods. Cooking deactivates goitrogen compounds in these foods.

Overview Iodine's only known function is the role it plays in the various thyroid hormones: diiodotyrosine, triiodothryonine (T3) and thyroxine (T4). Dietary iodine is converted to iodide in the GI tract where it is easily absorbed and transported to the thyroid gland. In the thyroid gland, iodine is stored on the tyrosine moiety of a protein complex called thyroglobulin.

Iodine metabolism and thyroid hormone production are regulated by a negative feedback hormonal control system. A decline in blood thyroid hormones triggers the hypothalamus to release thyroid releasing hormone (TRH) which in turn signals the anterior pituitary to release thyroid stimulating hormone (TSH). An increase in TSH stimulates the thyroid gland to increase the uptake of iodine and synthesize more thyroid hormones. TSH also stimulates the thyroid gland to produce enzymes, which cleave thyroglobulin to release the thyroid hormones into circulation for delivery to cells throughout the body.

Biological Function & Effect Iodine's effects are all related to activity and function of the thyroid hormones.

- **Cellular function:** Iodine-dependent thyroid hormones regulate cellular oxygen consumption, basal metabolism, and energy production throughout the body. As a result, thyroid hormones control a variety of biological and physiological activities including body temperature, physical growth, reproduction, neuromuscular function, synthesis of proteins, and skin and hair growth.
- **Fibrocystic breasts:** Iodine deficiency may be a contributing factor. Iodine supplementation has caused complete relief of symptoms in some women.
- **Mucolytic agents:** Iodine-containing prescription products such as SSKI (saturated solution of potassium iodide) and Organidin®, are frequently effective for loosening irritating mucous secretions.
- **Thyroid gland:** If the thyroid gland is damaged or absent, the basal metabolic rate can decline to as low as 55% of normal, resulting in impaired growth and development. When the thyroid gland is hyperactive, the basal metabolic rate can go up as high as 160% of normal, causing tachycardia, nervousness, and excitability.

Side Effects & Toxicity Iodine is a relatively benign trace element which generally causes no harm at dosages 10-20 times above normal daily needs. The thyroid gland absorbs more iodine, but thyroid synthesis remains normal. Chronic excessive intake of iodine can cause enlargement of the thyroid gland resembling a goiter. This condition is called an "iodine goiter."

RDA The RDA for iodine is 150 mcg/day.

Dosage Range 50-250 mcg/day. Pharmacologic doses for iodine in scientific studies are generally in the range of 3-6 mg/day, but these should only be taken under the supervision of a physician.

Dietary Sources Iodized salt is the most common source of iodine in the United States. Iodine-rich foods include seafood, sea vegetables (seaweed), and vegetables grown in iodine-rich soil.

Iron

Available Compounds Ferrous Sulfate; Ferrous Gluconate; Ferrous Fumarate; Ferrous Glycinate; Ferric Ammonium Citrate

Drugs That Deplete

See the Alphabetical Listing of Nutrients and the Drugs That Deplete *on page 273* for a complete listing.

Effects of Depletion Menstrual bleeding is the most common cause of iron deficiency. About 80% of iron in the body is in blood, so iron losses are greatest with blood loss. Menstruating women require approximately twice as much iron intake as men to replace their monthly losses. Individuals at risk include infants, adolescent girls, those who are pregnant or menstruating, people with bleeding ulcers, and vegetarians. Iron deficiency anemia is the classic condition where red blood cells contain less hemoglobin and consequently carry less oxygen. Symptoms of iron deficiency include anemia, weakness, fatigue, skin pallor, headache, hair loss, labored breathing upon exertion, spooning of fingernails, brittle nails, and greater susceptibility to infection.

Pagophagia is a term referring to an individual who deliberately consumes large quantities of ice. This condition is related to iron deficiency and is completely resolved with low level iron supplementation.

Hypochlorhydria: Gastric hydrochloric acid is necessary for iron absorption. A lack of hydrochloric acid, which occurs frequently in the elderly, can lead to iron deficiency.

The use of antacids and drugs that alter gastric acidity inhibit iron absorption. Complexing agents, such as phytates, oxalates, and phosphates, form insoluble iron complexes, which reduce absorption. Vitamin E also inhibits the absorption of iron. This is generally not a cause of iron deficiency, but it is not advisable to take supplemental doses of iron and vitamin E at the same time.

Diarrhea, intestinal inflammation, or other conditions that increase intestinal motility will also reduce absorption.

Iron deficiency is frequently overlooked as a cause of hair loss.

Overview Iron plays a central role in many vital biochemical pathways. The primary functions of iron involve oxygen transport within blood and muscle, electron transfer in relation to the cellular uptake of oxygen, and the conversion of blood sugar to energy. Iron is also a part of many enzymes that are involved in making new cells, amino acids, hormones, and neurotransmitters. Iron exists in various forms in the body: in functional forms (in hemoglobin and enzymes), and in transport and storage forms (ferritin, transferrin, and hemosiderin).

Biological Function & Effect

- **Oxygen transport:** The major function of iron is for oxygen transport by hemoglobin. Hemoglobin is the oxygen-carrying protein in red blood cells. The heme portion of hemoglobin contains 4 atoms of iron. Iron picks up the oxygen in the lungs where the concentration is high. Iron binds the oxygen and then transports it to the tissues and releases it wherever needed.

(Continued)

Iron *(Continued)*

- **Oxygen storage:** Myoglobin is an iron-containing protein in muscles that acts as an oxygen acceptor and oxygen storage reservoir in muscle.
- **Immune system:** Iron is one of the substances that is necessary for optimal immune response.
- **Metabolism:** Iron is necessary for the synthesis of the amino acid carnitine which plays an essential role in the metabolism of fatty acids.
- **Enzymatic:** Much of iron's functional activity in electron transport and energy production has to do with its ability to convert back and forth between its reduced, or ferrous state (Fe^{++}), and its oxidized ferric state (Fe^{+++}). This is how oxygen is either held or released. Iron plays an important role in the cytochrome P-450 liver detoxification enzymes. Iron is part of the enzymes that initiate the synthesis of the neurotransmitters serotonin and dopamine.
- **Collagen and elastin:** The synthesis of collagen and elastin require iron.

Side Effects & Toxicity When the body's iron stores are full, the body absorbs less iron. Therefore, iron toxicity is rare, but it can occur. Primary causes of iron toxicity include ingestion of too much iron and a genetic defect (hemochromatosis) usually occurring in men, which causes excessive iron absorption and results in damage to the heart, liver, spleen, and pancreas. Alcoholism can cause intestinal and liver damage which can lead to increased iron absorption.

RDA The RDA for iron is 15 mg/day for women and 10 mg/day for men. Pharmacologic doses in the scientific literature range from 10-50 mg/day.

Dosage Range 10-50 mg/day

Dietary Sources Liver is by far the richest iron-containing food. Other good sources of iron-rich foods include organ meats, fish, and poultry. Dried beans and vegetables are the best plant sources, followed by dried fruits, nuts, and whole grain breads and cereals. Fortification of cereals, flours, and bread with iron has contributed significantly to daily dietary iron consumption.

Forms Capsule; Capsule, time-release; Liquid; Tablet

Lactobacillus acidophilus

Drugs That Deplete

See the Alphabetical Listing of Nutrients and the Drugs That Deplete *on page 273* for a complete listing.

Effects of Depletion Gas, bloating, diarrhea or constipation, bad breath, and chronic vaginal yeast infections

Overview *Lactobacillus acidophilus* is the primary strain of beneficial bacteria that inhabit the small intestine. If the balance between the beneficial and pathological bacteria is disturbed, a condition known as dysbiosis develops. The use of antibiotics is a frequent cause of dysbiosis. When antibiotics are taken, most of the acidophilus bacteria are killed in addition to the pathological bacteria that are destroyed.

Products containing beneficial bacteria are frequently referred to as probiotics.

Biological Function & Effect

- **Antibiotic:** *Lactobacillus acidophilus* bacteria act as a barrier against infection by producing natural antibiotics in the GI tract that have been shown to inhibit the growth of over 20 types of harmful bacteria. Their metabolism produces lactic acid and hydrogen peroxide, which create an environment that is unfavorable for the growth of yeasts and other harmful organisms.

- **Digestion:** *L. acidophilus* bacteria promote healthy digestion. They produce enzymes that help digest fats, proteins, and dairy products.

- **Vitamin production:** *L. acidophilus* organisms also produce a wide range of B vitamins and vitamin K in the intestinal tract.

- **Immunity:** Oral ingestion of acidophilus has been shown to enhance the activity of several aspects of the immune system throughout the whole body.

- **Cholesterol metabolism:** *L. acidophilus* organisms also metabolize cholesterol.

Side Effects & Toxicity There is no toxicity associated with probiotics and they do not interfere with other medications.

RDA No RDA has been set; dosages for probiotics are measured in terms of cfu (colony forming units) which denote the number of live organisms per dose. Many probiotic products contain a combination of acidophilus and bifidobacteria.

Dosage range for prevention: Healthy people can take from 1-2 billion cfu/day

Patients with dysbiosis or after antibiotics: 10-15 billion cfu twice daily

Dosage Range 1-30 billion units

Dietary Sources The best food sources of *L. acidophilus* organisms are yogurt and acidophilus milk.

Forms Capsule; Powder

Magnesium

Available Compounds Oxide; Hydroxide; Gluconate; Glycinate; Sulfate; Chloride; Aspartate; maleate; Succinate; Fumarate; Ascorbate; Citrate

Drugs That Deplete

See the Alphabetical Listing of Nutrients and the Drugs That Deplete *on page 273* for a complete listing.

Effects of Depletion Although critical deficiency is rare in the U.S., marginal deficiency appears to be widespread. Some studies report that approximately 75% of Americans ingest less than the RDA. Deficiency symptoms include muscle cramps, weakness, insomnia, loss of appetite, GI disorders, kidney stones, osteoporosis, nervousness, restlessness, irritability, fear, anxiety, confusion, depression, fatigue, and high blood pressure.

Heart attacks: It is now known that many heart attacks occur in people with healthy hearts. Magnesium deficiency allows levels of calcium to increase, which can cause cardiac muscle spasm resulting in heart attack and frequently death.

(Continued)

Magnesium *(Continued)*

Food processing is a major cause of magnesium depletion. For example, up to 85% of magnesium is lost when whole wheat is refined to produce white flour. Modern farming techniques contribute to increasing soil depletion of magnesium. Artificial fertilizers used by farmers usually do not contain any magnesium. Poor food choices, excess calcium intake, intestinal malabsorption, alcohol abuse, liver and kidney disease, and diabetes can also cause deficiencies.

Hypomagnesemia occurs in approximately 25% of patients with diabetes. Low levels of magnesium have been reported in childhood type 1 diabetes and in adults with type 1 or type 2 diabetes.

Overview Magnesium is a cofactor in over 300 enzymatic reactions in the body. It is necessary for the transmission of nerve impulses, muscular activity, temperature regulation, detoxification reactions, and the formation of healthy bones and teeth. It also plays critical roles in energy production and the synthesis of DNA and RNA.

A U.S. Department of Agriculture survey revealed that many Americans do not ingest the RDA of magnesium, making it one of the most commonly deficient nutrients in our country. Suboptimal magnesium intake compromises all tissues, especially those of the heart, nerves, and kidneys.

Magnesium is a nutritional superstar when it comes to cardiovascular disease. Magnesium deficiency is associated with increased incidence of atherosclerosis, hypertension, strokes, and heart attacks. Low levels of magnesium can cause stiffness in the vasculature, which elevates blood pressure and contraction or spasm in the heart muscle, which can result in sudden death. Magnesium deficiency may play a key role in causing a cardiac spasm, which at times, results in death.

Magnesium single-handedly influences many of the activities associated with a wide variety of cardiac medications. For example, magnesium inhibits platelet aggregation (like aspirin), thins the blood (like Coumadin®), blocks calcium uptake (like calcium channel blocking drugs such as Procardia®), and relaxes blood vessels (like ACE inhibitors such as Vasotec®). Magnesium also increases oxygenation of the heart muscle by improving cardiac contractibility.

Biological Function & Effect

- **Carbohydrate metabolism:** In general, magnesium is required for the metabolism of carbohydrates, proteins, and fats, as well as activity related to calcium, phosphorus, and vitamin C. It is vital for the health of nervous and muscular tissues throughout the body.
- **Energy production:** Magnesium is a cofactor for oxidative phosphorylation in the production of ATP. As such, it is essential for the production and transfer of energy for protein and lipid synthesis, contractility of muscle, and nerve transmission.
- **Heart disease:** Adequate magnesium intake reduces the risk of cardiovascular disease and increases the rate of survival following a heart attack. If intravenous magnesium is given during the early stages of a heart attack, it results in a 70% decrease in deaths within one month following the event.

- **Cardiovascular function:** Magnesium influences many aspects of cardiovascular health. It acts to decrease platelet stickiness, helps thin blood, blocks calcium uptake, and relaxes blood vessels.
- **Blood pressure:** Over 30 reported clinical trials indicate that magnesium can lower elevated blood pressure. However, the effect is usually only moderate, thus magnesium should not be viewed as a primary product for hypertension.
- **PMS:** Numerous studies report that women with premenstrual syndrome have low levels of magnesium, and some studies report that magnesium helps to relieve PMS symptoms.
- **Asthma:** Various studies report low magnesium levels in asthma patients. Consuming adequate magnesium may reduce the risk of developing asthma and it is frequently useful as part of an overall management program.
- **Bone:** Magnesium may be more important than calcium for bone health. It is involved in calcium metabolism, the synthesis of vitamin D, and the integrity of skeletal bone-crystal formation.
- **Teeth:** Magnesium helps to bind calcium to tooth enamel, thus creating an effective barrier to tooth decay.

Side Effects & Toxicity Kidney excretion of excess magnesium makes magnesium toxicity rare. Excess magnesium intake frequently causes diarrhea.

RDA The RDA for magnesium is 400 mg/day. Pharmacologic doses in the scientific literature range from 500-1500 mg/day.

Dosage Range 400-1000 mg/day

Dietary Sources The magnesium content in foods varies widely, as does the soil content of magnesium. Good food sources include nuts, legumes, cereal grains, and dark green leafy vegetables.

Forms Capsule; Liquid; Powder; Spray; Tablet

Manganese

Drugs That Deplete

No medications were identified that deplete this nutrient.

Effects of Depletion Although widely involved in biological activities, manganese deficiency in humans is relatively uncommon because the mineral magnesium is capable of substituting for manganese in many of manganese's various enzyme-related functions.

The most notable symptoms of manganese deficiency are skeletal abnormalities such as loss of muscle coordination, sprains, strains, and weak ligaments. These problems develop due to the reduced synthesis of collagen and mucopolysaccharides. There is some indication that manganese deficiency impairs glucose metabolism and produces abnormalities in the secretion of insulin.

Low manganese levels are often found in people with epilepsy, hypoglycemia, schizophrenia, and osteoporosis. Women with osteoporosis have been shown to have low levels of manganese.

Manganese is necessary for the biosynthesis of cholesterol. Hypocholesterolemia may be associated with manganese deficiency. (Continued)

Manganese *(Continued)*

Intestinal absorption is hindered by ingestion of calcium, phosphate, iron, and phytate.

Overview Manganese is a cofactor that aids in the activation of a wide variety of enzymes. Manganese-containing enzymes influence many biological activities, including the synthesis of collagen, protein, mucopolysaccharides, cholesterol, and fatty acids. It is also necessary for normal bone growth and the metabolism of amino acids. The average human body only contains approximately 20 mg of manganese, most of which is stored in the bones. Smaller amounts concentrate in the pituitary, liver, pancreas, and intestinal mucosa. Absorption occurs throughout the entire small intestine and some competition exists.

Biological Function & Effect

- **Connective tissue and cartilage:** Manganese is necessary for the production of mucopolysaccharides, glycoproteins, and lipopolysaccharides, which are necessary for the growth and maintenance of connective tissue and cartilage.

- **Blood clotting:** In conjunction with vitamin K, manganese plays a role in the synthesis of prothrombin and the regulation of blood clotting.

- **Bone:** Manganese influences the activity of osteoblasts and osteoclasts, which makes it essential for normal bone growth and development.

- **Antioxidant:** Manganese is the central metal cofactor in mitochondrial superoxide dismutase, and as such, it is essential for optimal functioning of one of the body's most important antioxidant defense systems, protecting against the toxic effects of oxygen during energy production.

- **Thyroid:** Manganese is necessary in the synthesis of thyroxine, the principal hormone of the thyroid gland.

- **Production and synthesis:** Manganese is involved with the production of dopamine and melanin and in the synthesis of fatty acids.

Side Effects & Toxicity Manganese is quite safe and relatively large doses can be tolerated orally with no apparent adverse effects. Manganese toxicity has occurred in miners due to the inhalation of manganese dust. Toxicity can produce dementia, psychiatric disorders resembling schizophrenia, and neurologic disorders resembling Parkinson's disease.

RDA No RDA has been established for this mineral. The safe and adequate range for manganese is 2-5 mg/day. Pharmacologic doses in the scientific literature range from 2-50 mg/day.

Dosage Range 1-10 mg

Dietary Sources Manganese is widely distributed in foods of plant and animal origin. Best food sources include nuts, whole grain breads and cereals, dried beans and peas, vegetables, raisins, pineapple, and nuts.

Forms Injection; Tablet

Molybdenum

Drugs That Deplete

No medications were identified that deplete this nutrient.

Effects of Depletion Molybdenum deficiency in humans is rare because so little is needed. In a healthy state, body tissues contain <0.1 parts per million.

Molybdenum cofactor deficiency syndrome has recently been identified as a rare genetic condition that has caused previously unexplained seizures and developmental delays in neonates.

Molybdenum deficiency has occasionally developed in individuals who have been receiving prolonged total parenteral nutrition (TPN). The symptoms included tachycardia, headache, mental disturbances, and coma. Increased intake of sulfate or copper can cause excess excretion of molybdenum.

Overview Molybdenum is one of the rarest substances on earth, yet small amounts of this mineral are found in all tissues of the human body. Molybdenum is a component of several important metalloenzymes that participate in crucial liver detoxification pathways. Most biochemistry textbooks state that very little is known about this trace mineral beyond its role as a cofactor for several enzymes.

Biological Function & Effect Molybdenum is necessary for the function of the following three enzymes: xanthine oxidase, aldehyde oxidase, and sulfite oxidase.

- **Antioxidant:** Xanthine oxidase metabolizes xanthine to uric acid for urinary excretion. Uric acid is usually considered to be a negative substance because of its association to gouty arthritis. However, at appropriate levels, uric acid is a powerful antioxidant that neutralizes single oxygen and hydroxyl free radicals. Thus, molybdenum may play a role in regulating some important antioxidant functions.
- **Metabolism:** Sulfite oxidase catalyzes the last step in the metabolism of sulfur-containing amino acids. It is the liver detoxification pathway that converts sulfite, which is toxic to the nervous system, to sulfate for excretion.
- **Catalyst:** Aldehyde oxidase catalyzes the conversion of aldehydes to acids.
- **Absorption:** Molybdenum affects the absorption of iron, copper, and sulfate by competing for the same intestinal brush border receptor sites.

Side Effects & Toxicity Molybdenum toxicity is very rare. Excess intake of molybdenum (10-15 mg/day) can cause a gout-like syndrome due to an elevated production of uric acid.

RDA The National Academy of Sciences has determined that 10-500 mcg/day is a reasonable dietary level of molybdenum. Pharmacologic doses in the scientific literature range from 100-1000 mcg/day.

Dosage Range 200 mcg to 1 mg

Dietary Sources Good food sources of molybdenum include whole grains, organ meats, leafy green vegetables, legumes, and beans. The availability of molybdenum varies widely because of variations in the molybdenum content of the soil. Vegetables grown in molybdenum-
(Continued)

Molybdenum *(Continued)*

rich soil can contain up to 500 times more molybdenum than those grown in molybdenum-deficient soil.

Forms Injection; Tablet

♦ **Niacin** *see* Vitamin B₃ *on page 354*

Nickel

Drugs That Deplete
No medications were identified that deplete this nutrient.

Effects of Depletion Nickel is so common in the environment that deficiency is rare. Nickel deficiency depresses iron absorption. Low levels of nickel are associated with smaller litter sizes in animals. Nickel deficiency causes abnormal changes in the livers of laboratory animals. Rats raised on nickel-deficient diets develop anemia related to a reduction in iron absorption.

Overview Our knowledge that nickel is an essential nutrient is relatively recent. In 1974, nickel was discovered to be an essential nutrient in chicks. Since then it has been found to have an essential physiological role in the metabolism of other animals and in humans. However, its functions are still far from being understood at this time.

Nickel is present in the blood, various organs, teeth, bone, skin, and brain of humans, with the largest concentrations being found in skin and bone marrow. Nickel is so ubiquitous in nature (it occurs in air, plants, and animals) that scientists have only recently been able to effectively prepare nickel-deficient diets so that the biological effects of this mineral could start to be tested. To date, more is known about the effects of nickel in various animals than in man.

Biological Function & Effect Nickel has been found to be normally present in ribonucleic acid (RNA). Nickel is part of a protein called "nickeloplasmin" that is synthesized in the liver.

• **Metabolism:** It is thought that nickel's biological activities involve hormone, lipid, and cellular membrane metabolism.

• **Insulin:** Studies with rabbits and dogs have shown that nickel increases the hypoglycemic effect of insulin.

• **Stress:** Serum concentrations of nickel increase in response to stressful situations, such as heart attack, stroke, and even in women during labor.

• **Enzymes:** Nickel concentrations have been shown to influence the levels of a number of mitochondrial and liver enzymes.

Side Effects & Toxicity Under normal conditions, nickel is not a toxic element. Nickel sensitivity from jewelry is a relatively common occurrence in women who get their ears pierced. Some individuals with psoriasis and eczema have been found to have elevated levels of nickel in the blood and skin.

Occasionally, in industry, nickel combines with carbon monoxide to form a toxic compound called nickel carbonyl. Industrial exposure to this compound has caused hospitalizations and several deaths. Excess exposure to or ingestion of nickel and nickel carbonyl is suspected of causing cancer. These compounds are found in tobacco and cigarette smoke. Inhalation of large quantities of certain nickel compounds has been shown to cause lung cancer in laboratory animals. Long-term intake of excessive nickel causes degeneration of the heart, brains, lungs, liver, and kidney.

RDA There is no RDA for nickel. Nickel is so ubiquitous in the environment that studies on its supplementation have not been conducted.

Dosage Range None established.

Dietary Sources Grains and vegetable foods are the best dietary sources of nickel. Animal foods are relatively poor sources of nickel.

Forms This nutrient is not typically taken as a supplement. No supplement forms available.

♦ **Nutrient Depletion and Cancer Chemotherapy** *see page 515*

♦ **Pantothenic Acid** *see* Vitamin B₅ *on page 355*

Phosphorus
Drugs That Deplete
See the Alphabetical Listing of Nutrients and the Drugs That Deplete *on page 273* for a complete listing.

Effects of Depletion Phosphorus deficiency has been reported in animals, but it rarely occurs in humans. Long-term use of aluminum-containing antacids could lead to phosphate depletion.

Individuals who might be at risk for phosphorus depletion include alcoholics, people with kidney malfunction, individuals with intestinal malabsorption syndromes such as celiac disease or Crohn's disease, and individuals on starvation diets.

Overview Phosphorus, following calcium, is the second most abundant mineral in the human body. Approximately 80% of phosphorus is present in the skeleton while the other 20% is very active metabolically and plays a role in the metabolism of every cell in the body. In fact, phosphorus participates in more biological processes than any other mineral. A complete discussion of its functions would require delving into virtually every metabolic process in the body.

Biological Function & Effect
- **Bones and teeth:** Phosphorus, along with calcium, forms the insoluble calcium phosphate crystals, which provide the strength and rigidity in bones and teeth.
- **Phospholipids:** Unlike calcium, phosphorus is also an integral part of the structure of soft tissues. As part of phospholipids, such as phosphatidylcholine, it is a component of all cellular membranes. Phospholipids aid in transporting other lipids throughout the body and across cellular membranes.
- **Cellular energy:** ATP contains three phosphate groups and thus, phosphorus is an essential part of energy storage and production processes in every cell throughout the body.
- **Enzymes:** It is a part of many coenzymes and takes part in a wide variety of enzymatic reactions.
- **Buffer:** As phosphoric acid and its salts, phosphorous is part of one of the body's major buffer systems.

(Continued)

Phosphorus *(Continued)*

- **Cellular reproduction and protein synthesis:** It is part of DNA and RNA, and thus is necessary for all cellular reproduction and protein synthesis.

Side Effects & Toxicity Excessive consumption of high phosphorous-containing foods (eg, animal protein and cola soft drinks) may inhibit calcium absorption and contribute to skeletal problems such as osteoporosis. Excess phosphorous can increase hyperthyroidism, increase bone resorption, increase soft tissue calcium deposition, and decrease bone mass.

RDA The RDA for phosphorus is 800-1200 mg/day. Most Americans consume far too much phosphorus. Higher dosage recommendations are not appropriate.

Dosage Range See RDA above.

Dietary Sources Animal protein foods are the highest source of phosphorus for most people. Cola soft drinks contain a large amount of phosphorus.

Forms Injection; Tablet

♦ **Phytonadione** *see* Vitamin K *on page 367*

Potassium

Drugs That Deplete

See the Alphabetical Listing of Nutrients and the Drugs That Deplete *on page 273* for a complete listing.

Effects of Depletion In addition to the above-mentioned drugs, excessive diarrhea, kidney failure, diabetic acidosis, prolonged malnutrition, and vomiting can also cause potassium deficiency. Other factors that contribute to potassium depletion include alcohol, caffeine, excessive use of salt or sugar, and chronic stress. Symptoms associated with potassium deficiency include irregular heartbeat, poor reflexes, muscle weakness, fatigue, continuous thirst, edema, constipation, dizziness, mental confusion, and nervous disorders.

Overview Potassium is one of the body's three major electrolytes (the other two being sodium and chloride). They exist as fully dissociated ions and are the main particles responsible for osmotic pressure in body fluids. Potassium is the primary electrolyte functioning inside cells throughout the body. These substances are called electrolytes because they carry an electronic charge in their dissociated (ionic) states. Their ionic strength enables them to influence the solubility of proteins and other substances throughout the body.

Hormonal control of potassium and the other electrolytes is mediated through the hormones of the adrenal cortex and the anterior pituitary gland. Potassium is readily absorbed through the intestinal tract, and excess is efficiently excreted in urine via the kidneys.

Biological Function & Effect Potassium plays essential roles in many of the body's most important functions including nerve conduction, muscle contraction, and beating of the heart. Potassium is the primary cation in intracellular fluids throughout the body. Approximately 98% of total body potassium resides inside cells.

- **Water balance:** Potassium, along with sodium and chloride, helps maintain normal osmotic equilibrium by controlling the distribution and balance of water throughout the body.
- **High blood pressure:** Potassium has been shown to be effective in preventing hypertension and in some studies, potassium has been shown to help lower existing high blood pressure.
- **Stroke:** Potassium levels are inversely associated with the risk of stroke. One study reported that one serving of potassium-rich fruits or vegetables daily provided up to a 40% reduction in the risk of stroke.

Side Effects & Toxicity Potassium toxicity (hyperkalemia) usually results from kidney failure, in which case, serum levels rise because the kidneys cannot adequately excrete potassium. Malfunctioning adrenal glands can also cause hyperkalemia.

Symptoms of hyperkalemia include mental confusion, numbness of the extremities, labored breathing, and deteriorating cardiac activity.

RDA No RDA has been established for potassium because it is so readily available. The estimated safe and adequate intake of potassium for adults is from 1.8-5.6 g/day.

Dosage Range 60-99 mg OTC; dosages greater require a prescription.

Dietary Sources Potassium is plentiful in the diet. Potassium-rich foods include fresh fruits and vegetables, peanuts, meat, and milk. An average banana supplies over 600 mg, half a cantaloupe contains 885 mg, 3-4 ounces of raw spinach contain about 775 mg, 2 ounces of peanuts contain about 575 mg, and one large raw carrot contains about 330 mg of potassium.

Forms Capsule; Intravenous; Liquid; Powder; Tablet

- **Pyridoxine** *see* Vitamin B$_6$ *on page 357*
- **Retinol** *see* Vitamin A *on page 349*
- **Riboflavin** *see* Vitamin B$_2$ *on page 353*
- **S-Adenosyl Methionine** *see* SAMe *on page 341*

SAMe

Synonyms S-Adenosyl Methionine

Drugs That Deplete

See the Alphabetical Listing of Nutrients and the Drugs That Deplete *on page 273* for a complete listing.

Effects of Depletion A specific deficiency syndrome has not been adequately defined. As an essential cofactor in multiple biochemical pathways, a wide variety of symptoms are potentially related to a deficiency of SAMe.

Overview SAMe is formed from the essential amino acid methionine. It is a cofactor in three important biochemical pathways, and is synthesized throughout the body. Due to the nature and scope of biochemical reactions that it regulates, SAMe has been investigated for its effects in conditions such as depression, arthritis, fibromyalgia, and cardiovascular disease.

(Continued)

SAMe (Continued)

Biological Function & Effect

- **Methylation reactions:** SAMe functions as a methyl donor for the synthesis of nucleic acids (DNA and RNA), proteins, phospholipids, catecholamines, and various other neurotransmitters.
- **Transsulfuration:** SAMe is the precursor in the sulfur metabolic pathways for the synthesis of cysteine, glutathione, and taurine.
- **Polyamines:** SAMe is also necessary for the synthesis of a group of compounds collectively referred to as polyamines, which are spermidine, puescine, and spermine. These polyamines are essential for cellular growth and differentiation, gene expression, protein phosphorylation, neuron regeneration, and the repair of DNA.
- **Antioxidant production:** Because SAMe is necessary for the synthesis of glutathione, which is an antioxidant, it plays a role in protecting the body from free radical-induced aging damage.
- **Detoxification:** Glutathione is important for detoxification in the liver. Glutathione depletion is usually found in individuals with liver malfunction. SAMe supplementation promotes the synthesis of glutathione, which improves liver function and detoxification.
- **Healthy cellular membranes:** The ratio between phosphatidyl choline (PC) and cholesterol in cellular membranes determines their relative flexibility or stiffness; PC promotes flexibility whereas cholesterol promotes stiffness. Since SAMe is an important facilitator of phosphatidyl choline synthesis, it plays a role in promoting more pliant cellular menbranes. Stiffer cell membranes are not able to transmit cellular signals effectively and it is more difficult for neuropeptides and other messenger molecules to fit into receptor sites when cellular membranes are stiff.
- **Neuron protective:** Protects against neuronal death caused by lack of oxygen (anoxia). It regenerates nerves and provokes remyelination of nerve fibers.
- **Liver protection:** Protects the liver against alcohol, drugs, and cytokines. It protects against cholestasis (bile impairment or blockage). It may protect against chronic active hepatitis. It protects against chronic active hepatitis. It protects against liver damage caused by MAO inhibitors and anticonvulsants. It reverses hyperbilirubinemia.

Side Effects & Toxicity SAMe has no reported toxicity. A few minor side effects have been occasionally reported, which include dry mouth, nausea, and restlessness. Individuals are urged to consult with their physician before combining SAMe with other antidepressants, or with tryptophan or 5-HTP. People should also be careful about combining SAMe with antidepressants such as MAO inhibitors, tricyclic antidepressants, or SSRIs because they can potentiate the activities of each other.

RDA No RDA has been set for SAMe. The most common dosage used is 400 mg daily.

Dosage Range 200-1600 mg daily

Dietary Sources SAMe does not occur in the foods we consume.

Forms Capsule; Solution, intravenous; Tablet

Selenium

Drugs That Deplete

See the Alphabetical Listing of Nutrients and the Drugs That Deplete *on page 273* for a complete listing.

Effects of Depletion Symptoms of selenium deficiency include destructive changes to the heart and pancreas, sore muscles, increased red blood cell fragility, and a weakened immune system. Increased rates of various types of cancer are associated with low dietary intake of selenium.

The primary cause of selenium deficiency is insufficient dietary intake due to either poor food choices (as in junk foods and fast foods), or eating foods grown in selenium-depleted soils. Selenium is not an essential nutrient for plants and, therefore, many farmlands have become increasingly depleted of selenium because farmers see no need to add it to the soil. Food processing causes substantial loss of selenium. For example, whole wheat bread has twice the selenium as white bread, and brown rice has 15 times more selenium than white rice. Protein-calorie malnutrition can lead to selenium deficiency.

Human breast milk contains 6 times more selenium than cow's milk. A cow's milk diet for infants can contribute to low selenium levels and depressed immune systems in infants.

The Keshan district in China had extremely high rates of childhood cardiomyopathies until it was discovered that the soil was selenium deficient. Nutritional selenium supplementation has solved the problem.

Overview Until the late 1950s, selenium was thought to be toxic. Although it can be toxic at high doses, it is now recognized as one of the most important nutritional trace minerals. Selenium plays an important role in detoxification and antioxidant defense mechanisms in the body. Recent research has shown that selenium is one of the most powerful anticancer agents ever tested.

Biological Function & Effect

- **Antioxidant:** Selenium is an indispensable cofactor for glutathione peroxidase, which is one of the most important antioxidant enzymes in our immune system. Each molecule of this enzyme contains 4 atoms of selenium. As an antioxidant, selenium helps prevent lipid peroxidation and neutralizes destructive hydrogen peroxide. By neutralizing these types of free radicals, selenium works to prevent cancer and cardiovascular disease.

- **Cancer:** Selenium is a powerful anticancer nutrient. Numerous epidemiological studies have correlated low dietary selenium intake with higher rates of cancer.

- **Heart disease:** Selenium's antioxidant activities enable it to protect against heart attacks and strokes.

- **Immunity:** Selenium has antiviral activity, increases T lymphocytes, and enhances natural killer cell activity.

- **Detoxification:** Selenium is capable of detoxifying heavy metal toxins such as mercury and cadmium. Selenium greatly reduces the

(Continued)

343

Selenium *(Continued)*

toxicity of the anticancer drug Adriamycin® without reducing its anti-tumor activity.

- **Anti-inflammatory:** Selenium, as part of glutathione peroxidase, also has significant anti-inflammatory properties.

- **Thyroid hormone:** Recently, it was discovered that the deiodinase enzyme that converts thyroid hormone (T_4) to triiodothyronine (T_3, the active form) is a selenium-dependent enzyme.

- **Vitamin E:** Selenium potentiates the antioxidant activity of vitamin E.

Side Effects & Toxicity Selenium is a trace mineral that can be toxic. Although deaths from selenium toxicity have been reported in livestock, no deaths have occurred in humans. Symptoms of selenium toxicity include loss of hair and nails, skin lesions, nervous system abnormalities, digestive dysfunction, and a garlicky breath odor.

RDA The RDA for selenium is 70 mcg/day for men and 55 mcg/day for women. Pharmacologic doses in the scientific literature range from 50-500 mcg/day. Occasionally, physicians have used much higher doses in cancer therapy and for cases of acute inflammation.

Dosage Range 50-200 mcg

Dietary Sources Whole grains are the best dietary source of selenium followed by seafood, garlic, liver, eggs, dairy products, and some vegetables including cabbage, celery, cucumbers, and radishes. The selenium content of foods is directly dependent on the selenium content of the soil. Food grown in selenium-deficient soil in many areas of the United States has an inadequate selenium content.

Forms Injection; Tablet

Silicon

Drugs That Deplete

No medications were identified that deplete this nutrient.

Effects of Depletion Silicon is so abundant in the environment that outright deficiencies do not occur. On the other hand, the discovery of silicon's role as an essential nutrient is quite recent, and very little work has been done regarding its metabolic activity and optimal dosage ranges.

There is some indication that silicon deficiency might be associated with the development of osteoarthritis and some aspects of cardiovascular disease. Laboratory animals fed silicon-deficient diets exhibit growth retardation and incomplete and deformed development of the skeleton.

Overview Even though silicon is the most abundant mineral on earth, the fact that it is an essential trace mineral has only recently been discovered. The largest concentrations of silicon are found in the skin and cartilage, but it also occurs in connective tissue, bone, tendons, lymph nodes, trachea, aorta, and lungs. Inhalation of silicon from the environment is partially responsible for its high occurrence in lung tissue.

Preliminary studies have shown that there is an age-related decline in the silicon content of the skin, arteries, and thymus, while concentrations remain relatively stable in the heart, kidneys, muscles and tendons.

Biological Function & Effect

- **Connective tissues:** Silicon is an important component of the mucopolysaccharides and collagen of connective tissues. As such, it provides strength, rigidity, and flexibility to bones, teeth, tendons, ligaments, cell walls and membranes, nails, and skin.
- **Bones and teeth:** Silicon aids in building the organic matrix for the proper mineralization of bones and teeth.
- **Production:** Cell culture studies and work with chicks suggests that silicon somehow stimulates the production of mucopolysaccharides and collagen.
- **Atherosclerosis:** There is some indication that adequate levels of silicon may be associated with a decreased risk in the development of atherosclerosis.
- **Aluminum absorption:** Silicon may help to limit or inhibit the absorption of aluminum.

Side Effects & Toxicity Studies on silicon toxicity focus primarily on an occupational lung disease called silicosis. This is a respiratory disease caused by the inhalation of silicon dioxide dust which often occurs in mining or sandblasting, and in the manufacture of glass, ceramics, abrasives, and petroleum products. Silicosis is characterized by a degenerative fibrosis of the lung tissue.

RDA Nutritional guidelines for silicon have not been determined. Some researchers suggest that the recommended daily intake of silicon should be from 5-10 mg/day. It has been estimated that the average daily dietary intake of silicon is from 20-50 mg/day, so most people are getting sufficient silicon.

Dosage Range None established.

Dietary Sources None known.

Forms This nutrient is not typically taken as a supplement. No supplement forms known.

Sodium

Drugs That Deplete

See the Alphabetical Listing of Nutrients and the Drugs That Deplete *on page 273* for a complete listing.

Effects of Depletion Sodium deficiency is rare in humans. Conditions that could cause sodium deficiency include starvation, vomiting, severe diarrhea, and excess perspiration, in conjunction with a lack of water. Symptoms of sodium deficiency include muscle weakness, poor concentration, memory loss, dehydration, and loss of appetite.

Overview Sodium is one of the body's three major electrolytes (the other two being potassium and chloride). They exist as fully dissociated ions and are the main particles responsible for osmotic pressure in body fluids. Sodium is the primary extracellular electrolyte in body fluids. These substances are called electrolytes because they carry an electronic charge in their dissociated (ionic) state. Their ionic strength (Continued)

Sodium *(Continued)*

enables them to influence the solubility of proteins and other substances throughout the body.

Most Americans consume enormous amounts of sodium, from 10-35 times more than the recommended daily intake. Dietary sodium is easily absorbed from the intestine, carried by the blood to the kidneys where it is either filtered out and returned to the blood or excreted.

Biological Function & Effect

- **Blood pressure:** In regulating body fluids, sodium has a major role in the regulation of blood pressure.
- **Muscle and nerve action:** Sodium ions play a critical role in the transmission of electrochemical impulses for nerve function and muscle contraction.
- **Acid/alkaline balance:** Sodium helps regulate the acid/alkaline balance in the blood and lymph fluids.
- **Cellular permeability:** Sodium helps control and operate the sodium/potassium pump. This helps make the cell walls permeable and facilitates transport of materials across cell membranes.
- **CO_2 regulation:** Sodium helps regulate the transport and excretion of CO_2.

Side Effects & Toxicity High sodium intake is associated with edema and elevated blood pressure.

RDA There is no RDA for sodium. A reasonable dietary intake is from 1-3 g/day.

Dosage Range Amounts greater than the "reasonable dietary intake" should only be taken under the supervision of a healthcare provider.

Dietary Sources Table salt is the most concentrated source of sodium. Enormous amounts of sodium (and chloride) are used in cooking and food processing. This "hidden salt" often contributes more to an individual's daily diet than does the salt shaker. Protein foods generally contain more sodium than vegetables and grains. Fruits contain almost no sodium.

Forms Drops, nasal; Injection; Solution, oral; Tablet; Topical

- ◆ **Sodium Fluoride** *see* Fluoride *on page 323*
- ◆ **Stannous Fluoride** *see* Fluoride *on page 323*

Sulfur

Drugs That Deplete

No medications were identified that deplete this nutrient.

Effects of Depletion Deficiency symptoms related to sulfur are unknown. A diet severely lacking in protein (such as in starvation) could cause sulfur deficiency.

Overview Sulfur occurs in the body primarily as a component of the four sulfur-containing amino acids: cystine, cysteine, methionine, and taurine. All proteins contain sulfur, but it is most prevalent in the keratin of skin and hair, and in insulin. Joint tissues contain high levels of a sulfur-containing compound called chondroitin sulfate. Two B vitamins, thiamin and biotin, contain sulfur, as does heparin, an anticoagulant synthesized primarily in the liver. Small amounts of sulfur exist in the body as organic sulfates and sulfites.

Sulfur plays an important role in determining the shape, structure, and functionality of proteins. Sulfur-containing amino acids in protein can create crosslinks by forming disulfide bonds which act to strengthen and stabilize proteins. Sulfur exists in its reduced form in cysteine and in an oxidized form as a double molecule in cystine.

Sulfur has a characteristic odor. The smell from burning feathers, hair, skin, or nails is due to sulfur, and "smelly" foods such as onions and garlic contain significant amounts of sulfur.

Biological Function & Effect Sulfur-containing lipids (sulfolipids) are found in the liver, kidneys, and brain.

- **Structure:** Sulfur's major role, as part of amino acids, is to provide structure to proteins and mucopolysaccharides such as chondroitin sulfate and collagen.
- **Protein structure:** Sulfur, through disulfide (-S-S-) or sulfhydryl (-SH) bonds, gives proteins their different characteristic shapes. For example, hair curliness is due to the presence of disulfide bonds of cystine in hair.
- **Metabolism:** Sulfur plays an important metabolic role as a sulfhydryl group on the active site of coenzyme A. Sulfur, in conjunction with magnesium, takes part in the metabolic detoxification of sulfuric acid in the body for excretion in the urine.
- **Biological processes:** Sulfur is necessary for all of the biochemical processes involving thiamin, biotin, and lipoic acid.
- **Insulin:** The hormone insulin consists of 51 amino acids in 2 polypeptide chains. The two parallel chains are joined by two disulfide bridges.

Side Effects & Toxicity There is no toxicity associated with sulfur. Excesses are efficiently excreted in the urine.

RDA No RDA has been set for sulfur. The diets of most Americans are high in protein and provide more than adequate amounts of sulfur.

Dosage Range None established.

Dietary Sources Protein-rich foods are good sources of sulfur.

Forms Capsule; Tablet (as MSM products)

Note: Sulfur is not typically taken as a supplement in its pure form.

♦ **Thiamine** *see* Vitamin B$_1$ *on page 351*

Tyrosine

Drugs That Deplete

See the Alphabetical Listing of Nutrients and the Drugs That Deplete *on page 273* for a complete listing.

Effects of Depletion Depression and emotional disturbances; underactive thyroid and disturbed metabolism

Overview Tyrosine is classified as a nonessential amino acid because it can be synthesized from phenylalanine, an essential amino acid, in the body. However, tyrosine is a very important amino acid because it is part of the structure of almost all proteins in the body.

Biological Function & Effect Tyrosine plays a very important role in brain nutrition because it serves as a precursor for the synthesis of (Continued)

Tyrosine *(Continued)*

several neurotransmitters, including dopamine, norepinephrine, and epinephrine. These neurotransmitters regulate functions such as mood, stress response, mental function, and sex drive. Tyrosine is also necessary for the production of melanin, cholecystokinin (CCK), and the thyroid hormones.

Side Effects & Toxicity No known toxicities or serious side effects have been reported; however, it is not to be taken by individuals on MAO-inhibiting antidepressants. At extremely high doses, tyrosine may cause diarrhea, nausea, vomiting, and nervousness. These symptoms usually disappear when the dosage is lowered.

RDA There is no RDA for tyrosine. ODA: 1000-5000 mg/day.

Dosage Range 1000-5000 mg/day

Dietary Sources Eggs, wheat, corn, meats, soybeans, milk, poultry

Forms Capsule; Powder; Solution, oral; Tablet

Vanadium

Drugs That Deplete

No medications were identified that deplete this nutrient.

Effects of Depletion No known cases of vanadium deficiency have been recorded.

Overview How essential vanadium is in humans has yet to be established with certainty. In the late 60s, it was found to be an essential trace mineral for plant nutrition, and in the early 70s, it was discovered to be an essential nutrient for animals. It is probably essential for humans too, but there is still some debate. Nonetheless, interest in vanadium as a nutritional substance has been steadily building over the past twenty years.

Vanadium is a transition metal and, as such, it possesses biochemical properties similar to chromium, molybdenum, manganese, and iron. It exists in valences of 2, 3, 4, or 5, with the tetravalent and pentavalent forms being the most common. Vanadium primarily functions as a cofactor, which enhances or inhibits various enzymes. It accumulates primarily in organ tissues with the highest concentrations being found in the liver, kidneys, and bone. Bone appears to be the long-term storage site for vanadium, while storage of accessible vanadium is primarily in fat and serum lipids.

Biological Function & Effect

- **Diabetes:** The most significant research on vanadium to date involves its insulin-like properties and its possible role in diabetes. Vanadium and vanadyl salts stimulate glucose metabolism. When given to patients with Type 2 diabetes, it markedly decreases blood glucose levels. The insulin-like effect produced by vanadium compounds in the liver may be caused by the decreased activity of the gluconeogenesis enzyme, glucose-6-phosphatase, the increased activity of two glycolytic enzymes, glucokinase and phosphofructokinase, and increased glycogen production.
- **Bones and teeth:** Vanadium may have a functional role as a building material in bones and teeth.

- **Biological processes:** Vanadium's biochemical and physiological roles are not yet fully understood. However, it appears that it may be involved in the following processes: NADPH oxidation reactions, lipoprotein lipase activity, amino acid transport, and the growth of red blood cells.

- **Cholesterol:** At higher dosage levels, vanadium appears to be able to assist in lowering elevated serum cholesterol and triglyceride levels.

- **Inhibitor:** Vanadium is a potent inhibitor of $Na^+K^+ATPase$ enzymes.

Side Effects & Toxicity Vanadium has no known toxicity as a dietary nutrient in humans. Vanadium can be absorbed through inhalation, and excessive exposure could be toxic. It is used as a catalyst in a wide variety of industrial processes. Occasionally, industrial accidents occur where sufficient vanadium is inhaled so as to create a toxic situation.

Experimentally-induced vanadium toxicity in animal studies produces reproductive and developmental abnormalities, including decreased fertility, birth defects, and embryonic death.

RDA Dietary requirements for vanadium have not been established. To date, little is known about human nutritional needs for vanadium, and whether the amount or type absorbed by Americans is adequate. It is estimated that the daily requirement for vanadium might be on the order of 10 mcg/day. The average American diet contains from 15-30 mcg/day which is more than enough to satisfy nutritional needs.

Dosage Range 250 mcg to 15 mg

Dietary Sources Fats and vegetable oils are the richest food sources of vanadium. Vanadium also occurs in grains, meat, fish, and nuts. The following foods and spices also contain vanadium: dill seeds, parsley, black pepper, and mushrooms.

Forms Injection; Tablet

Vitamin A

Synonyms Retinol

Drugs That Deplete

See the Alphabetical Listing of Nutrients and the Drugs That Deplete *on page 273* for a complete listing.

Effects of Depletion Vitamin A deficiency can be caused by inadequate dietary intake or bodily dysfunction that interferes with absorption, storage, or transport of the vitamin. Deficiency of vitamin A is associated with the development and promotion of epithelial cell cancers in various glands and organs in the body.

Night blindness (nyctalopia) is the classic vision problem resulting from vitamin A deficiency. Xerophthalmia (a drying and hardening of the epithelial cell membranes in the eye) can also develop. This condition causes blindness in hundreds of thousands of infants and children yearly world wide, but seldom occurs in the United States.

Long-term vitamin A deficiency causes the skin to become dry, scaly, and rough. This is called keratinization where small hard bumps develop because hair follicles plug up with a hard protein called (Continued)

Vitamin A *(Continued)*

keratin. Vitamin A deficiency in infants and children hinders growth and development. Bone deformities and dental problems often occur.

Overview Vitamin A was the first fat-soluble vitamin to be recognized. It was discovered in 1913 as a result of its ability to prevent night blindness and xerophthalmia. In 1932, beta-carotene (pro-vitamin A) was discovered to be the precursor to vitamin A. Vitamin A is necessary for vision, the growth and maintenance of epithelial tissue, and the growth and development of bones. It also regulates immunity, reproduction, and has anticancer activity.

Vitamin A belongs to a class of compounds called retinoids, which only occur in animal products. Retinoids with vitamin A activity occur in nature in three different forms: 1) the alcohol, retinol, 2) the aldehyde, retinal or retinaldehyde, and 3) the acid, retinoic acid.

Beta-carotene and the other carotenoids are found exclusively in plant (fruit and vegetable) sources. Beta-carotene consists of two molecules of vitamin A linked head to head (A-A). Enzymes in the intestinal tract split beta-carotene into two molecules of vitamin A whenever the body needs it. Vitamin A requires fats as well as minerals in order to be properly absorbed from the digestive tract. Substantial amounts of vitamin A are stored in the liver and, therefore, it does not need to be supplied in the diet on a daily basis.

Biological Function & Effect

- **Eyes and vision:** Vitamin A plays an essential role in vision. Converted into 11-cis-retinal, it interacts with a photosensitive pigment in the retina that facilitates night vision.
- **Cancer:** Many studies show that adequate intake of vitamin A is associated with reduced risk of various epithelial-cell cancers (mouth, skin, lungs, bladder, breast, stomach, cervix, etc)
- **Epithelial tissue:** Vitamin A plays an important role in maintaining the integrity of all epithelial tissue. These are the mucous membrane-secreting cells that line all the glands and organs of the body.
- **Immune system:** By maintaining healthy epithelial cells (surface cells of many glands, organs, and skin), vitamin A facilitates in creating barriers to infections.
- **Growth and bone development:** Vitamin A is essential for the growth of bone and soft tissue. It is also necessary for the formation of tooth enamel in the development of teeth.

Side Effects & Toxicity Since vitamin A is fat-soluble, excesses can accumulate in fatty tissues to toxic levels. Signs of vitamin A toxicity include dry itchy skin, brittle nails, hair loss, bone pain, gingivitis, headaches, muscle and joint pains, anorexia, fatigue, diarrhea, increased infections, enlarged liver, and abnormal liver function.

There is no toxicity from ingestion of large doses of pro-vitamin A (beta-carotene), however, a harmless side effect called carotenosis can develop causing an orange coloring on the palms of the hands, soles of the feet, and in the eyes. Hypervitaminosis A has been reported in adults taking in excess of 50,000 international units (IU) daily for several years, and in a case of taking a water soluble synthetic vitamin A at 18,500-60,000 IU for several months.

RDA The RDA for vitamin A is 5000 international units/day; no RDA has been set for beta-carotene. Pharmacologic doses in the scientific literature usually range from 10,000-35,000 international units. However, occasional applications can go much higher, but should never be attempted without medical supervision. Dosages of vitamin A and beta-carotene are sometimes measured in terms of retinol equivalents (RE). One RE (equal to 1 mcg) is equivalent to 5 international units.

Dosage Range 2000-35,000 international units/day (400-7000 RE/day)

Dietary Sources Good food sources of vitamin A include liver, kidney, butter, egg yolk, whole milk and cream, and fortified skim milk. Good food sources of pro-vitamin A (beta-carotene) include yellow and dark leafy green vegetables (carrots, collards, spinach, sweet potatoes, squash), and yellow fruit (apricots, peaches, cantaloupe). Cod liver oil and halibut fish oil contain high levels of vitamin A and have been used therapeutically.

Forms Capsule; Liquid; Tablet

Vitamin B₁

Synonyms Thiamine

Available Compounds Thiamine Hydrochloride; Thiamine Mononitrate; Tetrahydrofurfuryl Disulfide (TTFD)

Drugs That Deplete

See the Alphabetical Listing of Nutrients and the Drugs That Deplete *on page 273* for a complete listing.

Effects of Depletion Deficiencies of vitamin B₁, manifest primarily as disorders of the neuromuscular, gastrointestinal, and cardiovascular systems. Deficiency symptoms include:

- Depression
- Irritability
- Memory loss
- Mental confusion
- Indigestion
- Weight loss
- Anorexia
- Edema
- Muscular weakness
- Sore calf muscles
- Heart palpitations
- Rapid pulse rate
- Loss of reflexes in legs
- Defective muscular coordination
- Nerve inflammation including "pins & needles" and numbness
- Fatigue

Thiamine is one of the most common nutritional deficiencies. In one U.S. Department of Agriculture study, it was reported that 45% of Americans consume less than the RDA of thiamine. Vitamin B₁ is (Continued)

Vitamin B₁ *(Continued)*

easily destroyed or lost during cooking because it is heat sensitive and water soluble.

Vitamin B₁ is also depleted by diuretic drugs and GI conditions such as diarrhea, and malabsorption occurs due to lactose intolerance and celiac disease (gluten or wheat sensitivity).

Alcohol interferes with the absorption of Vitamin B₁, yet the vitamin is necessary for the metabolism of alcohol. Severe deficiency associated with alcohol consumption produces a condition called Wernicke-Korsakoff syndrome, with symptoms ranging from mild confusion to severely impaired memory and cognitive function, and coma.

Overview Vitamin B₁, which is also known as thiamine, was the first of the B vitamins to be discovered. It was isolated in 1926 as a water-soluble, crystalline yellowish white powder with a salty, slightly nutty taste. In 1936, chemists accomplished the synthesis and determined its chemical formula.

Beriberi is the classic deficiency syndrome, resulting from a vitamin B₁ deficiency. It is more prevalent in Asian countries where polished rice is the staple diet. When beriberi occurs in the United States, it is most commonly seen in severely malnourished infants or elderly people. In adults, chronic dieting, alcoholism, and diets consisting primarily of highly processed, refined foods are causes of vitamin B₁ deficiency.

Biological Function & Effect

- **Cellular energy production:** Vitamin B₁ must be phosphorylated in order to be metabolically active. It combines with 2 molecules of phosphoric acid to form the important coenzyme thiamine pyrophosphate (TPP). As coenzyme TPP, it performs oxidative decarboxylation reactions (removal Of CO_2 groups) in the Krebs cycle and transketolation reactions (transfer of 2-carbon units) in the pentose phosphate shunt. Required by every cell in the body to make ATP, which is the fuel and energy source for the body.
- **Blood sugar conversion:** Plays a major role in the conversion of blood sugar (glucose) into biological energy.
- **Nerve function:** Necessary for the maintenance of nerve tissues, function, and transmission.
- **Muscle function:** Important in the maintenance of muscular function, especially the heart.
- **Thought and memory:** Required for the synthesis of acetylcholine, which is the primary neurotransmitter involved in thought and memory processes.
- **Fatty acid synthesis:** Involved in fatty acid synthesis.

Side Effects & Toxicity Since it is water-soluble, thiamine is not stored in the body. Accumulation to toxic levels is very unlikely. Overdose and toxicity would require very high doses (multiple gram range).

RDA The RDA for vitamin B₁ is 1.5 mg/day; therapeutic dosage ranges in the scientific literature vary from 10-100 mg/day in divided doses, although some applications use even larger doses.

Dosage Range 1.5-100 mg/day; occasionally doses from 200-600 mg/day have been used therapeutically

Dietary Sources All plant and animal foods contain vitamin B_1, but only in low concentrations. The richest sources are brewer's yeast and organ meats. Whole cereal grains comprise the most important dietary source of vitamin B_1 in human diets.

Forms Capsule; Liquid; Spray, liposomal; Tablet; Tablet, effervescent

Vitamin B₂

Synonyms Riboflavin

Available Compounds Riboflavin Hydrochloride; Riboflavin-5-Phosphate

Drugs That Deplete

See the Alphabetical Listing of Nutrients and the Drugs That Deplete *on page 273* for a complete listing.

Effects of Depletion Vitamin B_2 deficiencies primarily affect the skin, eyes, and mucous membranes of the GI tract. Deficiencies seldom occur alone, but rather as a component of multiple-nutrient deficiencies. Vitamin B_2 deficiency symptoms include:

- Cheilosis (cracks in the corners of the mouth); mucous membranes become inflamed; soreness & burning of the lips, mouth, and tongue (possible magenta-colored tongue).
- Reddening, tearing, burning, and itching of the eyes; eyes that tire easily and eyes that are very sensitive to light.
- Dry, itchy, scaly skin (seborrheic dermatitis) and scaling eczema of the face and genitals may develop. In severe long-term deficiency, damage to nerve tissue that can cause depression and hysteria.

Riboflavin is heat stable, but very sensitive to destruction by light. Because it is water-soluble, substantial amounts are lost by leaching into water when cooking. Since the vitamin exists in the germ and bran of grains, milling and processing of grains results in substantial losses.

Individuals at greatest risk for riboflavin deficiency include alcoholics, and infants and/or elderly persons on unbalanced, nutritionally deficient diets. A U.S. Department of Agriculture survey estimated that 34% of Americans get less than the RDA of vitamin B_2 daily. Oral contraceptives increase the need for vitamin B_2. Thorazine® and tricyclic antidepressants such as Elavil® and Tofranil® inhibit the absorption of riboflavin and can cause nutrient depletions.

Overview Vitamin B_2 is water-soluble and, like other B vitamins, it is not appreciably stored and, therefore, must be supplied daily. Vitamin B_2 is absorbed from the upper part of the small intestine, and better absorbed when taken with food. Only approximately 15% is absorbed if taken alone versus 60% absorption with food. Riboflavin belongs to a group of yellow fluorescent pigments called flavins. In its pure state, it is a yellow crystalline powder with a slight odor. When excreted, it gives the urine a characteristic bright yellow color.

Biological Function & Effect Riboflavin combines with phosphoric acid to become part of two important flavin coenzymes, FNfN (flavin mononucleotide) and FAD (flavin adenine dinucleotide). FNfN and FAD are known to bind to over 100 flavoprotein enzymes, which catalyze oxidation-reduction reactions in cells. These enzymes include the (Continued)

353

Vitamin B₂ *(Continued)*

oxidases, which function aerobically, and dehydrogenases, which function anaerobically.

- **Metabolism:** Riboflavin facilitates the metabolism of carbohydrates, fats, and proteins.
- **Cellular energy production:** Vitamin B₂ plays a critical role in the conversion of carbohydrates to ATP in the production of energy. In energy production, flavoprotein enzymes function as hydrogen carriers in the electron transport system resulting in the production of ATP and energy within the mitochondria.
- **Antioxidant:** Riboflavin has important antioxidant activity, both by itself, and as part of the enzyme glutathione reductase.
- **Growth and reproduction:** Necessary for growth and reproduction.
- **Hair and nails:** Necessary for the healthy growth of skin, hair, and nails.

Side Effects & Toxicity There is no known toxicity for riboflavin. Its negligible storage and easy excretion make it a very safe nutrient.

RDA The RDA for vitamin B₂ is 1.7 mg/day Pregnant women, nursing mothers, and individuals who exercise heavily will require somewhat higher intakes. High potency vitamin formulations and therapeutic dosages are in the range of 15-50 mg/day in divided doses.

Dosage Range 1.2-100 mg/day; occasionally higher doses have reportedly been used under medical supervision for certain conditions such as migraine headaches

Dietary Sources The best sources of vitamin B₂ are liver, milk, and dairy products. Moderate sources include meats, dark green vegetables, eggs, avocados, oysters, mushrooms, and fish (especially salmon and tuna).

Forms Capsule; Liquid; Powder; Spray, liposomal; Tablet; Tablet, effervescent

Vitamin B₃

Synonyms Niacin

Available Compounds Nicotinic Acid; Niacinamide (nicotinamide); Inositol Hexaniacinate

Drugs That Deplete

See the Alphabetical Listing of Nutrients and the Drugs That Deplete *on page 273* for a complete listing.

Effects of Depletion Severe deficiency is known as pellagra, which means rough skin. Pellagra is characterized by the "3 Ds:" dermatitis, dementia, and diarrhea. Pellagra occurs in areas where nutrition is meager and corn is the dietary staple. Tryptophan (an important chemical for niacin utilization) and niacin are poorly absorbed from corn. However, in Mexico, where corn is treated with lye before use, deficiency is less common because the alkali increases the absorption of tryptophan.

Overview Niacin is a water-soluble B vitamin that functions metabolically as a component of two important coenzymes: nicotinamide adenine dinucleotide (NAD) and nicotinamide adenine dinucleotide phosphate (NADP), known as the pyridine nucleotides.

Biological Function & Effect

- **Metabolism:** Niacin-containing coenzymes NAD and NADP are involved in more than 200 different reactions in the metabolism of carbohydrates, fatty acids, and amino acids, making it critical in supplying energy to, and maintaining the function of, every cell in the body.
- **Cellular energy production:** Niacin is especially important in the oxidation-reduction reactions in the Krebs cycle involving the production of energy from carbohydrates.
- **Cholesterol:** Niacin is useful in treating elevated blood cholesterol levels. It reduces LDL ("bad" cholesterol) and triglycerides, and increases HDL ("good" cholesterol).
- **Antianxiety:** Niacinamide has been shown to have antianxiety activity resembling benzodiazepines and Italian physicians report using it successfully to help addicted patients withdraw from benzodiazepines.
- **Histamine release:** Doses of niacin in the 75 mg range stimulate histamine release which causes temporary vasodilation and the characteristic "niacin flush."
- **Insulin:** Niacin has been identified as part of the glucose tolerance factor of yeast which enhances response to insulin.

Side Effects & Toxicity Large doses of niacin cause transient side effects such as tingling sensations, flushing of the skin, and head throbbing because of its vasodilating action. These effects disappear within 20 to 30 minutes. Research indicates the sustained release form of niacin can be hepatotoxic and people taking this form should be monitored appropriately by their healthcare provider.

RDA The RDA for adult males is 18 mg/day; for adult females, it is 13 mg/day. Therapeutic dosage ranges in the scientific literature vary from 30-2000 mg/day. However, some studies use dosages up to 6 g/day. Dosages >2 g/day should only be administered under medical supervision.

Dosage Range 15-2000 mg/day

Dietary Sources Both niacin and its precursor (tryptophan) are included when determining the niacin content of foods. Lean meats, poultry, fish, and peanuts are good sources of both niacin and tryptophan. Organ meats, brewer's yeast, milk, legumes, peanuts, and peanut butter are the best sources of niacin. Niacin is also synthesized by intestinal bacteria.

Forms Capsule; Liquid; Powder; Tablet; Tablet, effervescent

Vitamin B₅

Synonyms Pantothenic Acid

Available Compounds Calcium Pantothenate; Dexpanthenol

Drugs That Deplete
No medications were identified that deplete this nutrient.

Effects of Depletion Pantothenic acid is so widely available in foods that a deficiency in humans is virtually unknown. Experimentally-induced deficiencies manifest as problems related to the skin, liver, thymus, and nerves.
(Continued)

Vitamin B$_5$ *(Continued)*

Overview Dr Roger Williams discovered vitamin B$_5$ in 1933 and, since it is present in all cells, he named it pantothenic acid from the Greek word "pantothen" meaning "everywhere." Pantothenic acid plays a number of essential metabolic roles including the production of some hormones and neurotransmitters, and is involved in the metabolism of all carbohydrates, fats, and proteins.

It is most commonly available commercially as calcium pantothenate. After absorption, pantothenic acid is first converted to a sulfur-containing compound called pantotheine. Pantotheine is then converted into coenzyme A, which is its only known biologically active form of pantothenic acid.

Biological Function & Effect As a constituent of coenzyme A (CoA), pantothenic acid participates in a wide variety of enzymatic reactions transferring two-carbon units (acetyl groups) within cells throughout the body.

- **Energy:** CoA is involved in the release of energy from carbohydrates in the Krebs cycle.
- **Adrenal gland function:** Pantothenic acid can provide an antistress effect since CoA is necessary for the synthesis of steroid hormones and proper functioning of the adrenal glands.
- **Production:** CoA also functions in the production of fats, cholesterol, and bile acids.
- **Synthesis:** Pantothenic acid is necessary for the synthesis of acetyl-choline, phospholipids, and porphyrin in the hemoglobin of red blood cells.
- **Energy and athletic performance:** Pantothenic acid may help to boost energy and athletic ability because of its role in carbohydrate metabolism.
- **Detoxification:** Pantothenic acid helps to detoxify alcohol by participating in the metabolism of acetaldehyde.
- **Stress:** Pantothenic acid has been reported to improve the stress reactions of well-nourished individuals and to relieve "burning feet" syndrome.

Side Effects & Toxicity There are no known toxic effects from taking large doses of pantothenic acid. Ingestion of large amounts may cause diarrhea.

RDA The RDA for pantothenic acid is 10 mg/day. Pharmacologic doses in the scientific literature range from 50-1000 mg/day.

Dosage Range 10-1000 mg/day

Dietary Sources

- Pantothenic acid is present in all plant and animal tissues. Best sources of this vitamin include eggs, liver, fish, chicken, whole grain breads and cereals, and legumes.
- Other good sources are cauliflower, broccoli, lean beef, white and sweet potatoes, and tomatoes.

Forms Capsule; Liquid; Powder; Spray, liposomal; Tablet; Tablet, effervescent

Vitamin B$_6$

Synonyms Pyridoxine

Available Compounds Pyridoxine Hydrochloride; Pyridoxal Hydrochloride; Pyridoxal-5'-phosphate

Drugs That Deplete

See the Alphabetical Listing of Nutrients and the Drugs That Deplete on page 273 for a complete listing.

Effects of Depletion Deficiencies of vitamin B$_6$ manifest primarily as dermatologic, circulatory, and neurologic changes. Because of its many metabolic roles, there are a wide variety of deficiency symptoms, which include the following:

- Depression
- Sleep disturbances
- Nerve inflammation
- PMS
- Lethargy
- Decreased alertness
- Anemia
- Altered mobility
- Elevated homocysteine
- Nausea
- Vomiting
- Seborrheic dermatitis

Vitamin B$_6$ is one of the most commonly deficient nutrients in the United States. One U.S. Department of Agriculture study reported that approximately 80% of Americans consumed less than the RDA for vitamin B$_6$.

Vitamin B$_6$ is an essential cofactor for 5-hydroxytryptophan decarboxylase, which is an enzyme that catalyzes one of the steps in the conversion of tryptophan to serotonin. Thus, a vitamin B$_6$ deficiency can limit the brain's ability to synthesize serotonin. Low serotonin levels are associated with depression.

To date, no studies have been conducted to evaluate insomnia and other sleep disturbances in people taking drugs that deplete vitamin B$_6$. However, the metabolic pathways are well understood. Melatonin, which is our biochemical sleep trigger, is synthesized from serotonin in the brain. If a vitamin B$_6$ deficiency inhibits serotonin synthesis, there will be a corresponding decrease in the body's ability to synthesize melatonin.

Elevated homocysteine is now recognized as one of the most critical independent risk factors to cardiovascular disease. Homocysteine is a toxic intermediate metabolite in the metabolism of the amino acid methionine. It is capable of directly damaging the vascular system and initiating the process of atherosclerosis. Vitamin B$_6$ is one of the nutrients that is required to metabolize homocysteine so that it does not build up in the blood and begin to damage the lining of the blood vessels.

(Continued)

Vitamin B$_6$ *(Continued)*

Vitamin B$_6$ appears to influence estrogen-induced gene expression. A B$_6$ deficiency results in a substantial increase in estrogen gene expression. Under these conditions excess estrogen may be produced, which may cause symptoms such as heavy menstrual flow, tender breasts, irregular bleeding, and emotional mood swings.

Vitamin B$_6$ is water-soluble; substantial amounts are lost in cooking and food processing. In addition to the drugs that deplete vitamin B$_6$, there are numerous substances in the environment which antagonize vitamin B$_6$, such as alcohol, tobacco smoke, yellow dye #5 (tartrazine), PCBs, rancid fats in fried foods, the chemical used to accelerate the ripening process of fruits, to name a few.

Overview Vitamin B$_6$ is necessary for the proper functioning of over sixty enzymes. Many of its activities are related to the metabolism of amino acids and other protein-related compounds such as hemoglobin, serotonin, various hormones, and the prostaglandins.

After entering a cell, vitamin B$_6$ is phosphorylated, which converts it into its active form, pyridoxal phosphate (PLP).

Biological Function & Effect Many pyridoxal phosphate enzymes are involved with amino acid metabolism including: transamination (transfer of amino groups), deamination (removal of amino groups), desulfuration (transfer of sulfhydro groups), and decarboxylation (removal of COOH groups).

- **Hemoglobin:** Necessary for the formation of hemoglobin and the growth of red blood cells.
- **Tryptophan:** Essential for the synthesis of tryptophan, and the conversion of tryptophan to niacin.
- **Neurotransmitters:** Required for the production of neurotransmitters derived from amino acids such as serotonin, GABA, norepinephrine, acetylcholine, and histamine.
- **Energy production:** Facilitates conversion of glycogen to glucose for energy production.
- **Depression:** Useful in people with depression. Vitamin B$_6$ is involved in the synthesis of serotonin.
- **PMS:** Useful in people with premenstrual syndrome associated with oral contraceptives (estrogens inhibit the absorption of vitamin B$_6$).
- **Carpal tunnel syndrome:** May be beneficial in the prevention and support of repetitive motion injuries such as carpal tunnel syndrome.
- **Atherosclerosis:** Helps prevent atherosclerosis by metabolizing homocysteine.

Side Effects & Toxicity Vitamin B$_6$ can be neurotoxic when taken in large doses. Several cases have been reported in people taking 2 g or more per day. Symptoms included tingling in the hands and feet, decreased muscle coordination, and a stumbling gait. All recovered without problems.

RDA The RDA for vitamin B$_6$ is 2 mg/day. Therapeutic dosage ranges in the scientific literature vary from 10-100 mg/day, although some applications go higher.

Dosage Range 2-100 mg/day

Dietary Sources The best sources of pyridoxine are brewer's yeast, wheat germ, organ meats (especially liver), peanuts, legumes, potatoes, and bananas. Vitamin B$_6$ is also synthesized by the "friendly" intestinal bacteria.

Forms Capsule; Liquid; Powder; Spray, liposomal; Tablet; Tablet, effervescent

Vitamin B$_{12}$

Synonyms Cobalamin

Available Compounds Cyanocobalamin; Methylcobalamin

Drugs That Deplete

See the Alphabetical Listing of Nutrients and the Drugs That Deplete on page 273 for a complete listing.

Effects of Depletion Vitamin B$_{12}$ deficiencies manifest primarily as anemia and neurologic changes. Vitamin B$_{12}$ deficiency inhibits DNA synthesis, which affects the growth and repair of all cells. The symptoms of vitamin B$_{12}$ deficiency include:

- Fatigue
- Peripheral neuropathy
- Tongue and mouth irregularities
- Macrocytic anemia (abnormally enlarged red blood cells)
- Depression, confusion and memory loss (especially in the elderly)
- Poor blood clotting and easy bruising
- Dermatitis and skin sensitivity
- Loss of appetite
- Nausea
- Vomiting

Anemia is the first symptom of vitamin B$_{12}$ deficiency. Pernicious anemia results from either inadequate vitamin B$_{12}$ intake or reduced gastric secretion of intrinsic factor, which inhibits absorption.

The elderly are most susceptible to vitamin B$_{12}$ deficiency due to atrophy of gastric parietal cells causing inadequate production of intrinsic factor. Deficiencies in the elderly often cause varying degrees of neuropsychiatric symptoms such as moodiness, confusion, abnormal gait, memory loss, agitation, delusions, dizziness, dementia, and hallucinations.

Meatless diets are deficient in vitamin B$_{12}$. Strict vegetarians are urged to use a vitamin B$_{12}$ supplement.

Numerous drugs inhibit vitamin B$_{12}$ absorption and, when taken chronically, can lead to nutrient depletion. These include oral contraceptives, potassium medications, histamine-2 blockers (Axid®, Pepcid®, Tagamet®, Zantac®), proton pump inhibitors (Prevacid®, Prilosec™), and phenytoin (Dilantin®).

Overview Vitamin B$_{12}$ was isolated from liver extract in 1948 and shown to control pernicious anemia. Its structure was finally elucidated in 1955. Cobalamin is the generic name of vitamin B$_{12}$ because it contains the heavy metal cobalt. Vitamin B$_{12}$ is an essential growth factor and plays a vital role in the metabolism of all cells, especially those of the gastrointestinal tract, bone marrow, and nervous tissue. (Continued)

Vitamin B$_{12}$ *(Continued)*

Several different cobalamin compounds exhibit vitamin B$_{12}$ activity. Cyanocobalamin, the most stable and most active form of the vitamin, contains a cyanide group, which is well below toxic levels and totally safe.

Vitamin B$_{12}$ is a water-soluble, red crystalline substance. Its red color is due to the presence of cobalt in the molecule. A protein in gastric secretions called intrinsic factor binds to vitamin B$_{12}$ and facilitates its absorption. Without intrinsic factor, <1% of vitamin B$_{12}$ is absorbed. Relatively large amounts of vitamin B$_{12}$ are stored in the liver.

Biological Function & Effect

- **Growth factor:** Cobalamin coenzymes are necessary for reducing RNA to DNA. This means B$_{12}$ plays a central role in the replication of the genetic code, and makes it a critical growth factor in all cells of the body.
- **DNA synthesis:** Vitamin B$_{12}$ demethylates methylfolate and helps generate tetrahydrofolate in the synthesis of DNA.
- **Nervous system:** Vitamin B$_{12}$ is required for the synthesis of myelin, the insulation around nerves. Hence It plays a major role in the functioning and maintenance of the nervous system.
- **Synthesis and metabolism:** Vitamin B$_{12}$ transfers methyl groups in the synthesis of methionine and in folic acid metabolism. Vitamin B$_{12}$ is involved in various aspects of protein, fat, and carbohydrate metabolism.
- **Red blood cells:** Vitamin B$_{12}$ is necessary for the maturation of red blood cells.

Side Effects & Toxicity There are no known symptoms of toxicity for vitamin B$_{12}$, even at doses 1000 times greater than the U.S. RDA.

RDA The RDA for vitamin B$_{12}$ is 6 mcg (micrograms). Pharmacologic dosages in the scientific literature range from 100-2000 mcg. Oral supplements are not well absorbed. Intramuscular injection is the most effective route of administration, especially for the elderly.

Dosage Range 100-2000 mcg/day

Dietary Sources Vitamin B$_{12}$ is produced by microbial synthesis in the digestive tract of animals. Hence, animal protein products are the source of this nutrient. It does not occur in fruits, vegetables, grain, or legumes. Organ meats are the best source of vitamin B$_{12}$, followed by clams, oysters, beef, eggs, milk, chicken, and cheese.

Forms Capsule; Liquid; Lozenge, sublingual; Powder; Spray, intra-nasal; Spray, liposomal; Tablet; Tablet, effervescent

♦ **Vitamin Bw** *see Biotin on page 311*

Vitamin C

Synonyms Ascorbic Acid

Available Compounds Ascorbic Acid; Calcium Ascorbate; Magnesium Ascorbate; Sodium Ascorbate; Ester C; Ascorbyl Palmitate

Drugs That Deplete

See the Alphabetical Listing of Nutrients and the Drugs That Deplete *on page 273* for a complete listing.

Effects of Depletion Scurvy is rare in the United States, but subclinical deficiencies are common. Deficiency symptoms include:

- Capillary fragility
- Hemorrhage
- Muscular weakness
- Easy bruising
- Gums that bleed easily
- Poor wound healing
- Anemia
- Poor appetite and growth
- Tender and swollen joints

Stressful situations (both physical and emotional) tend to deplete the body's stores of vitamin C quickly. Individuals most likely to experience deficiencies include elderly individuals on poor diets, alcoholics, people who are severely ill or under chronic stress, and infants who are only fed cow's milk. Some studies have shown that up to 95% of the elderly in institutions, 75% of cancer patients, and 20% of healthy elderly individuals are deficient in vitamin C.

Overview Vitamin C is the vitamin that cures the world's oldest known nutritional deficiency disease, scurvy. In fact, the term "ascorbic" is derived from Latin (a = not, scorbutus = scurvy, meaning without scurvy). It was first isolated by Albert Szent-Györgyi in 1928 from pork adrenal glands and called hexuronic acid. In 1933, its correct structural formula was established, it was successfully synthesized, and the name was changed to ascorbic acid.

Vitamin C is a water-soluble vitamin that is easily absorbed from the small intestine. It is concentrated in many tissues throughout the body, but the adrenal glands contain the highest concentration.

Humans are one of the few species who cannot manufacture vitamin C and must depend on our diet, or nutritional supplements, as the primary source. Vitamin C exists in nature in both its reduced form, L-ascorbic acid, and in its oxidized form, L-dehydroascorbic acid. L-ascorbic acid is the most active form. However, they convert back and forth to each other in a reversible equilibrium, and both are antiscorbutic.

Biological Function & Effect Vitamin C participates in oxidation-reduction reactions, energy production, tyrosine metabolism, reduction and storage of iron, and the activation of folic acid. It is essential in the formation or synthesis of collagen, serotonin, norepinephrine, thyroxine, and some of the corticosteroids.

In his 1972 book, *The Healing Factor: Vitamin C Against Disease*, Irwin Stone, MD, discussed over 500 studies which reported the value of high doses of vitamin C in preventing and treating about 100 diseases. Research since then has continued to support the incredible importance of this nutrient.

Vitamin C plays a major role in the synthesis of collagen and elastin, the major structural components of skin, tendons, bone matrix, tooth (Continued)

Vitamin C *(Continued)*

dentin, blood vessels, and connective tissues between cells. Collectively, collagen is the most abundant protein in the body, comprising 25% to 30% of total body protein.

- **Antioxidant:** Vitamin C's ability to donate hydrogen atoms from its two hydroxyl (OH) positions to neutralize free radicals makes it one of the body's most powerful and important antioxidants. Being water-soluble, it provides protection in all body fluids, within every cell in the body, and is highly concentrated in the brain to protect against brain aging.
- **Stress:** Vitamin C helps the body handle all types of stress. It is required for the synthesis of the body's main stress response hormones in the adrenal glands, including adrenaline, noradrenaline, cortisol, and histamine. Stresses, such as fever, burns, exposure to cold, physical trauma, fractures, high altitude, and radiation all require larger doses of vitamin C.
- **Cancer:** Vitamin C prevents formation of nitrosamines, and dramatically reduces cervical dysplasia. Plasma levels of vitamin C are inversely correlated with the incidence of GI and cervical cancers. Vitamin C may prevent the formation of bladder tumors, inhibit hyaluronidase (an enzyme found in malignant tumors), slow down degradation of cellular tissue and decrease invasion of cancerous growth, stimulate production of phagocytic leukocytes which engulf and destroy cancer cells, and prevent free radical damage.
- **Cardiovascular:** Vitamin C has cardiovascular functions and include the following:
  - increases HDL
  - decreases elevated LDL and total cholesterol by conversion to bile acids for excretion
  - is necessary for synthesis of collagen and elastin which maintains strength and elasticity of blood vessels
  - decreases free radical oxidation of cholesterol
  - decreases levels of lipoprotein(a) or Lp(a) which is now known to form atherosclerotic plaques
- **Atherosclerotic plaques:** Vitamin C also helps to dissolve atherosclerotic plaques. Calcium/phospholipid/cholesterol plaque (insoluble) reacts with sodium ascorbate to form sodium/phospholipid/cholesterol (soluble) and calcium ascorbate (soluble).
- **Immunity:** Vitamin C also helps to boost the immune system by:
  - increasing the production of disease-fighting white blood cells (neutrophils, lymphocytes, and natural killer cells)
  - increasing levels of antibodies IgA, IgG, and IgM which fight infections
  - increasing body's production of interferon
  - modulating prostaglandin synthesis
- **Asthma:** Vitamin C functions as both a very mild antihistamine (it inhibits the release and enhances the degradation of histamine) and as a phosphodiesterase inhibitor (the same action as some asthma medications). Vitamin C reduces the frequency and intensity of bronchial spasms in asthmatics.

- **Antiviral:** Ascorbic acid may have some antiviral actions against most viruses (if enough is used) including herpes, shingles, viral hepatitis, polio, etc, by stimulating the production of interferons which are the proteins that protect cells against viral attack.
- **Common cold:** Vitamin C probably reduces the severity of symptoms associated with, and duration of, the common cold.
- **Wound healing:** Increases the healing of scars, broken bones, burns, etc.
- **Detoxification:** Vitamin C detoxifies heavy metal toxins such as mercury, lead, cadmium, and nickel.
- **Regeneration:** Vitamin C is capable of regenerating the antioxidant form of vitamin E.

Side Effects & Toxicity Vitamin C is nontoxic, excesses are excreted in the urine. Diarrhea is the only significant side effect from an overdose of vitamin C. Approximately 15% of people taking moderately high doses of vitamin C experience abdominal gas, bloating, and cramping. The mineral ascorbates such as calcium or magnesium ascorbate are much less acidic and will usually solve this problem.

While vitamin C has not been proven to cause kidney stones, in some individuals its metabolic pathway produces high amounts of oxalic acid, which could be a problem. Therefore, people with a history of gout, kidney stones, or kidney disease should not take amounts of vitamin C exceeding the RDA without medical supervision.

Large doses of vitamin C will interfere with:
- tests to determine occult blood in the stool
- tests to monitor blood glucose levels in diabetics

RDA The RDA for vitamin C is 60 mg/day. Pharmacologic doses in the scientific literature range from 500 mg up to 20 g; higher doses of vitamin C should be taken in 3 or 4 divided doses throughout the day. Any kind of physical or emotional stress calls for higher vitamin C intake.

Taking vitamin C to bowel tolerance (just below the diarrhea point) is a therapeutic technique that has gained some acceptance. The intake necessary to reach bowel tolerance varies from person to person.

Dosage Range 60-12,000 mg/day; some therapeutic applications go much higher

Dietary Sources Vitamin C is found in fresh fruits, especially citrus fruits, strawberries, cantaloupe, and currants. In addition, fresh vegetables, especially brussel sprouts, collard greens, lettuce, cabbage, peas, and asparagus, are good sources of vitamin C.

Forms Capsule; Powder; Spray, liposomal; Tablet; Tablet, effervescent

Vitamin D

Synonyms Calciferol

Drugs That Deplete

See the Alphabetical Listing of Nutrients and the Drugs That Deplete *on page 273* for a complete listing.

Effects of Depletion Rickets is the classic childhood vitamin D deficiency disease. Insufficient deposition of calcium phosphate into the bone matrix creates bones that are not strong enough to withstand the
(Continued)

Vitamin D *(Continued)*

ordinary stresses and strains of weight bearing. In adults, vitamin D deficiency can result in osteomalacia and osteoporosis. Symptoms of vitamin D deficiency include:

In children: Knock-knees, bowed legs, spinal curvature, pigeon breast, disfiguration of the skull, tooth decay, and dental problems.

In adults: Rheumatic pains, muscle weakness, increased incidence of fractures of the hip and pelvis, gradual loss of hearing

Vitamin D deficiency can result from several reasons including:
- inadequate dietary intake
- limited exposure to sunlight, which reduces the body's synthesis of vitamin D
- kidney or liver malfunctions which inhibit the conversion of vitamin D to its metabolically active forms

Vitamin D deficiency increases the risk of osteoporosis by reducing bone mass and density. However, there is no evidence that vitamin D supplementation is effective in treating osteoporosis.

Osteomalacia is the adult equivalent of rickets, where vitamin D deficiency causes softening of the bones which can lead to deformities. This condition occurs more frequently in the elderly. It can cause rheumatic pain, muscle weakness, and increases the likelihood of fractures of the hip and pelvis.

Vitamin D deficiency can also cause a gradual hearing loss because demineralization of the bones in the middle ear inhibit the transmission of vibrations to the nerves that communicate with the brain. Vitamin D deficiency also causes muscle weakness, severe tooth decay, and phosphorus retention in the kidneys.

Overview Vitamin D was isolated in 1930 and named calciferol. Since then, more metabolites have been found, and the two major forms of this vitamin are now known to be vitamin D_2 (ergocalciferol) and vitamin D_3 (cholecalciferol). Vitamin D is actually a hormone precursor, which can be manufactured by the body. Therefore, in a classical sense, it is not actually an essential nutrient. However, since the disease rickets is related to vitamin D deficiency, it has been traditionally classified as a vitamin.

Vitamin D is known as the "sunshine" vitamin. It is formed in the body by the action of the sun's ultraviolet rays on the skin, converting the biological precursor 7-dehydroergosterol (found in animals and humans) into vitamin D_3. Ultraviolet radiation converts the biological precursor ergosterol (found in plants) to vitamin D_2. Vitamin D is a fat-soluble nutrient that is stored in body fats, principally the liver.

Biological Function & Effect
- **Bones and teeth:** Vitamin D promotes the absorption of calcium and phosphorus for the growth of bones and teeth. For this reason, it is a very important growth nutrient for infants and children.
- **Calcitriol:** Vitamin D_3 is converted in the liver to 25-hydroxycholecalciferol (25-HCC) which is 5 times more active than vitamin D_3. 25-

HCC is then converted in the kidneys to 1,25-dihydroxycholecalciferol (1,25-HCC) which is ten times more potent than vitamin D_3. The active 1,25-HCC form of vitamin D is also called calcitriol. Since calcitriol is produced in the kidney and functions elsewhere in the body, it is considered a hormone, with the intestines and bone as its targets. It is the most active form of vitamin D, 1,25-dihydroxycholecalciferol, that acts in the intestines to promote absorption of calcium and phosphorus.

- **Bones:** Vitamin D is involved in both the formation (mineralization) of bone, as well as in the mobilization (demineralization) of bone mineral.
- **Cancer:** There is some indication that vitamin D might be helpful in some cancers. Geographic areas with the least amount of sunlight have the highest rates of colorectal and breast cancer. The active form of vitamin D, calcitriol, has some inhibitory activity against human melanoma, leukemia, breast, lymphoma, and colon cancer cells.
- **Regulation:** Active vitamin D (calcitriol) regulates serum levels of calcium and phosphorus.
- **Osteoporosis:** Vitamin D may help to prevent osteoporosis since it facilitates the absorption of calcium from the intestines. Low calcium levels stimulate the parathyroid gland which initiates pulling calcium out of the bone.
- **Psoriasis:** Sunlight and ultraviolet light are often helpful for individuals with psoriasis. This suggests the active form of vitamin D may also offer some support for these people.
- **Immunity:** The active form of vitamin D enhances the immune system by stimulating the activity of macrophages.

Side Effects & Toxicity Vitamin D can be toxic. Excessive intake of this nutrient causes hypercalcemia which causes calcium deposits in soft tissues such as kidneys, arteries, heart, ear, and lungs. Signs of vitamin D toxicity include headache, weakness, nausea and vomiting, and constipation.

RDA The RDA for vitamin D is 400 international units/day. Pharmacologic doses in the scientific literature range from 400-1000 international units/day.

Dosage Range 200-800 international units (IU) daily

Dietary Sources Vitamin D does not occur in significant amounts in many foods. It occurs in small and highly variable amounts in butter, cream, egg yolks, and liver. Milk fortified with vitamin D is the most common source of this nutrient in the United States.

Forms Capsule; Drops, oral; Injection; Tablet

Vitamin E

Synonyms Alpha Tocopherol

Drugs That Deplete
See the Alphabetical Listing of Nutrients and the Drugs That Deplete *on page 273* for a complete listing.

Effects of Depletion Vitamin E is destroyed by heat and oxidation during cooking or food processing. Therefore, reliance on processed foods and/or fast foods can contribute to depletion. Low levels of
(Continued)

Vitamin E *(Continued)*

selenium and high intake of polyunsaturated fatty acids both contribute to vitamin E depletion. Symptoms of vitamin E deficiency include:

- Dry skin
- Dull dry hair
- Rupturing of red blood cells resulting in anemia
- Easy bruising
- PMS
- Fibrocystic breasts
- Hot Flashes
- Eczema
- Psoriasis
- Cataracts
- Benign prostatic hyperplasia
- Poor wound healing
- Muscle weakness
- Sterility

Premature infants are likely to be deficient because very little vitamin E is transferred across the placenta. However, breast milk contains enough vitamin E to meet the infant's needs.

Overview In 1932, Evans and Bishop discovered that something in vegetable oils was necessary for reproduction in rats and named it vitamin E. They referred to it as the antisterility vitamin, which turned out to be an unfortunate designation since it was subsequently found to not have this activity in humans. The same researchers isolated the pure substance from wheat germ oil in 1936 and elucidated the structure in 1938, giving it the chemical name of tocopherol (after the Greek words "tokos", meaning offspring, and "phero", meaning to bring forth).

Vitamin E is actually a group of eight compounds including four tocopherols (alpha, beta, gamma, and delta) and four additional tocotrienol derivatives. Alpha tocopherol is the most common and most potent form and is what is usually meant by the term vitamin E. Pure vitamin E compounds are easily oxidized, so they are manufactured as acetate or succinate esters.

Natural vitamin E is d-alpha tocopherol, whereas synthetically produced vitamin E is a mixture consisting of both the d- and l-isomers as dl-alpha tocopherol. Different studies report that natural vitamin E has from 34% to 50% greater bioavailability than synthetic vitamin E.

Biological Function & Effect

- **Antioxidant:** Vitamin E is the body's most important fat-soluble antioxidant. As such, it ensures the stability and integrity of cellular tissues and membranes throughout the body by preventing free radical (lipid peroxidation) damage.
- **Cardiovascular disease:** Vitamin E decreases platelet stickiness, protecting blood vessels against developing atherosclerotic lesions, and protecting LDL-cholesterol against oxidation.
- **Cancer:** Low levels of vitamin E are associated with a greater risk for developing various forms of cancer, including lung, oral, colon,

rectal, cervical, pancreatic, and liver. This may be due to Vitamin E's ability to protect tissues against free radical damage and support the immune system.

- **Exercise:** During heavy exercise, vitamin E markedly reduces the amount of exercise-induced free radical damage to the blood and tissues, and also decreases the incidence of exercise-induced muscle injury.
- **Eyes:** Vitamin E protects the eyes against cataracts and macular degeneration through its antioxidant actions.
- **PMS:** Some studies have shown that vitamin E supplementation helps many women alleviate the symptoms of PMS, again through its antioxidant properties.

Side Effects & Toxicity Although it is fat-soluble, vitamin E is a relatively nontoxic nutrient. Approximately 60% to 70% of the daily dose is excreted in the feces. Vitamin E can potentiate an increase in blood clotting time, and therefore, high level supplementation is not advised for individuals taking anticoagulant drugs.

Most individuals studied while taking large doses of vitamin E have not shown toxic effects. However, symptoms reported from isolated cases where people were taking >1000 international units/day include headache, fatigue, nausea, double vision, muscular weakness, and GI distress.

RDA The RDA for vitamin E is 30 international units/day. Pharmacologic doses in the scientific literature range from 100-1000 international units/day. Natural vitamin E (d-alpha tocopherol) is more bioavailable and, therefore, better than synthetic vitamin E (dl-alpha tocopherol).

Dosage Range 30-1200 international units (IU) daily

Dietary Sources Vitamin E is one of the most widely available nutrients in commonly available foods. Sources of vitamin E include vegetable oils, wheat germ oil, seeds, nuts, and soy beans. Other adequate sources are leafy greens, brussel sprouts, whole wheat products, whole grain breads and cereals, avocados, spinach, and asparagus.

Forms Capsule; Injection; Liquid; Topical

♦ **Vitamin H** see Biotin on page 311

Vitamin K

Synonyms Phytonadione

Drugs That Deplete

See the Alphabetical Listing of Nutrients and the Drugs That Deplete on page 273 for a complete listing.

Effects of Depletion Vitamin K deficiency is rare except in newborn infants. However, it can cause hemorrhaging and death when it does occur. Deficiency symptoms include:

- Easy bleeding
- Skeletal disorders such as rickets, osteoporosis, and osteomalacia

Overview In 1935, a scientist in Copenhagen observed that newly hatched chickens receiving a diet containing all of the known essential nutrients were developing a hemorrhagic disease. The problem was thought to be related to a fall in prothrombin, a substance necessary
(Continued)

Vitamin K *(Continued)*

for normal clotting of blood. The Danish scientist named this newly discovered antihemorrhagic factor vitamin K or "Koagulationsvitamin."

Vitamin K refers to a group of three vitamins called the quinones. Phylloquinone (K_1) occurs in green plants, menaquinone (K_2) is synthesized by intestinal bacteria, and menadione (K_3) is manufactured synthetically. The vitamin Ks are fat-soluble nutrients. Bile and pancreatic juice are necessary for their absorption from the upper small intestine where they are then carried to the liver.

Biological Function & Effect

- **Blood clotting:** Vitamin K is an enzymatic cofactor that is necessary for the production of a number of blood clotting factors, including prothrombin, and factors VII, IX, and X.
- **Bones:** Vitamin K is also necessary for the synthesis of osteocalcin, a unique protein in bone, which attracts calcium to bone tissue. Osteocalcin modulates the deposition of calcium into bone matrix.
- **Osteoporosis:** Since vitamin K plays a significant role in the calcification of bone, it may play a role in the prevention and support of individuals with osteoporosis.

Side Effects & Toxicity Large doses of vitamin K can be toxic. Consequently, it is only available by prescription. Vitamin K can cause a fatal form of jaundice in infants.

RDA The RDA for vitamin K is 65 mcg for women and 80 mcg for men. Pharmacologic doses in the scientific literature range from 30-100 mcg. Patients receiving oral anticoagulants should not alter vitamin K intake without consultation with prescriber.

Dosage Range 0.5-25 mg daily under the supervision of a healthcare provider

Dietary Sources The best sources of vitamin K are liver, green leafy vegetables, and members of the cabbage family. Since intestinal bacteria synthesize vitamin K, we are not dependent upon food for this nutrient.

Forms Injection; Tablet

Zinc

Drugs That Deplete

See the Alphabetical Listing of Nutrients and the Drugs That Deplete *on page 273* for a complete listing.

Effects of Depletion Marginal zinc deficiencies are thought to be quite common in the United States. Because of its extensive range of biological activities, zinc deficiency can cause a wide range of deficiency symptoms. The symptoms of zinc deficiency include acne; impaired sense of smell and taste; delayed wound healing; anorexia; decreased immunity; frequent infections; depression; photophobia; night blindness; problems with skin, hair, and nails; menstrual problems; joint pain; and involuntary cyclical movements of the eyeball (nystagmus).

Zinc deficiency conditions were first reported in the 1960s in growing children and adolescent males from Egypt, Iran, and Turkey. Diets low in animal protein and high in phytate-containing grains produced symptoms of dwarfism, hypogonadism, and failure to mature sexually.

Pregnant women have greater zinc needs. Deficiency can cause impaired fetal development, low birth weight infants, and birth defects. Stretch marks during pregnancy are also partially due to zinc deficiency.

Zinc deficiency can be caused by inadequate dietary intake due to foods grown on zinc-depleted soils. Food processing also removes zinc, so fast foods and processed foods are also zinc depleted. Protein and/or calorie-restricted diets can also lead to zinc deficiency.

- Zinc depletion is frequently seen in the following medical conditions: alcoholism, macular degeneration, diabetes, malignant melanoma, liver and kidney diseases, malabsorption syndromes such as celiac sprue, and inflammatory bowel diseases such as Crohn's disease.

Overview Zinc is necessary for the functioning of well over 300 different enzymes and, as such, it plays a vital role in an enormous number of biological processes. Zinc is widely distributed in microorganisms, plants, and animals. In humans, the highest concentrations of zinc are found in the liver, pancreas, kidneys, bone, and voluntary muscles. Zinc is highly concentrated in parts of the eye, prostate gland, sperm, skin, hair, and nails.

Biological Function & Effect

- **Enzymatic:** A few of zinc's important enzymatic activities include alcohol dehydrogenase, which works in the liver to detoxify alcohol; alkaline phosphatase, which frees inorganic phosphates to be used in bone metabolism; carbonic anhydrase, which helps excrete carbon dioxide; zinc/copper-containing superoxide dismutase; cytochrome C, which is important in electron transport and energy production; and carboxypeptidase, which is necessary for the digestion of dietary proteins.
- **Cell division:** Zinc is necessary in the synthesis of DNA and RNA, protein synthesis, cellular division, and gene expression. Zinc protects DNA from damage.
- **Immunity:** Zinc helps regulate a wide variety of immune system activities, including T lymphocytes, CD4s, natural killer cells, interleukin 2, and Zn/Cu superoxide dismutase.
- **Wound healing:** Zinc facilitates wound healing, especially in burns, surgical incisions, and other types of scars.
- **Antiviral activity:** Zinc enhances immune function in AIDS patients.
- **Common cold:** Zinc lozenges may reduce the length and severity of colds.
- **Infertility:** Zinc is necessary for the maturation of sperm, for ovulation, and for fertilization.
- **Growth:** Zinc is necessary for normal growth and maturation.
- **Skin conditions:** Zinc is often useful in acne and eczema.
- **Senses:** Zinc is a critical regulator of the sensory perceptions of taste, smell, and vision. It controls salt-taste perception, and is necessary for dark adaptation and night vision.
- **Vitamin A regulation:** Zinc regulates vitamin A levels by controlling the release of stored vitamin A from the liver.

(Continued)

Zinc *(Continued)*

- **Arthritis:** Zinc has anti-inflammatory properties and has been used to support individuals with some types of arthritis.
- **Prostate:** Zinc is necessary for a healthy prostate gland and helps prevent benign prostatic hyperplasia (BPH).
- **Pancreas:** Although zinc is a component of insulin, it does not appear to be a regulator of insulin activity.
- **Thyroid:** Zinc promotes the conversion of thyroxine to triiodothyronine.

Side Effects & Toxicity Zinc is relatively nontoxic, and although toxicity has been reported in humans, it is uncommon. Ingestion of high levels of zinc can induce a copper deficiency. Doses of 45 mg/day are safe, but regular intakes >150 mg/day could be problematic. Zinc toxicity can cause diarrhea, dizziness, drowsiness, vomiting, muscle incoordination, and lethargy.

Inhalation of zinc oxide in certain industrial environments can also be a source of excess exposure.

Cooking acidic foods in galvanized cookware used to be a possible source of excess zinc intake. The widespread use of stainless steel and plastic materials to prepare and store foods has largely eliminated this problem. Galvanized pipes in older plumbing systems used to leach zinc into drinking water supplies, but modern plumbing has phased out the use of galvanized pipes.

RDA The RDA is 15 mg/day for adult men and 12 mg/day for adult women.

Dosage Range 10-50 mg daily

Dietary Sources The best dietary sources of zinc are lean meats, liver, eggs, and seafood (especially oysters). Whole grain breads and cereals are also good sources of zinc.

Forms Injection; Tablet

STUDIES AND ABSTRACTS

ANTACIDS

MAGNESIUM/ALUMINUM HYDROXIDE-CONTAINING ANTACIDS

Magnesium/Aluminum Hydroxide-Containing Antacids & Calcium Depletion

1. Spencer H and Lender M, "Adverse Effects of Aluminum-Containing Antacids on Mineral Metabolism," *Gastroenterology*, 1979, 76(3):603-606.

    Aluminum binds with phosphate and fluoride in the gut. Loss of phosphate results in lowering of serum phosphate levels, resulting in mobilization of calcium and phosphate from bone stores, and an accompanying loss of calcium in urine.

Magnesium/Aluminum Hydroxide-Containing Antacids & Phosphate Depletion

2. Balasa RW, Murray RL, Kondelis NP, et al, "Phosphate-Binding Properties and Electrolyte Content of Aluminum Hydroxide Antacids," *Nephron*, 1987, 45(1):16-21.

    Nineteen aluminum hydroxide gel antacids were studied to determine their phosphate binding capacities. Variations in sodium and potassium content were determined to be clinically insignificant. However, the differences in phosphate-binding properties were concluded to warrant clinical consideration, particularly in long-term aluminum hydroxide therapy.

3. Spencer H and Lender M, "Adverse Effects of Aluminum-Containing Antacids on Minerals Metabolism," *Gastroenterology*, 1979, 76(3):603:-6.

    In this review, the authors note that aluminum binds with phosphate and fluoride in the gastrointestinal tract. Due to effects on serum phosphate and calcium mobilization, loss of phosphate contributes to the development of osteomalacia during long-term aluminum-containing antacid therapy.

4. Baker LR, Ackrill P, Cattell WR, et al, "Iatrogenic Osteomalacia and Myopathy Due to Phosphate Depletion," *Br Med J*, 1974, 3(924):150-2.

    A case of osteomalacia and myopathy associated with long-term aluminum hydroxide therapy is reported. Phosphate depletion is proposed as the mechanism to explain these complications.

Magnesium/Aluminum Hydroxide-Containing Antacids & Vitamin D Depletion

5. D'Erasmo E, Ragno A, Raejntroph N, et al, "Drug-induced Osteomalacia," *Recenti Prog Med*, 1998, 89(10):529-33.

    In this review, drugs which are commonly associated with osteomalacia are discussed. Associated medications include cholestyramine, phenytoin, phenobarbital, isoniazid, aluminum-containing antacids, ferric oxide lead, bisphosphonates, fluoride, ammonium, and rifampicin. Pathophysiologic mechanisms related to drug-induced osteomalacia are discussed, including vitamin D metabolism, phosphorus homeostasis, and bone mineralization.

SODIUM BICARBONATE

Sodium Bicarbonate & Potassium Depletion

6. Rhodes J, "Side Effects of Antacids Treatments," *Antacids in the Eighties*, Halter F, ed, Munchen, Germany: Urban & Schwarzenberg, 1982, 99-102.

A sequence of events which begins with bicarbonate administration and results in excessive renal potassium excretion is described. The resulting hypokalemia may be severe enough to lead to cardiac irregularities.

ANTIBIOTICS

ANTIBIOTICS IN GENERAL

Advancements in technology in the past several decades have produced leaps in our understanding of human intestinal microflora. Previously, anaerobic bacteria could not be studied at all because exposure to an oxygen-containing environment was lethal to these organisms. We are now beginning to understand the important role these bacteria play in human nutrition. The development of germ-free laboratory animals has also been a breakthrough which facilitates investigation. Using germ-free animals and antibiotics, scientists were able to discover that intestinal bacteria are intimately involved in a wide range of human bodily functions. These include the synthesis and utilization of nutrients, resistance against infection, life expectancy, aging, the cause and/or prevention of various forms of cancer, as well as detoxification of pollutants, metabolism of cholesterol, and liver problems.

The use of antibiotics has grown enormously over the last few decades. Throughout the 1990s doctors in the United States have written between 200-250 million prescriptions for antibiotics each year. While the discovery and use of antibiotics has been a crucial development in the health and longevity of people living in the twentieth century, this widespread use has not been without its own serious health consequences. One of the main problems associated with antibiotic use is the disruption of bowel flora. Unfortunately, when an individual takes an antibiotic, beneficial bacteria are killed along with the pathologic species. When an individual does not re-inoculate their gastrointestinal tract with beneficial bacteria, other organisms are given the opportunity to grow and proliferate. This may result in a variety of health problems, both mental and physical. This condition is termed dysbiosis. The authors feel it is extremely important for healthcare professionals to educate patients about the importance of recolonizing the intestines with probiotics after a course of antibiotics.

The following studies document the fact that beneficial intestinal bacteria normally produce a wide range of vitamins in the human gastrointestinal tract.

Antibiotics & B Vitamins in the Gastrointestinal Tract

7. Cummings JH and Macfarlane G, "Role of Intestinal Bacteria in Nutrient Metabolism," *J Parenter Enteral Nutr*, 1997, 21(6):357-65.

    This paper summarizes the major functions of beneficial intestinal bacteria. When antibiotics are taken, a large majority of beneficial bacteria are destroyed. One consequence of this overall die-off is that it drastically reduces the normal bacterial production of vitamins B and K in the intestines. To date nobody has determined how important the vitamins produced by intestinal bacteria are to human nutritional status. However, a healthy intestinal microflora is extremely important to overall health, and problems associated with antibiotic use when beneficial microflora are not properly restored are responsible for a large number of health problems. Patients should be educated about the importance of consuming high doses of probiotics for 2-3 weeks during and after taking a course of antibiotics, in order to re-colonize the intestinal tract with the proper beneficial bacteria.

8. Honma N, "The Effect of Lactic Acid Bacteria, Part 1: Biological Significance," *New Medicines and Clinics*, 1986, 35(12):1-3.

    The author notes that intestinal bacteria flora produce a number of vitamins. These may include vitamins B_1, B_2, B_6, B_{12}, folic acid, nicotinic acid, pantothenic acid, biotin, inositol, vitamin K, and vitamin E. Not all bacterial species are equivalent in their capacity to synthesize these compounds, and their absorption into the human circulation is not necessarily complete. For example, *Steptococcus faecalis* does not synthesize vitamin B₁ while *L. acidophilus* does so. Administration of *faecalis* bacteria or *acidophilus* bacteria is useful for the host which carries aneurinase bacteria. It is known that the oral administration of *faecalis* bacteria promotes the growth of *bifidus* bacteria which synthesize vitamin B₁, which may be absorbed by the host. Based on the review, the author considers *Streptococcus faecalis* 129 BIO 3B and *L. acidophlius* KS-13 to be of value in the metabolism of vitamin B₁ due to their ability to suppress the growth of anerurinase bacteria. In addition *B. bifidum* G9-1 is a producer of vitamin B₁ which may be absorbed by the host.

9. Deguchi Y, et al, "Comparative Studies on Synthesis of Water-soluble Vitamins Among Human Species of Bifidobacteria," *Argic Biol Chem*, 1985, 19(1):13-19.

    The ability of bifidobacteria to synthesize six water-soluble vitamins (thiamine, folic acid, nicotinic acid, pyridoxine, vitamin B₁₂ and riboflavin) was investigated in multiple strains of five bacterial species found in human feces. Synthesis by many of the bacterial strains was confirmed for five of the vitamins, with the exception being riboflavin. The accumulation of vitamins varied widely among different species or strains. The authors identified a method to categorize *Bifidobacteria* strains into three general types according to their ability to synthesize and accumulate thiamine, nicotinic acid, and folic acid. These three vitamins were accumulated in all strains of *B. bifidum* and *B. infantis* as well as in many strains of *B. breve* and *B. longum*. These findings are discussed in relation to regulation of vitamin biosynthesis.

10. Ballongue J, "Bifidobacteria and Probiotic Action," *Lactic Acid Bacteria*, Salminen S and von Wright A, eds, New York, NY: Dekker Inc, 1993, 409.

    This publication discusses the importance of bacterial production of vitamins (B₁, B₆, B₁₂, and folic acid).

11. Stevens CE and Hume ID, "Contributions of Microbes in Vertebrate Gastrointestinal Tract to Production and Conservation of Nutrients," *Physiol Rev*, 1998, 78(2):393-427.

    This review discusses the contributions of gut microorganisms to nutrition in all vertebrates. Particular reference is made to the production of B vitamins. These vitamins are noted to be synthesized by beneficial bacteria in the intestinal tract of all vertebrates, including humans.

12. Gorbach SL, "Bengt E. Gustafsson Memorial Lecture. Function of the Normal Human Microflora," *Scand J Infect Dis Suppl*, 1986, 49:17-30.

    The role of normal microflora in the maintenance of homeostasis is emphasized. Certain metabolic functions and enzyme activities can be attributed to microflora, and these play a role in metabolizing nutrients and vitamins. In addition, roles in the metabolism of drugs, hormones, and carcinogens are discussed. Antibiotic administration is noted to suppress this metabolic activity. The author suggests manipulation of this microenvironment may maximize the beneficial effects of intestinal flora.

13. Shanhani KM and Chandan RC, "Nutritional and Healthful Aspects of Cultured and Culture-Containing Dairy Foods," *J Dairy Sci*, 1979, 62(10):1685-94.

    Nutritional and therapeutic aspects of fermented dairy products are discussed in this review. It is noted that organisms in these products, including *L. acidophilus*, synthesize important B vitamins. Other beneficial

ANTIBIOTICS *(Continued)*

effects of these organisms are presented. The authors suggest ingestion of a specific culture or strain may be considered for projected beneficial effects.

14. Krause LJ, Forsberg CW, and O'Connor DL, "Feeding Human Milk to Rats Increases *Bifidobacterium* in the Cecum and Colon Which Correlates With Enhanced Folate Status," *J Nutr*, 1996, 126(5):1505-11.

    In this rat study, the folate status of rats fed human milk-containing diets appeared to be improved. This was proposed to be due, at least in part, to increased folate synthesis by bifidobacteria and other intestinal folate-synthesizing microbes.

15. Noda H, Akasaka N, and Ohsugi M, "Biotin Production by Bifidobacteria," *J Nutr Sci Vitaminol*, 1994, 40(2):181-8.

    Biotin production and growth of *Bifidobacterium* strains were investigated. These were found to be dependent on the growth medium employed.

16. Hill MJ, "Intestinal Flora and Endogenous Vitamin Synthesis," *Eur J Cancer Prev*, 1997, 6(Suppl 1):S43-5.

    In this paper, evidence is presented that gut bacteria are a significant source of a range of vitamins, particularly those of the B group and vitamin K.

17. Shahani KM, and Ayebo AD, "Role of Dietary Lactobacilli in Gastrointestinal Microecology," *Am J Clin Nutr*, 1980, 33(11 Suppl):2448-57.

    Review. No abstract available.

18. Najjar VA and Holt LE Jr, "Biosynthesis of Thiamine in Man and Its Implications in Human Nutrition," *JAMA*, 1943, 123:683-4.

    This study reports that humans absorb and utilize thiamine (vitamin B_1) synthesized by intestinal bacteria.

19. Najjar VA, "Biosynthesis of Riboflavin in Man," *JAMA*, 1944, 126:357-8.

    This study reports that humans absorb and utilize riboflavin (vitamin B_2) synthesized by intestinal bacteria.

20. Ellenger P, et al, "Production and Release of Nicotinamide by the Intestinal Flora in Man," *Nature*, 1944, 154:270-271.

    This study reports that humans absorb and utilize nicotinamide (vitamin B_3) synthesized by intestinal bacteria.

Antibiotics & B Vitamins in the Gastrointestinal Tract - No Negative Studies

Antibiotics & Vitamin K Depletion in the Gastrointestinal Tract

21. Hill MJ, "Intestinal Flora and Endogenous Vitamin Synthesis," *Eur J Cancer Prev*, 1997, 6(Suppl 1):S43-5.

    In this paper evidence is presented that gut bacteria are a significant source of a range of vitamins, particularly those of the B group and vitamin K.

22. Conly J and Stein K, "Reduction of Vitamin K2 Concentrations in Human Liver Associated With the Use of Broad Spectrum Antimicrobials," *Clin Invest Med*, 1994, 17(6):531-9.

    This study evaluated the vitamin K content in postmortem liver samples from patients receiving broad spectrum antibiotics as compared to controls. There was a significant difference in the total menaquinone content. These findings are interpreted to suggest an association between broad spectrum antibiotics and a reduction in hepatic menaquione concentration. This observation lends support to the hypothesis that a reduction in gut microflora leads to reduced hepatic stores of this form of vitamin K.

23. Conly JM, Stein K, Worobetz L, et al, "The Contribution of Vitamin K_2 (Menaquinones) Produced by the Intestinal Microflora to Human Nutritional Requirements for Vitamin K," *Am J Gastroenterel*, 1994, 89(6): 915-23.

   After ileal administration of menaquinone to four normal volunteers, biochemical evidence of absorption and utilization in coagulation factor synthesis was identified. These data are proposed to represent evidence for the absorption of vitamin K_2 from the distal small bowel. This supports a role for bacterially synthesized vitamin K_2 as a contributing source of human vitamin K nutritional requirements.

24. Cordes I, Buchmann S, and Scheffner D, "Vitamin K Deficiency With Erythromycin. Observation of a Boy Treated With Valproate," *Monatsschr Kinderheilkd*, 1990, 138(2):85-7.

   This case report details the events in a 9 year old treated with long-term valproate who then received erythromycin. A vitamin K-reversible coagulopathy resulted. In this case, the simultaneous application of both valproic acid and erythromycin succinate appeared to suppress intestinal vitamin K production by bacteria.

25. Lipsky JJ, "Antibiotic-Associated Hypoprothrombinaemia," *J Antimicrob Chemother*, 1988, 21(3):281-300.

   This article reviews the mechanisms by which broad-scale antibiotics may alter prothrombin activity. Effects include disruption of colonic bacteria as well as the role of thiol-leaving groups in the inhibition of clotting factor synthesis.

26. Alitalo R, Ruutu M, Valtonen V, et al, "Hypoprothrombinaemia and Bleeding During Administration of Cefamandole and Cefoperazone. Report of Three Cases," *Ann Clin Res*, 1985, 17(3):116-9.

   The potential to develop a deficiency of vitamin K-dependent coagulation factors due to cephalosporins is discussed. Cefamandole, cefoperazone, and moxalactam are noted to be associated with this effect. Mechanisms include vitamin K deficiency caused by eradictation of the vitamin K producing intestinal bacteria or inhibition of action of vitamin K_1. The authors recommend prophylactic administration of vitamin K_1 during cefamandole or cefoperazone treatment in several patient groups.

27. Shimada K, Matsuda T, Inamatsu T, et al, "Bleeding Secondary to Vitamin K Deficiency in Patients Receiving Parenteral Cephem Antibiotics," *J Antimicrob Chemother*, 1984, 14(Suppl B):325-30.

   Thirteen patients treated with cephalosporin antibiotics were noted to develop coagulation disorders due to vitamin K deficiency. It is noted that the potential to alter prothrombin time varies with individual agents.

ANTIBIOTICS *(Continued)*

Antibiotics & Vitamin K Depletion in the Gastrointestinal Tract - No Negative Studies

AMINOGLYCOSIDES

Aminoglycosides & Magnesium, Calcium, Sodium, and Potassium Depletion

28. Bamford MF and Jones LF, "Deafness and Biochemical Imbalance After Burn Treatment With Topical Antibiotics in Young Children. Report of 6 Cases," *Arch Dis Child*, 1978, 53(4):326-9.

    Six cases are reported in which deafness followed treatment of full thickness burns with a neomycin-containing topical spray. Hypocalcemia, hypomagnesemia, and hypokalemia were noted. Hypocalcaemic tetany developed in 3 children. The authors emphasized the danger of treating burns with topical antibiotics which may be ototoxic and/or nephrotoxic.

29. Valdivieso A, Mardones JM, Loyola MS, et al, "Hypomagnesemia Associated With Hypokalemia, Hyponatremia, and Metabolic Alkalosis. Possible Complication of Gentamycin Therapy," *Rev Med Chil*, 1992, 120(8):914-9. (Article in Spanish)

    A case of a female patient developing hypomagnesemia after administration of gentamicin is reported. The hypomagnesemia was associated with severe hypokalemia, hyponatremia, and metabolic alkalosis. The authors discuss possible pathogenetic mechanisms and therapeutic measures.

30. Kes P and Reiner Z, "Symptomatic Hypomagnesemia Associated With Gentamicin Therapy," *Magnes Trace Elem*, 1990, 9(1):54-60.

    Seven patients (3 females, 4 males) developed symptomatic hypomagnesemia, hypocalcemia, and hypokalemia following gentamicin therapy. The excessive and inappropriate urinary excretion of magnesium and potassium in the presence of subnormal serum concentrations was noted. A significant correlation was found between the total cumulative dose of gentamicin and serum Mg concentration ($r = 0.76$, $p <0.05$), as well as between the renal wasting of Mg and the total cumulative dose of gentamicin administered ($r = 0.89$, $p <0.01$). The gentamicin-induced Mg depletion is a very rare, but important complication which is most likely to occur when the drug is given to older patients in large doses over extended periods of time.

31. Nanji AA and Denegri JF, "Hypomagnesemia Associated With Gentamicin Therapy," *Drug Intell Clin Pharm*, 1984, 18(7-8):596-8.

    The authors report two cases in which patients developed symptomatic hypomagnesemia in association with gentamicin therapy. Both patients had hypokalemia and hypocalcemia secondary to hypomagnesemia. Several mechanisms are postulated, including drug-induced hyperaldosteronism and tubular toxicity. Routine monitoring of serum magnesium, calcium, and potassium levels is proposed.

32. Goodhart GL, et al, "Gentamicin and Hypokalemia," *Ann Intern Med*, 1985, 103(4):645-6.

    No abstract available.

33. Kelnar CJ, Taor WS, Reynolds DJ, et al, "Hypomagnesaemic Hypocalcaemia With Hypokalaemia Caused by Treatment With High Dose Gentamicin," *Arch Dis Child*, 1978, 53(10):817-20.

A 12-year-old boy developed renal wasting of magnesium, calcium, and potassium, with secondary hypomagnesaemia, hypocalcaemia, and hypokalemia (without hyperaldosteronism) after treatment with 14,400 mg gentamicin over 4 months. Gentamicin should not be given for prolonged courses if less toxic antibiotics are suitable. If used, plasma magnesium, calcium, and potassium levels should be monitored both during and after treatment.

34. al-Ghamdi SM, Cameron EC, and Sutton RA, "Magnesium Deficiency: Pathophysiologic and Clinical Overview," *Am J Kidney Dis*, 1994, 24(5):737-52.

This review notes that many therapeutic agents cause renal magnesium wasting, potentially resulting in deficiency. These include loop and thiazide diuretics, aminoglycosides, cisplatin, pentamidine, and foscarnet. Due to a combination of factors, magnesium deficiency is seen frequently in alcoholics and diabetic patients. Symptoms of hypomagnesemia may include neuromuscular irritability, cardiac arrhythmias, and/or increased sensitivity to digoxin. Refractory hypokalemia and hypocalcemia may also be caused by concomitant hypomagnesemia. The very important point is made that serum magnesium levels can register as normal, and yet there can already be an intracellular depletion of magnesium present. Thus, a normal serum magnesium may fail to identify intracellular magnesium depletion.

Neomycin & Vitamin Depletion

35. Jacobson ED, et al, "Depletion of Vitamin B_{12}, Iron, Beta-Carotene, and Fat Malabsorptive Effects of Neomycin in Commonly Used Doses," *JAMA*, 1961, 175:187-190.

These authors report that the oral administration of large doses of neomycin produce symptoms such as diarrhea, fat malabsorption, and interference with the absorption of carotenoids, vitamin B_{12}, and iron. Smaller doses are qualitatively similar but less severe.

Neomycin & Vitamin A Depletion

36. Favaro RM, Silva HC, and Vannucchi H, "Bioavailability of Vitamin A in the Rat Following Ingestion of Neomycin Sulfate or Aluminium Hydroxide," *Int J Vitam Nutr Res*, 1994, 2: 98-103.

In a rat model, the bioavailability of vitamin A during neomycin therapy was investigated. Neomycin reduced the bioavailability by 13.9% in one assay and by 13.5% in a second assay.

37. Barrowman JA, Broomhall J, Cannon AM, et al, "Impairment of Vitamin A Absorption by Neomycin," *Clin Sci*, 1972, 42(4):17P.

No abstract available

ETHAMBUTOL

Ethambutol & Zinc and Copper Depletion

38. Solecki TJ, Aviv A, and Bogden, "Effect of a Chelating Drug on Balance and Tissue Distribution of Four Essential Metals," *Toxicology*, 1984, 31(304):207-16.

In this investigation conducted in rats, ethambutol produced significant decreases in heart copper, kidney zinc, plasma zinc, and liver copper and zinc. These were not due to reduced food intake. These results support the hypothesis that chelating drugs such as ethambutol may alter trace metal metabolism.

ANTIBIOTICS *(Continued)*

ISONIAZID

Isoniazid & Vitamin B₆ Depletion

39. Matsui MS and Rozovski SJ, "Drug-Nutrient Interaction," *Clin Ther*, 1982, 4(6):423-40.

    In this review, antituberculotic drugs such as INH and cycloserine, which interfere with vitamin B_6 metabolism, are noted to produce a secondary niacin deficiency.

40. Pellock JM, Howell J, Kendig El Jr, et al, "Pyridoxine Deficiency in Children Treated With Isoniazid," *Chest*, 1985, 87(5):658-61.

    Using a biologic assay, pyridoxine status was determined in children after 2-18 months of therapy with isoniazid. Although deficiency is normally regarded as rare in children, five patients (13%) were noted to be deficient. Children receiving isoniazid dosages >10 mg/kg/day had a higher incidence of deficiency. The authors note that recommendations for withholding pyridoxine prophylaxis in children receiving isoniazid should be re-evaluated. This risk is increased in children who are debilitated or have a poor nutritional history prior to therapy.

41. Snider DE Jr, "Pyridoxine Supplementation During Isoniazid Therapy," *Tubercle*, 1980, 61(4):191-6.

    In this review, the need for vitamin B_6 (pyridoxine) supplementation during isoniazid (INH) therapy to prevent the development of peripheral neuropathy is discussed. Routine prophylactic use of pyridoxine supplementation is recommended.

Isoniazid & Pyridoxine Depletion - Negative Studies

42. Nisar M, Watkin SW, Bucknall RC, et al, "Exacerbation of Isoniazid Induced Peripheral Neuropathy by Pyridoxine," *Thorax*, 1990, 45(5):419-20.

    Report of a patient noted to demonstrate subjective deterioration in peripheral neuropathy following withdrawal of isoniazid and pyridoxine supplementation is presented. The authors note improvement occurred only after pyridoxine withdrawal. In the authors' opinion, this case illustrates the need for caution in the use of this vitamin for the prevention and treatment of peripheral neuropathy.

Isoniazid & Niacin Depletion

43. Matsui MS and Rozovski SJ, "Drug-Nutrient Interaction," *Clin Ther*, 1982, 4(6):423-40.

    In this review, antituberculotic drugs such as INH and cycloserine, which interfere with vitamin B_6 metabolism, are noted to produce a secondary niacin deficiency.

Isoniazid & Niacin Depletion - No Negative Studies

Isoniazid & Vitamin D Depletion

44. Toppet M, Vanisel M, Vertongen F, et al, "Sequential Development of Vitamin D Metabolites Under Isoniazid and Rifampicin Therapy," *Arch Fr Pediatr*, 1988, 45(2):145-8.

    Biochemical evidence of a disturbance of vitamin D metabolism in a pediatric population receiving isoniazid is reported. The authors advocate biochemical supervision, even in the absence of clinical symptoms.

45. Brodie MJ, Boobis AR, Hillyard CJ, et al, "Effect of Isoniazid on Vitamin D Metabolism and Hepatic Monooxygenase Activity," *Clin Pharmacol Ther*, 1981, 30(3):363-7.

    In eight healthy subjects, the effects of isoniazid on a number of metabolic parameters was evaluated. Calcium and phosphate levels were noted to decline. The concentration of alpha-,25-dihydroxyvitamin D, the most active metabolite of vitamin D, fell by 47% after the initial dose and was reduced throughout the study. Levels of 25-hydroxyvitamin D, the major circulating form of the vitamin, also declined in all subjects. Isoniazid-inhibited hepatic mixed-function oxidase activity, measured by antipyrine and cortisol oxidation, was reduced. The authors note that a similar inhibition of hepatic 25-hydroxylase and renal 1-alpha-hydroylase would explain the observed reduction in vitamin D metabolites.

46. D'Erasmo E, Ragno A, Raejntroph N, et al, "Drug-induced Osteomalacia," *Recenti Prog Med*, 1998, 89(10):529-33.

    In this review, drugs which are commonly associated with osteomalacia are discussed. Associated medications include cholestyramine, phenytoin, phenobarbital, isoniazid, aluminum-containing antacids, ferric oxide lead, bisphosphonates, fluoride, ammonium, and rifampicin. Pathophysiologic mechanisms related to drug-induced osteomalacia are discussed, including vitamin D metabolism, phosphorus homeostasis, and bone mineralization.

47. Bengoa JM, Bolt MJ, and Rosenberg IH, "Hepatic Vitamin D 25-Hydroxylase Inhibition by Cimetidine and Isoniazid," *J Lab Clin Med*, 1984, 104(4):546-52.

    This *in vitro* study evaluated the effect of cimetidine and isoniazid on hepatic vitamin D 25-hydroxylase activity. Whole liver homogenates from rats deficient in vitamin D were used. Cimetidine and isoniazid both inhibited *in vitro* vitamin D 25-hydroxylase activity. The authors conclude that the long-term effect of cimetidine on vitamin D metabolism warrants further investigation.

Isoniazid & Vitamin D Depletion - Negative Studies

48. Williams SE, Wardman AG, Taylor GA, et al, "Long Term Study of the Effect of Rifampicin and Isoniazid on Vitamin D Metabolism," *Tubercle*, 1985, 66(1):49-54.

    In this long-term study of eight patients, no significant change in either 1,25(OH)2D or 25 OH D occurred during the study. The authors conclude that the combined effects of these drugs are not likely to cause clinically significant derangement of vitamin D metabolism over a 9-month treatment period.

PENICILLINS

Penicillins (Penicillin, Ampicillin, Carbenicillin, Oxacillin, Amoxicillin, Ticarcillin, Nafcillin, Cloxacillin) & Potassium Depletion

49. Gill MA, DuBe JE, and Young WW, "Hypokalemic, Metabolic Alkalosis Induced by High-Dose Ampicillin Sodium," *Am J Hosp Pharm*, 1977, 34(5):528-31.

    High-dose, intravenous ampicillin was reported to be the cause of hypokalemic metabolic alkalosis in this case report. Possible mechanisms of antibiotic-induced hypokalemic metabolic alkalosis are discussed.

50. Morck HI and Linde J, "Hypokalemia During Carbenicillin Treatment," *Ugeskr Laeger*, 1980, 142(11):702-3.

    No abstract available.

ANTIBIOTICS *(Continued)*

51. Lipner HI, Ruzany F, Dasgupta M, et al, "The Behavior of Carbenicillin as a Nonreabsorbable Anion," *J Lab Clin Med*, 1975, 86(2):183-94.

    Renal clearance experiments were conducted in rats to determine the mechanism of hypokalemic alkalosis observed in some patients receiving carbenicillin. In addition, observations on electrical changes in isolated toad bladders were studied. The observations in both the rat and toad bladder experiments were consistent with the activity of an anion which is not reabsorbed in the nephron. Hypokalemic alkalosis may be the result of increased electrical negativity of the distal nephron, and subsequent increases in potassium and hydrogen ion excretion.

52. Klastersky J, Vanderklen B, Daneau D, et al, "Carbenicillin and Hypokalemia," *Ann Intern Med*, 1973, 78(5):774-5.

    No abstract available.

53. Garcia Diaz B, Plaza S, Garcia Benayas E, et al, "Hypopotassemia Caused by Cloxacillin: A New Case," *Rev Clin Esp*, 1997, 197(11):792-3.

    No abstract available.

54. Schlaeffer F, "Oxacillin-Associated Hypokalemia," *Drug Intell Clin Pharm*, 1988, 22(9):695-6.

    The authors report a case in which a patient treated with high-dose oxacillin developed severe hypokalemia. It is noted that this is a rare phenomenon, and although ureidopenicillins have been previously associated with hypokalemia, this case represents the first report in association with oxacillin.

55. Nanji AA and Lindsay J, "Ticarcillin Associated Hypokalemia," *Clin Biochem*, 1982, 15(2):118-9.

    The degree and frequency of ticarcillin-associated hypokalemia was evaluated in 16 patients. Frequency correlated to dosage, with four patients receiving <10 grams of ticarcillin failing to demonstrate this abnormality, while 6 of 9 patients receiving >18 grams per day had significant hypokalemia. Mean urinary potassium was elevated in the high-dose group. Degree of hypokalemia correlated with volume status.

56. Mohr JA, Clark RM, Waack TM, et al, "Nafcillin-Associated Hypokalemia," *JAMA*, 1979, 242(6):544.

    No abstract available.

57. Stapleton FB, Nelson B, Vats TS, et al, "Hypokalemia Associated With Antibiotic Treatment. Evidence in Children With Malignant Neoplasms," *Am J Dis Child*, 1976, 130(10):1104-8.

    In a review of 33 children with malignant neoplasms, it was found that 24 of 48 antibiotic courses were associated with hypokalemia. These cases could not be explained by gastrointestinal fluid losses. Combination therapy with carbenicillin, gentamicin, and methicillin or nafcillin was associated with hypokalemia in 23 of 35 courses. No correlation between hypokalemia and the stage of disease or antineoplastic agents was identified. The authors propose carbenicillin as a cause, speculating that it produces hypokalemia through its activity as a non-absorbed anion within the renal tubule. Frequent monitoring of electrolytes is recommended in children.

PENTAMIDINE

Pentamidine & Magnesium Depletion

58. al-Ghamdi SM, Cameron EC, and Sutton RA, "Magnesium Deficiency: Pathophysiologic and Clinical Overview," *Am J Kidney Dis*, 1994, 24(5):737-52.

   This article reviews the causes and consequences of magnesium deficiency. It is noted that hypomagnesemia may arise from various disorders of the gastrointestinal tract, conditions affecting renal magnesium excretion, or cellular redistribution of magnesium. Drugs which cause renal magnesium wasting are noted to include loop and thiazide diuretics, aminoglycosides, cisplatin, pentamidine, and foscarnet.

RIFAMPICIN

Rifampicin & Vitamin D Depletion

59. Brodie MJ, Boobis AR, Dollery CT, et al, "Rifampicin and Vitamin D Metabolism," *Clin Pharmacol Ther*, 1980, 27(6):810-4

   In eight male subjects, a 2-week course of oral rifampicin resulted in a consistent fall in plasma 25-hydroxycholecalciferol levels. Decreases were approximately 70%. The authors conclude that the fall in 25-hydroxychole-calciferol may represent evidence of possible drug-induced osteomalacia.

60. D'Erasmo E, Ragno A, Raejntroph N, et al, "Drug-induced Osteomalacia," *Recenti Prog Med*, 1998, 89(10):529-33.

   In this review, drugs which are commonly associated with osteomalacia are discussed. Associated medications include cholestyramine, phenytoin, phenobarbital, isoniazid, aluminum-containing antacids, ferric oxide lead, bisphosphonates, fluoride, ammonium, and rifampicin. Pathophysiologic mechanisms related to drug-induced osteomalacia are discussed, including vitamin D metabolism, phosphorus homeostasis, and bone mineralization.

Rifampicin & Vitamin D Depletion - Negative Studies

61. Williams SE, Wardman AG, Taylor GA, et al, "Long-term Study of the Effect of Rifampicin and Isoniazid on Vitamin D Metabolism," *Tubercle*, 1985, 66(1):49-54.

   In this long-term study of eight patients, no significant change in either 1,25(OH)2D or 25 OH D occurred during the study. The authors conclude that the combined effects of these drugs are not likely to cause clinically significant derangement of vitamin D metabolism over a 9-month treatment period.

TETRACYCLINES

Tetracyclines & Calcium Depletion

62. Lambs I, Brion M, and Berthon G, "Metal Ion-Tetracycline Interactions in Biological Fluids. Part 3. Formation of Mixed-Metal Ternary Complexes of Tetracycline, Oxytetracycline, Doxycycline and Minocycline With Calcium and Magnesium, and Their Involvement in the Bioavailability of These Antibiotics in Blood Plasma," *Agents Actions*, 1984, 14(5-6):743-50.

   Tetracycline compounds which form mixed-metal chelates are investigated. Specific complexes include magnesium and calcium. The impact on bioavailability of tetracyclines is discussed.

ANTIBIOTICS *(Continued)*

63. Neuvonen PJ, "Interactions With the Absorption of Tetracyclines," *Drugs*, 1976, 11(1):45-54.

   Tetracyclines are noted to have a potential to form chelates with multivalent cations including iron, aluminum, magnesium, and calcium. The impact on bioavailability of tetracyclines is discussed. Milk and other dairy products are noted to lead to a potentially significant decrease in bioavailability.

64. Jung H, Peregrina AA, Rodriguez JM, et al, "The Influence of Coffee With Milk and Tea on the Bioavailability of Tetracycline," *Biopharm Drug Dispos*, 1997, 18(5):459-63.

   The addition of milk to tea or coffee demonstrated a significant impact on absorption of tetracycline. The authors suggest care in administration of tetracyclines to avoid concurrent calcium.

65. Hurwitz S, "On the Inhibition of Tetracycline Absorption of Dietary Calcium," *Poult Sci*, 1970, 49(5):1183-7.

   No abstract available

Tetracyclines & Calcium Depletion - No Negative Studies

Tetracyclines & Iron Depletion

66. Neuvonen PJ, "Interactions With the Absorption of Tetracyclines," *Drugs*, 1976, 11(1):45-54.

   Tetracyclines are noted to have a potential to form chelates with multivalent cations, including iron, aluminum, magnesium, and calcium. The impact on bioavailability of tetracyclines is discussed. Milk and other dairy products are noted to lead to a potentially significant decrease in bioavailability.

Tetracyclines & Magnesium Depletion

67. Berthon G, Brion M, and Lambs L, "Metal Ion-Tetracycline Interactions in Biological Fluids. Part 2. Potentiometric Study of Magnesium Complexes With Tetracycline, Oxytetracycline, Doxycycline, and Minocycline, and Discussion of Their Possible Influence on the Bioavailability of These Antibiotics in Blood Plasma," *J Inorg Biochem*, 1983, 19(1):1-18.

   The complexes formed between magnesium and four tetracycline derivatives were investigated. The impact on bioavailability of tetracyclines is discussed.

68. Neuvonen PJ, "Interactions With the Absorption of Tetracyclines," *Drugs*, 1976, 11(1):45-54.

   Tetracyclines are noted to have a potential to form chelates with multivalent cations, including iron, aluminum, magnesium and calcium. The impact on bioavailability of tetracyclines is discussed. Milk and other dairy products are noted to lead to a potentially significant decrease in bioavailability.

TRIMETHOPRIM

Trimethoprim & Folic Acid Depletion

69. Kahn SB, Fein SA, and Brodsky I, "Effects of Trimethoprim on Folate Metabolism in Man," *Clin Pharmacol Ther*, 1968, 9(5):550-60.

   These authors report a mild folate deficiency may develop in humans after long-term or high-dose therapy with trimethoprim.

70. Schulz R, "Inhibition of Rat Folic Acid Reductase Activity by Trimethoprim During the Later Stages of Gestation," *Naunyn Schmiedebergs Arch Pharmacol*, 1973, 278(2):227-30.

   No abstract available

Trimethoprim & Folic Acid Depletion - Negative Studies

71. Pelliniemi TT, Junnila SY and Kasanen A, "Trimethoprim Does Not Cause Folic Acid Deficiency," *Duodecim*, 1984, 100(23-24):1618-23.

   No abstract available

ANTICONVULSANTS

Anticonvulsants & Folic Acid Depletion

72. Leary PM, "Folate Studies in Underprivileged Children With Epilepsy," *S Afr Med J*, 1973, 47(46):2245-6.

   A significantly lower level of serum folate was demonstrated when comparison was made with other children in the community. The study reports that all of these children were being treated with anticonvulsants: 30 were taking Pb; 3 were taking phenytoin; 3 were being treated with primidone; and 2 were taking a combination of Pb and phenytoin. Levels of serum folate were found to significantly lower in the epileptic group compared to controls (P = 0.0005).

BARBITURATES

Barbiturates & Calcium Depletion

73. Foss MC, Meneghelli UG, and Tabosa Verissimo IM, "The Effect of the Anticonvulsants Phenobarbital and Diphenylhydantoin on Intestinal Absorption of Calcium," *Acta Physiol Lat Am*, 1979, 29(4-5):223-8.

   In a rat model, phenobarbital and diphenylhydantoin produced an increase in fecal excretion of calcium and a decrease of intestinal absorption of calcium. Both effects were more intense in rats treated with phenobarbital. This suggests that anticonvulsant drugs affect the intestinal active transport of calcium.

74. Young RE, Ramsay LE, and Murray TS, "Barbiturates and Serum Calcium in the Elderly," *Postgrad Med J*, 1977, 53(618):212-5.

   In a retrospective biochemical survey of people aged 65 and over, subjects taking a barbiturate preparation for indications other than epilepsy had a significantly lower serum calcium concentration than did those taking two types of benzodiazepines. The authors concluded that ordinary doses of barbiturates may adversely affect vitamin D metabolism in the elderly.

75. Gough H, Goggin T, Bissessar A, et al, "A Comparative Study of the Relative Influence of Different Anticonvulsant Drugs, UV Exposure and Diet on Vitamin D and Calcium Metabolism in Out-Patients With Epilepsy," *Q J Med*, 1986, 59(230):569-77.

   Biochemical parameters associated with calcium and vitamin D metabolism were assessed in 226 outpatients with epilepsy. Patients were grouped depending on drug treatment; monotherapy with either carbamazepine, phenytoin, phenobarbitone or sodium valproate, and combinations of these drugs as polytherapy. Hypocalcemia was more severe in the phenobarbitone monotherapy group than the carbamazepine or phenytoin groups. No patient on sodium valproate monotherapy had subnormal levels of calcium. The carbamazepine, phenytoin, and phenobarbitone groups were found to have reduced 25-hydroxy vitamin D levels, with no reduction in the sodium valproate group. The most severe alterations occurred in the polytherapy group. This study confirms biochemical evidence for anticonvulsant osteomalacia when enzyme-inducing anticonvulsants are used, with the degree of severity depending on the drug regimen.

Barbiturates & Calcium Depletion - No Negative Studies

Barbiturates & Folic Acid Depletion

76. Kishi T, Fujita N, Eguchi T, et al, "Mechanism for Reduction of Serum Folate by Antiepileptic Drugs During Prolonged Therapy," *J Neurol Sci*, 1997, 145(1):109-12.

    Serum folate concentrations were measured in age-matched control subjects and in epileptic outpatients treated with a single antiepileptic drug. Two of the four drugs being administered were enzyme inducers. Compared with controls, mean serum folate levels were reduced significantly in patients treated with phenobarbitone and carbamazepine. In contrast, folate levels in patients treated with the non-enzyme-inducer valproate did not differ significantly from controls. These data suggest the induction of microsomal liver enzymes may be critical to depletion of folate by antiepileptic drugs.

77. Formiggini G, Bovina C, Marchi-Marchetti M, et al, "Pteroylpolyglutamates in Liver of Phenobarbitone-Treated Rats," *Int J Vitam Nutr Res*, 1983, 53(4):390-3.

    In a rat model, the administration of two doses of phenobarbitone caused a severe depletion in the folate pool, free folate, and percentage of longer-chain polyglutamates, while protein-bound folates were unchanged. Possible mechanisms by which phenobarbitone might interfere with the synthesis of coenzymic forms of folic acid are discussed.

78. Formiggini G, Bovina C, Marchi-Marchetti M, et al, "Effect of Phenobarbitone on Folic Acid Metabolism in the Rat," *Pharmacol Res Commun*, 1984, 16(5):467-78.

    In a rat model, phenobarbitone demonstrated strong interference with folic acid metabolism, particularly with hepatic pteroylpolyglutamate synthesis.

79. Reynolds EH and Trimble MR, "Adverse Neuropsychiatric Effects of Anticonvulsant Drugs," *Drugs*, 1985, 29(6):570-81.

    Peripheral neuropathy may result from long-term treatment or prolonged toxic exposure to phenytoin or barbiturates, especially in combination. In addition, all the major anticonvulsant drugs can produce occasional subacute cognitive or behavioral syndromes, especially in combination. Possible mechanisms are discussed, including metabolic disturbances involving folic acid, monoamines, or hormones, which may potentially result in neuronal damage.

Barbiturates & Folic Acid Depletion - No Negative Studies

Barbiturates & Vitamin D Depletion

80. Zerwekh JE, Homan R, Tindall R, et al, "Decreased Serum 24,25-Dihydroxyvitamin D Concentration During Long-Term Anticonvulsant Therapy in Adult Epileptics," *Ann Neurol*, 1982, 12(2):184-6.

    Serum concentrations of 25-hydroxyvitamin D (25-OHD), 24,25-dihydroxyvitamin D [24,25-(OH)2D], and 1α, 25-dihydroxyvitamin D [1,25-(OH)2D] were measured in 30 ambulatory adult epileptic patients. All were receiving long-term anticonvulsant treatment with phenytoin, phenobarbital, or carbamazepine. The drugs appear to exert different effects on vitamin D metabolism. All three caused a significant reduction of serum 24,25-(OH)2D concentrations. A significant decrease in serum 25-OHD was observed only for the phenobarbital-treated patients. A deficiency of 24,25-(OH)2D may

ANTICONVULSANTS *(Continued)*

play an important role in the development of anticonvulsant-induced osteo-malacia.

81. Baran DT, "Effect of Phenobarbital Treatment on Metabolism of Vitamin D by Rat Liver," *Am J Physiol*, 1983, 245(1):E55-9.

The effect of phenobarbital on hepatic vitamin D metabolism was investigated using a hepatic perfusion system in rats. Intraperitoneal phenobarbital (75 mg/kg/day) administered to D-replete rats increased circulating 25(OH)D blood levels after 4 weeks, but levels after 6 and 8 weeks were decreased. Although total production was unaffected, efficiency of production was decreased after 8 weeks of phenobarbital treatment, and the release of 25(OH)D was inhibited after both 4 and 8 weeks of treatment. The author proposes that chronic phenobarbital therapy decreases both the release of [3H]25(OH)D from the liver and the efficiency of hepatic [3H]25(OH)D production. Phenobarbital-induced inhibition of 25(OH)D release from the liver may be another mechanism for low 25(OH)D levels noted in humans after long-term phenobarbital therapy.

82. Liakakos D, Papadopoulos Z, Vlachos P, et al, "Serum Alkaline Phosphatase and Urinary Hydroxyproline Values in Children Receiving Phenobarbital With and Without Vitamin D," *J Pediatr*, 1975, 87(2):291-6.

The effect of phenobarbital on concentrations of serum alkaline phosphatase and total urinary hydroxyproline was measured in 36 children to study the development of rickets in patients receiving prolonged anticonvulsive therapy. The results are believed to support the concept that phenobarbital administration is implicated in the development of rickets. The need for simultaneous daily administration of supplements of vitamin D in subjects receiving anticonvulsive drugs is stressed.

83. Hathcock JN, "Metabolic Mechanisms of Drug-Nutrient Interactions," *Fed Proc*, 1985, 44(1 Pt 1):124-9.

This review discusses the metabolic mechanisms of nutrition and drug interactions, including the effects of diet on drug metabolism and action, and the effects of drugs on nutritional processes. Phenobarbital and other anticonvulsants are inducers of cytochrome P-450 and the mixed-function oxidase system. Long-term treatment with these inducers can cause excessive metabolism and deficiency of vitamin D. The range of metabolic interactions of drugs and nutrients includes the full scope of physiological processes to which drugs and nutrients are subject.

84. Chung S and Ahn C, "Effects of Anti-Epileptic Drug Therapy on Bone Mineral Density in Ambulatory Epileptic Children," *Brain Dev*, 1994, 16(5):382-5.

In an effort to determine the effect of long-term antiepileptic drug (AED) therapy, 78 epileptic children and 78 control subjects were scanned to determine bone mineral densities (BMDs) of the arms, legs, ribs, pelvis, spine, and the whole body. There were significant differences in the rib and spine BMDs in patients receiving anticonvulsants for 24 months or more. The authors propose that the measurement of BMDs in the ribs and spine is necessary for the early detection of subtle bone loss, and it is recommended that vitamin D be administered to children with epilepsy receiving AEDs over 24 months.

85. Gough H, Goggin T, Bissessar A, Baker M, et al, "A Comparative Study of the Relative Influence of Different Anticonvulsant Drugs, UV Exposure and

Diet on Vitamin D and Calcium Metabolism in Outpatients With Epilepsy," *Q J Med*, 1986, 59(230):569-77.

Biochemical parameters associated with calcium and vitamin D metabolism were assessed in 226 outpatients with epilepsy. Patients were grouped depending on drug treatment; monotherapy with either carbamazepine, phenytoin, phenobarbitone or sodium valproate and combinations of these drugs as polytherapy. Hypocalcemia was more severe in the phenobarbitone monotherapy group than the carbamazepine or phenytoin groups. No patient on sodium valproate monotherapy had subnormal levels of calcium. The carbamazepine, phenytoin, and phenobarbitone groups were found to have reduced 25-hydroxy vitamin D levels, with no reduction in the sodium valproate group. The most severe alterations occurred in the polytherapy group. This study confirms biochemical evidence for anticonvulsant osteomalacia when enzyme-inducing anticonvulsants are used, with the degree of severity depending on the drug regimen.

86. D'Erasmo E, Ragno A, Raejntroph N, et al, "Drug-induced Osteomalacia," *Recenti Prog Med*, 1998, 89(10):529-33.

In this review, drugs which are commonly associated with osteomalacia are discussed. Associated medications include cholestyramine, phenytoin, phenobarbital, isoniazid, aluminum-containing antacids, ferric oxide lead, bisphosphonates, fluoride, ammonium, and rifampicin. Pathophysiologic mechanisms related to drug-induced osteomalacia are discussed, including vitamin D metabolism, phosphorus homeostasis, and bone mineralization.

Barbiturates & Vitamin D Depletion - Negative Studies

87. Camfield CS, Delvin EE, Camfield PR, et al, "Normal Serum 25-Hydroxyvitamin D Levels in Phenobarbital-Treated Toddlers," *Dev Pharmacol Ther*, 1983, 6(3):157-61.

Serum 25-hydroxyvitamin D (25-OHD) levels were measured in 74 children treated after a single febrile seizure in a randomized, double-blind fashion with either phenobarbital or placebo. Phenobarbital treatment had no effect over a 5- to 12-month period on the 25-OHD levels. However, vitamin D supplementation in both groups significantly increased the serum 25-OHD concentration.

88. Stoffer SS, Zaka-Ur-Rahman, Meier DA, et al, "Prompt Resolution of Osteomalacia by Switching From Phenytoin to Phenobarbital," *Arch Intern Med*, 1980, 140(6):852.

In a phenytoin-treated patient with osteomalacia, switching the drug regimen to phenobarbital led to prompt resolution of her symptoms, along with restoration of normal serum calcium and 25-hydroxyvitamin D levels. The authors suggest that a change in therapy may obviate the need for supplemental vitamin D and calcium administration.

Barbiturates & Biotin Depletion

89. Mock DM, Mock NI, Nelson RP, et al, "Disturbances in Biotin Metabolism in Children Undergoing Long-Term Anticonvulsant Therapy," *J Pediatr Gastroenterol Nutr*, 1998, 26(3):245-50.

To determine whether biotin catabolism was accelerated in children receiving long-term treatment with certain anticonvulsants and to assess biotin status, seven children treated with carbamazepine and/or phenytoin and six treated with phenobarbital were evaluated. Sixteen healthy children receiving no

ANTICONVULSANTS *(Continued)*

anticonvulsants served as controls. Bisnorbiotin excretion was increased significantly in both groups receiving anticonvulsant medications. Biotin sulfoxide excretion was significantly increased in the carbamazepine/phenytoin group, but not in the phenobarbital group. 3-Hydroxyisovaleric acid excretion was increased significantly in the carbamazepine/phenytoin group. However, only one child (carbamazepine/phenytoin group) had decreased urinary excretion of biotin. These data are interpreted to suggest the long-term administration of some anticonvulsants can accelerate biotin catabolism.

90. Krause KH, Bonjour JP, Berlit P, et al, "Biotin Status of Epileptics," *Ann N Y Acad Sci*, 1985, 447:297-313.

Plasma biotin levels in 404 epileptics under long-term treatment with anticonvulsants were markedly lower than in 112 controls. Epileptics treated with valproate sodium in monotherapy showed considerably higher biotin levels than epileptics with monotherapy of primidone, carbamazepine, phenytoin, or phenobarbital. Four epileptics treated with anticonvulsants had increased urinary excretion of organic acids, as found in patients with deficiency of biotin-dependent carboxylases. In 37 epileptics who had measurements of plasma lactate concentrations, a higher mean concentration was noted. The authors propose the lowering of biotin in epileptics is caused by intake of anticonvulsants, and has a biochemical effect in these patients which could be a factor in the mode of action of anticonvulsants.

91. Krause KH, Kochen W, Berlit P, et al, "Excretion of Organic Acids Associated With Biotin Deficiency in Chronic Anticonvulsant Therapy," *Int J Vitam Nutr Res*, 1984, 54(2-3):217-22.

Urinary organic acids were determined in 7 patients with epilepsy receiving long-term therapy with anticonvulsants and in 3 control subjects. These acids are known to be elevated in children with biotin deficiency. A total of 4 patients (each receiving phenytoin, primidone, phenobarbital, or carbamazepine as monotherapy or in combination) had reduced plasma biotin levels and an elevated excretion of organic acids. The authors speculate that decreased activity of propionyl CoA carboxylase (3-OH-propionate, methylcitrate) and 3-methylcrotonyl CoA carboxylase (3-methylcrotonate and the glycine conjugate, 3-OH-isovalerate) are involved. In contrast, two patients receiving sodium valproate alone had normal circulating biotin levels and no change in urinary acid excretion.

Barbiturates & Biotin Depletion - No Negative Studies

Barbituates & Vitamin K Depletion

92. Keith DA, Gundberg CM, Japour A, et al, "Vitamin K-Dependent Proteins and Anticonvulsant Medication," *Clin Pharmacol Ther*, 1983, 34(4):529-32.

Interference with vitamin K metabolism, as indicated by a raised serum osteocalcin level, is associated with certain anticonvulsant drugs (particularly phenobarbital and phenytoin). This finding is believed to be of importance in the pathogenesis of side effects of these medications.

CARBAMAZEPINE

Carbamazepine & Biotin Depletion

93. Said HM, Redha R, and Nylander W, "Biotin Transport in the Human Intestine: Inhibition by Anticonvulsant Drugs," *Am J Clin Nutr*, 1989, 49(1):127-31.

The effect of the anticonvulsant drugs carbamazepine and primidone on the transport of biotin in human intestine was examined *in vitro*. Results indicate that carbamazepine and primidone are competitive inhibitors of biotin transport in human intestine. The inhibitory effect is localized to the substrate transport system of the brush border membrane. The authors conclude impairment of biotin status may occur in patients receiving anticonvulsant agents for long periods.

94. Krause KH, Bonjour JP, Berlit P, et al, "Biotin Status of Epileptics," *Ann N Y Acad Sci*, 1985, 447:297-313.

Plasma biotin levels in 404 epileptics under long-term treatment with anticonvulsants were markedly lower than in 112 controls. Epileptics treated with valproate sodium in monotherapy showed considerably higher biotin levels than epileptics with monotherapy of primidone (PRM), carbamazepine (CBZ), phenytoin (PHT), or phenobarbital (PB). Four epileptics treated with PHT, PB, PRM, or CBZ had increased urinary excretion of organic acids, as found in patients with a deficiency of biotin-dependent carboxylases. In 37 epileptics who had measurements of plasma lactate concentrations, a higher mean concentration was noted. The authors conclude a lowering of biotin in epileptics is caused by intake of anticonvulsants and has a biochemical effect in these patients, and could be a factor in the mode of action of anticonvulsants.

95. Krause KH, Berlit P, and Bonjour JP, "Impaired Biotin Status in Anticonvulsant Therapy," *Ann Neurol*, 1982, 12(5):485-6.

In 264 epileptics undergoing long-term therapy with anticonvulsants, reduced plasma biotin levels were found compared with a normal control group. Mean plasma biotin levels in patients treated with valproate were higher than those in patients treated with phenytoin, primidone, or carbamazepine. The observed reduction in biotin levels is proposed to contribute to the efficacy of these three anticonvulsants.

96. Mock DM, Mock NI, Nelson RP, et al, "Disturbances in Biotin Metabolism in Children Undergoing Long-Term Anticonvulsant Therapy," *J Pediatr Gastroenterol Nutr*, 1998, 26(3):245-50.

To determine whether biotin catabolism was accelerated in children receiving long-term treatment with certain anticonvulsants and to assess biotin status, seven children treated with carbamazepine and/or phenytoin and six treated with phenobarbital were evaluated. Sixteen healthy children receiving no anticonvulsants served as controls. Bisnorbiotin excretion was increased significantly in both groups receiving anticonvulsant medications. Biotin sulfoxide excretion was significantly increased in the carbamazepine/phenytoin group, but not in the phenobarbital group. 3-Hydroxyisovaleric acid excretion was increased significantly in the carbamazepine/phenytoin group. However, only one child (carbamazepine/phenytoin group) had decreased urinary excretion of biotin. These data are interpreted to suggest the long-term administration of some anticonvulsants can accelerate biotin catabolism.

Carbamazepine & Biotin Depletion - No Negative Studies

Carbamazepine & Folic Acid Depletion

97. Kishi T, Fujita N, Eguchi T, et al, "Mechanism for Reduction of Serum Folate by Antiepileptic Drugs During Prolonged Therapy," *J Neurol Sci*, 1997, 145(1):109-12.

Serum folate concentrations were measured in age-matched control subjects and in epileptic outpatients treated with a single antiepileptic drug. Two of the

ANTICONVULSANTS *(Continued)*

four drugs being administered were enzyme inducers. Compared with serum folate levels in controls, mean serum folate levels were reduced significantly in patients treated with phenobarbitone and carbamazepine. In contrast, folate levels in patients treated with the non-enzyme-inducer valproate did not differ significantly from controls. The authors conclude that the induction of microsomal liver enzymes may be critical to the depletion of folate by antiepileptic drugs.

98. Froscher W, Maier V, Laage M, et al, "Folate Deficiency, Anticonvulsant Drugs, and Psychiatric Morbidity," *Clin Neuropharmacol*, 1995, 18(2):165-82.

Serum and erythrocyte folic acid levels were determined in 100 epileptic patients and 100 controls. Folic acid levels were significantly lower in the epileptic patients than in controls. In patients who took carbamazepine, folic acid serum and erythrocyte concentrations were significantly lower than in the group who took phenytoin. Supplementation with 5 mg folinic acid in four patients with folic acid deficiency demonstrated an improvement in some measurements of cognitive performance.

99. Goggin T, Gough H, Bissessar A, et al, "A Comparative Study of the Relative Effects of Anticonvulsant Drugs and Dietary Folate on the Red Cell Folate Status of Patients With Epilepsy," *Q J Med*, 1987, 65(247):911-9.

In a survey of 200 epileptic patients, median red cell folate levels were reduced significantly in patients treated with phenytoin or carbamazepine monotherapy, as compared to a control population. Patients taking more than one drug also had reduced levels. However, in patients treated with sodium valproate alone there was no significant decrease in red cell folate levels compared to controls. A significant correlation between red cell folate levels and dietary folate was not established. Significant negative relationships were established between carbamazepine dose or serum level and red cell folate level. The correlation between dose or serum level of phenytoin and red cell folate level was also negative, but did not reach statistical significance.

100. Isojarvi JI, Pakarinen AJ, and Myllyla VV, "Basic Haematological Parameters, Serum Gamma-glutamyl-transferase Activity, and Erythrocyte Folate and Serum Vitamin B_{12} Levels During Carbamazepine and Oxcarbazepine Therapy," *Seizure*, 1997, 6(3):207-11.

A prospective 5-year study of 25 patients with newly diagnosed epilepsy demonstrated that the mean white blood cell count and red blood cell count decreased after 2 months and remained low over the remaining 5 years. Mean erythrocyte volume and serum GGT activity increased progressively during carbamazepine treatment. Parameters normalized after replacing carbamazepine with oxcarbazepine. These data indicate the hematologic changes during carbamazepine medication are possibly related to changes in folate and vitamin B_{12} metabolism.

101. Hendel J, Dam M, Gram L, et al, "The Effects of Carbamazepine and Valproate on Folate Metabolism in Man," *Acta Neurol Scand*, 1984, 69(4):226-31.

The effect of carbamazepine and valproate treatment on folate metabolism was studied in 11 epileptic patients. After 2 months' treatment, the AUC for folic acid was decreased and time of maximal plasma concentration was significantly delayed. Inhibition of intestinal folate deconjugation was not observed, and hepatic metabolism of folic acid was not found to be affected by treatment. The authors concluded an inhibition of intestinal folic acid absorption may be caused by these antiepileptic agents.

102. Traccis S, Monaco F, Sechi GP, et al, "Long-term Therapy With Carbamazepine: Effects on Nerve Conduction Velocity," *Eur Neurol*, 1983, 22(6):410-6.

Electrophysiological data indicated a mild progressive reduction of both motor and sensory conduction velocity in 30 patients receiving long-term treatment with carbamazepine. The degree of nerve function impairment was associated with the duration of therapy. Folic acid levels were below normal in approximately 50% of the subjects. Folate deficiency is proposed to play some role in the development of peripheral nerve dysfunction in carbamazepine-treated patients.

103. Reynolds EH and Trimble MR, "Adverse Neuropsychiatric Effects of Anticonvulsant Drugs," *Drugs*, 1985, 29(6):570-81.

In this review, peripheral neuropathy is noted to potentially result from long-term treatment or prolonged toxic exposure to phenytoin or barbiturates, especially in combination. In addition, all the major anticonvulsant drugs can produce occasional subacute cognitive or behavioral syndromes, especially in combination. Possible mechanisms include metabolic disturbances of folic acid, monoamines, or hormones, potentially resulting in neuronal damage.

Carbamazepine & Folic Acid - Negative Studies

104. Tomson T, Lindbom U, Sundqvist A, et al, "Red Cell Folate Levels in Pregnant Epileptic Women," *Eur J Clin Pharmacol*, 1995, 48(3-4):305-8.

In a prospective study, red cell folate concentrations were determined in 74 epileptic women in early pregnancy. All patients were treated continuously with antiepileptic drugs since before conception. Sixty-four of the patients were on monotherapy. The most frequently used drugs were carbamazepine (n=39) and phenytoin (n=26). Blood samples for red cell folate and antiepileptic drug concentrations were drawn before folate supplementation. Red cell folate levels in patients did not differ from those in nonepileptic, drug-free, pregnant women, or from those in non-pregnant age-matched healthy controls. No correlation was found between red cell folate concentrations and doses or plasma levels of phenytoin or carbamazepine.

Carbamazepine & Vitamin D Depletion

105. Zerwekh JE, Homan R, Tindall R, et al, "Decreased Serum 24,25-Dihydroxyvitamin D Concentration During Long-term Anticonvulsant Therapy in Adult Epileptics," *Ann Neurol*, 1982, 12(2):184-6.

Serum concentrations of 25-hydroxyvitamin D (25-OHD), 24,25-dihydroxyvitamin D [24,25-(OH)2D], and 1α, 25-dihydroxyvitamin D [1,25-(OH)2D] were measured in 30 ambulatory adult epileptic patients. All were receiving long-term anticonvulsant treatment with phenytoin, phenobarbital, or carbamazepine. The drugs appear to exert different effects on vitamin D metabolism. All three caused a significant reduction of serum 24,25-(OH)2D concentrations. A significant decrease in serum 25-OHD was observed only for the phenobarbital-treated patients. A deficiency of 24,25-(OH)2D is proposed to play an important role in the development of anticonvulsant-induced osteomalacia.

106. Hoikka V, Alhava EM, Karjalainen P, et al, "Carbamazepine and Bone Mineral Metabolism," *Acta Neurol Scand*, 1984, 70(2):77-80.

Bone mineral metabolism was studied in 21 epileptic patients receiving carbamazepine monotherapy as compared to a control population. Serum

ANTICONVULSANTS *(Continued)*

25-hydroxyvitamin D values were significantly lower in patients than in controls, but no statistically significant difference in bone mineral density was observed. Histomorphometric analysis did not reveal a statistically significant difference in the amount of trabecular bone or osteoid bone, but the patients had an increased amount of trabecular resorption surfaces. An increased amount of osteoid, suggesting histological osteomalacia, was found in 2 of the 18 biopsies. The authors conclude that epileptic patients receiving carbamazepine therapy may have vitamin D deficiency, potentially leading to the development of osteomalacic skeletal changes.

107. Rajantie J, Lamberg-Allardt C, and Wilska M, "Does Carbamazepine Treatment Lead to a Need of Extra Vitamin D in Some Mentally Retarded Children?" *Acta Paediatr Scand*, 1984, 73(3):325-8.

Biochemical parameters of vitamin D metabolism in 40 institutionalized mentally retarded patients were measured. Twenty were receiving carbamazepine monotherapy and 20 had no antiepileptic drugs. Patients receiving carbamazepine demonstrated significantly lower serum calcium and 25-hydroxyvitamin D. Alkaline phosphatase was significantly higher. Dietary supplementation with vitamin D in carbamazepine treated patients abolished the observed differences.

108. Gough H, Goggin T, Bissessar A, et al, "A Comparative Study of the Relative Influence of Different Anticonvulsant Drugs, UV Exposure and Diet on Vitamin D and Calcium Metabolism in Outpatients With Epilepsy," *Q J Med*, 1986, 59(230):569-77.

Biochemical parameters associated with calcium and vitamin D metabolism were assessed in 226 outpatients with epilepsy. Patients were grouped depending on drug treatment; monotherapy with either carbamazepine, phenytoin, phenobarbitone or sodium valproate, and combinations of these drugs as polytherapy. Hypocalcemia was more severe in the phenobarbitone monotherapy group than the carbamazepine or phenytoin groups. No patient on sodium valproate monotherapy had subnormal levels of calcium. Carbamazepine, phenytoin, and phenobarbitone groups were found to have reduced 25-hydroxy vitamin D levels, with no reduction in the sodium valproate group. The most severe alterations occurred in the polytherapy group. This study confirms biochemical evidence for anticonvulsant osteomalacia when enzyme-inducing anticonvulsants are used, with the degree of severity depending on the drug regimen.

109. Valimaki MJ, Tiihonen M, Laitinen K, et al, "Bone Mineral Density Measured by Dual-Energy X-Ray Absorptiometry and Novel Markers of Bone Formation and Resorption in Patients on Antiepileptic Drugs," *J Bone Miner Res*, 1994, 9(5):631-7.

A total of 38 epileptic patients (24 women and 14 men) who were using either carbamazepine or phenytoin, or both, were studied. Bone mineral density at the lumbar spine and three femoral sites was measured by dual-energy x-ray absorptiometry (DXA). Serum and urine markers of bone and mineral metabolism were also determined. In female patients on phenytoin, bone mineral density was reduced at the femoral neck and Ward's triangle. This value was similar to control levels at all four measurement sites in the other patient groups. Compared with controls, serum concentrations of 25-hydroxyvitamin D and 1,25-dihydroxyvitamin D were reduced in female patients. These changes were independent of the therapy used and were not noted in male patients. For both genders the serum levels of vitamin D binding protein were normal. Both female and male patients had hypocalcemia, but only women showed hypocalciuria.

Carbamazepine & Vitamin D Depletion - Negative Studies

110. Ala-Houhala M, Korpela R, Koivikko M, et al, "Long-term Anticonvulsant Therapy and Vitamin D Metabolism in Ambulatory Pubertal Children," *Neuropediatrics*, 1986, 17(4):212-6.

Parameters of calcium metabolism were evaluated in 28 adolescents receiving long-term anticonvulsant therapy and in 10 controls. Serum calcium, inorganic phosphorus, parathyroid hormone, and alkaline phosphatase levels did not differ from the control group. There was no correlation between anticonvulsant serum free fraction levels and vitamin D metabolites. Bone mineral content was not significantly decreased in the epileptic patients. Long-term anticonvulsant therapy did not induce 'anticonvulsant rickets' in this ambulatory adolescent population. These data do not indicate that anticonvulsant drugs alter vitamin D metabolism significantly. Thus, the authors conclude routine vitamin D supplementation is not indicated in children on anticonvulsant therapy.

111. Gough H, Goggin T, Bissessar A, et al, "A Comparative Study of the Relative Influence of Different Anticonvulsant Drugs, UV Exposure and Diet on Vitamin D and Calcium Metabolism in Out-Patients With Epilepsy," *Q J Med*, 1986, 59(230):569-77.

No abstract available.

PHENYTOIN

Phenytoin & Biotin Depletion

112. Mock DM, Mock NI, Nelson RP, et al, "Disturbances in Biotin Metabolism in Children Undergoing Long-Term Anticonvulsant Therapy," *J Pediatr Gastroenterol Nutr*, 1998, 26(3):245-50.

To determine whether biotin catabolism was accelerated in children receiving long-term treatment with certain anticonvulsants and to assess biotin status, seven children treated with carbamazepine and/or phenytoin and six treated with phenobarbital were evaluated. Sixteen healthy children receiving no anticonvulsants served as controls. Bisnorbiotin excretion was increased significantly in both groups receiving anticonvulsant medications. Biotin sulfoxide excretion was significantly increased in the carbamazepine/phenytoin group but not in the phenobarbital group. 3-Hydroxyisovaleric acid excretion was increased significantly in the carbamazepine/phenytoin group. However, only one child (carbamazepine/phenytoin group) had a decreased urinary excretion of biotin. The authors conclude that the long-term administration of some anticonvulsants can accelerate biotin catabolism.

113. Krause KH, Bonjour JP, Berlit P, et al, "Biotin Status of Epileptics," *Ann N Y Acad Sci*, 1985, 447:297-313.

Plasma biotin levels in 404 epileptics under long-term treatment with anticonvulsants were markedly lower than in 112 controls. Epileptics treated with valproate sodium monotherapy showed considerably higher biotin levels than epileptics with monotherapy of primidone (PRM), carbamazepine (CBZ), phenytoin (PHT) or phenobarbital (PB). Four epileptics treated with PHT, PB, PRM or CBZ had an increased urinary excretion of organic acids, as found in patients with a deficiency of biotin-dependent carboxylases. In 37 epileptics who had measurements of plasma lactate concentrations, a higher mean concentration was noted. The authors conclude a lowering of biotin in epileptics is caused by intake of anticonvulsants and has a biochemical

ANTICONVULSANTS *(Continued)*

effect in these patients which could contribute to the action of anticonvulsants.

114. Krause KH, Berlit P, and Bonjour JP, "Impaired Biotin Status in Anticonvulsant Therapy," *Ann Neurol*, 1982, 12(5):485-6.

In 264 epileptics undergoing long-term therapy with anticonvulsants, reduced plasma biotin levels were found compared with a normal control group. Mean plasma biotin levels in patients treated with valproate were higher than those in patients treated with phenytoin, primidone, or carbamazepine. The observed reduction in biotin levels is proposed to contribute to the efficacy of these three anticonvulsants.

Phenytoin & Biotin Depletion - No Negative Studies

Phenytoin & Calcium Depletion

115. Shafer RB and Nuttall FQ, "Calcium and Folic Acid Absorption in Patients Taking Anticonvulsant Drugs," *J Clin Endocrinol Metab*, 1975, 41(06):1125-9.

Calcium and folic acid absorption were studied in 28 adult male epileptics on chronic anticonvulsant therapy. Calcium absorption was abnormal in 9 of 16 patients on diphenylhydantoin alone. Calcium absorption was abnormal in 3 of 12 patients on both diphenylhydantoin and phenobarbital. Folic acid absorption was normal in all but 1 patient. Serum folate was reduced in all patients. Hypocalcemia occurred in only 2 patients, while serum alkaline phosphatase was elevated in 7 patients. The effect of these drugs appears to be acceleration of the metabolism of vitamin D and an increase in excretion of polar metabolites. This may result in reduced levels of 25-hydroxycholecalciferol and 1,25-dihydroxycholecalciferol which are necessary for normal absorption of calcium. Rickets and osteomalacia reported in patients on chronic anticonvulsant therapy may result from reduced calcium absorption. A supplemental increase in vitamin D intake by patients on anticonvulsant drugs is recommended.

116. Foss MC, Meneghelli UG, and Tabosa Verissimo JM, "The Effect of the Anticonvulsants Phenobarbital and Diphenylhydantoin on Intestinal Absorption of Calcium," *Acta Physiol Lat Am*, 1979, 29(4-5):223-8.

An *in situ* model was used to evaluate the effect of anticonvulsant drugs on the metabolic balance of calcium and on its intestinal absorption in rats. The administration of phenobarbital and diphenylhydantoin produced an increase in fecal excretion of calcium and a decrease in the intestinal absorption of calcium. Both effects were more intense in rats treated with phenobarbital. These data are interpreted to suggest that anticonvulsant drugs affect intestinal active transport of calcium.

117. Reunanen MI, Sotaniemi EA, and Hakkarainen HK, "Serum Calcium Balance During Early Phase of Diphenylhydantoin Therapy," *Int J Clin Pharmacol Biopharm*, 1976, 14(1):15-9.

The timing of anticonvulsant-induced disturbances of calcium metabolism was investigated in ten epileptics. One month after the initiation of therapy, there was a significant decrease in average serum calcium and an increase in average serum alkaline phosphatase. These values remained constant thereafter. The findings suggest that prophylactic vitamin D supplementation to prevent bone disease is indicated from the earliest phase of anticonvulsant therapy.

Phenytoin & Folic Acid Depletion - CAUTION

118. Ch'ien LT, Krumdieck CL, Scott CW Jr, et al, "Harmful Effect of Megadoses of Vitamins: Electroencephalogram Abnormalities and Seizures Induced by Intravenous Folate in Drug-Treated Epileptics," *Am J Clin Nutr*, 1975, 28(1):51-8.

Folic acid was administered intravenously during constant EEG monitoring to eight epileptic subjects who had received diphenylhydantoin therapy for more than 1 year. Six patients received folate intravenously without clinical effect of EEG change. One patient exhibited an increase in spike discharges on the EEG in comparison to the baseline pattern, but no clinical change or seizure. One patient displayed EEG changes, followed by tonic-clonic seizure, after the infusion of folate. The authors note there appears to be wide variation in the response to folic acid in drug-treated epileptic subjects, which may help to explain conflicting reports concerning the effect of folic acid administration on seizure control. The authors conclude megadoses of folic acid should be employed with great caution in all subjects, but particularly among epileptics.

Phenytoin & Folic Acid Depletion

119. Lewis DP, Van Dyke DC, Willhite LA, et al, "Phenytoin-Folic Acid Interaction," *Ann Pharmacother*, 1995, 29(7-8):726-35.

Available human studies examining the effects of phenytoin on serum folate concentrations and of folic acid supplementation on serum phenytoin concentrations were evaluated. When phenytoin therapy is initiated serum folate decreases. Folic acid supplementation in folate-deficient patients with epilepsy may change phenytoin pharmacokinetics. This usually leads to lower serum phenytoin concentrations and possible seizure breakthrough. Concurrent initiation of phenytoin and folic acid therapy prevents the decrease in folate and achieves steady-state concentrations sooner. The authors recommend that folic acid supplementation should be initiated at the onset of phenytoin therapy. This may prevent folate deficiency, facilitate a hypothesized cofactor mechanism, and improve seizure control without altering phenytoin pharmacokinetics.

120. Berg MJ, Stumbo PJ, Chenard CA, et al, "Folic Acid Improves Phenytoin Pharmacokinetics," *J Am Diet Assoc*, 1995, 95(3):352-6.

Six fertile women participated in a randomized crossover study of two treatments. Treatment 1 consisted of phenytoin alone, while treatment 2 consisted of phenytoin plus 1 mg of folic acid/day. Dietary folic acid intake was calculated daily. During treatment 1, the serum folate level decreased and the serum PHT concentration was in the low therapeutic range. During treatment 2, the serum folate level increased, and the serum PHT level was similar to that in treatment 1. Only one subject attained PHT steady state during treatment 1, but four subjects achieved steady state during treatment 2. This study suggests an interdependence between PHT and folic acid and supports the observation that fertile women treated with PHT require folic acid supplementation to maintain a normal serum folate level.

121. Berg MJ, Fincham RW, Ebert BE, et al, "Phenytoin Pharmacokinetics: Before and After Folic Acid Administration," *Epilepsia*, 1992, 33(4):712-20.

Phenytoin pharmacokinetics were investigated before and after folic acid supplementation in 13 healthy male volunteers. The measured total serum phenytoin concentration was always greater than the calculated concentration, and t90% was always longer than the calculated t90% before folic acid.

ANTICONVULSANTS *(Continued)*

The authors conclude that if folate is a cofactor in phenytoin metabolism, depletion of the vitamin would result in less folate to be used in the metabolism of phenytoin, resulting in higher total serum PHT concentrations and a longer time to reach steady state.

122. Carl GF, Hudson FZ, and McGuire BS Jr, "Phenytoin-Induced Depletion of Folate in Rats Originates in Liver and Involves a Mechanism That Does Not Discriminate Folate Form," *J Nutr*, 1997, 127(11):2231-8.

To study the mechanism of folate depletion in epileptic patients, phenytoin was administered to rats for up to 8 weeks. At selected times during phenytoin administration the composition of folate pools of intestinal mucosa, liver, bile, and brain were determined. Phenytoin administration had minimal effect on either folate concentration or composition of the folate pool in intestinal mucosa. Phenytoin administration did, however, cause a depletion of total hepatic folate to about 50% of control. Phenytoin appears to inhibit the formation of polyglutamyl folates in rat liver.

123. Carl GF and Smith ML, "Phenytoin-Folate Interactions: Differing Effects of the Sodium Salt and the Free Acid of Phenytoin," *Epilepsia*, 1992, 33(2):372-5.

It has been suggested that pH changes in the gut associated with phenytoin may be responsible for decreased folate uptake, either by direct inhibition of intestinal folate transport or by inhibition of folate conjugase. To examine these possibilities, rats were gavaged with phenytoin using either the sodium salt or the free acid in the presence of folic acid. The sodium salt caused a greater depletion of folate in liver and brain and a significant increase in methylenetetrahydrofolate reductase activity in liver. The free acid caused a significantly decreased weight gain over the 8 weeks of treatment and resulted in a much higher hepatic phenytoin concentration and a slightly lower plasma concentration. These data support the hypothesis that changes in pH in the gut affect enterohepatic folate circulation induced by phenytoin.

124. Rivey MP, Schottelius DD, and Berg MJ, "Phenytoin-Folic Acid: A Review," *Drug Intell Clin Pharm*, 1984, 18(4):292-301.

Although folate deficiency resulting from long-term phenytoin therapy is a common occurrence, megaloblastic anemia is rare. There are data to suggest that nonanemic folate deficiency may be detrimental. Folic acid supplementation in folate-deficient patients results in lowered serum concentrations of phenytoin. This may result in loss of seizure control. Folate appears to be associated with the hepatic metabolism of phenytoin.

125. Shafer RB and Nuttall FQ, "Calcium and Folic Acid Absorption in Patients Taking Anticonvulsant Drugs," *J Clin Endocrinol Metab*, 1975, 41(06):1125-9.

Calcium and folic acid absorption were studied in 28 adult male epileptics on chronic anticonvulsant therapy. Calcium absorption was abnormal in 9 of 16 patients on diphenylhydantoin alone. Calcium absorption was abnormal in 3 of 12 patients on both diphenylhydantoin and phenobarbital. Folic acid absorption was normal in all but 1 patient. Serum folate was reduced in all patients. Hypocalcemia occurred in only 2 patients, while serum alkaline phosphatase was elevated in 7 patients. The authors note that the effect of these drugs appears to be acceleration of metabolism of vitamin D and an increase in excretion of polar metabolites. This may result in reduced levels of 25-hydroxycholecalciferol and 1,25-dihydroxycholecalciferol which are necessary for normal absorption of calcium. Rickets and osteomalacia reported in patients on chronic anticonvulsant therapy may result from reduced calcium absorption. A supplemental increase in vitamin D intake by patients on anticonvulsant drugs is recommended

126. Latham J, Gill DS, and Wickramasinghe SN, "Effects of Phenytoin Sodium on Doubling Time, Deoxyuridine Suppression, 3H-Methotrexate Uptake and 57 Co-cyanocobalamin Uptake in HL60 Cells," *Clin Lab Haematol*, 1990, 12(1):67-75.

Phenytoin caused a dose-dependent prolongation of the doubling time of the human promyelocytic leukemia cell line, HL60. The data indicate that the effects of phenytoin on the proliferation of HL60 cells may have been partly mediated by a reduced uptake of folate, and possibly vitamin B_{12}. One of the mechanisms underlying the undesirable effects of long-term phenytoin therapy may be a drug-related impairment of both folate and vitamin B_{12} uptake by hemapoietic and neural cells.

127. Goggin T, Gough H, Bissessar A, et al, "A Comparative Study of the Relative Effects of Anticonvulsant Drugs and Dietary Folate on the Red Cell Folate Status of Patients With Epilepsy," *Q J Med*, 1987, 65(247):911-9.

In a survey of 200 epileptic patients, median red cell folate levels were reduced significantly in patients treated with phenytoin or carbamazepine monotherapy as compared to a control population. Patients taking more than one drug also had reduced levels. However, in patients treated with sodium valproate alone, there was no significant decrease in red cell folate levels compared to controls. A significant correlation between red cell folate levels and dietary folate was not established. Significant negative relationships were established between carbamazepine dose or serum level and red cell folate level. Correlation between dose or serum level of phenytoin and red cell folate level was also negative, but did not reach statistical significance.

128. Reynolds EH and Trimble MR, "Adverse Neuropsychiatric Effects of Anticonvulsant Drugs," *Drugs*, 1985, 29(6):570-81.

This review notes peripheral neuropathy may result from long-term treatment or prolonged toxic exposure to phenytoin or barbiturates, especially in combination. In addition, all the major anticonvulsant drugs can produce occasional subacute cognitive or behavioral syndromes, especially in combination. Proposed mechanisms include metabolic disturbances of folic acid, monoamines, or hormones, potentially resulting in neuronal damage.

129. Haghshenass M and Rao DB, "Serum Folate Levels During Anticonvulsant Therapy With Diphenylhydantoin," *J Am Geriatr Soc*, 1973, 21(6):275-7.

No abstract available.

130. Mallek HM and Nakamoto T, "Dilantin and Folic Acid Status. Clinical Implications for the Periodontist," *J Periodontol*, 1981, 52(5):255-9.

No abstract available.

Phenytoin & Folic Acid Depletion - Negative Studies

131. Tomson T, Lindbom U, Sundqvist A, et al, "Red Cell Folate Levels in Pregnant Epileptic Women," *Eur J Clin Pharmacol*, 1995, 48(3-4):305-8.

In a prospective study, red cell folate concentrations were determined in 74 epileptic women in early pregnancy. All patients were treated continuously with antiepileptic drugs since before conception. Sixty-four of the patients were on monotherapy. The most frequently used drugs were carbamazepine (n=39) and phenytoin (n=26). Blood samples for red cell folate and antiepileptic drug concentrations were drawn before folate supplementation. Red cell folate levels in patients did not differ from those in nonepileptic, drug-

ANTICONVULSANTS *(Continued)*

free, pregnant women, or from those in non-pregnant age-matched healthy controls. No correlation was found between red cell folate concentrations and doses or plasma levels of phenytoin or carbamazepine.

Phenytoin & Vitamin B$_1$ Depletion

132. Botez MI, Botez T, Ross-Chouinard A, et al, "Thiamine and Folate Treatment of Chronic Epileptic Patients: A Controlled Study With the Wechsler IQ Scale," *Epilepsy Res*, 1993, 16(2):157-63.

In a 6-month clinical trial, 72 epileptic patients receiving phenytoin alone or in combination with phenobarbital, for more than 4 years, were divided into four groups. At baseline, 31% of the patients had subnormal blood thiamine levels and 30% had low folate levels. Groups received either 2 placebo tablets per day; folate plus placebo; placebo plus thiamine; or both vitamins. It was found that thiamine improved both verbal and nonverbal IQ testing. Folate treatment was ineffective. The authors conclude thiamine may improve neuropsychological function in epileptics chronically treated with phenytoin.

133. Botez MI, Joyal C, Maag U, et al, "Cerebrospinal Fluid and Blood Thiamine Concentrations in Phenytoin-Treated Epileptics," *Can J Neurol Sci*, 1982, 9(1):37-9.

Thiamine and folate levels in blood and cerebrospinal fluid (CSF) were determined by microbiological assays in 23 control subjects and 11 phenytoin-treated epileptics. There was no significant difference between the two groups for serum and CSF folate levels. There was, however, a statistically significant difference between the groups for both whole blood thiamine and CSF thiamine levels. Epileptic patients being treated with phenytoin had lower values of thiamine than control subjects.

134. Patrini C, Perucca E, Reggiani C, et al, "Effects of Phenytoin on the *In Vivo* Kinetics of Thiamine and Its Phosphoesters in Rat Nervous Tissues," *Brain Res*, 1993, 628(1-2):179-86.

The *in vivo* effects of either 30-day or 10-day intragastric treatment with phenytoin, on the uptake and metabolism of thiamine (T), T monophosphate (TMP) and T pyrophosphate (TPP), were evaluated in rat nervous regions by determining the radioactivity of thiamine and its phosphoesters in plasma and tissues at fixed time intervals. Compared with vehicle-treated controls, animals treated chronically with PHT exhibited lower levels of radiolabelled T compounds in all nervous regions except for the cerebral cortex. These alterations were not found in animals receiving 10 days of treatment. Phenytoin-induced effects on thiamine metabolism differed depending on the length of treatment and the nervous region considered. Since all changes in thiamine uptake and metabolism were observed in the absence of overt toxicity, the authors believe these findings may have clinical relevance.

Phenytoin & Vitamin B$_1$ Depletion - No Negative Studies

Phenytoin & Vitamin B$_{12}$ Depletion

135. Latham J, Gill DS, and Wickramasinghe SN, "Effects of Phenytoin Sodium on Doubling Time, Deoxyuridine Suppression, 3H-Methotrexate Uptake and 57Co-cyanocobalamin Uptake in HL60 Cells," *Clin Lab Haematol*, 1990, 12(1):67-75.

Phenytoin caused a dose-dependent prolongation of the doubling time of the human promyelocytic leukaemia cell line, HL60. The data indicate that the effects of phenytoin on the proliferation of HL60 cells may have been partly mediated by a reduced uptake of folate, and possibly vitamin B_{12}. The authors propose that one of the mechanisms underlying the undesirable effects of long-term phenytoin therapy may be a drug-related impairment of both folate and vitamin B_{12} uptake by hemapoietic and neural cells.

Phenytoin & Vitamin B_{12} Depletion - Negative Studies

136. Reynolds EH, Hallpike JF, Phillips BM, et al, "Reversible Absorptive Deficits in Anticonvulsant Megaloblastic Anemia," *J Clin Pathol*, 1965, 18:593-98.

The authors of this study reported that the vitamin B_{12} levels in epileptics using anticonvulsants were almost always within the normal range.

Phenytoin & Vitamin D Depletion

137. D'Erasmo E, Ragno A, Raejntroph N, et al, "Drug-induced Osteomalacia," *Recenti Prog Med*, 1998, 89(10):529-33.

In this review, drugs which are commonly associated with osteomalacia are discussed. Associated medications include cholestyramine, phenytoin, phenobarbital, isoniazid, aluminum-containing antacids, ferric oxide lead, bisphosphonates, fluoride, ammonium, and rifampicin. Pathophysiologic mechanisms related to drug-induced osteomalacia are discussed, including vitamin D metabolism, phosphorus homeostasis, and bone mineralization.

138. Stoffer SS, Zaka-Ur-Rahman, Meier DA, et al, "Prompt Resolution of Osteomalacia by Switching From Phenytoin to Phenobarbital," *Arch Intern Med*, 1980, 140(6):852.

In a phenytoin-treated patient with osteomalacia, switching the drug regimen to phenobarbital led to prompt resolution of her symptoms, along with restoration of normal serum calcium and 25-hydroxyvitamin D levels. The authors suggest that a change in therapy may obviate the need for supplemental vitamin D and calcium administration.

139. Zerwekh JE, Homan R, Tindall R, et al, "Decreased Serum 24,25-Dihydroxyvitamin D Concentration During Long-Term Anticonvulsant Therapy in Adult Epileptics," *Ann Neurol*, 1982, 12(2):184-6.

Serum concentrations of 25-hydroxyvitamin D (25-OHD), 24,25-dihydroxyvitamin D [24,25-(OH)2D], and 1α, 25-dihydroxyvitamin D [1,25-(OH)2D] were measured in 30 ambulatory adult epileptic patients. All were receiving long-term anticonvulsant treatment with phenytoin, phenobarbital, or carbamazepine. The drugs appear to exert different effects on vitamin D metabolism. All three caused a significant reduction of serum 24,25-(OH)2D concentrations. A significant decrease in serum 25-OHD was observed only for the phenobarbital-treated patients. A deficiency of 24,25-(OH)2D may play an important role in the development of anticonvulsant-induced osteomalacia.

140. Chung S and Ahn C, "Effects of Anti-Epileptic Drug Therapy on Bone Mineral Density in Ambulatory Epileptic Children," *Brain Dev*, 1994, 16(5):382-5.

In an effort to determine the effect of long-term anticonvulsant therapy, 78 epileptic children and 78 control subjects were scanned to determine bone mineral densities (BMDs) of the arms, legs, ribs, pelvis, spine, and the whole body. There were significant differences in the rib and spine BMDs in patients receiving anticonvulsants for 24 months or more. The authors propose that the measurement of BMDs in the ribs and spine is necessary

ANTICONVULSANTS *(Continued)*

for the early detection of subtle bone loss, and it is recommended that vitamin D be administered to children with epilepsy receiving AEDs over 24 months.

141. Bell RD, Pak CY, Zerwekh J, et al, "Effect of Phenytoin on Bone and Vitamin D Metabolism," *Ann Neurol,* 1979, 5(4):374-8.

Five adult epileptic patients were evaluated before and during treatment with phenytoin for effects on calcium and vitamin D metabolism. Significant decreases occurred in serum concentrations of calcium, albumin, and 25-hydroxycholecalciferol. Significant increases occurred in serum alkaline phosphatase and 1α, 25-dihydroxycholecalciferol, in urinary hydroxyproline, and in the fractional gastrointestinal absorption of calcium. These data suggest that the bone disease associated with phenytoin therapy may be due to a deficiency of 25-hydroxycholecalciferol and not of 1α, 25-dihydroxycholecalciferol.

142. Somerman MJ, Rifkin BR, Pointon-Miska S, et al, "Effect of Phenytoin on Rat Bone Resorption *In Vitro,*" *Arch Oral Biol,* 1986, 31(4):267-8.

Effects of phenytoin on parathyroid hormone and 1,25-dihydroxyvitamin D3(1,25DHCC)-mediated bone resorption were examined in bone organ culture. Phenytoin inhibited the actions of both, however, PTH tended to overcome the initial effects of phenytoin. In contrast, bone resorption due to 1,25DHCC remained depressed as if phenytoin treatment had continued. Phenytoin-induced abnormalities in bone are concluded to involve a greater direct effect on 1,25DHCC than on PTH.

143. Gascon-Barre M, Villeneuve JP, and Lebrun LH, "Effect of Increasing Doses of Phenytoin on the Plasma 25-Hydroxyvitamin D and 1,25-Dihydroxyvitamin D Concentrations," *J Am Coll Nutr,* 1984, 3(1):45-50.

Circulating levels of 25-hydroxyvitamin D [25(OH)D] and 1,25-dihydroxyvitamin D [1,25-(OH)2D] concentrations were studied in a patient who received sequentially increasing doses of phenytoin. The plasma 1,25(OH)2D concentrations were independent of the phenytoin dose and plasma concentrations However, plasma 25(OH)D concentrations were increased by low phenytoin concentration and declined when the phenytoin dose of phenytoin was increased. This effect also occurred as the length of time of exposure to the drug increased. These data suggest that chronic phenytoin administration may have a dose-related effect on the circulating 25(OH)D concentrations.

144. Shafer RB and Nuttall FQ, "Calcium and Folic Acid Absorption in Patients Taking Anticonvulsant Drugs," *J Clin Endocrinol Metab,* 1975, 41(06):1125-9.

Calcium and folic acid absorption were studied in 28 adult male epileptics on chronic anticonvulsant therapy. Calcium absorption was abnormal in 9 of 16 patients on diphenylhydantoin alone. Calcium absorption was abnormal in 3 of 12 patients on both diphenylhydantoin and phenobarbital. Folic acid absorption was normal in all but one patient. Serum folate was reduced in all patients. Hypocalcemia occurred in only 2 patients, while serum alkaline phosphatase was elevated in 7 patients. The effect of these drugs appears to be the acceleration of the metabolism of vitamin D and an increase in the excretion of polar metabolites. This may result in reduced levels of 25-hydroxycholecalciferol and 1,25-dihydroxycholecalciferol which are necessary for normal absorption of calcium. Rickets and osteomalacia reported in patients on chronic anticonvulsant therapy may result from reduced calcium absorption. A supplemental increase in vitamin D intake by patients on anticonvulsant drugs is recommended.

145. Valimaki MJ, Tiihonen M, Laitinen K, et al, "Bone Mineral Density Measured by Dual-Energy X-Ray Absorptiometry and Novel Markers of Bone Formation and Resorption in Patients on Antiepileptic Drugs," *J Bone Miner Res*, 1994, 9(5):631-7.

A total of 38 epileptic patients (24 women and 14 men) who were using either carbamazepine or phenytoin, or both, were studied. Bone mineral density at the lumbar spine and three femoral sites was measured by dual-energy x-ray absorptiometry (DXA). Serum and urine markers of bone and mineral metabolism were also determined. In female patients on phenytoin, bone mineral density was reduced at the femoral neck and Ward's triangle. This value was similar to control levels at all four measurement sites in the other patient groups. Compared with controls, serum concentrations of 25-hydroxyvitamin D and 1,25-dihydroxyvitamin D were reduced in female patients. These changes were independent of the therapy used and were not noted in male patients. For both genders serum levels of vitamin D binding protein were normal. Both female and male patients had hypocalcemia, but women only showed hypocalciuria.

146. Gough H, Goggin T, Bissessar A, et al, "A Comparative Study of the Relative Influence of Different Anticonvulsant Drugs, UV Exposure and Diet on Vitamin D and Calcium Metabolism in Outpatients With Epilepsy," *Q J Med*, 1986, 59(230):569-77.

Biochemical parameters associated with calcium and vitamin D metabolism were assessed in 226 outpatients with epilepsy. Patients were grouped depending on drug treatment; monotherapy with either carbamazepine, phenytoin, phenobarbitone, or sodium valproate and combinations of these drugs as polytherapy. Hypocalcemia was more severe in the phenobarbitone monotherapy group than the carbamazepine or phenytoin groups. No patient on sodium valproate monotherapy had subnormal levels of calcium. Carbamazepine, phenytoin, and phenobarbitone groups were found to have reduced 25-hydroxy vitamin D levels, with no reduction in the sodium valproate group. The most severe alterations occurred in the polytherapy group. This study confirms biochemical evidence for anticonvulsant osteomalacia when enzyme-inducing anticonvulsants are used, with the degree of severity depending on the drug regimen.

Phenytoin & Vitamin D Depletion - Negative Studies

147. Ala-Houhala M, Korpela R, Koivikko M, et al, "Long-Term Anticonvulsant Therapy and Vitamin D Metabolism in Ambulatory Pubertal Children," *Neuropediatrics*, 1986, 17(4):212-6.

Parameters of calcium metabolism were evaluated in 28 adolescents receiving long-term anticonvulsant therapy and in 10 controls. Serum calcium, inorganic phosphorus, parathyroid hormone, and alkaline phosphatase levels did not differ from the control group. There was no correlation between anticonvulsant serum free fraction levels and vitamin D metabolites. Bone mineral content was not significantly decreased in the epileptic patients. Long-term anticonvulsant therapy did not induce 'anticonvulsant rickets' in this ambulatory adolescent population. These data do not indicate that anticonvulsant drugs alter vitamin D metabolism significantly. The authors conclude that routine vitamin D supplementation does not appear to be indicated in children on anticonvulsant therapy.

ANTICONVULSANTS (Continued)

Phenytoin & Vitamin K Depletion

148. Keith DA and Gallop PM, "Phenytoin, Hemorrhage, Skeletal Defects and Vitamin K in the Newborn," *Med Hypotheses*, 1979, 5(12):1347-51.

    Evidence for a sequence of events leading to fetal vitamin K deficiency after maternal ingestion of anticonvulsants is discussed. These agents may result in a greater risk of neonatal hemorrhagic disease, possibly as a result of induction of fetal microsomal enzymes, and a resultant increase in the oxidative degradation of vitamin K. Vitamin K deficiency may have the potential for other clinical effects such as skeletal defects.

149. Keith DA, Gundberg CM, Japour A, et al, "Vitamin K-Dependent Proteins and Anticonvulsant Medication," *Clin Pharmacol Ther*, 1983, 34(4):529-32.

    Interference with vitamin K metabolism, as indicated by a raised serum osteocalcin level, is associated with certain anticonvulsant drugs (particularly phenobarbital and phenytoin). This finding is believed to be of importance in the pathogenesis of side effects of these medications.

150. Solomon GE, Hilgartner MW, and Kutt H, "Anticonvulsant-Induced Depression of Clotting Factors in Children," *Neurol Neurocir Psiquiatr*, 1977, 18(2-3 Suppl):277-84.

    Anticonvulsants were observed to produce clotting defects in 9 children, 2 weeks to 8 years of age. Six patients were on drug combination including two or more of the following: phenytoin, phenobarbital, primidone, carbamazepine, diazepam, ethosuximide. Elevated levels of anticonvulsants were documented, as well as clinical symptoms of toxicity. Clotting defects included elevated prothrombin time, elevated partial thromboplastin time, diminished factors V, VII, or X. Clotting factors returned to normal after lowering serum concentrations of the anticonvulsants. These data suggest elevated levels of anticonvulsants may be associated with clotting defects in neonates and young children.

Phenytoin & Vitamin K Depletion - No Negative Studies

PRIMIDONE

Primidone & Biotin Depletion

151. Said HM, Redha R, and Nylander W, "Biotin Transport in the Human Intestine: Inhibition by Anticonvulsant Drugs," *Am J Clin Nutr*, 1989, 49(1):127-31.

    The effect of the anticonvulsant drugs carbamazepine and primidone on the transport of biotin in human intestine was examined *in vitro*. Results indicate that carbamazepine and primidone are competitive inhibitors of biotin transport in human intestine. The inhibitory effect is localized to the substrate transport system of the brush border membrane. These findings indicate that impairment of biotin status may occur in patients receiving anticonvulsant agents for long periods.

152. Krause KH, Bonjour JP, Berlit P, et al, "Biotin Status of Epileptics," *Am N Y Acad Sci*, 1985, 447:297-313.

    Plasma biotin levels in 404 epileptics under long-term treatment with anticonvulsants were markedly lower than in 112 controls. Epileptics treated with valproate sodium in monotherapy showed considerably higher biotin levels than epileptics with monotherapy of primidone, carbamazepine, phenytoin, or phenobarbital. Four epileptics treated with anticonvulsants had increased urinary excretion of organic acids, as found in patients with a deficiency of biotin-dependent carboxylases. In 37 epileptics who had measurements of plasma lactate concentrations, a higher mean concentration was noted. The lowering of biotin in epileptics is caused by intake of anticonvulsants and has a biochemical effect in these patients. This could be a factor in the mode of action of anticonvulsants.

153. Krause KH, Berlit P, and Bonjour JP, "Impaired Biotin Status in Anticonvulsant Therapy," *Ann Neurol*, 1982, 12(5):485-6.

In 264 epileptics undergoing long-term therapy with anticonvulsants, reduced plasma biotin levels were found compared with a normal control group. Mean plasma biotin levels in patients treated with valproate were higher than those in patients treated with phenytoin, primidone, or carbamazepine. The observed reduction in biotin levels is proposed to contribute to the efficacy of these three anticonvulsants.

Primidone & Biotin Depletion - No Negative Studies

Primidone & Folic Acid Depletion

154. Carl GF, Gill MW, and Schatz RA, "Effect of Chronic Primidone Treatment on Folate-Dependent One-Carbon Metabolism in the Rat," *Biochem Pharmacol*, 1987, 36(13):2139-44.

The effects of chronic primidone on brain and liver one-carbon metabolism were evaluated in rats. These data support the hypothesis that chronic primidone treatment leads to folate depletion by disruption of folate metabolism.

155. Carl GF, Eto I, and Krumdieck CL, "Chronic Treatment of Rats With Primidone Causes Depletion of Pteroylpentaglutamates in Liver," *J Nutr*, 1987, 117(5):970-5.

The effects of chronic primidone treatment on folates in the rat were investigated. Within 1 week, primidone caused a decrease of pteroylpentaglutamates in the liver to less than half the control value. Total liver folacin concentration decreased by 30% in the first week followed by a further, gradual decline. Plasma folacin exhibited a similar pattern, however, no effect was observed on brain folacin concentration. These data lend support to the hypothesis that the anticonvulsants (primidone and/or phenobarbital) cause folate depletion due to an interaction with folate metabolism.

156. Taliani U, Camellini A, Bernardi P, et al, "A Clinical Case of Severe Megaloblastic Anemia During Treatment With Primidone," *Acta Biomed Ateneo Parmense*, 1989, 60(5-6):245-8.

A case of a patient who developed megaloblastic anemia caused by folate deficiency during treatment with primidone is reported. Anemia was completely reversed by oral supplementation of folic acid. The authors conclude a concomitant nutritional deficiency is required to precipitate frank megaloblastic anemia during therapy with antiepileptic drugs.

Primidone & Folic Acid Depletion - No Negative Studies

VALPROIC ACID

Valproic Acid & Carnitine Depletion

157. Farkas V, Bock I, Cseko J, et al, "Inhibition of Carnitine Biosynthesis by Valproic Acid in Rats — The Biochemical Mechanism of Inhibition," *Biochem Pharmacol*, 1996, 52(9):1429-33.

ANTICONVULSANTS *(Continued)*

Valproic acid inhibits the biosynthesis of carnitine, and may contribute to carnitine deficiency. In a rat model, conversion of [3H]-butyrobetaine into [3H]-carnitine and total carnitine in the liver were decreased, whereas the precursor butyrobetaine was increased. VPA also reduced conversion of an unlabeled loading amount of butyrobetaine. These data prove that VPA reduces the flux through butyrobetaine hydroxylase, but did not appear to inhibit the enzyme directly. VPA decreased the level of alpha-ketoglutarate (alpha-KG; a cofactor of butyrobetaine hydroxylase), and the level of 1-glutamate showed a dramatic decrease in the liver. Moreover, alpha-KG proved to have a protective role against VPA induced changes.

158. Van Wouwe JP, "Carnitine Deficiency During Valproic Acid Treatment," *Int J Vitam Nutr Res*, 1995, 65(3):211-4.

In 13 children, paired samples of plasma were drawn at initiation and after 9 months of valproic acid treatment. After 9 months mean plasma free carnitine decreased by 40%, plasma total carnitine decreased by 20%, and the esterified/free carnitine ratio increased by 40%. In 6 out of 13 patients, a biochemical deficiency was found. Clinical symptoms, including fatigue, were also observed in 2 patients. In 4 others only biochemical deficiency was found. A dose of 15 mg/kg body weight is effective to reverse the clinical symptoms of carnitine deficiency within a week. The dose to prevent deficiency has not been established.

159. Matsuda I, Ohtani Y, and Ninomiya N, "Renal Handling of Carnitine in Children With Carnitine Deficiency and Hyperammonemia Associated With Valproate Therapy," *J Pediatr*, 1986, 109(1):131-4.

Five patients with hyperammonemia associated with anticonvulsant therapy including valproate were evaluated. Three patients had a Reye-like syndrome. All had considerable reduction in serum free carnitine and a slight increase of acylcarnitine concentrations, suggesting increased conversion of free to acylcarnitine by valproate administration. The authors note that a combination of several factors may be responsible for carnitine deficiency in patients with valproate-associated hyperammonemia.

160. Ohtani Y, Endo F, and Matsuda I, "Carnitine Deficiency and Hyperammonemia Associated With Valproic Acid Therapy," *J Pediatr*, 1982, 101(5):782-5.

Plasma carnitine and blood ammonia concentrations were measured in 25 severely handicapped patients, 3-21 years of age, and 27 age-matched control subjects. Fourteen of the handicapped patients were treated with valproic acid. Plasma carnitine concentrations were lower and blood ammonia values were higher in patients treated with valproic acid. Plasma carnitine concentrations and the dosage of valproic acid demonstrated an inverse relationship, along with plasma carnitine and blood ammonia values. Oral administration of D,L-carnitine (50 mg/kg/day) for 4 weeks corrected both carnitine deficiency and hyperammonemia.

161. Tein I, DiMauro S, Xie ZW, et al, "Valproic Acid Impairs Carnitine Uptake in Cultured Human Skin Fibroblasts. An *In Vitro* Model for the Pathogenesis of Valproic Acid-Associated Carnitine Deficiency," *Pediatr Res*, 1993, 34(3):281-7.

The authors discuss controversial aspects concerning mechanisms of valproate-associated carnitine deficiency. They note that urinary excretion of valproylcarnitine is insufficient to account for tissue carnitine depletion. For this reason, the effects of valproic acid (VPA) on carnitine uptake in cultured human skin fibroblasts were evaluated. There was an exponential dose-dependent decrease in carnitine uptake with increasing VPA concentrations, implicating a potential contribution by this mechanism.

162. Opala G, Winter S, Vance C, et al, "The Effect of Valproic Acid on Plasma Carnitine Levels," *Am J Dis Child*, 1991, 145(9):999-1001.

Plasma total, free, and acyl carnitine levels were determined in four groups of children: (1) valproic acid monotherapy, (2) valproic acid plus other antiepileptics as polytherapy, (3) other antiepileptic drugs alone, and (4) normal patients. The mean free carnitine level was significantly lower in both the valproic acid monotherapy and polytherapy groups compared with normal subjects. Levels were also significantly lower than in patients treated with other antiepileptic drugs. The authors conclude a general decrease in the carnitine pool should be anticipated in patients taking valproic acid polytherapy and, to a lesser extent, monotherapy.

163. Melegh B, Kerner J, Kispal G, et al, "Effect of Chronic Valproic Acid Treatment on Plasma and Urine Carnitine Levels in Children: Decreased Urinary Excretion," *Acta Paediatr Hung*, 1987, 28(2):137-42.

Plasma levels and urinary carnitine excretion rates were determined in children treated with valproic acid and in age- and sex-matched controls. The plasma level of total and free carnitine was significantly lower in the treated group. There was no significant alteration in the acylcarnitine fraction. A significant reduction in the plasma beta-hydroxybutyrate level was noted, indicating limited fatty acid utilization. Urinary total and free carnitine decreased; the acyled fraction was not significantly reduced.

164. De Vivo DC, Bohan TP, Coulter DL, et al, "L-carnitine Supplementation in Childhood Epilepsy: Current Perspectives," *Epilepsia*, 1998, 39(11):1216-25.

This article reports the recommendations of a panel of pediatric neurologists which met in 1996 to update the 1989 consensus statement concerning L-carnitine supplementation in childhood epilepsy. Intravenous L-carnitine supplementation is indicated for valproate (VPA)-induced hepatotoxicity, overdose, and other acute metabolic crises associated with carnitine deficiency. Oral supplementation is indicated for primary plasmalemmal carnitine transporter defect. In addition, the panelists concurred that oral L-carnitine supplementation is strongly suggested for the following groups: patients with certain secondary carnitine-deficiency syndromes, symptomatic VPA-associated hyperammonemia, multiple risk factors for VPA hepatotoxicity, or renal-associated syndromes; infants and young children taking VPA; patients with epilepsy using the ketogenic diet who have hypocarnitinemia; patients receiving dialysis; and premature infants who are receiving total parenteral nutrition. An oral L-carnitine dosage of 100 mg/kg/day, up to a maximum of 2 g/day was recommended. It was noted that intravenous supplementation for medical emergency situations usually exceeds this dosage.

165. Coulter DL, "Carnitine, Valproate, and Toxicity," *J Child Neurol*, 1991, 6(1):7-14.

In a detailed discussion, the role of carnitine and carnitine deficiency are presented. Carnitine is noted to function to assist long-chain fatty acid metabolism and to regulate the ratio of free coenzyme A to acylcoenzyme A in the mitochondrion. Carnitine deficiency is noted to occur in genetic metabolic disorders, nutritional deficiency, and various other disorders. In addition, valproate therapy is noted to be frequently associated with decreased carnitine levels. Occasionally this manifests as a true carnitine deficiency. Although some experimental and clinical evidence links carnitine deficiency with valproate hepatotoxicity, this evidence is inconclusive. Limited data

ANTICONVULSANTS *(Continued)*

suggest carnitine supplementation may be useful. Young children with neurologic disabilities taking multiple antiepileptic drugs may be at greatest risk for carnitine deficiency. Measurement of carnitine levels appears warranted in patients with signs and symptoms of possible carnitine deficiency and in high-risk patients.

Valproic Acid & Carnitine Depletion - Negative Studies

166. Hirose S, Mitsudome A, Yasumoto S, et al, "Valproate Therapy Does Not Deplete Carnitine Levels in Otherwise Healthy Children," *Pediatrics*, 1998, 101(5):E9.

A population of 45 otherwise healthy epileptic children receiving valproate were randomly selected, along with an age-matched control group (n=45) without epilepsy (control group). Total and free serum carnitine, serum valproate concentration, and plasma ammonia level were measured. There was no significant difference in total or free carnitine levels between the valproate-treated and control groups. Plasma ammonia levels were the same in the two groups. There was no significant correlation between blood ammonia and either total or free carnitine. The authors state that children on a regular diet ingest a sufficient amount of carnitine that meets their daily requirement, and the usefulness of supplementation of carnitine in this population must be carefully evaluated.

ANTIDIABETIC DRUGS

SULFONYLUREAS

Sulfonylureas & Coenzyme Q_{10} Depletion

167. Kishi T, Kishi H, Watanabe T, et al, "Bioenergetics in Clinical Medicine. XI. Studies on Coenzyme Q and Diabetes Mellitus," *J Med*, 1976, 7(3-4):307-21.

The activity of coenzyme Q_{10} enzymes was evaluated in 120 diabetic patients. Succinate dehydrogenase-coenzyme Q_{10} reductase was deficient in diabetic patients. The antidiabetic medications acetohexamide, glyburide, phenformin, and tolazamide inhibited the CoQ_{10}-enzyme, NADH-oxidase. Tolbutamide, glipizide, and chlorpropamide do not inhibit succinoxidase and NADH-oxidase. Patients receiving tolazamide and phenformin showed a higher incidence of CoQ_{10}-deficiency than controls or patients controlled by diet alone. This review emphasized that diabetic individuals are CoQ_{10} deficient and the drugs used in treatment further deplete CoQ_{10}. This deficiency may create a pancreatic energy deficit which could impair insulin synthesis and/or secretion, worsening the diabetic condition.

Sulfonylureas & Coenzyme Q_{10} Depletion - No Negative Studies

BIGUANIDES

Biguanides & Folic Acid Depletion

168. Hermann LS, "Metformin: A Review of Its Pharmacological Properties and Therapeutic Use," *Diabete Metab*, 1979, 5(3):233-45.

A review of metformin pharmacologic and therapeutic properties is presented. These data mention two possible nutrient-depletion situations that may be induced by long-term metformin therapy: folic acid and vitamin B_{12}.

169. Carlsen SM, Folling I, Grill V, et al, "Metformin Increases Total Serum Homocysteine Levels in Nondiabetic Male Patients With Coronary Heart Disease," *Scand J Clin Lab Invest*, 1997, 57(6):521-7.

The premise for this evaluation was the theory that folic acid, vitamin B_{12}, and vitamin B_6 all play a significant role in homocysteine metabolism. The authors studied 60 patients with cardiovascular disease in an open, prospective, randomized trial to evaluate the effects of metformin on total homocysteine levels. Their results demonstrated a significant increase of total homocysteine levels after 40 weeks of treatment, and concomitant decreases in vitamin B_{12} and folic acid levels. They were unable to identify a direct relationship between the increased homocysteine levels and any specific nutrient depletion, as the increase could have been caused by either or a combination of the two.

Biguanides & Vitamin B_{12} Depletion

170. Adams JF, Clark JS, Ireland JT, et al, "Malabsorption of Vitamin B_{12} and Intrinsic Factor Secretion During Biguanide Therapy," *Diabetologia*, 1983, 24(1):16-8.

A random survey of 46 diabetic patients receiving biguanide therapy demonstrated that 30% had malabsorption of vitamin B_{12}. Normalization on drug withdrawal occurred in only half of those with malabsorption. Therefore, the authors concluded biguanides may induce malabsorption by two different mechanisms; a temporary form unrelated to intrinsic factor secretion, and a permanent form mediated by depressed secretion of intrinsic factor. This

ANTIDIABETIC DRUGS *(Continued)*

study reports that about 50% of individuals who develop biguanide-related vitamin B_{12} deficiency have actually developed a permanent inability to produce intrinsic factor. These people will require vitamin B_{12} therapy indefinitely.

171. Berger W, "Incidence of Severe Side Effects During Therapy With Sulfonylureas and Biguanides," *Horm Metab Res Suppl*, 1985, 15:111-5.

In this review of severe side effects of anti-diabetic agents, it is noted that both biguanides, phenformin and metformin, may cause vitamin B_{12}-malabsorption in about one-third of the cases. Despite this observation, symptomatic vitamin B_{12}-deficiency is noted to be extremely rare.

172. Rieder HP, Berger W, and Fridrich R, "Vitamin Status in Diabetic Neuropathy," *Z Ernahrungswiss*, 1980, 19(1):1-13.

Blood concentrations of vitamins were measured in 119 diabetic patients (53 with neuropathies and 66 without neuropathy). The occurrence of neuropathy was strongly correlated with the duration of the diabetic state, but did not correlate with sex or concomitant diseases including adipositas, hypertension, heart, and circulatory diseases. There was no statistically significant difference between diabetic controls and those with neuropathy in their vitamin profiles. Patients receiving biguanide therapy demonstrated a higher proportion of low or subnormal B_{12} values. An increased frequency of neuropathy in patients treated with sulfonylureas approaching the level of statistical significance was noted.

173. Carpentier JL, Bury J, Luyckx A, et al, "Vitamin B_{12} and Folic Acid Serum Levels in Diabetics Under Various Therapeutic Regimens," *Diabete Metab*, 1976, 2(4):187-90.

Evaluations were performed in diabetics treated with insulin, metformin, or sulfonylureas. Results indicated that mean serum levels of vitamin B_{12} were significantly lower in patients receiving metformin than in both other groups. No difference was found in mean serum folic acid levels, red blood cell counts, volumes, or hemoglobin concentration, or in mean values of serum iron and lacticodeshydrogenase levels. Since the hematologic and neurologic complications of vitamin B_{12} deficiency may only appear after 10-15 years, the authors suggest monitoring hematological values and vitamin B_{12} levels at regular intervals in diabetic patients treated with metformin.

174. Berchtold P, Dahlquist A, Gustafson A, et al, "Effects of a Biguanide (Metformin®) on Vitamin B_{12} and Folic Acid Absorption and Intestinal Enzyme Activities," *Scand J Gastroenterol*, 1971, 6(8):751-4.

No abstract available

175. Keiser G, Berchtold P, Bolli P, et al, "Disorder of the Vitamin B_{12} Absorption After Biguanide Therapy," *Schweiz Med Wochenschr*, 1970, 100(7):351-3.

No abstract available

176. Berchtold P, Bolli P, Arbenz U, et al, "Disturbance of Intestinal Absorption Following Metformin Therapy (Observations on the Mode of Action of Biguanides)," *Diabetologia*, 1969, 5(6):405-12.

No abstract available

Biguanides & Vitamin B_{12} Depletion - No Negative Studies

ANTIFUNGAL DRUGS

AMPHOTERICIN B

Note: Formulation may impact potential for depletion.

Amphotericin B & Sodium, Calcium, Potassium, and Magnesium Depletion

177. Gulati M, Bajad S, Singh S, et al, "Development of Liposomal Amphotericin B Formulation," *J Microencapsul*, 1998, 15(2):137-51.

     The authors review adverse effects of amphotericin B which led to the use of liposomal dosage forms. Included in these reports were cases of hypokalemia, renal dysfunction, and hematological abnormalities. The article focused on *in vitro*, *in vivo*, and clinical studies, mechanism of action, distribution, and formulation considerations of liposomal amphotericin. In addition, clinical experience is reviewed.

178. Kline S, Larsen TA, Fieber L, et al, "Limited Toxicity of Prolonged Therapy With High Doses of Amphotericin B Lipid Complex," *Clin Infect Dis*, 1995, 21(5):1154-8.

     Six patients with invasive fungal infections who received large cumulative doses of amphotericin B lipid complex were monitored. Over the course of therapy, two patients had sustained serum creatinine levels ≥2 mg/dL. Several patients were noted to require replacement therapy with oral or intravenous potassium.

Amphotericin B & Potassium Depletion

179. Oravcova E, Mistrik M, Sakalova A, et al, "Amphotericin B Lipid Complex to Treat Invasive Fungal Infections in Cancer Patients: Report of Efficacy and Safety in 20 Patients," *Chemotherapy*, 1995, 41(6):473-6.

     Amphotericin B lipid complex was administered in 20 patients (due to preexisting renal disease or after failure with conventional amphotericin B). Persistent hypokalemia was noted with conventional amphotericin B in 5 patients, but no serious reactions were noted in patients receiving amphotericin B lipid complex. The authors concluded the lipid complex is a promising, well-tolerated, and effective drug for the therapy of fungal infections after the failure of a previous antifungal therapy or after toxic reactions due to conventional amphotericin B

180. Bernardo JF, Murakami S, Branch RA, at al, "Potassium Depletion Potentiates Amphotericin-B-Induced Toxicity to Renal Tubules," *Nephron*, 1995, 70(2):235-41.

     The acute nephrotoxic response to amphotericin B was investigated in a murine model to determine the role of hypokalemia in the development of this toxicity. The authors concluded that potassium depletion does not influence the acute renovascular effects of amphotericin B but potentiates its tubular toxicity. The authors noted that potassium depletion is a frequent complication of amphotericin B therapy, suggesting these findings may have important clinical implications.

181. Cruz JM, Peacock JE Jr, Loomer L, et al, "Rapid Intravenous Infusion of Amphotericin B: A Pilot Study," *Am J Med*, 1992, 93(2):123-30.

ANTIFUNGAL DRUGS *(Continued)*

A prospective, nonrandomized study to determine the safety and toxicity of rapid infusions was conducted in patients with clinical indications for antifungal therapy. Serum potassium levels dropped below the normal limit of 3.5 mEq/L in all patients, but no patient had potassium levels <2.5 mEq/L. Temperatures >38 C occurred in 64% of patients, but only two had temperatures >40°C. Chills were observed in 56% of patients, but only one had severe symptoms. Serum creatinine increased more than 0.5 mg/dL above the pretreatment baseline in 68% of patients, and the absolute creatinine level was greater than or equal to ≥2.0 mg/dL in 40% of patients. Rapid infusions of amphotericin B were concluded to have toxicity similar to prolonged infusions.

ANTI-INFLAMMATORY DRUGS

CORTICOSTEROIDS (Glucocorticoids)

Corticosteroids & Calcium Depletion

182. Lems WF, Van Veen GJ, Gerrits MI, et al, "Effect of Low-Dose Prednisone (With Calcium and Calcitriol Supplementation) on Calcium and Bone Metabolism in Healthy Volunteers," *Br J Rheumatol*, 1998, 37(1):27-33.

The effect of low-dose prednisone on calcium and bone metabolism was evaluated in healthy volunteers to determine a possible mitigating effect on calcium and 1.25 (OH)2 vitamin D (calcitriol). Prednisone was noted to have a negative effect on bone metabolism. Bone formation decreased while bone resorption remained unchanged or decreased slightly. The increase in parathyroid hormone during prednisone therapy could be prevented by calcitriol combined with calcium supplementation.

183. Reid DM, Kennedy NS, Smith MA, et al, "Total Body Calcium in Rheumatoid Arthritis: Effects of Disease Activity and Corticosteroids Treatment," *Br Med J (Clin Res Ed)*, 1982, 285(6338):330-2.

The influence of corticosteroid treatment on bone loss was evaluated in 63 patients with rheumatoid arthritis and compared to normal controls. There were significant reductions in mean total body calcium in groups treated with either NSAIDs or corticosteroids, however, greater reductions occurred in corticosteroid-treated patients. Reduction correlated with disease duration and activity in the patients treated with nonsteroid anti-inflammatory drugs alone, but this relationship was less than predicted in the corticosteroid-treated patients. These data suggest that increased bone loss in RA patients treated with corticosteroids is attributable to drug treatment rather than disease activity. These patients are likely to be at risk from the complications of osteoporosis.

184. Lems WF, Jacobs JW, Netelenbos JC, et al, "Pharmacological Prevention of Osteoporosis in Patients on Corticosteroid Medication," *Ned Tijdschr Geneeskd*, 1998, 142(34):1904-8.

Mechanisms by which corticosteroids lead to osteoporosis are reviewed. These include an increase of renal calcium excretion and a decrease in intestinal calcium absorption, bone formation by osteoblasts, and serum levels of sex hormones. In spite of guidelines advising sufficient calcium and cholecalciferol, only about one-tenth of patients at risk take any form of medication to prevent osteoporosis. In patients taking 7.5 mg of prednisone or more per day, the authors advise additional anti-osteoporosis medication, which may include bisphosphonates in patients with low bone mineral density or hormonal replacement.

185. Gennari C, "Differential Effect of Glucocorticoids on Calcium Absorption and Bone Mass," *Br J Rheumatol*, 1993, 32 (Suppl 2):11-4.

A 15-day study was conducted to compare bone loss and changes in calcium absorption induced by prednisone, deflazacort (DFZ), and betamethasone. Betamethasone (at both dosages studied) and high doses of prednisone induced a significant decrease in intestinal calcium absorption. These changes were not observed with deflazacort. Levels of 1,25-dihydroxycholecalciferol were unchanged throughout the study. Therefore, it appears that glucocorticoids alter calcium absorption through a mechanism which does not involve this hormone. A long-term study of equipotent doses showed that all three glucocorticoids caused a decrease in calcium absorption and a

ANTI-INFLAMMATORY DRUGS *(Continued)*

progressive decrease in lumbar spine bone mineral content. However, changes were least with deflazacort.

186. Need AG, Philcox JC, Hartley TF, et al, "Calcium Metabolism and Osteoporosis in Corticosteroid-Treated Postmenopausal Women," *Aust N Z J Med*, 1986, 16(3):341-6.

Osteoporosis is a complication of corticosteroid therapy. Radiocalcium absorption, fasting urinary calcium/creatinine, and hydroxyproline/creatinine ratios were measured in 30 postmenopausal women receiving prednisolone therapy. These were compared to patients with normal spine radiographs (n=14) and with those whose spine radiographs showed osteoporosis (n=16). The osteoporotic cases had lower radiocalcium absorption, higher fasting urinary calcium, and higher fasting urinary hydroxyproline excretion. In addition, a derived variable evaluating the difference between calcium absorption and excretion (radiocalcium absorption--fasting urinary calcium/creatinine) disclosed a greater difference in the osteoporotic group.

187. Nielsen HK, Charles P, and Mosekilde L, "The Effect of Single Oral Doses of Prednisone on the Circadian Rhythm of Serum Osteocalcin in Normal Subjects," *J Clin Endocrinol Metab*, 1988, 67(5):1025-30.

In a double-blind placebo-controlled study, the effects of 2.5 mg and 10 mg oral prednisone on the circadian variation of serum osteocalcin (a sensitive marker of bone formation) was determined in 15 normal subjects. Both doses of prednisone inhibited and even reversed the nocturnal rise in serum osteocalcin levels. The duration of inhibition was significantly shorter after 2.5 mg than after 10 mg of prednisone. Serum osteocalcin appears to be sensitive to small doses of prednisone. The authors propose that serial serum osteocalcin measurements may be a sensitive marker of the effect of exogenous glucocorticoids on osteoblastic activity *in vivo*. Even short-term glucocorticoid treatment is noted to alter this parameter. Comment: Although not directly attributed to calcium loss, an effect on osteocalcin levels is indicative of disturbances in calcium metabolism.

188. Reid IR and Ibbertson HK, "Calcium Supplements in the Prevention of Steroid-Induced Osteoporosis," *Am J Clin Nutr*, 1986, 44(2):287-90.

The value of calcium supplementation (1 g/day) in preventing osteoporosis in patients receiving glucocorticoids was assessed. After 2 months, the fasting urine hydroxyproline-creatinine ratio decreased and there was an increase in fasting urine-calcium excretion. Serum alkaline phosphatase and osteocalcin showed no change. Calcium supplementation suppressed bone resorption without detectable suppression of indices of bone formation. This was felt to likely result in increased bone mass. Calcium supplementation appears to be a low-cost strategy to address corticosteroid-induced alteration in the normal metabolism and utilization of calcium in the body.

189. Walker GS, Peacock M, Marshall DH, et al, "Factors Influencing the Intestinal Absorption of Calcium and Phosphorus Following Renal Transplantation," *Nephron*, 1980, 26(5):225-9.

The authors describe mechanisms by which malabsorption of calcium and phosphorus may continue despite successful renal transplantation. This is due in part to the action of steroids on calcium and phosphorus absorption, particularly in the first 18 months. Calcium and phosphorus malabsorption can be improved by exogenous 1,25-dihydroxy vitamin D (oral 1α-OH D3 or 1,25-[OH]2D3).

Corticosteroids & Calcium Depletion - Negative Studies

190. Cosman F, Nieves J, Herbert J, et al, "High-Dose Glucocorticoids in Multiple Sclerosis Patients Exert Direct Effects on the Kidney and Skeleton," *J Bone Miner Res*, 1994, 9(7):1097-105.

    In 56 patients with multiple sclerosis, the effects of a total of 38 days of steroid treatment on skeletal and mineral metabolism were assessed. During and after steroid administration, there were no changes in ionized calcium, 25(OH)D, urinary hydroxyproline, or pyridinoline. Serum osteocalcin decreased to below assay sensitivity limits within 3 days of steroid administration. This value later increased but remained at 50% of baseline values. PTH(1-84) increased to a peak at week 2. Tartrate-resistant acid phosphatase, urinary calcium, and urinary cyclic AMP all increased above baseline in a manner which paralleled that of PTH.

191. Leboff MS, Wade JP, Mackowiak S, et al, "Low Dose Prednisone Does Not Affect Calcium Homeostasis or Bone Density in Postmenopausal Women With Rheumatoid Arthritis," *J Rheumatol*, 1991, 18(3):339-44.

    Indices of calcium metabolism and bone mineral density (BMD) were measured in postmenopausal women with RA treated with prednisone (6.6 mg/day). This was compared to a control population which did not receive steroids. Low-dose prednisone did not adversely affect indices of mineral metabolism or bone density in RA.

Corticosteroids & Vitamin D Depletion

NOTE: Corticosteroid drug treatment does not directly cause a depletion of vitamin D. However, by causing a depletion of calcium, corticosteroids create a greater need for vitamin D in order to increase calcium absorption. Thus, by creating an indirect need for more vitamin D, corticosteroids can create a relative vitamin D deficiency.

192. Weryha G, Klein M, Guillemin F, et al, "Corticosteroids Osteoporosis in the Adult," *Presse Med*, 1998, 27(32):1641-6.

    This article reviews bone loss due to supra-physiologic corticosteroid therapy, noting this loss is greatest during the first months of treatment. The rate of loss then declines but persists throughout the duration of treatment due to depressed osteoblast activity. Corticosteroid-induced osteoporosis is multifactorial. It may depend in part on the duration and dose of treatment. In addition, prior bone status and underlying disease contribute. Young subjects may partially or completely recover bone mass after withdrawal of the corticosteroid. Postmenopausal women not taking hormone replacement therapy are at high risk. The authors recommend preventive measures against corticosteroid-induced osteoporosis beginning at the onset of treatment. This may include calcium and vitamin D supplements, hormone replacement therapy (in postmenopausal women) or androgens (in hypogonadic men), and biphosphonates (for young patients at risk or when bone mass declines despite other prophylactic therapy).

193. Hachulla E and Cortet B, "Prevention of Glucocorticoid-Induced Osteoporosis," *Rev Med Interne*, 1998, 19(7):492-500.

    The authors present a rationale and recommendations for optimal management strategies to prevent bone loss during glucocorticoid treatment. Use of the lowest effective steroid dose is encouraged, while noting that alternate-day dosing and bolus dosing do not provide effective protection. Prevention

ANTI-INFLAMMATORY DRUGS *(Continued)*

should include adequate calcium intake and supplemental vitamin D. Life-style modification and additional drug therapy, when necessary, may be used to prevent or slow the development of osteoporosis.

194. Gerster JC, So AK, and Burckhardt P, "Systemic Corticosteroid Therapy in Rheumatology, Advantages and Risks," *Schweiz Rundsch Med Prax*, 1998, 87(33):1024-7.

Long-time corticosteroid therapy has been associated with a higher incidence of bone demineralization, especially in postmenopausal women. Systematic prevention with calcium and vitamin D must be implemented. The authors note that demineralization can be limited by the use of deflazacort, a corticosteroid, which decreases the loss of calcium.

195. Buckley LM, Leib ES, Cartularo KS, et al, "Calcium and Vitamin D₃ Supplementation Prevents Bone Loss in the Spine Secondary to Low-Dose Corticosteroids in Patients With Rheumatoid Arthritis. A Randomized, Double-Blind, Placebo-Controlled Trial," *Ann Intern Med*, 1996, 125(12):961-8.

In 96 patients with rheumatoid arthritis, the effects of supplemental calcium and vitamin D_3 on bone mineral density was assessed. In addition, the relationship between the effects of supplementation and corticosteroid use was evaluated. Supplementation included calcium carbonate (1000 mg/day) and vitamin D_3 (500 IU/day) or a placebo. Calcium and vitamin D_3 prevented loss of bone mineral density in the lumbar spine and trochanter in rheumatoid arthritis patients treated with low-dose corticosteroids.

196. Frauman AG, "An Overview of the Adverse Reactions to Adrenal Corticosteroids," *Adverse Drug React Toxicol Rev*, 1996, 15(4):203-6.

The author notes that recent evidence suggests that calcium and vitamin D coadministration may offset the chronic effects of glucocorticoids in inducing bone loss. They assert a greater understanding of the molecular and cellular basis of glucocorticoid action is necessary to optimize safety in order to minimize the long-term effects of glucocorticoids while retaining efficacy. In addition, the development of newer glucocorticoids which have lesser effects on bone metabolism is encouraged.

197. Sambrook PN, "Corticosteroid Induced Osteoporosis," *J Rheumatol Suppl*, 1996, 45:19-22.

The author defines the consequences of corticosteroid therapy in terms of fracture sites. Fractures are noted to occur in the spine and, to a lesser extent, the ribs. These are uncommon sites of fracture in other forms of osteoporosis. Therefore, the author states that the most important consideration in the selection of therapy for corticosteroid-induced osteoporosis is the effect of particular agents on spine bone mineral density. Calcitriol and the bisphosphonates are noted to be effective in treatment of corticosteroid-induced spinal bone loss.

198. Dechant KL and Goa KL, "Calcitriol. A Review of Its use in the Treatment of Postmenopausal Osteoporosis and Its Potential in Corticosteroid-Induced Osteoporosis," *Drugs Aging*, 1994, 5(4):300-17.

Although this review notes the results of small studies have been conflicting, it presents data to support that the most physiologically active metabolite of vitamin D, calcitriol, has shown benefit in the treatment of postmenopausal osteoporosis. In addition, calcitriol has shown some efficacy in corticosteroid-induced osteoporosis. A clinical trial in 622 women with mild to moderate postmenopausal osteoporosis demonstrated that patients receiving calcitriol

(0.25 mcg twice daily) had a 3-fold lower rate of new vertebral fractures after 3 years of treatment as compared to patients receiving elemental calcium 1000 mg/day. In patients commencing long-term treatment with prednisone or prednisolone, calcitriol 0.5-1.0 mcg/day, plus calcium 1000 mg/day, prevented steroid-induced bone loss when administered with or without intranasal calcitonin. The authors state that the narrow 'therapeutic window' of calcitriol requires appropriate monitoring, including serum calcium and creatinine levels.

Corticosteroids & Vitamin D Depletion - Negative Studies

199. Lund B, Storm TL, Lund B, et al, "Bone Mineral Loss, Bone Histomorphometry and Vitamin D Metabolism in Patients With Rheumatoid Arthritis on Long-Term Glucocorticoid Treatment," Clin Rheumatol, 1985, 4(2):143-9.

In 50 patients with rheumatoid arthritis on long-term corticosteroids, serum concentrations of 25-OHD were significantly reduced. Circulating levels of 1,25-(OH)2D were normal. Bone mineral density in the forearm was significantly reduced, however, the degree of bone loss did not correlate with dose or duration of treatment. Except for a significant correlation between serum 25-OHD and the fractional volume of trabecular bone, no relationships were observed between bone histomorphometry and vitamin D metabolites or serum iPTH. These data indicate that bone loss was due to decreased osteoblastic activity rather than impaired vitamin D metabolism.

200. Hahn TJ, Halstead LR, and Baran DT, "Effects of Short-Term Glucocorticoid Administration on Intestinal Calcium Absorption and Circulating Vitamin D Metabolite Concentrations in Man," J Clin Endocrinol Metab, 1981, 52(1):111-5.

The effect of glucocorticoids on the suppression of intestinal calcium absorption relative to circulating concentrations of biologically active vitamin D metabolites was investigated. Reduced intestinal calcium absorption after glucocorticoid administration could not be attributed to decreased circulating concentrations of the major known vitamin D metabolites.

201. Nielsen HK, Thomsen K, Eriksen EF, et al, "The Effects of High-Dose Glucocorticoid Administration on Serum Bone Gamma Carboxyglutamic Acid-Containing Protein, Serum Alkaline Phosphatase and Vitamin D Metabolites in Normal Subjects," Bone Miner, 1988, 4(1):105-13.

The effects of 40 mg of prednisone given daily for 5 days to normal individuals was evaluated in a double-blind, controlled study to evaluate the relationship between multiple indicators of bone metabolism. The data suggest a direct inhibition of osteoblast number and/or function by short-term glucocorticoid administration. Bone resorption remained unchanged, resulting in a negative bone mineral balance. An observed increase in serum 1,25-dihydroxyvitamin D was judged to be due to direct stimulation of renal 1 alpha-hydroxylase by glucocorticoids. However, the effects of the vitamin D metabolite appear to be blunted.

Corticosteroids & Potassium Depletion

202. Widmer P, Maibach R, Kunzi UP, et al, "Diuretic-Related Hypokalaemia: The Role of Diuretics, Potassium Supplements, Glucocorticoids and Beta 2-Adrenoceptor Agonists. Results From the Comprehensive Hospital Drug Monitoring Programme, Berne (CHDM)," Eur J Clin Pharmacol, 1995, 49(1-2):31-6.

In a large-scale survey of 5047 patients who had received diuretic therapy, 2429 were found to have taken either a potassium-sparing diuretic, or a

ANTI-INFLAMMATORY DRUGS *(Continued)*

combination of potassium-wasting and potassium-sparing diuretics. The overall incidence of hypokalemia was evaluated in the different groups. The data showed patients on the combination of diuretics with no potassium substitution had a higher incidence of hypokalemia than the group who took potassium-wasting diuretics who received potassium supplements. In addition, the use of oral or parenteral glucocorticoids was found to increase risk of low potassium. Finally, patients who used 12 or more medications, (and possibly female gender), were found to be the greatest risk factor for this problem.

203. Shenfield GM, Knowles GK, Thomas N, et al, "Potassium Supplements in Patients Treated With Corticosteroids," *Br J Dis Chest*, 1975, 69:171-6.

Eight patients with lung disease were given prednisone with or without potassium supplementation. There were no abnormalities of plasma potassium, but there was a relationship between the dose of prednisone and the urinary excretion of potassium when potassium supplements were not administered. The effect was also related to duration of therapy. Patients who had been on treatment for a short period retained more of their supplements than did those who had been on treatment for several years. In conclusion, control of potassium homeostasis is altered during prolonged steroid treatment.

204. Stanton B, Giebisch G, Klein-Robbenhaar G, et al, "Effects of Adrenalectomy and Chronic Adrenal Corticosteroid Replacement on Potassium Transport in Rat Kidney," *J Clin Invest*, 1985, 75(4):1317-26.

The long-term effects of adrenalectomy and selective physiologic adrenal corticosteroid replacement on renal potassium transport were investigated in rats. It was concluded that physiological levels of both classes of adrenal corticosteroids stimulate renal potassium excretion. However, mineralocorticoids stimulate tubular potassium excretion directly, whereas glucocorticoids augment excretion indirectly through an increase in distal fluid and sodium delivery.

205. Adam WR, Goland GJ, and Wellard RM, "Renal Potassium Adaptation in the Rat: Role of Glucocorticoids and Aldosterone," *Am J Physiol*, 1984, 246:3(Pt 2):F300-8.

This study examined the role of adrenocortical hormones in potassium urinary excretion. Adrenalectomized rats receiving high potassium diets had a greater kaliuretic response to dexamethasone and aldosterone than control animals. These results demonstrate a role for glucocorticoids in potassium excretion and illustrate the importance of increased responsiveness to both glucocorticoids and mineralocorticoids in potassium adaptation.

Corticosteroids & Potassium Depletion - Negative Studies

206. Jackson SH, Beevers DG, and Myers K, "Does Long-Term Low-Dose Corticosteroid Therapy Cause Hypertension?" *Clin Sci*, 1981, 61(Suppl 7):381s-3s.

The effect of prednisone or prednisolone on blood pressure and electrolytes was investigated in 195 patients prior to treatment and after 1 year. There was no relationship between increase in blood pressure and either dose or duration of corticosteroid therapy. Blood pressure prior to treatment was the main determinant of change in blood pressure. Mean serum sodium levels rose slightly but serum potassium levels did not change. There was no significant weight gain. These results indicate that treatment with predniso-lone or prednisolone in low dose does not cause hypertension or biochemical features suggestive of mineralocorticoid excess.

Corticosteroids & Zinc Depletion

207. Goldberg ED, Eshchenko VA, Bovt VD, et al, "[The Effect of Immunosup-pressive Substances on the Zinc Content in Cells]," *Biull Eksp Biol Med*, 1993, 116(10):412-3.

Decreases in cellular zinc levels were observed in mice receiving cyclo-sporine A and sodium diethyldithiocarbamate. Glucocorticoid therapy induced a decrease of zinc levels in human peripheral granulocytes. This paper discusses the role of alterations in zinc metabolism in the mechanism of action of immunosuppressive drugs.

208. Hempe JM, Carlson JM, and Cousins RJ, "Intestinal Metallothionein Gene Expression and Zinc Absorption in Rats are Zinc-Responsive but Refractory to Dexamethasone and Interleukin 1 Alpha," *J Nutr*, 1991, 121(9):1389-96.

Plasma zinc concentrations decreased in rats given dexamethasone or inter-leukin 1 alpha and increased in those given zinc, but they were not related to 65Zn absorption. Intestinal metallothionein gene expression and 65Zn absorption appear to be refractory to glucocorticoid hormone and interleukin 1 alpha.

209. Fontaine J, Neve J, Peretz A, et al, "Effects of Acute and Chronic Predniso-lone Treatment on Serum Zinc Levels in Rats With Adjuvant Arthritis," *Agents Actions*, 1991, 33(3-4):247-53.

This study evaluated the relative importance of inflammation or glucocorti-coid administration on serum zinc concentrations. Acute steroid administra-tion caused a rapid drop in serum zinc followed by a quick recovery, whether these concentrations were normal or previously reduced by the inflammatory process. Chronic steroid administration had a more complex effect. In animals with induced arthritis, the early steroid treatment promoted a further decrease in the serum zinc level.

210. Yunice AA, Czerwinski AW, and Lindeman RD, "Influence of Synthetic Corti-costeroids on Plasma Zinc and Copper Levels in Humans," *Am J Med Sci*, 1981, 282(2):68-74.

Intravenous administration of either methylprednisolone or dexamethasone initially increased plasma zinc and copper levels. However, by 12 hours, plasma zinc concentrations had decreased below control levels. Extent and duration of the change depended on the steroid dose. No significant decrease was noted beyond 48 hours. Plasma copper levels did not decrease until after zinc levels began returning toward normal, reaching a nadir at 48 hours and persisting as long as 96 hours. The different timing of the change suggests different control mechanisms for the two metals. The authors propose serum zinc levels may depend on the adrenal axis, while copper levels may depend on changes in ceruloplasmin.

211. Fodor L, Ahnefeld FW, and Fazekas AT, "Studies on the Glucocorticoid Control of Zinc Metabolism," *Infusionsther Klin Ernahr*, 1975, 2(3):210-3.

Under stress, physiologic cortisol release occurs, while serum zinc concen-trations decrease significantly. Zinc metabolism may be linked to glucocorti-coid regulation. This review evaluates this relationship.

ANTI-INFLAMMATORY DRUGS *(Continued)*

Corticosteroids & Zinc Depletion - Negative Studies

212. Nair N, Bedwal RS, and Mathur RS, "Zinc, Copper and Hydrolytic Enzymes in Epididymis of Hydrocortisone Treated Rat," *Indian J Exp Biol*, 1998, 36(1):22-33.

In a rat model, zinc tissue levels increased statistically after hydrocortisone treatment while copper increased. The authors believed these changes to be the result of cellular degeneration leading to impairment of metabolic/secretory activity of the epididymal cells studied. A possible involvement of pituitary-testis axis in hydrocortisone-induced epididymal degeneration and functional inhibition is discussed.

213. Weismann K and Hoyer H, "Serum Zinc Levels During Oral Glucocorticoid Therapy," *J Invest Dermatol*, 1986, 86(6):715-6.

A population of 14 hospitalized patients receiving glucocorticoid therapy was monitored for changes in several parameters, including serum zinc and plasma albumin. Within 3 days serum zinc decreased slightly, then rose and remained elevated, but within the normal range for the next 2 weeks. Plasma albumin level paralleled these fluctuations. The serum zinc-to-plasma albumin ratio increased. The authors discuss a possible role of ACTH in the regulation of serum zinc concentrations.

Corticosteroids & Magnesium Depletion

214. Atkinson SA, Halton JM, Bradley C, et al, "Bone and Mineral Abnormalities in Childhood Acute Lymphoblastic Leukemia: Influence of Disease, Drugs, and Nutrition," *Int J Cancer Suppl*, 1998, 11:35-9.

This study attempted to define the etiology of abnormalities in mineral and bone metabolism observed in acute lymphocytic leukemia. A group of children with acute lymphocytic leukemia was studied to evaluate the impact of the leukemic process, chemotherapeutic drugs such as steroids, and aminoglycosides. At diagnosis, 70% of children had abnormally low plasma 1,25-dihydroxyvitamin D, 73% had low osteocalcin and 64% had hypercalciuria. Treatment with high-dose steroid during induction resulted in further reduction in plasma osteocalcin and an increase in parathyroid hormone. During 24 months of remission maintained by chemotherapy, reduction in bone mineral content occurred in 64% of children. A reduction in bone mineral content during the first 6 months was predictive of subsequent fracture risk. After 2 years, fractures occurred in 39% of children and radiographic evidence of osteopenia was found in 3% of the entire study group. Hypomagnesemia developed in 84% of children and 52% were hypermagnesuric. Plasma 1,25-dihydroxyvitamin D remained abnormally low in 70% after 6 months of treatment. Magnesium depletion due to renal wastage was attributed to prednisone and aminoglycoside treatment. Magnesium intake and absorption were normal. Supplemental magnesium for up to 16-20 weeks normalized magnesium in only half of the treated patients.

215. Simeckova A, Neradilova M, and Reisenauer R, "Effect of Prednisolone on the Rat Bone Calcium, Phosphorus, and Magnesium Concentration," *Physiol Bohemoslov*, 1985, 34(2):155-60.

Adult male rats given prednisolone demonstrated a statistically significant decrease in bone magnesium content. Bone calcium content was reduced only in the initial phase of the experiment.

216. Rolla G, Bucca C, Bugiani M, et al, "Hypomagnesemia in Chronic Obstructive Lung Disease: Effect of Therapy," *Magnes Trace Elem*, 1990, 9(3):132-6.

The impact of drug therapy on serum magnesium was evaluated in 95 patients with severe chronic airway obstruction. Multiple-regression analysis showed that the use of diuretics was associated with a significantly lower serum magnesium level. There was a significant negative correlation between serum magnesium and the length of oral steroid therapy. Theophylline, inhaled steroids, or beta 2-agonists did not have an effect. Routine serum magnesium monitoring is recommended in patients with chronic obstructive lung disease who are taking diuretic drugs or corticosteroids, due to a potential impact on respiratory function.

Corticosteroids & Magnesium Depletion - No Negative Studies

Corticosteroids & Vitamin C Depletion

217. Chowdhury AR and Kapil N, "Interaction of Dexamethasone and Dehydroepiandrosterone on Testicular Ascorbic Acid and Cholesterol in Prepubertal Rat," *Arch Androl*, 1984, 12(1):65-7.

After treatment with dexamethasone, a decline in cholesterol and ascorbic acid was observed in the immature testicular tissues of rats. Although a 20 mcg dose was found to be ineffective, concurrent administration of 80 mcg dehydroepiandrosterone reversed these effects.

218. Levine MA and Pollard HB, "Hydrocortisone Inhibition of Ascorbic Acid Transport by Chromaffin Cells," *FEBS Lett*, 1983, 158(1):134-8.

In adrenal chromaffin cells, hydrocortisone was found to inhibit the saturable high affinity mechanism for ascorbic acid uptake in a reversible manner. Control of ascorbic acid uptake by hydrocortisone was noted to represent an unexpected aspect of the adrenal stress response.

219. Mehra KS, Kumar A, Duey SS, et al, "The Effect of Vitamin A and Cortisone on Ascorbic Acid Content in the Aqueous Humor," *Ann Ophthalmol*, 1982, 14(11):1013-5.

Cortisone ophthalmic drops reduce the concentration of ascorbic acid in the aqueous humor. This effect could be neutralized by simultaneous administration of vitamin A drops. The authors note that ophthalmologists have hesitated to use cortisone locally for prolonged periods due to concerns that this practice may either precipitate glaucoma or cataract, an effect which may be related to lowering of ascorbic acid concentration in the aqueous humor and lens. Administration of vitamin A drops along with cortisone drops may limit these concerns.

Corticosteroids & Vitamin C Depletion - No Negative Studies

Corticosteroids & Folic Acid Depletion

220. Frequin ST, Wevers RA, Braam M, et al, "Decreased Vitamin B_{12} and Folate Levels in Cerebrospinal Fluid and Serum of Multiple Sclerosis Patients After High-Dose Intravenous Methylprednisolone," *J Neurol*, 1993, 240(5):305-8.

Twenty-one patients (15 women, 6 men) with definite multiple sclerosis were treated with methylprednisolone for 10 days. A significant decrease in CSF and serum folate as well as a decrease in the CSF vitamin B_{12} levels were demonstrated after methylprednisolone treatment. The authors speculate that low or reduced vitamin B_{12}/folate levels found in MS patients may be

ANTI-INFLAMMATORY DRUGS *(Continued)*

related to corticosteroid treatments, although a causal relationship to MS cannot be excluded.

Corticosteroids & Folic Acid Depletion - No Negative Studies

Corticosteroids & Selenium Depletion

221. Peretz A, Neve J, Vertongen F, et al, "Selenium Status in Relation to Clinical Variables and Corticosteroid Treatment in Rheumatoid Arthritis," *J Rheumatol*, 1987, 14(6):1104-7.

     Corticosteroid treatment, particularly at doses between 20 and 60 mg of prednisolone daily, was significantly related to depressed plasma selenium levels in some patients with rheumatoid arthritis, relative to controls.

Corticosteroids & Selenium Depletion - Negative Studies

222. Marano G, Fischioni P, Graziano C, et al, "Increased Serum Selenium Levels in Patients Under Corticosteroid Treatment," *Pharmacol Toxicol*, 1990, 67(2):120-2.

     Corticosteroid treatment was significantly associated with increased serum selenium levels. A dose-dependent relationship was found in subjects treated with methylprednisolone. The authors speculated that renal excretion of selenium could be affected by the corticosteroid therapy.

223. Koskelo EK, "Serum Selenium in Children During Anti-Cancer Chemotherapy," *Eur J Clin Nutr*, 1990, 44(11):799-802.

     During corticosteroid treatment, serum selenium levels increased in children with acute leukemia. Results were interpreted to suggest redistribution of endogenous selenium stores. For this reason, measurement of serum selenium was not felt to be a valid indicator of selenium status in these cases.

SALICYLATES

Salicylates & Vitamin C Depletion

224. Loh HS, Watters K, Wilson CW, et al, "The Effects of Aspirin on the Metabolic Availability of Ascorbic Acid in Human Beings," *J Clin Pharmacol*, 1973, 13(11):480-6.

     These authors state that aspirin is the drug most likely to create ascorbic acid tissue depletion in normal individuals. Their study showed that the usual therapeutic dose of aspirin, which is either 600 mg in a single dose or at 6-hour intervals, significantly alters the availability of ascorbic acid. *In vivo* experiments confirmed that the presence of aspirin can completely inhibit the uptake of ascorbic acid into leukocytes. These authors also confirmed earlier publications, which reported that aspirin causes an increased urinary excretion of ascorbic acid.

225. Daniels AL and Everson GJ, "Influence of Acetylsalicylic Acid (Aspirin) on Urinary Excretion of Ascorbic Acid," *Proc Soc Exp Biol N Y*, 1936, 35:20-24.

     This is the first published report of vitamin C depletion by salicylates. The authors reported that administration of acetylsalicylic acid to three children was followed by an increased elimination of ascorbic acid in urine.

226. Keith JD and Hickmans EM, "Vitamin C Excretion in Children With Particular Reference to Rheumatic Fever," *Arch Dis Childhood*, 1938, 13:125-136.

The authors report that children treated with acetylsalicylic acid were found to have increased urinary excretion of ascorbic acid.

227. Sahud MA and Cohen RJ, "Effect of Aspirin Ingestion on Ascorbic-acid Levels in Rheumatoid Arthritis," *Lancet*, 1971, 1(7006):937-8.

In 34 patients with rheumatoid arthritis, plasma ascorbic acids were decreased only in those patients who were taking 12 or more tablets per day of aspirin. Aspirin was concluded to cause a depletion of tissue ascorbic acid in rheumatoid arthritis patients.

228. Ioannides C, Stone An, Breacker PJ, et al, "Impairment of Absorption of Ascorbic Acid Following Ingestion of Aspirin in Guinea Pigs," *Biochem Pharmacol*, 1982, 31(24):4035-8.

The interaction between ascorbic acid and aspirin was investigated in guinea pigs. Coadministration of vitamin C with aspirin resulted in lower peak plasma concentrations of aspirin. In addition, the bioavailability of ascorbic acid was reduced. These observations are believed to indicate that aspirin impairs the gastrointestinal absorption of ascorbic acid in guinea pigs. An effect on active intestinal transport is proposed to explain these findings.

Salicylates & Vitamin C Depletion - Negative Studies

229. Youmans JB, et al, "Failure of Acetylsalicylic Acid to Effect Excretion of Ascorbic Acid (Vitamin C) in Urine," *Proc Soc Exp Biol*, 1937, 36:73-76.

These authors were not able to demonstrate an increase in urinary excretion of vitamin C in children with rheumatic fever who were treated with aspirin.

230. Van Ecklen M, "Effect of Acetylsalicylic Acid on Urinary Excretion of Ascorbic Acid," *Acta Brev Neerl Physiol*, 1937, 7:69-70.

The author was not able to demonstrate an increase in urinary excretion of vitamin C in children with rheumatic fever who were treated with aspirin.

Salicylates & Folic Acid Depletion

231. Lawrence VA, Loewenstein JE, and Eichner ER, "Aspirin and Folate Binding *In Vivo* and *In Vitro* Studies of Serum Binding and Urinary Excretion of Endogenous Folate," *J Lab Clin Med*, 1984, 103(6):944-8.

In one healthy female subject, aspirin induced a brisk, significant, but reversible fall in total and bound serum folate and a small, but insignificant rise in urinary folate excretion. Aspirin *in vitro* also displaced significant amounts of bound serum folate. Thus, aspirin in therapeutic doses can contribute to subnormal serum folate values, and if it increases urinary folate excretion even slightly, may impair folate balance.

232. Alter HJ, Zvaifler NJ, and Rath CE, "Interrelationship of Rheumatoid Arthritis, Folic Acid, and Aspirin," *Blood*, 1971, 38(4):405-16.

It was discovered that patients who were taking aspirin had a decreased ability to bind folic acid and a coinciding increase in urinary excretion of folic acid.

Salicylates & Folic Acid Depletion - No Negative Studies

Salicylates & Iron Depletion

233. Leonards JR and Levy G, "Gastrointestinal Blood Loss From Aspirin and Sodium Salicylate Tablets in Man," *Clin Pharmacol Ther*, 1973, 14(1):62-6.

In 13 healthy volunteers, sodium salicylate tablets and aspirin tablets caused gastrointestinal blood loss. The blood loss in subjects receiving aspirin

ANTI-INFLAMMATORY DRUGS *(Continued)*

tablets was appreciably greater (5.6 mL vs 1.2 mL per day above control values).

234. Palme G and Koeppe P, "Comparative Experimental Studies in Animals and Humans on Gastrointestinal Blood Loss Following Antirheumatic Pharmacotherapy," *Arzneimittelforschung*, 1978, 28(3):426-8.

   Based on studies in rats and humans which evaluated total body iron retention, the daily iron loss caused by aspirin is higher by nearly a factor of 2 than a comparison antirheumatic drug (benorilate).

235. Cook JD, "Iron-Deficiency Anaemia," *Baillieres Clin Haematol*, 1994, 7(4):787-804.

   Iron-deficiency anemia is identified as a complication of aspirin therapy.

Salicylates & Iron Depletion - No Negative Studies

Salicylates & Sodium and Potassium Depletion

236. Nain CK, Kaur U, Singh V, et al, "Acetylsalicylic Acid-Induced Biochemical Changes in Gastric Juice: A Failure of Adaptation?" *Indian J Gastroenterol*, 1998, 17(1):4-5.

   After 4 weeks of aspirin ingestion in 18 subjects with irritable bowel syndrome, gastric acid secretion was unchanged but sodium and potassium loss was increased via gastric secretion.

Salicylates & Sodium and Potassium Depletion - No Negative Studies

SULFASALAZINE

Sulfasalazine & Folic Acid Depletion

237. Krogh Jensen M, Ekelund S, and Svendsen L, "Folate and Homocysteine Status and Haemolysis in Patients Treated With Sulphasalazine for Arthritis," *Scand J Clin Lab Invest*, 1996, 56(5):421-9.

   In a group of 25 outpatients with arthritis treated with sulfasalazine, hematological measurements including plasma total homocysteine (which is a sensitive marker of folate deficiency, serum folate, erythrocyte folate, S-cobalamin, and routine indices of hemolysis) were performed. Folate deficiency and hemolysis were found to occur in a considerable number of patients receiving treatment. Measurements of plasma total homocysteine suggest a substantial number of treated patients had tissue folate deficiency.

238. Zimmerman J, "Drug Interactions in Intestinal Transport of Folic Acid and Methotrexate. Further Evidence for the Heterogeneity of Folate Transport in the Human Small Intestine," *Biochem Pharmacol*, 1992, 44(9):1839-42.

   The effects of sulfasalazine and olsalazine on the transport of folic acid and methotrexate (MTX) were investigated in organ-cultured endoscopic biopsy specimens of small intestinal mucosa. Both drugs inhibited the transport of folic acid. Uptake of MTX was only partially inhibited by sulfasalazine and was unaffected by olsalazine. These data corroborate findings concerning heterogeneous transport mechanisms in human small intestinal mucosa.

239. Logan EC, Williamson LM and Ryrie DR, "Sulphasalazine Associated Pancytopenia May be Caused by Acute Folate Deficiency," *Gut*, 1986, 27(7):868-72.

A report of three patients who, after taking sulphasalazine for over 2 years, suddenly developed severe pancytopenia with gross megaloblastic changes in the marrow. Two patients responded to oral folic acid while a third required folinic acid. Folic acid deficiency, as well as an inhibition of folate metabolism in one case, appear to be responsible. High dosage and slow acetylator status appear to be associated.

240. Grieco A, Caputo S, Bertoli A, et al, "Megaloblastic Anaemia Due to Sulphasalazine Responding to Drug Withdrawal Alone," *Postgrad Med J*, 1986, 62(726):307-8.

A 60-year-old man with ulcerative colitis treated with sulphasalazine, presented with severe megaloblastic anemia caused by folate deficiency. The drug was stopped and the anemia recovered promptly without recurrence.

241. Baggott JE, Morgan SL, Ha T, et al, "Inhibition of Folate-Dependent Enzymes by Nonsteroidal Anti-Inflammatory Drugs," *Biochem J*, 1992, 282(Pt 1):197-202.

Many nonsteroidal anti-inflammatory drugs (including sulphasalazine, sulindac, indomethacin, naproxen, salicylic acid, ibuprofen, piroxicam, and mefenamic acid) were found to be competitive inhibitors of avian and bovine folate pathways. In contrast, aspirin, acetaminophen, and antipyrine were weak inhibitors of these enzymes. The NSAIDs also inhibited the folate-coenzyme-mediated biosynthesis of serine from glycine and formate, by human blood mononuclear cells. These data appear to demonstrate the antifolate activity of NSAIDs and resultant cytostatic effects.

242. "Sulfasalazine Inhibits Folate Absorption," *Nutr Rev*, 1988, 46(9):320-3.

No abstract available

243. Halsted CH, Gandhi G, and Tamura T, "Sulfasalazine Inhibits the Absorption of Folates in Ulcerative Colitis," *N Engl J Med*, 1981, 305(25):1513-7.

No abstract available

244. Schneider RE and Beeley L, "Megaloblastic Anaemia Associated With Sulphasalazine Treatment," *Br Med J*, 1977, 1(6077):1638-9.

No abstract available

Sulfasalazine & Folic Acid Depletion - Negative Studies

245. Schoeman M and Bezuidenhout DJ, "Folate Levels in Patients With Ulcerative Colitis Receiving Sulphasalazine," *S Afr Med J*, 1984, 66(11):415.

No significant lowering of folate levels could be determined in a random sample of patients with ulcerative colitis treated with sulphasalazine.

INDOMETHACIN

Indomethacin & Folic Acid Depletion

246. Baggott JE, Morgan SL, Ha T, et al, "Inhibition of folate-Dependent Enzymes by Nonsteroidal Anti-Inflammatory Drugs," *Biochem J*, 1992, 282(Pt 1):197-202.

Many nonsteroidal anti-inflammatory drugs (including sulphasalazine, sulindac, indomethacin, naproxen, salicylic acid, ibuprofen, piroxicam and mefenamic acid) were found to be competitive inhibitors of avian and bovine folate pathways. In contrast, aspirin, acetaminophen, and antipyrine were weak inhibitors of these enzymes. The NSAIDs also inhibited the folate-

ANTI-INFLAMMATORY DRUGS *(Continued)*

coenzyme-mediated biosynthesis of serine from glycine and formate, by human blood mononuclear cells. These data appear to demonstrate the antifolate activity of NSAIDs and resultant cytostatic effects, are important to anti-inflammatory activity. Aspirin appears to exert its anti-inflammatory effects after its conversion into salicylic acid, which possesses greater antifolate activity.

Indomethacin & Folic Acid Depletion - No Negative Studies

Indomethacin & Iron Depletion

247. Peterson DA, Gerrard JM, Rao GH, et al, "Inhibition of Ferrous Iron Induced Oxidation of Arachidonic Acid by Indomethacin," *Prostaglandins Med*, 1979, 2(2):97-108.

    This study explored the possibility that indomethacin might interact with ferrous ion to produce its inhibitory effect. The results suggest indomethacin may inhibit prostaglandin endoperoxide synthetase by complexing ferrous ion in the enzyme. Ibuprofen and tolmetin, two other prostaglandin synthetase inhibitors, also inhibit the interaction of ferrous ion with arachidonic acid. Therefore, this may be a general mechanism for nonsteroidal anti-inflammatory drugs.

248. Ganchev T, Negrev N, and Mileva V, "Effects of Indomethacin on Erythropoiesis and Plasma Iron in Rats," *Acta Physiol Pharmacol Bulg*, 1989, 15(2):53-7.

    The effect of indomethacin on erythropoiesis and plasma iron was investigated in rats. After a 3-day treatment, a decrease in erythrocytes, hemoglobin, and plasma iron was observed. In addition, an increase in reticulocytes and 59Fe incorporated in the newly-formed erythrocytes was demonstrated. Results were felt to be compatible with a regeneratory anemia. The authors concluded prostaglandins may be necessary for normal iron metabolism and erythropoiesis. However, their absence does not prevent the process of erythroid regeneration.

249. Collins AJ, Reid J, Soper CJ, et al, "Characteristics of Ulcers of the Small Bowel Induced by Nonsteroidal Anti-Inflammatory Drugs in the Rat: Implications for Clinical Practice," *Br J Rheumatol*, 1995, 34(8)727-31.

    Small bowel ulcers were created in the rat after oral administration of nonsteroidal anti-inflammatory drugs (NSAIDs). Of the six NSAIDs tested, indomethacin and diclofenac were associated with damage which did not occur in a simple dose-related fashion. Anatomically, NSAID-induced ulcers were found throughout the length of the bowel, although more abundant in the proximal half. Aerobic and anaerobic bacteria were identified which may have an important role in ulcer production in this model. The NSAID-induced gastrointestinal toxicity demonstrated in this rat model is discussed in relation to the human disease. The model was felt to be pertinent to patients who take NSAIDs and develop an iron-deficiency anemia and blood in their feces, without lesions in either the upper or lower bowel.

250. Boardman PL and Hart FD, "Side-Effects of Indomethacin," *Ann Rheum Dis*, 1967, 26(2):127-32.

    This study reports that indomethacin can cause iron deficiency via the mechanism of blood loss, which results in a decreased serum iron concentration.

Indomethacin & Iron Depletion - Negative Studies

251. Cremades A, Garcia-Penarrubia P, Garcia F, et al, "Effect of Different Treatments of the Endotoxin-Induced Modifications in Serum Iron Levels," *Gen Pharmacol*, 1986, 17(5):573-6.

   The effects of hyperthermia, injection of endotoxin, and different antipyretics (ketoprofen, indomethacin, and polymyxin B) on serum iron levels were determined in a rabbit model. The antipyretics induced a rise in serum iron concentration. Hyperthermia did not alter serum iron levels.

OTHER NSAIDs

Other NSAIDS & Folic Acid Depletion

252. Baggott JE, Morgan SI, Ha T, et al, "Inhibition of Folate-Dependent Enzymes by Nonsteroidal Anti-Inflammatory Drugs," *Biochem J*, 1992, 282(Pt 1):197-202.

   Many nonsteroidal anti-inflammatory drugs (including sulphasalazine, sulindac, indomethacin, naproxen, salicylic acid, ibuprofen, piroxicam and mefenamic acid) were found to be competitive inhibitors of avian and bovine folate pathways. In contrast, aspirin, acetaminophen, and antipyrine were weak inhibitors of these enzymes. The NSAIDs also inhibited the folate-coenzyme-mediated biosynthesis of serine from glycine and formate, by human blood mononuclear cells. These data appear to demonstrate the antifolate activity of NSAIDs and resultant cytostatic effects, are important to anti-inflammatory activity. Aspirin appears to exert its anti-inflammatory effects after its conversion into salicylic acid, which possesses greater antifolate activity.

Other NSAIDs & Folic Acid Depletion - No Negative Studies

ANTIVIRALS

FOSCARNET

Foscarnet & Potassium, Magnesium, Phosphorus, and Calcium Depletion

253. "Morbidity and Toxic Effects Associated With Ganciclovir or Foscarnet Therapy in a Randomized Cytomegalovirus Retinitis Trial. Studies of Ocular Complications of AIDS Research Group, in Collaboration With the AIDS Clinical Trials Group," *Arch Intern Med*, 1995, 155(1):65-74.

In the Foscarnet-Ganciclovir Cytomegalovirus Retinitis Trial, the use of either ganciclovir or foscarnet for the initial treatment of cytomegalovirus retinitis was compared in patients with the acquired immunodeficiency syndrome. Patients assigned to foscarnet reported more infusion-related symptoms, nephrotoxic effects, and electrolyte abnormalities. Included in these electrolyte abnormalities were the depletion of potassium, magnesium, phosphorus, and calcium.

254. Gearhart MO and Sorg TB, "Foscarnet-Induced Severe Hypomagnesemia and Other Electrolyte Disorders," *Ann Pharmacother*, 1993, 27(3):285-9.

The authors report a case of possible foscarnet-induced severe hypomagnesemia and other electrolyte disorders. Electrolyte disorders associated with foscarnet, including hypocalcemia, hypokalemia, and hypophosphatemia are reviewed.

255. Malin A and Miller RF, "Foscarnet-Induced Hypokalaemia," *J Infect*, 1992, 25(3):329-30.

No abstract available.

256. al-Ghamdi SM, Cameron EC, and Sutton RA, "Magnesium Deficiency: Pathophysiologic and Clinical Overview," *Am J Kidney Dis*, 1994, 24(5):737-52.

This article reviews the causes and consequences of magnesium deficiency. It is noted that hypomagnesemia may arise from various disorders of the gastrointestinal tract, conditions affecting renal magnesium excretion, or cellular redistribution of magnesium. Drugs which cause renal magnesium wasting are noted to include loop and thiazide diuretics, aminoglycosides, cisplatin, pentamidine, and foscarnet.

Foscarnet & Calcium Depletion

257. Omar RF, Dusserre N, Desormeaux A, et al, "Liposomal Encapsulation of Foscarnet Protects Against Hypocalcemia Induced by Free Foscarnet," *Antimicrob Agents Chemother*, 1995, 39(9):1973-8.

The potential protective role of liposome-encapsulated foscarnet on metabolic abnormalities was investigated in an animal model. Significant, rapid decreases in the serum levels of calcium and phosphorus were noted within minutes of foscarnet injection. However, liposome-encapsulated foscarnet did not cause these changes. Liposomal encapsulation of this drug seems appropriate to protect against abnormalities in calcium and phosphorus levels caused by the free drug.

258. Jacobson MA, Gambertoglio JG, Aweeka FT, et al, "Foscarnet-Induced Hypocalcemia and Effects of Foscarnet on Calcium Metabolism," *J Clin Endocrinol Metab*, 1991, 72(5):1130-5.

The investigators noted plasma ionized calcium concentrations decreased acutely following foscarnet administration. *In vitro* experiments demonstrated a linear, inverse relationship between foscarnet concentration and ionized calcium. No correlation was found between foscarnet and total calcium or phosphate concentration. Dialysis experiments suggested that the complexity of foscarnet with ionized calcium may be a cause of ionized hypocalcemia. Physicians were encouraged to monitor serum ionized during foscarnet therapy (ideally at the end of a foscarnet infusion) whenever neurologic or cardiac abnormalities occur.

259. MacGregor RR, Graziani AL, Weiss R, et al, "Successful Foscarnet Therapy for Cytomegalovirus Retinitis in an AIDS Patient Undergoing Hemodialysis: Rationale for Empiric Dosing and Plasma Level Monitoring," *J Infect Dis*, 1991, 164(4):785-7.

Foscarnet administration to a hemodialysis patient over a 14-week period resulted in a decrease in both serum calcium and phosphorus levels. Neither had an effect on response to therapy.

ZIDOVUDINE

Zidovudine & Vitamin B_{12} Depletion

260. Paltiel O, Falutz J, Veilleux M, et al, "Clinical Correlates of Subnormal Vitamin B_{12} Levels in Patients Infected With the Human Immunodeficiency Virus," *Am J Hematol*, 1995, 49(4):318-22.

In an outpatient referral clinic, 200 HIV infected patients were evaluated to determine the prevalence of subnormal cobalamin levels. In addition, the relationship to immunosuppression by the virus and/or antiviral treatment was evaluated. In 61 patients, subnormal serum B_{12} levels were found. The patients who were deficient in B_{12} were more likely to be receiving zidovudine treatment. In addition, evidence of B_{12} malabsorption is found among those with more advanced disease and gastrointestinal symptoms.

Zidovudine & Vitamin B_{12} Depletion - No Negative Studies

Zidovudine & Carnitine Depletion

261. Dalakas MC and Leon-Monzon ME, "Zidovudine-Induced Mitochondrial Myopathy is Associated With Muscle Carnitine Deficiency and Lipid Storage," *Ann Neurol*, 1994, 35(4):482-7.

The degree of neutral fat accumulation and muscle carnitine levels was analyzed from muscle biopsy specimens of 21 patients with AZT-induced myopathy. Based on the analysis, the authors concluded that the impairment of mitochondrial function in muscle, which may be caused by AZT, results in several pathologic changes. These include the accumulation of lipid secondary to decreased utilization of long-chain fatty acids, reduction of muscle carnitine levels, and depletion of muscle fiber energy stores. The authors note these observations may have potential therapeutic implications regarding the use of oral carnitine supplementation in the treatment of AZT-induced myopathy.

Zidovudine & Carnitine Depletion - No Negative Studies

Zidovudine & Copper and Zinc Depletion

262. Baum MK, Javier JJ, Mantero-Atienza E, et al, "Zidovudine-Associated Adverse Reactions in a Longitudinal Study of Asymptomatic HIV-1-Infected Homosexual Males," *J Acquir Immune Defic Syndr*, 1991, 4(12):1218-26.

ANTIVIRALS *(Continued)*

This study examined and compared the nutritional, immunological, and hematological status of fifteen asymptomatic, CDC stage III, HIV-1-seropositive males. Those receiving zidovudine (500-1200 mg/day) were compared with nontreated, CD4-matched HIV-1-seropositive controls. Hematologic and nutrient levels were similar in both groups prior to zidovudine treatment. Zidovudine-treated subjects demonstrated alterations in hematological and nutritional parameters, including decreased levels of zinc and copper. In contrast, a significant increase in red cell folate was noted in treated patients. Plasma zinc levels were observed to have a potential relationship to the maintenance of immune function. The authors concluded that nutritional monitoring should be performed in patients treated with medications such as zidovudine.

Zidovudine & Copper Depletion - No Negative Studies

Zidovudine & Zinc - No Negative Studies

BRONCHODILATORS / DECONGESTANTS

THEOPHYLLINE

Theophylline & Vitamin B_6 Depletion

263. Martinez de Haas MG, Poels PJ, de Weert CJ, et al, "Subnormal Vitamin B_6 Levels in Theophylline Users," *Ned Tijdschr Geneeskd*, 1997, 141(45):2176-9.

In a descriptive study on the effect of theophylline use on the vitamin B_6 status, a higher prevalence of subnormal vitamin B_6 was found in patients receiving theophylline than in patients who did not. Of the nontheophylline users, between 56% to 70% were found to have subnormal vitamin B_6 levels. These values were 94% and 96% respectively, in geriatric and nongeriatric patients with COPD who were receiving theophylline.

264. Shimizu T, Maeda S, Arakawa H, et al, "Relation Between Theophylline and Circulating Vitamin Levels in Children With Asthma," *Pharmacology*, 1996, 53(6):384-9.

The effect of theophylline administration on circulating vitamin levels was investigated in children with asthma. Circulating vitamin B_1 and B_6 levels were depressed in asthmatic children treated with theophylline compared to those not receiving the agent. Theophylline did not affect circulating vitamin A, B_2, B_{12}, or C levels. The authors concluded that theophylline induces depression of circulating vitamin B_1 and B_6 in asthmatic children. However, a relationship between theophylline dose and vitamin B_1 was not apparent.

265. Tanaka I, Ito Y, Hiraga Y, et al, "Serum Concentrations of the Pyridoxal and Pyridoxal-5'-Phosphate in Children During Sustained-Release Theophylline Therapy," *Arerugi*, 1996, 45(10):1098-105.

The effect of sustained-release theophylline on circulating vitamin B_6 concentrations was evaluated in asthmatic children. The serum vitamin B_6 level correlated with serum theophylline concentrations. Serum vitamin B_6 concentrations were significantly lower in children treated for more than 5 weeks compared with those treated for less than 4 weeks. Vitamin B_6 concentrations in children with theophylline serum concentrations between 5 and 15 mcg/mL, were significantly lower than those with <5 mcg/mL. The results suggest that long-term theophylline therapy or serum theophylline concentration within the therapeutic range can depress serum vitamin B_6 concentration in asthmatic children. The authors hypothesize that theophylline-induced seizures may be caused by a decrease in brain gamma-aminobutyric acid concentrations which may result from a decrease in vitamin B_6 concentration as theophylline concentrations rise above the recommended therapeutic range.

266. Shimizu T, Maeda S, Mochizuki H, et al, "Theophylline Attenuates Circulating Vitamin B_6 Levels in Children With Asthma," *Pharmacology*, 1994, 49(6):392-7.

This study evaluated the effect of theophylline on circulating vitamin B_6 levels in asthmatic children. A depression of serum pyridoxal-5-phosphate (PLP) levels existed in asthmatic children treated with theophylline compared to those not receiving theophylline. A significant negative correlation between the serum levels of PLP and theophylline was demonstrated. The authors concluded that theophylline induces a depression of circulating PLP levels in asthmatic children.

BRONCHODILATORS / DECONGESTANTS *(Continued)*

267. Delport R, Ubbink JB, Serfontein WJ, et al, "Vitamin B$_6$ Nutritional Status in Asthma: The Effect of Theophylline Therapy on Plasma Pyridoxal-5'-Phosphate and Pyridoxal Levels," *Int J Vitam Nutr Res*, 1988, 58(1):67-72.

Plasma pyridoxal-5'-phosphate concentrations were significantly lower in asthmatic women when compared to controls. Plasma pyridoxal levels were not different. Theophylline was administered to a group of 17 volunteers and resulted in reductions in plasma pyridoxal-5'-phosphate levels. Plasma pyridoxal levels and urinary 4-pyridoxic acid excretion were not affected.

268. Laine-Cessac P, Cailleaux A, and Allain P, "Mechanisms of the Inhibition of Human Erythrocyte Pyridoxal Kinase by Drugs," *Biochem Pharmacol*, 1997, 54(8):863-70.

This study evaluated the relationship between drugs and vitamin B$_6$ metabolism. Drugs were selected for study based on their clinical neurotoxicity or chemical structure and were screened to determine their potential inhibitory effect on pyridoxal kinase. Based on the results of this trial, the drugs were divided into three groups. The first group, including theophylline and progabide, were true inhibitors of pyridoxal kinase which did not form covalent complexes. The second group, which included cycloserine, dopamine, isoniazid, and thiamphenicol glycinate, were able to form covalent complexes with pyridoxal or pyridoxal-5'-phosphate. Pyridoxal kinase inhibition by these drugs appeared to be due to complex formation. A third group, including levodopa, D-penicillamine, and muzolimine, formed chemical derivatives that probably had no inhibitory effect on pyridoxal kinase. The clinical consequences of inhibition are discussed and compared with results of previous studies.

Theophylline & Vitamin B$_6$ Depletion - No Negative Studies

CARDIOVASCULAR DRUGS

ACE INHIBITORS

ACE Inhibitors & Zinc Depletion

269. Golik A, Zaidenstein R, Dishi V, et al, "Effects of Captopril and Enalapril on Zinc Metabolism in Hypertensive Patients,"*J Am Coll Nutr*, 1998, 17(1):75-8.

Patients with newly diagnosed essential hypertension were randomly divided into two treatment groups. The first included patients treated with captopril monotherapy (n=16) while the second included patients treated with enalapril (n=18). Ten healthy subjects served as controls. An increase in the 24-hour urinary zinc excretion was observed after 6 months only in the captopril group. Intramonocytic zinc levels decreased significantly in both of the treated groups. It was concluded that treatment of hypertensive patients with captopril or enalapril may result in zinc deficiency.

270. Golik A, Modai D, Averbukh Z, et al, "Zinc Metabolism in Patients Treated With Captopril Versus Enalapril," *Metabolism*, 1990, 39(7):665-7.

Zinc parameters were assessed in 13 patients with essential hypertension receiving captopril (6 subjects) or enalapril (7 subjects) monotherapy. Two control populations included 6 untreated hypertensives and 9 healthy controls. Pretreatment serum zinc levels were comparable in all groups. Twenty-four-hour urinary zinc excretion was significantly increased only in the captopril-treated patients. The zinc:creatinine ratio in 24-hour urine was significantly increased in both captopril and enalapril groups, but the magnitude was far greater in patients receiving captopril. Red blood cell zinc values were significantly decreased in the captopril group.

ACE Inhibitors & Zinc Depletion - Negative Studies

271. O'Connor DT, Strause L, Saltman P, et al, "Serum Zinc is Unaffected by Effective Captopril Treatment of Hypertension," *J Clin Hypertens*, 1987 3(4):405-8.

Serum zinc and copper concentrations were evaluated in a group of 14 essential hypertensive subjects before treatment and after 5-6 months of antihypertensive oral monotherapy with captopril. A control population received either propranolol or alphamethyldopa. Serum zinc and copper were unaltered by any study regimen. Zinc depletion was concluded to be an unlikely consequence of long-term exposure to commonly used doses of captopril.

CHLORTHALIDONE

Chlorthalidone & Zinc Depletion

272. Reyes AJ, Leary WP, Lockett CJ, et al, "Diuretics and Zinc," *S Afr Med J*, 1982 62(11):373-5.

This review discusses the effects of diuretics on zinc homeostasis. Distal tubule diuretics increase urinary zinc output by mechanisms involving both direct and hormone-mediated processes. Zinc depletion is noted to be a possibility during long-term administration of distal tubule diuretics. This may be detrimental in conditions associated with diminished total body zinc levels (hepatic cirrhosis, diabetes mellitus, gastrointestinal disorders and many renal diseases). Attention to the early symptoms of zinc deficiency such as hypogeusia, hyposmia, abnormal dark adaptation, and impotence, and the

CARDIOVASCULAR DRUGS *(Continued)*

monitoring of serum zinc levels are advisable during long-term treatment with these agents.

273. Wester PO, "Zinc Balance Before and During Treatment With Bendroflume-thiazide," *Acta Med Scand*, 1980, 208(4):265-7.

Full balance data for zinc was determined in two healthy individuals before and during treatment with chlorthalidone. Prior to therapy, positive zinc balances were noted in both subjects. Balances became negative during chlorthalidone treatment. The normal or slightly increased serum zinc values observed during diuretic treatment despite increased urinary losses cannot be explained by increased zinc absorption. The author concludes depletion of tissue zinc concentrations may offer an explanation.

Chlorthalidone & Zinc Depletion - No Negative Studies

CLONIDINE

Clonidine & Coenzyme Q_{10} Depletion

274. Kishi H, Kishi T, and Folkers K, "Bioenergetics in Clinical Medicine. III. Inhibition of Coenzyme Q_{10}-Enzymes by Clinically Used Antihypertensive Drugs," *Res Commun Chem Pathol Pharmacol*, 1975, 12(3):533-40.

Eight antihypertensive drugs were tested for inhibition of two mitochondrial coenzyme Q_{10}-enzymes of heart tissue, succinoxidase and NADH-oxidase. These enzymes are important to the bioenergetics of cardiac function. Diazoxide and propranolol significantly inhibited both enzymes. Metoprolol did not inhibit succinoxidase, and was one-fourth as active as propranolol for inhibition of NADH-oxidase. Hydrochlorothiazide, hydralazine, and clonidine also inhibited CoQ$_{10}$-NADH-oxidase. Reserpine did not inhibit either CoQ$_{10}$-enzyme, and methyldopa was a very weak inhibitor of succinoxidase. The authors conclude some of the clinical side-effects of propranolol may be due, in part, to inhibition of CoQ$_{10}$-enzymes. Pre-existing deficiencies of coenzyme Q_{10} in the myocardium of hypertensives may be exacerbated.

Clonidine &Coenzyme Q_{10} Depletion - No Negative Studies

HYDRALAZINE

Hydralazine & Coenzyme Q_{10} Depletion

275. Kishi H, Kishi T, and Folkers K, "Bioenergetics in Clinical Medicine. III. Inhibition of Coenzyme Q_{10}-Enzymes by Clinically Used Antihypertensive Drugs," *Res Commun Chem Pathol Pharmacol*, 1975, 12(3):533-40.

Eight antihypertensive drugs were tested for inhibition of two mitochondrial coenzyme Q_{10}-enzymes of heart tissue, succinoxidase and NADH-oxidase. These enzymes are important to the bioenergetics of cardiac function. Diazoxide and propranolol significantly inhibited both enzymes. Metoprolol did not inhibit succinoxidase, and was one-fourth as active as propranolol for inhibition of NADH-oxidase. Hydrochlorothiazide, hydralazine, and clonidine also inhibited CoQ$_{10}$-NADH-oxidase. Reserpine did not inhibit either CoQ$_{10}$-enzyme, and methyldopa was a very weak inhibitor of succinoxidase. The authors conclude that some clinical side-effects of propranolol may be due, in part, to inhibition of CoQ$_{10}$-enzymes. In particular, pre-existing deficiencies of coenzyme Q_{10} in the myocardium of hypertensive patients could be exacerbated by treatment with propranolol.

Hydralazine &Coenzyme Q$_{10}$ Depletion - No Negative Studies

HYDRALAZINE

Hydralazine & Vitamin B$_6$ Depletion

276. Vidrio H, "Interaction With Pyridoxal as a Possible Mechanism of Hydralazine Hypotension," *J Cardiovasc Pharmacol*, 1990, 15(1):150-6.

The author presents information related to hydralazine's impact on pyridoxal metabolism. Hydralazine interacts with pyridoxal and can attribute to B$_6$ deficiency. It also inhibits a number of enzymes requiring pyridoxal as a cofactor. There is no apparent relation between its enzymatic and blood pressure effects. Hydralazine hypotension in anesthetized rats was reduced by pyridoxal pretreatment. These observations suggest that part of hydralazine-induced hypotension may be related to interaction with pyridoxal. This is proposed to be caused by interference, with an effect of the vitamin on calcium and/or sodium transport in vascular smooth muscle.

277. Shigetomi S and Kuchel O, "Defective 3,4-Dihydroxyphenylalanine Decarboxylation to Dopamine in Hydralazine-Treated Hypertensive Patients May be Pyridoxine Remediable," *Am J Hypertens*, 1993, 6(l):33-40.

Defective dopamine generation can be seen in patients treated with hydralazine, which has been suspected to be related to pyridoxine depletion. Eleven hydralazine-treated stable essential hypertensive (EH) patients, initially found to have a defect in the DOPA decarboxylation to dopamine pathway were retested 4 days after pyridoxine pretreatment. Pyridoxine pretreatment accelerated dopamine generation and attenuated the DOPA-induced increases in plasma and urinary DOPA and its metabolite 3-0-methyl-DOPA, but accentuated the increase in free dopamine and its main metabolites. Other parameters including blood pressure remained unchanged. Urinary sodium excretion was attenuated by pyridoxine pretreatment. This effect exceeded that of dopamine excretion, suggesting that pyridoxine acted by a mechanism independent of atrial natriuretic factor or aldosterone.

278. Rosen F, et al, "Selective Metabolic and Chemotherapeutic Effects of Vitamin B$_6$ Antimetabolites," *Vitamins and Hormones*, Harris RS, Wool IG, and Loraine JA, eds, New York, NY: Academic Press, 1964, 609-41.

In summarizing the types of compounds that interfere with vitamin B$_6$ metabolism, the authors discuss hydralazine as one of the drugs that combines with pyridoxal phosphate, forming an inactive complex.

279. Raskin NH and Fishman RA, "Pyridoxine-Deficiency Neuropathy Due to Hydralazine," *N Engl J Med*, 1965, 273(22):1182-5.

No abstract available.

Hydralazine & Vitamin B$_6$ Depletion - No Negative Studies

LOOP DIURETICS

Loop Diuretics & Calcium Depletion

280. Suki WN, Yium JJ, Von Minden M, et al, "Acute Treatment of Hypercalcemia With Furosemide," *N Engl J Med*, 1970, 283(16):836-40.

This study reports that I.V. furosemide was used successfully as a temporary measure to control hypercalcemia.

281. *Physicians Desk Reference*, 49th ed, Montvale, NJ: Medical Economics Co, 1995, 1133.

CARDIOVASCULAR DRUGS *(Continued)*

Under Precautions: All patients receiving Lasix® therapy should be observed for signs of fluid or electrolyte imbalance (hyponatremia, hypochloremic alkalosis, hypokalemia, hypomagnesemia or hypocalcemia).

Loop Diuretics & Calcium Depletion - No Negative Studies

Loop Diuretics & Magnesium Depletion

282. Rolla G, Bucca C, Bugiani M, et al, "Hypomagnesemia in Chronic Obstructive Lung Disease: Effect of Therapy," *Magnes Trace Elem*, 1990, 9(3):132-6.

The impact of drug therapy on serum magnesium was evaluated in 95 patients with severe chronic airway obstruction. Multiple-regression analysis showed that the use of diuretics was associated with a significantly lower serum magnesium level. There was a significant negative correlation between serum magnesium and the length of oral steroid therapy. Theophylline, inhaled steroids, or beta 2-agonists did not have an effect. Routine serum magnesium monitoring is recommended in patients with chronic obstructive lung disease who are taking diuretic drugs or corticosteroids, due to a potential impact on respiratory function.

283. Quamme GA, "Renal Magnesium Handling: New Insights in Understanding Old Problems," *Kidney Int*, 1997, 52(5):1180-95.

In this extensive review, the author notes that loop diuretics such as furosemide increase magnesium excretion by an effect on the transepithelial voltage, inhibiting passive magnesium absorption. Distally acting diuretics, like amiloride and chlorothiazide, enhance Mg2+ entry into cells of the distal convoluted tubule. While amiloride may be used as a magnesium-conserving diuretic, potassium depletion from chlorothiazide may lead to potassium-depletion which may compromise renal magnesium absorption.

284. Schwinger RH and Erdmann E, "Heart Failure and Electrolyte Disturbances," *Methods Find Exp Clin Pharmacol*, 1992, 14(4):315-25.

Electrolyte abnormalities are noted to be a frequent and potentially hazardous complication in patients with heart failure. This may be due to the pathophysiological alterations leading to neurohumoral activation as well as complications of therapy. Loop diuretics (eg, furosemide) may cause a substantial loss of both magnesium and potassium. The authors emphasize the need to consider preventing depletion of electrolytes, as well as replacement, when treating patients with congestive heart failure.

285. Ryan MP, "Magnesium and Potassium-Sparing Diuretics," *Magnesium*, 1986, 5(5-6):282-92.

The magnesium wasting effects of loop diuretics are reviewed based on data from experimental and clinical studies. These findings are noted to be consistent with micropuncture studies in laboratory animals which indicate the loop of Henle to be the major site of magnesium reabsorption.

286. al-Ghamdi SM, Cameron EC, and Sutton RA, "Magnesium Deficiency: Pathophysiologic and Clinical Overview," *Am J Kidney Dis*, 1994, 24(5):737-52.

This review notes that many therapeutic agents cause renal magnesium wasting, potentially resulting in deficiency. These include loop and thiazide diuretics, aminoglycosides, cisplatin, pentamidine, and foscarnet. Due to a combination of factors, magnesium deficiency is seen frequently in alcoholics and diabetic patients. Symptoms of hypomagnesemia may include neuro-muscular irritability, cardiac arrhythmias, and/or increased sensitivity to digoxin. Refractory hypokalemia and hypocalcemia may also be caused by concomitant hypomagnesemia. The very important point is made that serum magnesium levels can register as normal, and yet there can already be an intracellular depletion of magnesium present. Thus, a normal serum magnesium may fail to identify intracellular magnesium depletion.

287. Wong NL, Sutton RA, and Dirks JH, "Is Lymphocyte Magnesium Concentration a Reflection of Intracellular Magnesium Concentration?" *J Lab Clin Med*, 1988, 112(6):721-6.

Studies were conducted in male Wistar rats given daily furosemide for 19 weeks. Fractional excretion of magnesium was modestly elevated in the furosemide-treated group. After 7 weeks of furosemide treatment, lympho-cyte magnesium concentration decreased significantly. After 11 weeks, furo-semide-treated rats developed a lower plasma magnesium concentration compared with controls. This difference persisted through week 19.

288. Iseri LT, Freed J, and Bures AR, "Magnesium Deficiency and Cardiac Disorders," *Am J Med*, 1975, 58(6):837-46.

Magnesium deficiency is noted to occur following diuresis with furosemide, ethacrynic acid, and mercurials. Two cases of serious ventricular arrhyth-mias associated with magnesium depletion are described. In addition to clinical manifestations such as weakness, tremors, stupor, coma, nausea, vomiting, and anorexia, serious cardiac arrhythmias are noted to occur with magnesium depletion. The article encourages frequent monitoring of serum magnesium concentrations.

289. Lucker PW and Witzmann HK, "Influence of Magnesium and Potassium Deficiency on Renal Elimination and Cardiovascular Function Demonstrated by Impedance Cardiography," *Magnesium*, 1984, 3(4-6):265-73.

In an open controlled trial involving 6 male human volunteers, magnesium and potassium intake was reduced to 32% to 35% of normal for a 5- and 4-day period, respectively. Furosemide was administered during the second period in order to induce magnesium and potassium wasting. Reduced magnesium and potassium intake induced depletion of intracellular stores which was enhanced by furosemide. Magnesium renal elimination was 54% to 60% of intake, but potassium elimination exceeded intake. This was related to magnesium depletion. Changes in cardiovascular function could be reversed in part by a single intravenous infusion of potassium, magnesium, and L-aspartate.

290. Ryan MP, Devane J, Ryan MF, et al, "Effects of Diuretics on the Renal Handling of Magnesium," *Drugs*, 1984, 28 (Suppl 1):167-81.

Congestive heart failure patients being treated with furosemide were found to be both potassium- and magnesium-deficient. Amiloride reduced urinary magnesium and potassium, increased plasma magnesium and potassium, and also increased lymphocyte magnesium and potassium. The effects of amiloride were believed to involve enhanced reabsorption of magnesium.

291. Cohen N, Golik A, Dishi V, et al, "Effect of Furosemide Oral Solution Versus Furosemide Tablets on Diuresis and Electrolytes in Patients With Moderate Congestive Heart Failure," *Miner Electrolyte Metab*, 1996, 22(4):248-52.

The effects of oral furosemide tablets versus oral furosemide solution on serum levels, as well as on 4- and cumulative 24-hour urinary volume, and multiple electrolyte excretions, were evaluated in 10 patients with moderate congestive heart failure due to ischemic heart disease. Oral furosemide

CARDIOVASCULAR DRUGS *(Continued)*

solution was found to provide a more potent 24-hour diuretic and natriuretic effect than an identical dosage in tablet form. Urinary losses of potassium, calcium, magnesium, and zinc were not different.

Loop Diuretics & Magnesium Depletion - Negative Studies

292. Brucato A, Bonati M, Gaspari F, et al, "Tetany and Rhabdomyolysis Due to Surreptitious Furosemide-Importance of Magnesium Supplementation," *J Toxicol Clin Toxicol*, 1993, 31(2):341-4.

The authors note symptomatic hypokalemia has been reported in patients with surreptitious ingestion of diuretics, and in one case hypocalcemia was observed, but magnesium depletion was not noted in these patients.

Loop Diuretics & Potassium Depletion

293. Lindeman RD, "Hypokalemia: Causes, Consequences, and Correction," *Am J Med Sci*, 1976, 272(1):5-17.

This review details multiple factors which may contribute to hypokalemia. Diuretic therapy (loop diuretics, thiazides) is identified as the most common cause of a potassium deficit. The author also emphasizes consideration of abnormalities of the pituitary-adrenal axis, renal disorders including tumors, other drugs, and a variety of less well-defined entities. Potassium deficiency is noted to produce both functional and structural defects in the kidneys, myocardium, skeletal muscle, central nervous system, and gastrointestinal tract. Treatment is aimed at potassium replacement or prevention of further potassium loss.

294. Schwinger RH and Erdmann E, "Heart Failure and Electrolyte Disturbances," *Methods Find Exp Clin Pharmacol*, 1992, 14(4):315-25.

Electrolyte abnormalities are noted to be a frequent and potentially hazardous complication in patients with heart failure. This may be due to the pathophysiological alterations leading to neurohumoral activation, as well as complications of therapy. Loop diuretics (eg, furosemide) may cause a substantial loss of both magnesium and potassium. The authors emphasize preventing the depletion of electrolytes, as well as replacement in treating congestive heart failure patients.

295. *Physicians Desk Reference*, 49th ed, Montvale, NJ: Medical Economics Co, 1995, 1133.

Under Precautions: All patients receiving Lasix® therapy should be observed for signs of fluid or electrolyte imbalance (hyponatremia, hypochloremic alkalosis, hypokalemia, hypomagnesemia or hypocalcemia).

296. Rastogi S, Bayliss JM, Nascimento L, et al, "Hyperkalemic Renal Tubular Acidosis: Effect of Furosemide in Humans and in Rats," *Kidney Int*, 1985, 28(5):801-7.

To gain insight into the mechanism whereby furosemide increases urinary acidification, control and amiloride-treated rats pretreated with mineralocorticoid were studied. In response to furosemide, control rats had a significantly lower urine pH and higher net acid and K excretion than that observed in amiloride-treated rats. These data suggest that furosemide may increase H+ and K excretion by creating a gradient for secretion of these ions.

297. Nuutinen LS, "The Effect of Furosemide on Potassium Balance in Open Heart Surgery," *Ann Chir Gynaecol*, 1976, 65(4):277-81.

Potassium balance was investigated in 45 patients who underwent open-heart surgery. On the day of operation, patients in the short perfusion group with furosemide prophylaxis had a more negative potassium balance as compared to controls, although serum potassium level declined slightly in all the groups.

298. *Physicians Desk Reference*, 49th ed, Montvale, NJ: Medical Economics Co, 1995, 2032.

In Clinical Pharmacology section: Potassium excretion is also increased by Bumex® in a dose-related fashion.

299. *Physicians Desk Reference*, 49th ed, Montvale, NJ: Medical Economics Co, 1995, 1547.

In Clinical Pharmacology section: With prolonged administration, chloride excretion declines, and potassium and hydrogen ion excretion may increase.

300. Cohen N, Golik A, Dishi V, et al, "Effect of Furosemide Oral Solution Versus Furosemide Tablets on Diuresis and Electrolytes in Patients With Moderate Congestive Heart Failure," *Miner Electrolyte Metab*, 1996, 22(4):248-52.

The effects of oral furosemide tablets versus oral furosemide solution on serum levels, as well as on 4- and cumulative 24-hour urinary volume, and multiple electrolyte excretions, were evaluated in ten patients with moderate congestive heart failure due to ischemic heart disease. Oral furosemide solution was found to provide a more potent 24-hour diuretic and natriuretic effect than an identical dosage in tablet form. Urinary losses of potassium, calcium, magnesium, and zinc were not different.

301. Valmin K, Hansen T, and Ronsted P, "Treatment of Benign Essential Hypertension With Furosemide in Different Doses," *Pharmatherapeutica*, 1980, 2(5):296-304.

A total of 26 hypertensive patients were evaluated in a double-blind, randomized, crossover trial. Hypotensive effects, urine output, and effects on serum potassium of three different furosemide dosages were studied. Mean arterial blood pressure fell about 10 mm Hg within the first 2 weeks and was independent of furosemide dosage. Increase in urinary output was dose-dependent. There was correlation between the fall in serum potassium and the diuretic effect, but this was not correlated to the fall in blood pressure.

Loop Diuretics & Potassium Depletion - No Negative Studies

Loop Diuretics & Vitamin B₁ (Thiamine) Depletion

302. Brady JA, Rock CL, and Horneffer MR, "Thiamine Status, Diuretic Medications, and the Management of Congestive Heart Failure," *J Am Diet Assoc*, 1995, 95(5):541-4.

Thirty-eight patients with heart failure were recruited to assess the prevalence of thiamine deficiency when treated with diuretics. Biochemical evidence of thiamine deficiency was found in 21% of patients. Evidence of risk for inadequate dietary thiamine intake was found in 25% of patients. The possibility of potential adverse side effects, including nutrition problems, associated with diuretic therapy in the management of congestive heart failure has prompted a few small laboratory and human studies. Results from these investigations suggest that there may be an increased risk of thiamine deficiency in patients with congestive heart failure who are treated with long-term loop diuretic therapy. It has been postulated that thiamine deficiency may be promoted by excessive urinary losses of thiamine secondary to

CARDIOVASCULAR DRUGS *(Continued)*

diuretic therapy. Inadequate dietary intake was cited as a contributor to thiamine deficiency in patients with heart failure.

303. Yui Y, Itokawa Y, and Kawai C, "Furosemide-Induced Thiamine Deficiency," *Cardiovasc Res*, 1980, 14(9):537-40.

    In male Wistar rats, 4 weeks of therapy with furosemide resulted in the following: thiamine concentration and transketolase activity were significantly decreased. The intraperitoneal administration of various concentrations of furosemide resulted in a significant increase in urinary thiamine excretion. Thus, it is assumed that long-term administration of furosemide could induce a thiamine deficiency.

304. Seligmann H, Halkin H, Rauchfleisch S, et al, "Thiamine Deficiency in Patients With Congestive Heart Failure Receiving Long-term Furosemide Therapy: A Pilot Study," *Am J Med*, 1991, 91(2):151-5.

    Twenty-three patients with chronic CHF receiving furosemide, and 16 age-matched control patients with heart failure and not taking diuretics were studied. Biochemical evaluation of thiamine status was performed. In addition, the effects of intravenous thiamine on cardiac performance was studied in a subset of six patients with CHF. In these patients, a 7-day course of intravenous thiamine was administered. An indication of thiamine deficiency was found in 21 of 23 furosemide-treated patients and in 2 of 16 controls. Values normalized in the 6 patients treated with intravenous thiamine. Left ventricular ejection fraction increased in 4 of 5 of these patients. These preliminary findings suggest that long-term furosemide therapy may be associated with clinically significant thiamine deficiency. The authors believe this may be explained by urinary loss and may contribute to impaired cardiac performance in patients with CHF. The deficit may be prevented or corrected by appropriate thiamine supplements.

305. Yui Y, Itokawa Y, and Kawai C, "Furosemide-Induced Thiamine Deficiency," *Cardiovasc Res*, 1980, 14(9):537-40.

    In a rat model, the intraperitoneal administration of various concentrations of furosemide resulted in a significant increase in urinary thiamine excretion. Based on these data, the authors note long-term administration of furosemide could induce a thiamine deficiency.

306. Shimon I, Almog S, Vered Z, et al, "Improved Left Ventricular Function After Thiamine Supplementation in Patients With Congestive Heart Failure Receiving Long-Term Furosemide Therapy," *Am J Med*, 1995, 98(5):485-90.

    The effect of thiamine repletion on thiamine status, functional capacity, and left ventricular ejection fraction (LVEF) was studied in patients with moderate to severe CHF who had received furosemide for at least 3 months. Thiamine repletion was shown to improve left ventricular function and biochemical evidence of thiamine deficiency in some patients with moderate-to-severe CHF who were receiving long-term furosemide therapy.

Loop Diuretics & Vitamin B₁ (Thiamine) Depletion - Negative studies

307. Yue QY, Beermann B, Lindstrom B, et al, "No Difference in Blood Thiamine Diphosphate Levels Between Swedish Caucasian Patients With Congestive Heart Failure Treated With Furosemide and Patients Without Heart Failure," *J Intern Med*, 1997, 242(6):491-5.

    Thiamine deficiency was not found to be a complication of furosemide therapy in a selected population of patients with congestive heart failure.

Loop Diuretics & Vitamin B$_6$ (Pyridoxine) Depletion

308. Mydlik M, Derzsiova K, Zemberova E, et al, "The Effect of Furosemide on Urinary Excretion of Oxalic Acid, Vitamin C and Vitamin B$_6$ in Chronic Kidney Failure," *Vnitr Lek*, 1998, 44(3):127-31.

    A single dose of furosemide increased urinary excretion of oxalic acid, vitamin C and vitamin B$_6$ during the first 3 hours after furosemide administration. The effect of furosemide persisted for 6 hours in patients with chronic renal failure without dialysis. The authors recommend monitoring of vitamin C and vitamin B$_6$ in plasma during long-term high-dose administration of furosemide in patients with chronic renal failure.

309. Mydlik M, Derzsiova K, and Zemberova E, "Metabolism of Vitamin B$_6$ and Its Requirement in Chronic Renal Failure," *Kidney Int Suppl*, 1997, 62:S56-9.

    A daily oral dose of pyridoxine 6 mg was optimal for replacement in patients without erythropoietin treatment during the period of 12 months of CAPD. Indirect evidence has shown that higher amounts of erythrocyte vitamin B$_6$ is consumed by hemoglobin synthesis during erythropoietin treatment in hemodialysis patients. For prevention of vitamin B$_6$ deficiency in hemodialysis and CAPD patients, the authors recommend pyridoxine according to the following schedule: without erythropoietin treatment: 5 mg/day; with treatment: 20 mg/day. A dose of 50 mg/day in hemodialysis patients has also been found to improve several parameters of cellular immunity.

Loop Diuretics & Vitamin B$_6$ (Pyridoxine) Depletion - No Negative Studies

Loop Diuretics & Vitamin C Depletion

310. Mydlik M, Derzsiova K, Zemberova E, et al, "The Effect of Furosemide on Urinary Excretion of Oxalic Acid, Vitamin C and Vitamin B$_6$ in Chronic Kidney Failure," *Vnitr Lek*, 1998, 44(3):127-31.

    A single dose of furosemide increased urinary excretion of oxalic acid, vitamin C and vitamin B$_6$ during the first 3 hours after furosemide administration. The effect of furosemide persisted for 6 hours in patients with chronic renal failure without dialysis. The authors recommend monitoring of vitamin C and vitamin B$_6$ in plasma during long-term high-dose administration of furosemide in patients with chronic renal failure.

Loop Diuretics & Vitamin C Depletion - No Negative Studies

Loop Diuretics & Zinc Depletion

311. Valmin K, Hansen T, and Ronsted P, "Treatment of Benign Essential Hypertension With Frusemide in Different Doses," *Pharmatherapeutica*, 1980, 2(5):296-304.

    A total of 26 hypertensive patients were evaluated in a double-blind, randomized, crossover trial. Hypotensive effects, urine output, and effects on serum potassium of three different dosages of furosemide were studied. Mean arterial blood pressure fell about 10 mm Hg within the first 2 weeks and was independent of the furosemide dosage. The increase in urinary output was dose-dependent. There was a correlation between the fall in serum potassium and the diuretic effect, but this was not correlated to the fall in blood pressure.

CARDIOVASCULAR DRUGS *(Continued)*

METHYLDOPA

Methyldopa & Coenzyme Q_{10} Depletion

312. Kishi H, Kishi T, and Folkers K, "Bioenergetics in Clinical Medicine. III. Inhibition of Coenzyme Q_{10}-Enzymes by Clinically Used Antihypertensive Drugs," *Res Commun Chem Pathol Pharmacol*, 1975, 12(3):533-40.

Eight antihypertensive drugs were tested for inhibition of two mitochondrial coenzyme Q_{10}-enzymes of heart tissue, succinoxidase, and NADH-oxidase. These enzymes are important to the bioenergetics of cardiac function. Diazoxide and propranolol significantly inhibited both enzymes. Metoprolol did not inhibit succinoxidase, and was one-fourth as active as propranolol for inhibition of NADH-oxidase. Hydrochlorothiazide, hydralazine, and clonidine also inhibited CoQ_{10}-NADH-oxidase. Reserpine did not inhibit either CoQ_{10}-enzyme, and methyldopa was a very weak inhibitor of succinoxidase. The authors note some of the clinical side-effects of propranolol may be due, in part, to inhibition of CoQ_{10}-enzymes. Pre-existing deficiencies of coenzyme Q_{10} in the myocardium of hypertensive patients could be exacerbated by treatment with propranolol.

Methyldopa & Coenzyme Q_{10} Depletion - No Negative Studies

POTASSIUM-SPARING DIURETICS

Potassium-Sparing Diuretics & Calcium Depletion

313. Hanze S and Seyberth H, "Studies of the Effect of the Diuretics Furosemide, Ethacrynic Acid, and Triamterene on Renal Magnesium and Calcium Excretion," *Klin Wochenschr*, 1967, 45(6):313-4.

This study reports that orally administered triamterene results in an increased clearance of calcium.

314. D'Arcy PF and Griffin JP, *Iatrogenic Diseases*, New York, NY: Oxford University Press, 1972.

The authors report that the oral diuretics furosemide, ethacrynic acid, and triamterene each produce significant increase in urinary calcium excretion.

Potassium-Sparing Diuretics & Calcium Depletion - No Negative Studies

Potassium-Sparing Diuretics & Folic Acid Depletion

315. Lambie DG and Johnson RH, "Drugs and Folate Metabolism," *Drugs*, 1985, 30(2):145-55.

This article reviews data concerning the impact of many drug classes on folate metabolism. Drugs such as aminopterin, methotrexate (amethopterin), pyrimethamine, trimethoprim, and triamterene act as folate antagonists. Other drugs such as anticonvulsants, antituberculosis drugs, alcohol, and oral contraceptives produce low serum and tissue folate concentrations, although the mechanism of these effects is uncertain. Treatment with folic acid antagonists causes megaloblastic anemia which may be prevented by supplemental folinic acid. Megaloblastic anemia occurs in less than 0.75% of patients receiving anticonvulsants. The authors suggest a trial of therapy with folic or folinic acid in patients with folate deficiency who have neuropsychiatric symptoms including neuropathy or myelopathy despite normal vitamin B_{12} levels.

316. Zimmerman J, Selhub J, and Rosenberg IH, "Competitive Inhibition of Folic Acid Absorption in Rat Jejunum by Triamterene," *J Lab Clin Med*, 1986, 108(4):272-6.

The effect of triamterene on folic acid absorption in rat jejunum was investigated by an *in vivo* intestinal loop method. Triamterene inhibited the intestinal absorption of folic acid in a dose-dependent fashion. Because therapeutic doses can result in luminal concentrations equal to or greater than the inhibitory constant, the authors believe this interaction is of potential clinical interest.

317. Joosten E and Pelemans W, "Megaloblastic Anaemia in an Elderly Patient Treated With Triamterene," *Neth J Med*, 1991, 38(5-6):209-11.

The case is presented of an elderly woman in whom megaloblastic anemia due to folate deficiency was diagnosed. It is speculated that this disorder was induced by treatment with triamterene.

318. Corcino J, Waxman S, and Herbert V, "Mechanism of Triamterene-Induced Megaloblastosis," *Ann Intern Med*, 1970, 73(3):419-24.

No abstract available

Potassium-Sparing Diuretics & Folic Acid Depletion - Negative Studies

319. Mason JB, Zimmerman J, Otradovec CL, et al, "Chronic Diuretic Therapy With Moderate Doses of Triamterene is Not Associated With Folate Deficiency," *J Lab Clin Med*, 1991, 117(5):365-9.

The folate status of triamterene users was compared to those not taking the drug. The hemoglobin concentration, RBC count, MCV, serum folate values, and RBC folate values were not found to differ significantly between users and hypertensive controls.

THIAZIDE DIURETICS

Thiazide Diuretics & Coenzyme Q_{10} Depletion

320. Kishi H, Kishi T, and Folkers K, "Bioenergetics in Clinical Medicine. III. Inhibition of Coenzyme Q_{10}-Enzymes by Clinically Used Antihypertensive Drugs," *Res Commun Chem Pathol Pharmacol*, 1975, 12(3):533-40.

Eight antihypertensive drugs were tested for inhibition of two mitochondrial coenzyme Q_{10}-enzymes of heart tissue, succinoxidase, and NADH-oxidase. These enzymes are important to the bioenergetics of cardiac function. Diazoxide and propranolol significantly inhibited both enzymes. Metoprolol did not inhibit succinoxidase, and was one-fourth as active as propranolol for inhibition of NADH-oxidase. Hydrochlorothiazide, hydralazine, and clonidine also inhibited CoQ_{10}-NADH-oxidase. Reserpine did not inhibit either CoQ_{10}-enzyme, and methyldopa was a very weak inhibitor of succinoxidase. The authors note that the clinical side-effects of propranolol may be due, in part, to inhibition of CoQ_{10}-enzymes. Pre-existing deficiencies of coenzyme Q_{10} in the myocardium of hypertensive patients could be exacerbated by treatment with propranolol.

Thiazide Diuretics & Coenzyme Q_{10} Depletion - No Negative Studies

Thiazide Diuretics & Magnesium Depletion

321. al-Ghamdi SM, Cameron EC, and Sutton RA, "Magnesium Deficiency: Pathophysiologic and Clinical Overview," *Am J Kidney Dis*, 1994, 24(5):737-52.

CARDIOVASCULAR DRUGS *(Continued)*

In this extensive review, it is noted that many therapeutic agents have the potential to cause renal magnesium wasting and subsequent deficiency. Loop and thiazide diuretics, aminoglycosides, cisplatin, pentamidine, and foscarnet are identified with magnesium wasting. Hypomagnesemia is noted to produce a wide variety of clinical symptoms, including neuromuscular irritability, cardiac arrhythmias, and increased sensitivity to digoxin.

322. Dai LJ, Friedman PA, and Quamme GA, "Cellular Mechanisms of Chlorothiazide and Cellular Potassium Depletion on Mg2+ Uptake in Mouse Distal Convoluted Tubule Cells," *Kidney Int*, 1997, 51(4):1008-17.

The effect of chlorothiazide on cellular mechanisms which alter magnesium uptake was investigated in immortalized mouse distal convoluted tubule cells. Acute chlorothiazide was found to stimulate magnesium transport in these cells. The ability of chlorothiazide to stimulate magnesium uptake was concentration-dependent and related to the diuretic-induced hyperpolarization of the plasma membrane. These studies support the notion that acute chlorothiazide administration enhances renal magnesium conservation through its effects on Mg2+ transport within the distal convoluted tubule. The authors postulate that chronic chlorothiazide use may lead to hypokalemia, which diminishes magnesium transport in the distal tubule resulting in urinary magnesium-wasting. The basis for diminished uptake may be, in part, due to membrane depolarization.

323. Malini PL, Strocchi E, Valtancoli G, et al, "Angiotensin-Converting Enzyme Inhibitors, Thiazide Diuretics and Magnesium Balance. A Preliminary Study," *Magnes Res*, 1990, 3(3):193-6.

In a cross-sectional study, serum and mononuclear cell magnesium content was determined in four groups of hypertensive patients on chronic treatment. Groups include patients treated with atenolol (n=11), enalapril (n=10), thiazide diuretics (n=12), or enalapril + thiazides (n=11). Mononuclear cell magnesium was decreased in patients treated with the thiazides alone, in spite of normal serum potassium and magnesium levels. These results indicate that thiazides may induce a depletion of magnesium body stores which may not be detectable by monitoring serum levels.

324. Nicholls MG, "Interaction of Diuretics and Electrolytes in Congestive Heart Failure," *Am J Cardiol*, 1990, 65(10):17E-21E; discussion 22E-23E.

The author discusses the effects of diuretics on electrolytes in the context of alterations in electrolyte balance caused by heart failure itself. The natriuretic effect of loop diuretics is noted to be greater in edematous patients than in healthy volunteers. However, the initial kaliuresis is minimal. The author speculates that low aldosterone levels may account for this observation. With continued treatment (or after the edema has been reduced), the natriuretic action of loop diuretics is less than controls, but loss of potassium occurs. Concomitant thiazide and loop diuretic therapy enhances the natriuretic effect. Depletion of magnesium may be caused by both loop and thiazide diuretics. While potassium-sparing diuretics augment natriuresis from loop or thiazide diuretics, they may limit or prevent potassium or magnesium loss. However, they may contribute to hyponatremia.

325. Hollifield JW, "Potassium and Magnesium Abnormalities: Diuretics and Arrhythmias in Hypertension," *Am J Med*, 1984, 77(5A):28-32.

Thirty-eight patients with moderate diastolic hypertension were treated with hydrochlorothiazide. Dose escalation was discontinued when either normal blood pressure was attained or a dose of 200 mg was reached, then maintained for 24 weeks of continuous thiazide monotherapy. During dose escalation and long-term maintenance therapy, serum potassium and magnesium levels fell in a step-wise, dose-dependent fashion. In a separate study, the occurrence of premature ventricular contractions correlated significantly with decrease in serum potassium and serum magnesium in patients receiving thiazide diuretics. The author concluded that thiazide therapy causes both potassium and magnesium depletion, and these decreases correlate well with the occurrence of ventricular ectopy.

326. Dyckner T and Wester PO, "Potassium/Magnesium Depletion in Patients With Cardiovascular Disease," Am J Med, 1987, 82(3A):11-7.

This article discusses the impact of diuretic-induced deficiencies in potassium and magnesium in patients with cardiovascular disease. Hypokalemia is noted to be found in up to 50% of patients receiving thiazide therapy. It is associated with a greater frequency of serious arrhythmias and increased mortality in patients with acute myocardial infarction. In addition, hypomagnesemia has been identified in 42% of patients with hypokalemia. Depressed muscle magnesium levels have been found in 43% of congestive heart failure patients receiving diuretics. Magnesium is noted to be important for maintenance of cellular potassium concentrations, and infusions of magnesium have increased both muscle potassium and magnesium levels. This, in turn, significantly decreased the frequency of ventricular ectopic beats. Both potassium and magnesium are noted to be conserved by potassium-sparing agents. The authors advise prevention of electrolyte abnormalities, noting that correlations between serum and tissue concentrations of these electrolytes are weak.

327. Petri M, Cumber P, Grimes L, et al, "The Metabolic Effects of Thiazide Therapy in the Elderly: A Population Study," Age Ageing, 1986, 15(3):151-5.

Plasma and intracellular electrolytes and plasma glucose were measured in an elderly population to quantify the risk of metabolic abnormalities. Reductions in both plasma and cellular magnesium and potassium were found in the thiazide-treated subjects. Hypomagnesemia occurred in 48% of the thiazide-treated group, and 28% were hypokalemic. The authors conclude that magnesium and potassium depletion are commonly associated with thiazide therapy in the elderly.

Thiazide Diuretics & Magnesium Depletion - Negative Studies

328. Cohen L, Kitzes R, and Shnaider H, "The Myth of Long-Term Thiazide-Induced Magnesium Deficiency," Magnesium, 1985, 4(4):176-81.

In a population of patients treated with 50 mg hydrochlorothiazide daily for a period of 3-10 years, magnesium concentrations in serum, erythrocyte, lymphocyte, skeletal muscle, bone, and urine were found to be within the normal range. In addition, all patients retained a normal percentage of a loading dose of magnesium. The authors conclude that long-term thiazide therapy does not appear to lead to magnesium depletion.

Thiazide Diuretics & Potassium Depletion

329. Gettes LS, "Electrolyte Abnormalities Underlying Lethal and Ventricular Arrhythmias," Circulation, 1992, 85(1 Suppl):I70-6.

The author reviews the contribution of electrolyte abnormalities to arrhythmogenesis. Changes in serum potassium contribute to ventricular arrhythmias as a result of electrophysiologic changes in single fibers. The author notes that hypokalemia induced by thiazide and loop diuretics may

CARDIOVASCULAR DRUGS *(Continued)*

contribute to the incidence of sudden cardiac death in some populations. In addition, hypokalemia appears to be an independent risk factor for lethal ventricular arrhythmias in the setting of acute myocardial infarction. Hypomagnesemia is also believed to be arrhythmogenic, and magnesium depletion is thought to contribute to arrhythmias associated with hypokalemia. Changes in intracellular calcium contribute to arrhythmias associated with acute ischemia and reperfusion. Calcium may also be important in the genesis of ventricular tachycardia induced by exercise and by digitalis. The author emphasizes that electrolyte and metabolic abnormalities should be routinely considered as potential etiologic factors in hypertensive and congestive heart failure patients with life-threatening ventricular arrhythmias, particularly those receiving thiazide and loop diuretics.

330. Petri M, Cumber P, Grimes L, et al, "The Metabolic Effects of Thiazide Therapy in the Elderly: A Population Study," *Age Ageing,* 1986, 15(3):151-5.

Plasma and intracellular electrolytes and plasma glucose were measured in an elderly population to quantify the risk of metabolic abnormalities. Reductions in both plasma and cellular magnesium and potassium were found in the thiazide-treated subjects. Hypomagnesemia occurred In 48% of the thiazide-treated group, and 28% were hypokalemic. The authors conclude that magnesium and potassium depletion are commonly associated with thiazide therapy in the elderly.

331. Hollifield JW, "Potassium and Magnesium Abnormalities: Diuretics and Arrhythmias in Hypertension," *Am J Med,* 1984, 77(5A):28-32.

Thiazide diuretics are widely accepted as the cornerstone of antihypertensive treatment programs. Thirty-eight patients with moderate diastolic hypertension were treated with hydrochlorothiazide. Dose escalation was discontinued when either normal blood pressure was attained or a dose of 200 mg was reached, then maintained for 24 weeks of continuous thiazide monotherapy. During dose escalation and long-term maintenance therapy, the serum potassium and magnesium levels fell in a step-wise, dose-dependent fashion. In a separate study, the occurrence of premature ventricular contractions correlated significantly with the decrease in serum potassium and serum magnesium in patients receiving thiazide diuretics. The author concluded that thiazide therapy causes both potassium and magnesium depletion, and these decreases correlate well with the occurrence of ventricular ectopy.

332. Robertson JI, "Diuretics, Potassium Depletion and the Risk of Arrhythmias," *Eur Heart J,* 1984, 5(Suppl A):25-8.

The author reviews evidence which suggests that the use of thiazide diuretics in the treatment of essential hypertension causes a fall in both plasma and total body potassium. The incidence of ventricular arrhythmias is noted to correlate to the potassium deficit and may be exacerbated by concomitant magnesium deficiency. To reduce the potential risk of rhythm disturbance, the author recommends careful maintenance of serum potassium levels above 3.5 mmol/L.

Thiazide Diuretics & Potassium Depletion - No Negative Studies

Thiazide Diuretics & Sodium Depletion

333. Clark BA, Shannon RP, Rosa RM, et al, "Increased Susceptibility to Thiazide-Induced Hyponatremia in the Elderly," *J Am Soc Nephrol*, 1994, 5(4):1106-11.

To determine the relationship between age and susceptibility to thiazide-induced changes in serum osmolality, three groups were studied. Eleven healthy young volunteers, eight healthy elderly volunteers, and five elderly patients with a history of thiazide-induced hyponatremia were each evaluated with respect to their handling of a water load following 3 days of thiazide ingestion. There were no differences in minimum urinary osmolality between young and old. However, healthy older patients demonstrated lower hourly free water clearances and greater declines in serum osmolality in response to water loading. Greater impairment was noted in elderly subjects in minimum urine osmolality and free water clearance, as well as a delayed recovery of serum osmolality following hydrochlorothiazide. Restudy of a subset of the subjects following ibuprofen administration suggested a role for renal prostaglandins in modulating hyponatremia.

334. Friedman E, Shadel M, Halkin H, et al, "Thiazide-Induced Hyponatremia. Reproducibility by Single Dose Rechallenge and an Analysis of Pathogenesis," *Ann Intern Med*, 1989, 110(1):24-30.

In a prospective controlled study, patients with a history of thiazide-induced hyponatremia were compared to two control groups (10 young healthy volunteers and 11 elderly hypertensive patients). A single dose of hydrochlorothiazide, 50 mg, and amiloride, 5 mg was administered to each subject. The difference in the decrease in serum sodium within 6-8 hours and serum osmolality was significantly greater in the elderly patients as compared to the young controls. The response of patients to drug administration did not differ from both control groups regarding sodium and potassium urinary excretion, osmolar and free water clearance, and antidiuretic hormone blood levels. The authors concluded the response to a single dose of a thiazide diuretic may predict the development of hyponatremia. Further, they noted an increase in body weight (apparently due to polydipsia) may play a role in the pathogenesis of thiazide-induced hyponatremia.

335. Kone B, Gimenez L, and Watson AJ, "Thiazide-Induced Hyponatremia," *South Med J*, 1986, 79(11):1456-7.

A case of severe acute hyponatremia following long-term thiazide treatment is reported. The hyponatremia developed after 8 months of previously uneventful therapy, when the patient was instructed to increase his water intake. The hydration apparently unmasked an impairment of water excretion. Withdrawal of the thiazide promptly resulted in a diuresis and rapid correction of the hyponatremia.

336. Oles KS and Denham JW, "Hyponatremia Induced by Thiazide-Like Diuretics in the Elderly," *South Med J*, 1984, 77(10):1314-5.

In three elderly patients, five episodes of hydrochlorothiazide-induced hyponatremia are described. Thiazide diuretic use was linked to each event. The authors note that the nonspecific nature of hyponatremia symptoms warrant close monitoring of elderly patients receiving thiazide diuretics.

337. Johnson JE and Wright LF, "Thiazide-Induced Hyponatremia," *South Med J*, 1983, 76(11):1363-7.

CARDIOVASCULAR DRUGS *(Continued)*

A case report of a 54-year-old woman who experienced seizures and a focal neurologic deficit associated with thiazide-induced hyponatremia. Following the episode, the patient was rechallenged with hydrochlorothiazide and metabolic balance studies were undertaken. The patient's hyponatremia could not be explained solely on the basis of changes in external water and electrolyte balance. The authors concluded that the rapidity of the induced changes suggests osmolar inactivation and that this phenomena may contribute to the severe alteration in tonicity observed in some patients.

Thiazide Diuretics & Phosphate Depletion

338. Itescu S, Haskell LP, and Tannenberg AM, "Thiazide-Induced Clinically Significant Hypophosphatemia," *Clin Nephrol*, 1987, 27(3):161-2.

No abstract available.

Thiazide Diuretics & Zinc Depletion

339. Reyes AJ, Olhaberry JV, Leary WP, et al, "Urinary Zinc Excretion, Diuretics, Zinc Deficiency and Some Side-effects of Diuretics," *S Afr Med J*, 1983, 64(24):936-41.

This article notes that hyperzincuria caused by common distal tubular diuretics such as thiazides and chlorthalidone can cause zinc deficiency, particularly when factors such as alcoholism, renal insufficiency and pregnancy are also present. Symptoms of zinc deficiency are discussed.

340. Reyes AJ, Leary WP, Lockett CJ, et al, "Diuretics and Zinc," *S Afr Med J*, 1982, 62(11):373-5.

Distal tubule diuretics increase urinary zinc output. This review describes mechanisms which could involve both direct and hormone-mediated processes. As a consequence, significant zinc depletion may occur during long-term administration of distal tubule diuretics. This may be detrimental in conditions associated with diminished total body zinc levels (hepatic cirrhosis, diabetes mellitus, gastrointestinal disorders, and many renal diseases). Attention to the early symptoms of zinc deficiency such as hypogeusia, hyposmia, abnormal dark adaptation, and impotence, and the monitoring of serum zinc levels are advisable during long-term treatment with these agents.

341. Mountokalakis T, Dourakis S, Karatzas N, et al, "Zinc Deficiency in Mild Hypertensive Patients Treated With Diuretics," *J Hypertens Suppl*, 1984, 2(3):S571-2.

In mild hypertensive patients treated with thiazides for 6-36 months, mean hair zinc was found to be significantly lower than in similar patients who had not been given diuretics. Mean serum zinc did not differ between the two groups. The authors note that chronic diuretic treatment can result in zinc deficiency through enhanced urinary zinc excretion.

342. Cohanim M and Yendt ER, "The Effects of Thiazides on Serum and Urinary Zinc in Patients With Renal Calculi," *Johns Hopkins Med J*, 1975, 136(3):137-41.

Urine zinc excretion was found to be significantly higher in male patients with renal calculi than in normal male subjects. However, there was no significant difference between female patients. There is a possibility that lower urine zinc excretion may contribute to the formation of renal calculi in some patients. Hydrochlorothiazide was noted to produce a large and sustained increase in urinary zinc excretion, which might contribute to the efficacy of this drug in the prevention of calcific renal stones. The authors noted that serum zinc levels remained normal in the majority of subjects on long-term thiazide therapy. However, the occasional finding of subnormal levels suggests a risk of zinc deficiency.

Thiazide Diuretics & Zinc Depletion - No Negative Studies

CARDIAC GLYCOSIDES

Cardiac Glycosides & Calcium Depletion

343. Kupfer S and Kosovsky JD, "Effects of Cardiac Glycosides on Renal Tubular Transport of Calcium, Magnesium, Inorganic Phosphate and Glucose in the Dog," *J Clin Investig*, 1965, 44:1143.

    In a dog model, the authors report that digoxin causes increased renal excretion of calcium, magnesium, and inorganic phosphate.

Cardiac Glycosides & Calcium Depletion - No Negative Studies

Cardiac Glycosides & Magnesium Depletion

344. Schwinger RH and Erdmann E, "Heart Failure and Electrolyte Disturbances," *Methods Find Exp Clin Pharmacol*, 1992, 14(4):315-25.

    This review notes that electrolyte abnormalities are a common and potentially hazardous complication of heart failure and its treatment. The roles of calcium, magnesium, and potassium are discussed. The authors note that digoxin directly limits reabsorption of magnesium in the renal tubule, leading to magnesium excretion. Low magnesium and potassium concentrations may enhance toxicity from digitalis glycosides. The authors encourage prevention of electrolyte abnormalities in addition to repletion in deficiency.

345. Kupfer S and Kosovsky JD, "Effects of Cardiac Glycosides on Renal Tubular Transport of Calcium, Magnesium, Inorganic Phosphate and Glucose in the Dog," *J of Clin Investig*, 1965, 44:1143.

    In a dog model, the authors report that digoxin causes increased renal excretion of calcium, magnesium, and inorganic phosphate.

Cardiac Glycosides & Magnesium Depletion - No Negative Studies

Cardiac Glycosides & Phosphorus Depletion

346. Kupfer S and Kosovsky JD, "Effects of Cardiac Glycosides on Renal Tubular Transport of Calcium, Magnesium, Inorganic Phosphate and Glucose in the Dog," *J Clin Investig*, 1965, 44:1143.

    In a dog model, the authors report that digoxin causes increased renal excretion of calcium, magnesium, and inorganic phosphate.

Cardiac Glycosides & Phosphorus Depletion - No Negative Studies

Cardiac Glycosides & Thiamine Depletion

347. Zangen A, Botzer D, Zangen R, et al, "Furosemide and Digoxin Inhibit Thiamine Uptake in Cardiac Cells," *Eur J Pharmacol*, 1998, 361(1):151-5.

    In an *in vitro* model, cardiac cells demonstrated a loss of intracellular thiamine after treatment with furosemide or digoxin. In addition, cells grown in thiamine-free media for 7 days demonstrated decreased thiamine uptake in the presence of either furosemide or digoxin. This effect was dose-

CARDIOVASCULAR DRUGS *(Continued)*

dependent, and the effects were additive when furosemide and digoxin were combined. The authors suggest thiamine deficiency may occur in patients receiving chronic treatment with these agents.

BETA-BLOCKERS

Beta-Blockers & Coenzyme Q_{10} Depletion

348. Kishi H, Kishi T, and Folkers K, "Bioenergetics in Clinical Medicine. III. Inhibition of Coenzyme Q_{10}-Enzymes by Clinically Used Antihypertensive Drugs," *Res Commun Chem Pathol Pharmacol*, 1975, 12(3):533-40.

    Eight antihypertensive drugs were tested for inhibition of two mitochondrial coenzyme Q_{10}-enzymes of heart tissue, succinoxidase, and NADH-oxidase. These enzymes are important to the bioenergetics of cardiac function. Diazoxide and propranolol significantly inhibited both enzymes. Metoprolol did not inhibit succinoxidase, and was one-fourth as active as propranolol for inhibition of NADH-oxidase. Hydrochlorothiazide, hydralazine, and clonidine also inhibited CoQ_{10}-NADH-oxidase. Reserpine did not inhibit either CoQ_{10}-enzyme, and methyldopa was a very weak inhibitor of succinoxidase. The authors conclude that some clinical side-effects of propranolol may be due, in part, to inhibition of CoQ_{10}-enzymes. In particular, pre-existing deficiencies of coenzyme Q_{10} in the myocardium of hypertensive patients could be exacerbated by treatment with propranolol.

349. Kishi T, Watanabe T, Folkers K, "Bioenergetics in Clinical Medicine XV. Inhibition of Coenzyme Q_{10}-Enzymes by Clinically Used Adrenergic Blockers of Beta-Receptors," *Res Commun Chem Pathol Pharmacol*, 1977, 17(1):157-64.

    A number of beta-blockers were evaluated for their effect on myocardial CoQ_{10} enzymes. It was noted that myocardial depression could be related to these bioenergetic enzymes. Propranolol was noted to have the greatest effect, while metoprolol was less inhibitory against myocardial CoQ_{10} enzymes. Timolol was noted to have negligible effects on these enzymes, and was proposed to be a preferred agent due to this property.

Beta- Blockers & Coenzyme Q_{10} Depletion - No Negative Studies

CHOLESTEROL-LOWERING AGENTS

GEMFIBROZIL

Gemfibrozil Depletes Vitamin E & Coenzyme Q$_{10}$ Depletion

350. Aberg F, Appelkvist EL, Broijersen A, et al, "Gemfibrozil-Induced Decrease in Serum Ubiquinone and Alpha- and Gamma-Tocopherol Levels in Men With Combined Hyperlipidaemia," *Eur J Clin Invest*, 1998, 28(3):235-42.

In a randomized, placebo-controlled cross-over study of 21 men with combined hyperlipidaemia, the effect of 10-12 weeks of gemfibrozil treatment on the serum concentrations of ubiquinone-10 or alpha- or gamma-tocopherol was evaluated. Median levels of each antioxidant decreased during gemfibrozil treatment. However, the values decreased only to levels encountered in normal control subjects. The authors concluded that gemfibrozil treatment of men with combined hyperlipidaemia reduces serum antioxidant levels to the levels seen in healthy normolipidaemic men. The authors note that the mechanisms and relevance of their findings are unclear and propose further investigation.

HMG-CoA REDUCTASE INHIBITORS

HMG-CoA Reductase Inhibitors & Coenzyme Q$_{10}$ Depletion

351. Folkers K, Langsjoen P, Willis R, et al, "Lovastatin Decreases Coenzyme Q Levels in Humans," *Proc Natl Acad Sci U S A*, 1990, 87(22):8931-4.

Inhibition of 3-hydroxy-3-methylglutaryl-coenzyme A reductase may inhibit the biosynthesis of coenzyme Q$_{10}$, an enzyme which is important for cardiac function. This article reports on three protocols (one described in more detail in this section; see Willis, et al) which were designed to determine whether lovastatin inhibited the biosynthesis of coenzyme Q$_{10}$. Data from the three protocols demonstrated that lovastatin does indeed lower levels of CoQ$_{10}$. An increase in cardiac disease from lovastatin, particularly in patients with class IV cardiomyopathy was proposed. Oral administration of CoQ$_{10}$ increased blood levels of CoQ$_{10}$ and improved cardiac function in most patients. The authors also speculate that some cases of lovastatin-induced liver dysfunction may be attributed to a deficiency of CoQ$_{10}$.

352. Mortensen SA, Leth A, Agner E, et al, "Dose-Related Decrease of Serum Coenzyme Q$_{10}$ During Treatment With HMG-CoA Reductase Inhibitors," *Mol Aspects Med*, 1997, 18(Suppl):S137-44.

In a randomized, double-blind trial, 45 hypercholesterolemic patients were treated with increasing dosages of either lovastatin (20-80 mg/day) or pravastatin (10-40 mg/day). Serum levels of coenzyme Q$_{10}$ and cholesterol were measured over 18 weeks of treatment. A significant, dose-related decrease in the serum level of coenzyme Q$_{10}$ was found in both the pravastatin and lovastatin groups at the end of the study. The decrease after lovastatin therapy was more pronounced. The authors note that HMG-CoA reductase inhibitors are generally safe and effective over a limited time, but patients should be monitored for possible adverse consequences of coenzyme Q$_{10}$ reductions during long-term therapy.

353. Ghirlanda G, Oradei A, Manto A, et al, "Evidence of Plasma CoQ$_{10}$-Lowering Effect by HMG-CoA Reductase Inhibitors: A Double-Blind, Placebo-Controlled Study," *J Clin Pharmacol*, 1993, 33(3):226-9.

This article reports two studies of the effects of pravastatin and simvastatin on coenzyme Q$_{10}$ levels. One study included healthy volunteers treated with

CHOLESTEROL-LOWERING AGENTS *(Continued)*

20 mg/day of pravastatin or simvastatin for a month. The second was a double-blind, controlled study of 30 hypercholesterolemic patients treated with pravastatin, simvastatin, or placebo for 3 months. Significant changes in total cholesterol and coenzyme Q_{10} levels were observed in the volunteer group. Coenzyme Q_{10} reductions of approximately 40% were noted. As compared to placebo, similar reductions were observed in hypercholesterolemic patients treated with pravastatin or simvastatin. It was concluded that treatment with HMG-CoA reductase inhibitors lowers both total cholesterol and coenzyme Q_{10} plasma levels.

354. Willis RA, Folkers K, Tucker JL, et al, "Lovastatin Decreases Coenzyme Q Levels in Rats," *Proc Natl Acad Sci U S A*, 1990, 87(22):8928-30.

This study, conducted in rats, was designed to determine whether lovastatin treatment decreases coenzyme Q_{10} levels. In addition, the possibility that decreases may be prevented by coenzyme Q_{10} supplementation was investigated. Coenzyme Q_{10} concentrations decreased in all tissues analyzed in the lovastatin-treated rats. Lovastatin-treated animals which received coenzyme Q_{10} supplementation had blood, heart, and liver CoQ_{10} concentrations approximately equal to or higher than those of control animals. The authors conclude that lovastatin lowered tissue concentrations of coenzyme Q_{10}, and this depletion may be prevented by supplementation.

355. Morand OH, Aebi JD, Dehmlow H, et al, "Ro 48-8.071, A New 2,3-Oxidosqualene:lanosterol Cyclase Inhibitor Lowering Plasma Cholesterol in Hamsters, Squirrel Monkeys, and Minipigs: Comparison to Simvastatin," *J Lipid Res*, 1997, 38(2):373-90.

In an *in vitro* as well as several animal models, two cholesterol lowering drugs were evaluated with respect to efficacy and impact on enzyme levels. In contrast to a cholesterol-lowering drug which did not inhibit HMG CoA reductase, simvastatin stimulated an increased production of several enzymes while reducing coenzyme Q_{10} levels in liver and heart tissue.

356. De Pinieux G, Chariot P, Ammi-Said M, et al, "Lipid-Lowering Drugs and Mitochondrial Function: Effects of HMG-CoA Reductase Inhibitors on Serum Ubiquinone and Blood Lactate/Pyruvate Ratio," *Br J Clin Pharmacol*, 1996, 42(3):333-7.

The effect of lipid-lowering drugs on coenzyme Q_{10} serum levels and mitochondrial function as assessed by blood lactate/pyruvate ratio was evaluated in 80 hypercholesterolaemic patients (40 treated by statins, 20 treated by fibrates, and 20 control untreated patients). All patients had a total cholesterol level >6.0 mmol/L. Twenty healthy controls were also evaluated. Lactate/pyruvate ratios were significantly higher in patients treated with statins as compared to untreated hypercholesterolemic patients or healthy controls. Coenzyme Q_{10} serum levels were lower in statin-treated patients than in untreated hypercholesterolemic patients. The authors conclude that statin therapy can be associated with suggestive evidence of mitochondrial dysfunction. Low serum levels of ubiquinone could potentially contribute to mitochondrial dysfunction.

357. Bargossi AM, Grossi G, Fiorella PL, et al, "Exogenous CoQ_{10} Supplementation Prevents Plasma Ubiquinone Reduction Induced by HMG-CoA Reductase Inhibitors," *Mol Aspects Med*, 1994, 15 (Suppl):187-93.

The CoQ polyisoprenoid side chain and cholesterol share the same pathway starting from acetyl-CoA and proceeding through mevalonate and isopentenylpyrophosphate. The authors performed this study to evaluate whether vastatins (hypocholesterolemic drugs that inhibit HMG-CoA reductase) modify blood levels of ubiquinone. Thirty-four outpatients with type IIa hypercholesterolemia were treated for six months with simvastatin (20 mg) or simvastatin plus coenzyme Q_{10} (100 mg). There was a marked decrease in total cholesterol and LDL-C and in plasma and platelet coenzyme Q_{10} levels in patients receiving simvastatin alone. In contrast, in the supplemented group, a significant increase in plasma and platelet coenzyme Q_{10} was observed. The hypocholesterolemic effect was comparable in both groups. The authors conclude this study demonstrates simvastatin lowers both LDL-C and apo B plasma levels along with plasma and platelet levels of coenzyme Q_{10}. In addition, coenzyme Q_{10} supplementation prevents both plasma and platelet coenzyme Q_{10} depletion without negating the cholesterol-lowering effects of simvastatin.

358. Watts GF, Castelluccio C, Rice-Evans C, et al, "Plasma Coenzyme Q (Ubiquinone) Concentrations in Patients Treated With Simvastatin," *J Clin Pathol*, 1993, 46(11):1055-7.

Twenty hyperlipidemic patients treated with diet and simvastatin were compared to patients treated with diet alone and a control population of normal volunteers. Patients treated with simvastatin had a significantly lower plasma coenzyme Q_{10} than patients receiving diet alone or normal controls. There was a significant inverse association between coenzyme Q_{10} and dose of simvastatin. The authors concluded that simvastatin may lower the plasma coenzyme Q_{10} concentration. Further, this may exceed the reduction in cholesterol. The authors propose further investigation.

359. Belichard P, Pruneau D, and Zhiri A, "Effect of a Long-Term Treatment With Lovastatin or Fenofibrate on Hepatic and Cardiac Ubiquinone Levels in Cardiomyopathic Hamster," *Biochem Biophys Acta*, 1993, 1169(1):98-102.

The effect of long-term oral administration of lovastatin (50 mg/kg/day) or fenofibrate (200 mg/kg/day) was evaluated with respect to their impact on ubiquinone levels in the heart and the liver of cardiomyopathic hamsters. Lovastatin significantly decreased ubiquinone concentrations, as compared to controls, in the heart, but not in the liver. Fenofibrate did not alter these parameters.

360. Hanaki Y, Sugiyama S, Ozawa T, et al, "Coenzyme Q_{10} and Coronary Artery Disease," *Clin Investig*, 1993, 71(8 Suppl):S112-5.

Plasma levels of ubiquinone, total cholesterol, high-density lipoprotein (HDL) cholesterol, and triglycerides were measured in 29 patients receiving pravastatin, 245 normal subjects and in 104 patients with coronary artery disease not receiving pravastatin. Ubiquinone concentrations were significantly lower in the patient groups as compared to normal subjects. The authors conclude that the HMG CoA reductase inhibitor decreased plasma cholesterol level, but did not improve either the ubiquinone level or the LDL/ubiquinone ratio. Further, they propose that the LDL/ubiquinone ratio is likely to be a risk factor for atherogenesis, and administration of ubiquinone to patients at risk may be necessary.

361. Appelkvist EL, Edlund C, Low P, et al, "Effects of Inhibitors of Hydroxymethylglutaryl Coenzyme A Reductase on Coenzyme Q and Dolichol Biosynthesis," *Clin Investig*, 1993, 71(8 Suppl):S97-102.

In a rat model, oral administration of mevinolin was found to decrease dolichol, dolichyl-P, and coenzyme Q levels in heart and skeletal muscle. In addition, an increase in the dolichol level with a decrease in the coenzyme Q content was noted in the liver. The amounts of dolichyl-P decreased in heart and muscle and increased in brain. Both up-regulation and down-regulation

CHOLESTEROL-LOWERING AGENTS *(Continued)*

of different proteins was noted to occur in various tissues, resulting in modifications in lipid synthesis. Hypercholesterolemic patients were found to have high blood coenzyme Q levels, which decreased upon pravastatin treatment (although they remained above control values). The authors concluded that HMG-coenzyme A reductase inhibitors do not selectively lower cholesterol levels, but also modify dolichol and coenzyme Q content and synthesis.

HMG-CoA Reductase Inhibitors &Coenzyme Q_{10} Depletion - Negative Studies

362. Human JA, Ubbink JB, Jerling JJ, et al, "The Effect of Simvastatin on the Plasma Antioxidant Concentrations in Patients With Hypercholesterolaemia," *Clin Chim Acta*, 1997, 263(1):67-77.

Forty-seven patients, treated with 10 mg or 20 mg of simvastatin per day for 14 weeks were monitored for changes in antioxidant levels. The results of this study were interpreted to suggest that the significant decline in circulating alpha-tocopherol and coenzyme Q_{10} concentrations were primarily a function of the decline in total serum cholesterol.

BILE ACID SEQUESTRANTS (CHOLESTYRAMINE)

NOTE: Cholestyramine causes the malabsorption of many nutrients. Rather than report each nutrient individually, a note at the beginning of each abstract will indicate which nutrient depletions are reported in that particular study.

Bile Acid Sequestrants (Cholestyramine) & Nutrient Depletions

363. Hathcock JN, "Metabolic Mechanisms of Drug-Nutrient Interactions," *Fed Proc*, 1985, 44(1 Pt 1):124-9.

This review reports depletion of fat-soluble vitamins A, D, E, K, and beta-carotene by bile acid sequestrants and some laxatives.

364. West RJ and Lloyd JK, "The Effect of Cholestyramine on Intestinal Absorption," *Gut*, 1975, 16(2):93-8.

This study reports depletion of folic acid, vitamin A, vitamin E, and phosphorus in 18 children with familial hypercholesterolemia treated with cholestyramine for 1-1.5 years. In addition, prolonged treatment resulted in folate deficiency. Oral folic acid supplementation (5 mg daily) reversed this depletion. A significant decrease in the concentrations of vitamins A and E and of inorganic phosphorus was noted over the first 2 years of treatment, although values remained within the normal range. The authors suggest that vitamin supplementation may not be necessary, yet a steady decrease in vitamins A and E was observed.

365. Cywes C and Millar AJ, "Assessment of the Nutritional Status of Infants and Children With Biliary Atresia," *S Afr Med J*, 1990, 77(3):131-5.

Eleven infants and children with biliary atresia (age range 1, 5 months to 7 years) were studied. All patients with cholestasis showed evidence of fat-soluble vitamin deficiency and zinc deficiency, but had raised serum copper levels. In spite of supplementation, 3 of 4 patients receiving cholestyramine had very low levels of vitamin E.

366. Elinder LS, Hadell K, Johansson J, et al, "Probucol Treatment Decreases Serum Concentrations of Diet-Derived Antioxidants," *Arterioscler Thromb Vasc Biol*, 1995, 15(8):1057-63.

In a 3-year, double-blind, randomized trial of 303 hypercholesterolemic subjects, the progression of femoral atherosclerosis and antioxidant concentrations were investigated. Both serum and lipoprotein antioxidant levels were measured. Cholestyramine lowered serum concentrations of vitamin E, beta-carotene, and lycopene. This was attributed to impaired gastrointestinal absorption and lowering of serum cholesterol. Probucol reduced serum vitamin E secondary to a lowering of cholesterol and triglyceride. The carotenoids were also reduced by probucol, an effect which was likely due to a reduction in lipoprotein particle size. The authors conclude this study demonstrates that these drugs may have unfavorable effects on blood levels of antioxidants derived from the diet.

367. Hoppner K and Lampi B, "Bioavailability of Folate Following Ingestion of Cholestyramine in the Rat," *Int J Vitam Nutr Res*, 1991, 61(2):130-4.

Using a rat bioassay, the effect of cholestyramine ingestion on the intestinal deconjugation and absorption of folic acid and brewers yeast folate was investigated. Ingestion of cholestyramine significantly reduced the bioavailability of folic acid as compared to brewers yeast folate in rats.

368. Knodel LC and Talbert RL, "Adverse Effects of Hypolipidaemic Drugs," *Med Toxicol*, 1987, 2(1):10-32.

In this review, large doses of cholestyramine (>32 g/day) are noted to be associated with malabsorption of fat-soluble vitamins. The authors observe that osteomalacia and, on rare occasions, hemorrhagic diathesis are reported with cholestyramine impairment of vitamin D and vitamin K absorption.

369. Watkins DW, Khalafi R, Cassidy MM, et al, "Alterations in Calcium, Magnesium, Iron, and Zinc Metabolism by Dietary Cholestyramine," *Dig Dis Sci*, 1985, 30(5):477-82.

The influence of cholestyramine on dietary balance of four mineral elements was investigated in rats. Cholestyramine-fed rats had a net negative balance for calcium and, although a net positive balance for magnesium, iron, and zinc was maintained, these values were lower than controls. Other effects of cholestyramine included increased urinary excretion of calcium and magnesium, decreased urinary zinc, and alkalinization of urine. A reduction in serum magnesium was observed. The authors speculate that alterations in calcium, magnesium, and zinc metabolism could be explained by inadequate gastrointestinal vitamin D absorption, with a resultant increase in secretion of parathyroid hormone. Resin binding of iron could account for the changes in iron balance.

370. Matsui MS and Rozovski SJ, "Drug-Nutrient Interaction," *Clin Ther*, 1982, 4(6):423-40.

In this review, cholestyramine is noted to be associated with malabsorption of vitamins. Reports suggesting that cholestyramine affects absorption of the fat-soluble vitamins K and D and folic acid are discussed.

Bile Acid Sequestrants (Cholestyramine) & Nutrient Depletion - No Negative Studies

BILE ACID SEQUESTRANTS - COLESTIPOL

Bile Acid Sequestrants (Colestipol) & Vitamins A and E Depletion

371. Schwarz KB, Goldstein PD, Witztum JL, et al, "Fat-Soluble Vitamin Concentrations in Hypercholesterolemic Children Treated With Colestipol," *Pediatrics*, 1980, 65(2):243-50.

CHOLESTEROL-LOWERING AGENTS *(Continued)*

During 24 months of colestipol therapy plus diet, serum vitamin A and E concentrations decreased in patients who were compliant with therapy. However, concentrations remained within normal limits.

Bile Acid Sequestrants (Colestipol) & Folic Acid, Vitamin D, Vitamin E, and Carotenoids Depletion

372. Tonstad S, Sivertsen M, Aksnes L, et al, "Low Dose Colestipol in Adolescents With Familial Hypercholesterolaemia," *Arch Dis Child*, 1996, 74(2):157-60.

    The effects of orange colestipol granules in children with familial hypercholesterolemia were examined initially in an 8-week, double-blind, placebo-controlled protocol, followed by a period of open treatment for 44-52 weeks. Levels of serum folate, vitamin E, and carotenoids were reduced in the colestipol group, but not the vitamin E/cholesterol and carotenoid/cholesterol ratios, or serum concentrations of vitamins A and D. Although no adverse effects on weight gain or linear growth velocity were observed, folate and possibly vitamin D supplementation were recommended.

Bile Acid Sequestrants & Vitamin B_{12}, Folic Acid, and Iron Depletion

373. Leonard JP, Desager JP, Beckers C, et al, "*In vitro* Binding of Various Biological Substances by Two Hypocholesterolaemic Resins, Cholestyramine and Colestipol," *Arzneimittelforschung*, 1979, 29(7):979-81.

    The *in vitro* binding of several compounds, including vitamin B_{12}, vitamin B_{12}-intrinsic factor complex, folic acid, iron citrate and calcium chloride, with cholestyramine and colestipol, was investigated. Both resins demonstrated extensive binding of vitamin B_{12}-intrinsic factor complex, folic acid, and iron citrate. Cholestyramine also bound calcium. These data were interpreted to emphasize the necessity of regular nutritional monitoring during chronic treatment with these two resins.

Edetate Calcium Disodium (EDTA)

EDTA & Calcium Depletion

374. Desmecht DJ, Linden AS, Godeau JM, et al, "Experimental Production of Hypocalcemia by EDTA Infusion in Calves: A Critical Appraisal Assessed From the Profile of Blood Chemicals and Enzymes," *Comp Biochem Physiol A Physiol*, 1995, 110(2):115-30.

EDTA infusion in bovine calves allowed effective chelation of blood calcium, leading to progressive hypocalcemia. Magnesium levels remained constant and concentrations of other ions remained within the normal range. Monitoring of systemic arterial pressure provided a valuable tool to estimate the degree of hypocalcemia.

375. Hotz J, Minnie H, and Ziegler R, "Behavior of Gastric Secretion in Acute EDTA-Hypocalcemia in Man," *Verh Dtsch Ges Inn Med*, 1971, 77:501-4.

No abstract available.

ELECTROLYTE REPLACEMENT

POTASSIUM CHLORIDE

Potassium Chloride & Vitamin B_{12} Depletion

376. Palva IP, Salokannel SJ, Timonen T, et al, "Drug-Induced Malabsorption of Vitamin B_{12}. IV. Malabsorption and Deficiency of B_{12} During Treatment With Slow-Release Potassium Chloride," *Acta Med Scand*, 1972, 191(4):355-7.

No abstract available.

377. Salokannel SJ, Palva IP, Takkunen JT, et al, "Malabsorption of Vitamin B_{12} During Treatment With Slow-Release Potassium Chloride. Preliminary Report," *Acta Med Scand*, 1970, 187(5):431-2.

No abstract available.

Potassium Chloride & Vitamin B_{12} Depletion - No Negative Studies

FEMALE HORMONES

ESTROGEN REPLACEMENT THERAPY

A substantial body of research has been published on the nutritional depletions caused by orally ingested estrogen in the form of oral contraceptives. Unfortunately, very little research has been done on the estrogen-containing medications used for estrogen replacement therapy (ERT) and hormone replacement therapy (HRT). Although there may be similarities, this text can only report what has been scientifically documented.

Estrogen Replacement Therapy & Vitamin B₆ Depletion

378. Haspels AA, Bennink HJ, and Schreurs WH, "Disturbance of Tryptophan Metabolism and Its Correction During Oestrogen Treatment in Postmenopausal Women," *Maturitas*, 1978, 1(1):15-20.

A relative pyridoxine deficiency was found in all women studied who were using conjugated estrogens. This was related to disturbed tryptophan metabolism. The authors note that the intake of synthetic estrogens such as ethinyl estradiol has already been found to lead to a disturbance of tryptophan metabolism and to a deficiency of vitamin B_6. Alteration of tryptophan metabolism based on xanthurenic acid excretion was only slightly increased in three women who used concurrent progestins. The biochemical changes were felt to be easily corrected by administration of vitamin B_6.

Estrogen Replacement Therapy & Magnesium Depletion

379. Seelig MS, "Interrelationship of Magnesium and Estrogen in Cardiovascular and Bone Disorders, Eclampsia, Migraine, and Premenstrual Syndrome," *J Am Coll Nutr*, 1993, 12(4):442-58.

Estrogen's enhancement of magnesium utilization and uptake by soft tissues and bone may explain resistance of young women to heart disease and osteoporosis. This may also explain the increased prevalence of these diseases when estrogen secretion ceases. However, estrogen-induced magnesium shifts can be deleterious when estrogen levels are high and magnesium intake is low. The resultant lowering of blood magnesium can increase the calcium/magnesium ratio. This alteration may favor coagulation. The author expresses that calcium supplementation in the face of low magnesium intake may increase the risk of thrombosis.

ORAL CONTRACEPTIVES

Oral Contraceptives & Folic Acid Depletion

380. Webb JL, "Nutritional Effects of Oral Contraceptive Use: A Review," *J Reprod Med*, 1980, 25(4):150-6.

This review notes that oral contraceptives have been shown to affect a number of metabolic and nutritional processes. Oral contraceptives were shown to depress the physiologic levels of six nutrients (riboflavin, pyridoxine, folacin, vitamin B_{12}, ascorbic acid, and zinc). Levels of three others (vitamin K, iron, and copper) were elevated. Little or no change was noted in alpha tocopherol and questionable increases in vitamin A were noted. The author emphasized that females consuming oral contraceptives should pay particular attention to vitamin and mineral intake. If warranted, supplements of needed nutrients may be used.

FEMALE HORMONES *(Continued)*

381. Prasad AS, Lei KY, Moghissi KS, et al, "Effect of Oral Contraceptives on Nutrients. III. Vitamins B_6, B_{12}, and Folic Acid," *Am J Obstet Gynecol*, 1976, 125(8):1063-9.

    The interactions of oral contraceptive agents with vitamins was studied in a large population. As compared to controls, a higher incidence of abnormal clinical signs related to vitamin deficiencies was seen in the upper socioeconomic group. Plasma pyridoxal phosphate and red cell and serum folate levels were lower in subjects using contraceptive agents. With respect to vitamins B_6 and folic acid, a relative deficiency is suggested in oral contraceptive users. No significant effect on serum vitamin B_{12} was observed.

382. Shojania AM, "Oral Contraceptives: Effect of Folate and Vitamin B_{12} Metabolism," *Can Med Assoc J*, 1982, 126(3):244-7.

    As shown by slightly but significantly lower levels of folate in serum and erythrocytes, and an increased urinary excretion of formiminoglutamic acid, women who use oral contraceptives have impaired folate metabolism. The vitamin B_{12} level in their serum is also significantly lower than in controls. However, there is no evidence of associated tissue depletion of vitamin B_{12}. Of particular importance, clinicians are advised to ensure that women who stop taking "the pill" in order to become pregnant have adequate folate stores prior to conception.

383. Matsui MS and Rozovski SJ, "Drug-Nutrient Interaction," *Clin Ther*, 1982, 4(6):423-40.

    In this review, the effect of certain drugs on nutrient metabolism is discussed. Oral contraceptives interfere with the metabolism of folic acid and ascorbic acid. They also seem to interfere with riboflavin in nutritional deficiency. Simultaneous supplementation with folate has been recommended in some cases.

384. Ahmed F, Bamji MS, and Iyengar L, "Effect of Oral Contraceptive Agents on Vitamin Nutrition Status," *Am J Clin Nutr*, 1975, 28(6):606-15.

    The effects of low estrogen oral contraceptives on some of the biochemical markers of vitamin status were investigated. Two groups were evaluated, a group of women who had used the pill for 6-12 months and a group followed from an initial exam through the first 6 months of treatment. Observed changes included an increased excretion of kynurenic acid and xanthurenic acid following tryptophan load, increased vitamin A levels, a fall in erythrocyte folate levels, a fall in erythrocyte transketolase activity, and a fall in erythrocyte riboflavin concentration. Most of these changes were observed during the first few cycles of oral contraceptive treatment.

385. Butterworth CE Jr, Hatch KD, Gore H, et al, "Improvement in Cervical Dysplasia Associated With Folic Acid Therapy in Users of Oral Contraceptives," *Am J Clin Nutr*, 1982, 35(1):73-82.

    In a double-blind study, 47 young women with mild or moderate dysplasia of the uterine cervix received oral supplements of folic acid or a placebo daily for 3 months. All had used a combination-type oral contraceptive agent for at least 6 months. These agents were continued over the period of evaluation. Subjects returned monthly for follow-up examinations, smears, and a biopsy obtained at the end of the trial period. Mean biopsy scores from folate-supplemented subjects were significantly better than in folate-unsupplemented subjects. Final versus initial cytology scores were also improved in supplemented subjects while these were unchanged in patients receiving the placebo. Before treatment, the mean red cell folate concentration was lower in oral contraceptive agent users than in controls, and even lower among users with dysplasia. Megaloblastosis was associated with dysplasia and also improved with folate supplementation. This study indicated that a reversible, localized derangement in folate metabolism may sometimes be misdiagnosed as cervical dysplasia. Alternatively, such a derangement may be an integral component of the dysplastic process. This process may be arrested or reversed by oral folic acid supplementation.

386. Li X, Ran J, and Rao H, "Megaloblastic Changes in Cervical Epithelium Associated With Oral Contraceptives and Changes After Treatment With Folic Acid," *Chung Hua Fu Chan Ko Tsa Chih*, 1995, 30(7):410-3.

The morphology of cervical epithelium, serum folate, and red blood cell folate levels were studied in 101 women who had used oral contraceptives for over 6 months. The mean nuclear diameter of cervical epithelial cells was larger in the oral contraceptive group than in the control group. There was a significant difference in the occurrence of cervical megaloblastic changes between the two groups. The level of red blood cell folate was lower in the oral contraceptive group than that in the control group. There was no difference in serum folate, hemoglobin, and neutrophil nuclear index between the two groups. Twenty-nine women using oral contraceptives with cervical megaloblastic changes were treated with folic acid. The mean nuclear diameter of cervical epithelial cells decreased significantly and multinuclear and vacuolar changes disappeared in 26 treated women. The authors concluded that oral contraceptives reduced folate storage in the body and resulted in megaloblastic changes in cervical epithelium. Folate supplementation reversed these changes.

387. Kornberg A, Segal R, Theitler J, et al, "Folic Acid Deficiency, Megaloblastic Anemia and Peripheral Polyneuropathy Due to Oral Contraceptives," *Isr J Med Sci*, 1989, 25(3):142-5.

After 4 years of oral contraceptive use, a 34-year-old woman developed megaloblastic anemia and peripheral polyneuropathy. Low levels of folic acid and vitamin B_{12} were documented. Based on response to vitamin replacement, the authors provide a rationale to support that oral contraceptive use results in a primary folate deficiency with a secondary depletion of vitamin B_{12}.

388. Harper JM, Levine AJ, Rosenthal DL, et al, "Erythrocyte Folate Levels, Oral Contraceptive Use and Abnormal Cervical Cytology," *Acta Cytol*, 1994, 38(3):324-30.

The initial hypothesis of this study was that folate depletion is a risk factor for human papillomavirus infection and cervical epithelial cell abnormalities, including dysplasia. The prevalence of low erythrocyte folate levels was determined in 250 UCLA students. Among oral contraceptive users, low erythrocyte folate was a risk factor for an abnormal cytologic smear (both benign atypia and squamous intraepithelial lesions). In oral contraceptive users, low erythrocyte folate was a risk factor for a positive Virapap® result. The authors speculate that folate levels should be higher in oral contraceptive users than in nonusers to protect against an abnormal cytologic smear.

Oral Contraceptives & Folic Acid Depletion - Negative Studies

389. Spray GH, "Oral Contraceptives and Serum Folate Levels," *Lancet*, 1968, 2:110-11.

This study found no difference in serum and red cell folate levels among 19 women taking oral contraceptives compared to 34 healthy controls.

FEMALE HORMONES *(Continued)*

390. McLean FW, Heine MW, Held B, et al, "Relationship Between the Oral Contraceptive and Folic Acid Metabolism. Serum Folate Concentrations," *Am J Obstet Gynecol*, 1969, 104(5):745-7.

This study found no difference in serum and red cell folate levels among 39 women taking oral contraceptives compared to 17 controls.

Oral Contraceptives & Vitamin B_6 (Pyridoxine) Depletion

391. Webb JL, "Nutritional Effects of Oral Contraceptive Use: A Review," *J Reprod Med*, 1980, 25(4):150-6.

This review notes that oral contraceptives have been shown to affect a number of metabolic and nutritional processes. Oral contraceptives were shown to depress the physiologic levels of six nutrients (riboflavin, pyridoxine, folacin, vitamin B_{12}, ascorbic acid, and zinc). Levels of three others (vitamin K, iron, and copper) were elevated. Little or no change was noted in alpha tocopherol and questionable increases in vitamin A were noted. The author emphasized that females consuming oral contraceptives should pay particular attention to vitamin and mineral intake. If warranted, supplements of needed nutrients may be used.

392. Prasad AS, Lei KY, Moghissi KS, et al, "Effect of Oral Contraceptives on Nutrients. III. Vitamins B_6, B_{12}, and Folic Acid," *Am J Obstet Gynecol*, 1976, 125(8):1063-9.

Interactions of oral contraceptive agents with vitamins were studied in a large population. As compared to controls, a higher incidence of abnormal clinical signs related to vitamin deficiencies were seen in the upper socioeconomic group. Plasma pyridoxal phosphate and red cell and serum folate were lower in subjects using contraceptive agents. With respect to vitamins B_6 and folic acid, a relative deficiency is suggested in oral contraceptive users. No significant effect on serum vitamin B_{12} was observed.

393. Ahmed F, Bamji MS, and Iyengar L, "Effect of Oral Contraceptive Agents on Vitamin Nutrition Status," *Am J Clin Nutr*, 1975, 28(6):606-15.

The effects of low estrogen oral contraceptives on some of the biochemical markers of vitamin status were investigated. Two groups were evaluated, a group of women who had used the pill for 6-12 months and a group followed from an initial exam through the first 6 months of treatment. Observed changes included an increased excretion of kynurenic acid and xanthurenic acid following tryptophan load, increased EGOT activity (also an increase in vitro stimulation of EGOT with added PALP), increased vitamin A levels, a fall in erythrocyte folate levels, a fall in erythrocyte transketolase activity, and a fall in erythrocyte riboflavin concentration. Most of these changes were observed during the first few cycles of oral contraceptive treatment.

394. Bhagavan HN and Brin M, "Drug-Vitamin B_6 Interaction," *Curr Concepts Nutr*, 1983, 12:1-12.

This review notes that there are several drug types that can interfere with vitamin B_6 metabolism. The mechanisms of this interaction are detailed. Oral contraceptives are cited as an example of an interacting medication group.

395. Shaarawy M, Fayad M, Nagui AR, et al, "Serotonin Metabolism and Depression in Oral Contraceptive Users," *Contraception*, 1982, 26(2):193-204,

Thirty women using oral contraceptives for 2-5 years were evaluated to characterize their tryptophan metabolism. Results indicated the alterations in tryptophan metabolism are usually well compensated in non-depression patients, but these alterations may accentuate or precipitate the development of depression in susceptible women.

396. Haspels AA, Bennink HJ, and Schreurs WH, "Disturbance of Tryptophan Metabolism and Its Correction During Oestrogen Treatment in Postmenopausal Women," *Maturitas*, 1978, 1(1):15-20.

A relative pyridoxine deficiency was found in all women studied who were using conjugated estrogens. This was related to disturbed tryptophan metabolism. The authors note that the intake of synthetic estrogens such as ethinyl estradiol has already been found to lead to a disturbance of tryptophan metabolism and to a deficiency of vitamin B_6. Slight alteration of tryptophan metabolism based on xanthurenic acid excretion was noted in three women who used concurrent progestins. The biochemical changes were felt to be easily corrected by administration of vitamin B_6

397. Bermond P, "Therapy of Side Effects of Oral Contraceptive Agents With Vitamin B_6," *Acta Vitaminol Enzymol*, 1982, 4(1-2):45-54.

The author states that use of contraceptive hormones may be accompanied by increased urinary excretion of tryptophan metabolites similar to pyridoxine deficiency. Assessment of vitamin B_6 in humans have confirmed an impairment in women using hormonal contraception. Disturbances in the metabolism of tryptophan have been shown to be responsible for such symptoms as depression, anxiety, decrease of libido and impairment of glucose tolerance in some of the oral contraceptive users. Administration of 40 mg of vitamin B_6 daily not only restores normal biochemical values but also relieves the clinical symptoms in those vitamin B_6 deficient women. The need for further studies to clarify whether vitamin B_6 supplementation may contribute to improving depression in other situations associated with hyperoestrogenism (pregnancy, puerperium, estroprogestational treatments, etc), is noted.

398. Slap GB, "Oral Contraceptives and Depression: Impact, Prevalence and Cause," *J Adolesc Health Care*, 1981, 2(1):53-64.

This review describes the association between oral contraceptive use and depression. Trends in adolescent pregnancy, contraceptive use, and compliance are discussed. In an analysis of 12 clinical studies, 9 reported depression in 16% to 56% of women using oral contraceptives. The author notes that current biochemical research suggests oral contraceptives induce tryptophan oxygenase, which may lead to pyridoxine deficiency. However, the author states that further study is needed concerning the use of pyridoxine to prevent or treat depression in women taking oral contraceptives.

399. Kishi H, Kishi T, Williams RH, et al, "Deficiency of Vitamin B_6 in Women Taking Contraceptive Formulations," *Res Commun Chem Pathol Pharmacol*, 1997, 17(2):283-93.

The specific activities of glutamic oxaloacetic transaminase from erythrocytes of 75 women taking oral contraceptive formulations were determined. Data from this study indicate that 1-5 mg of pyridoxine is inadequate for women on contraceptives. The appropriate daily dosage is projected to be 50-100 mg. In addition, a period of 5-12 weeks of supplementation with pyridoxine can be required to reach stabilization.

Oral Contraceptives & Vitamin B_6 Depletion - Negative Studies

400. Villegas-Salas E, Ponce de Leon R, Juarez-Perez MA, et al, "Effect of Vitamin B_6 on the Side Effects of a Low-Dose Combined Oral Contraceptive," *Contraception*, 1997, 55(4):245-8.

FEMALE HORMONES *(Continued)*

A randomized, triple-blind, controlled trial of 124 women was performed to evaluate the effect of vitamin B_6 (150 mg daily) on the severity of nausea, headache, vomiting, dizziness, depression, and irritability associated with initiation of a low-dose oral contraceptive. Reductions in symptoms were observed in both the treatment group and a placebo control group. There was no statistically significant difference in reductions found in the vitamin B_6 and placebo groups, although reductions in the severity of headache and dizziness were greater in the B_6 group. The authors concluded that the decrease in severity of all oral contraceptive side effects can be explained more by a placebo effect than by a marginal pharmacological effect of vitamin B_6.

401. Masse PG, van den Berg H, Duguay C, et al, "Early Effect of a Low Dose (30 Micrograms) Ethinyl Estradiol-Containing Triphasil on Vitamin B_6 Status. A Follow-Up Study on Six Menstrual Cycles," *Int J Vitam Nutr Res*, 1996, 66(1):46-54.

By using multiple evaluation techniques, only one case (7%) of deficiency due to an oral contraceptive was evidenced. Short-term use of a relatively low-dose estrogen-containing oral contraceptive (30 mcg) did not alter parameters in plasma and erythrocytes in the majority of young subjects consuming adequate diets. However, a disturbance in vitamin B_6 metabolism was detected by some indicators. The authors concluded the use of a single measurement of vitamin B_6 may be misleading, and note this approach has been used by several investigators. Additional functional enzymatic testing may be necessary to fully establish and comprehend hormone-induced adverse effects on this metabolism.

Oral Contraceptives & Vitamin B_{12} Depletion

402. Webb JL, "Nutritional Effects of Oral Contraceptive Use: A Review," *J Reprod Med*, 1980, 25(4):150-6.

This review notes that oral contraceptives have been shown to affect a number of metabolic and nutritional processes. Oral contraceptives were shown to depress the physiologic levels of six nutrients (riboflavin, pyridoxine, folacin, vitamin B_{12}, ascorbic acid, and zinc). Levels of three others (vitamin K, iron, and copper) were elevated. Little or no change was noted in alpha tocopherol and questionable increases in vitamin A were noted. The author emphasized that females consuming oral contraceptives should pay particular attention to vitamin and mineral intake. If warranted, supplements of needed nutrients may be used.

403. Shojania AM, "Oral Contraceptives: Effect of Folate and Vitamin B_{12} Metabolism," *Can Med Assoc J*, 1982, 126(3):244-7.

As shown by slightly but significantly lower levels of folate in serum and erythrocytes, and an increased urinary excretion of formiminoglutamic acid, women who use oral contraceptives have impaired folate metabolism. The vitamin B_{12} level in their serum is also significantly lower than in controls. However, there is no evidence of associated tissue depletion of vitamin B_{12}. Of particular importance, clinicians are advised to ensure that women who stop taking "the pill" in order to become pregnant have adequate folate stores prior to conception.

404. Hjelt K, Brynskov J, Hippe E, et al, "Oral Contraceptives and the Cobalamin (Vitamin B_{12}) Metabolism," *Acta Obstet Gynecol Scand*, 1985, 64(1):59-63.

Mean concentrations of vitamin B_{12} and S-unsaturated B_{12} binding capacity were significantly decreased in 101 women taking combination oral contraceptives as compared to 113 controls. The incidence of extremely low concentrations was not increased in oral contraceptive users. Absorption and excretion of radiolabeled cobalamin and concentrations of erythrocyte-folate, S-iron and S-transferrin were no different between the groups. The authors concluded routine measurement of S-cobalamin in women taking oral contraceptives was not justified.

405. Prasad AS, Lei KY, Moghissi KS, et al, "Effect of Oral Contraceptives on Nutrients. III. Vitamins B_6, B_{12}, and Folic Acid," *Am J Obstet Gynecol*, 1976, 125(8):1063-9.

Interactions of oral contraceptive agents with vitamins were studied in a large population. As compared to controls, a higher incidence of abnormal clinical signs related to vitamin deficiencies were seen in the upper socioeconomic group. Plasma pyridoxal phosphate and red cell and serum folate were lower in subjects using contraceptive agents. With respect to vitamins B_6 and folic acid, a relative deficiency is suggested in oral contraceptive users. No significant effect on serum vitamin B_{12} was observed.

Oral Contraceptives & Vitamin B_2 Depletion

406. Webb JL, "Nutritional Effects of Oral Contraceptive Use: A Review," *J Reprod Med*, 1980, 25(4):150-6.

This review notes that oral contraceptives have been shown to affect a number of metabolic and nutritional processes. Oral contraceptives were shown to depress the physiologic levels of six nutrients (riboflavin, pyridoxine, folacin, vitamin B_{12}, ascorbic acid, and zinc). Levels of three others (vitamin K, iron, and copper) were elevated. Little or no change was noted in alpha tocopherol and questionable increases in vitamin A were noted. The authors emphasized that females consuming oral contraceptives should pay particular attention to vitamin and mineral intake. If warranted, supplements of needed nutrients may be used.

407. Matsui MS and Rozovski SJ, "Drug-Nutrient Interaction," *Clin Ther*, 1982, 4(6):423-40.

In this review, the effect of certain drugs on nutrient metabolism is discussed. Oral contraceptives are noted to interfere with the metabolism of folic acid and ascorbic acid. They also seem to interfere with riboflavin in nutritional deficiency. In addition, drugs used to treat tuberculosis such as INH and cycloserine interfere with vitamin B_6 metabolism and may produce a secondary niacin deficiency. Anticonvulsants can act as folate antagonists and precipitate folic acid deficiency. Simultaneous supplementation with folate has been recommended in some cases. Cholestyramine therapy has been associated with malabsorption of vitamins. In addition, several reports suggest that cholestyramine affects absorption of the fat-soluble vitamins K and D, as well as water-soluble vitamins including folic acid.

408. Ahmed F, Bamji MS, and Iyengar L, "Effect of Oral Contraceptive Agents on Vitamin Nutrition Status," *Am J Clin Nutr*, 1975, 28(6):606-15.

The effects of low estrogen oral contraceptives on some of the biochemical markers of vitamin status were investigated. Two groups were evaluated, a group of women who had used the pill for 6-12 months and a group followed from an initial exam through the first 6 months of treatment. Observed changes included an altered metabolic response following tryptophan load, increased specific enzymatic activity (EGOT), increased vitamin A levels, a

FEMALE HORMONES (Continued)

fall in erythrocyte folate levels, a fall in erythrocyte transketolase activity, and a fall in erythrocyte riboflavin concentration. Most of these changes were observed during the first few cycles of oral contraceptive treatment.

409. Sanpitak N and Chayutimonkul L, "Oral Contraceptives and Riboflavine Nutrition," *Lancet*, 1974, 1(7862):836-7.

This study evaluated 42 women on oral contraceptives compared to 31 controls. The erythrocyte reductase activity, which is an accurate index of riboflavin nutrition, was found to be significantly lower in the women taking oral contraceptives compared the controls.

410. Briggs M and Briggs M, "Letter: Oral Contraceptives and Vitamin Nutrition," *Lancet*, 1974, 1(7868):1234-5.

Three groups of healthy women were studied; one as controls, one using oral contraceptives of the combination type, and the third was taking Upjohn's long-acting medroxyprogesterone contraceptive, Depo-Provera®. Women using the combination-type oral contraceptive (but not the other groups) were found to have highly significant decreases in riboflavin as well as decreases in plasma levels of ascorbate and vitamin B_{12}.

411. Newman LJ, Lopez R, Cole HS, et al, "Riboflavin Deficiency in Women Taking Oral Contraceptive Agents," *Am J Clin Nutr*, 1978, 31(2).247-9.

The effect of oral contraceptive agents on riboflavin status of women in a low socioeconomic population was studied. Eleven of 100 women in the control group had biochemical evidence of deficiency compared to 24 of 56 oral contraceptive users. The frequency of deficiency was associated with prolonged use. This study demonstrated that riboflavin deficiency is a problem of women in the lower socioeconomic level who are of child-bearing age. Furthermore, the use of oral contraceptives appears to increase the prevalence of deficiency.

Oral Contraceptives & Riboflavin Depletion - Negative Studies

412. Roe DA, Bogusz S, Sheu J, et al, "Factors Affecting Riboflavin Requirements of Oral Contraceptive Users and Nonusers," *Am J Clin Nutr*, 1982, 35(3):495-501.

This study was conducted to compare the riboflavin requirements of healthy oral contraceptive users and nonusers when diets were controlled by preparation in metabolic unit. Assay values and urinary riboflavin excretion showed intersubject and interperiod differences but no significant differences between oral contraceptive users and controls. The authors concluded that when dietary intake is controlled, oral contraceptives do not significantly impact riboflavin status.

413. Vir SC and Love AH, "Riboflavin Nutriture of Oral Contraceptive Users," *Int J Vitam Nutr Res*, 1979, 49(3):286-90.

A cross-sectional and follow-up study of young women taking oral contraceptive agents revealed no significant adverse effect of oral contraceptives on riboflavin status.

Oral Contraceptives & Tryptophan and Tyrosine Depletion

414. Moller SE, "Effect of Oral Contraceptives on Tryptophan and Tyrosine Availability: Evidence for a Possible Contribution to Mental Depression," *Neuropsychobiology*, 1981, 7(4):192-200.

Plasma concentrations of several metabolic parameters were determined in oral contraceptive users and control subjects. Combination estrogen-progestogen users were found to have higher plasma levels of total tryptophan and decreased levels of tyrosine. The authors noted a correlation between the incidence of adverse reactions and the decrease in tyrosine levels. Additional analysis suggested a decreased brain tyrosine concentration. The author suggests that a substrate-limited reduction in brain noradrenaline synthesis may contribute to the occurrence of depressive symptoms in some individuals receiving combination estrogen-progestogen contraceptives.

415. Moller SE, Maach-Moller B, Olesen M, et al, "Tyrosine Metabolism in Users of Oral Contraceptives," *Life Sci*, 1995, 56(9):687-95.

Tyrosine metabolism was evaluated in users of combination oral contraceptives and comparable controls at various stages of the menstrual cycle. Users of oral contraceptives demonstrated significantly increased plasma tyrosine transaminase activity, and significantly decreased plasma tyrosine at mid-cycle and luteal phase. The authors suggest that the decreased tyrosine availability to the brain may result in a substrate-limited reduction of brain norepinephrine formation in oral contraceptive users. Further, they propose this reduction may contribute to disturbances of mood and appetite in some patients.

Oral Contraceptives & Vitamin C Depletion

416. Webb JL, "Nutritional Effects of Oral Contraceptive Use: A Review," *J Reprod Med*, 1980, 25(4):150-6.

This review notes that oral contraceptives have been shown to affect a number of metabolic and nutritional processes. Oral contraceptives were shown to depress the physiologic levels of six nutrients (riboflavin, pyridoxine, folacin, vitamin B_{12}, ascorbic acid, and zinc). Levels of three others (vitamin K, iron, and copper) were elevated. Little or no change was noted in alpha tocopherol and questionable increases in vitamin A were noted. The author emphasized that females consuming oral contraceptives should pay particular attention to vitamin and mineral intake. If warranted, supplements of needed nutrients may be used.

417. Matsui MS and Rozovski SJ, "Drug-Nutrient Interaction," *Clin Ther*, 1982, 4(6):423-40.

In this review, the effect of certain drugs on nutrient metabolism is discussed. Oral contraceptives interfere with the metabolism of folic acid and ascorbic acid. They also seem to interfere with riboflavin in nutritional deficiency. In addition, drugs used to treat tuberculosis such as INH and cycloserine interfere with vitamin B_6 metabolism and may produce a secondary niacin deficiency. Anticonvulsants can act as folate antagonists and precipitate folic acid deficiency. Simultaneous supplementation with folate has been recommended in some cases. Cholestyramine therapy has been associated with malabsorption of vitamins. In addition, several reports suggest that cholestyramine affects absorption of the fat-soluble vitamins K and D as well as watersoluble vitamins including folic acid.

418. Nash AL, Cornish EJ, and Hain R, "Metabolic Effects of Oral Contraceptives Containing 30 Micrograms and 50 Micrograms of Oestrogen," *Med J Aust*, 1979, 2(6):277-81.

Biochemical data were collected from women on oral contraceptives before and during the first 3 or 4 months of therapy. An increase in serum concentration of triglycerides, beta-lipoproteins, and ceruloplasmin, along with a

FEMALE HORMONES *(Continued)*

decrease in serum levels of antithrombin III and ascorbic acid, were observed. Serum cholesterol and phospholipid concentrations were unchanged. However, the proportion of serum cholesterol carried by high density lipoproteins decreased, while that carried by low density and very low density lipoproteins increased.

419. Rivers JM, "Oral Contraceptives and Ascorbic Acid," *Am J Clin Nutr*, 1975, 28(5):550-4.

This review notes that plasma, leukocyte, and platelet ascorbic acid levels are decreased in women ingesting oral contraceptive steroids. The estrogenic component of the oral contraceptive agents appears to be responsible for the decreased ascorbic acid concentrations. Urinary excretion of ascorbic acid does not appear to be increased. Although serum levels of copper are increased by estrogens and oral contraceptives, ascorbic acid catabolism does not appear to be increased. The author reports preliminary data on tissue uptake of ascorbic acid which suggests that changes in tissue distribution are one possible answer for the observed effects of the steroids on blood levels of ascorbic acid.

420. Weininger J and King JC, "Effect of Oral Contraceptive Agents on Ascorbic Acid Metabolism in the Rhesus Monkey," *Am J Clin Nutr*, 1982, 35(6):1408-16.

Ascorbic acid metabolism was studied in female rhesus monkeys with normal menstrual cycles before and during oral contraceptive administration. Serum copper and ceruloplasmin were significantly elevated during oral contraceptive treatment. There were no significant changes in plasma or leukocyte ascorbic acid values. However, urinary ascorbic acid excretion decreased significantly. Urinary excretion of radioactive ascorbic acid indicated a significantly faster turnover rate during oral contraceptive use. These data suggest women using oral contraceptives may have an increased dietary requirement for ascorbic acid.

Oral Contraceptives & Vitamin C Depletion - Negative Studies

421. Hudiburgh NK and Milner AN, "Influence of Oral Contraceptives on Ascorbic Acid and Triglyceride Status," *J Am Diet Assoc*, 1979, 75(1):19-22.

With adequate intake of ascorbic acid, no threat to ascorbic acid status was demonstrated from using oral contraceptives for periods of 6 months to 7 years.

422. Tyrer LB, "Nutrition and the Pill," *J Reprod Med*, 1984, 29(7 Suppl):547-50.

This review notes that the use of contraceptive pills has been shown to decrease the physiologic levels of six nutrients (riboflavin, pyridoxine, folacin, vitamin B_{12}, ascorbic acid,and zinc) and to increase the levels of four others (vitamin C, iron, copper, and vitamin A). The author asserts that women who take oral contraceptives and have adequate diets need little or no supplemental vitamins.

423. Horwitt MK, Harvey CC, and Dahm CH Jr, "Relationship Between Levels of Blood Lipids, Vitamins C, A, and E, Serum Copper Compounds, and Urinary Excretions of Tryptophan Metabolites in Women Taking Oral Contraceptive Therapy," *Am J Clin Nutr*, 1975, 28(4):403-12.

Biochemical alterations were evaluated in women taking oral contraceptives and several control populations. The most consistent changes due to oral contraceptive agents were in serum levels of copper, triglycerides, and vitamin A, and in the urinary excretion of xanthurenic acid and niacin derivatives before and after a tryptophan load test. Decrease in serum vitamin C when ceruloplasmin levels were high was not statistically significant. The highest blood pressures and serum triglycerides and vitamin A levels were obtained in those women who ingested the highest doses of estrogens. Oral contraceptive agent users had the lowest average levels of carotenoids corresponding to the highest average serum levels of vitamin A. It was concluded that estrogens not only increase the rate of change of tryptophan to niacin but may also increase the rate of conversion of carotene to vitamin A.

Oral Contraceptives & Magnesium Depletion

424. Muneyvirci-Delale O, Nacharaju VL, Altura BM, et al, "Sex Steroid Hormones Modulate Serum Ionized Magnesium and Calcium Levels Throughout the Menstrual Cycle in Women," *Gertil Steril*, 1998, 69(5):958-62.

Concentrations of estrogen, progesterone, and testosterone, as well as ionized calcium and magnesium levels, were measured in the serum of normal cycling women during the menstrual, early follicular, late follicular, ovulatory, and luteal phases. Patterns of magnesium fluctuation were observed to correlate to specific phases of the menstrual cycle. Changes in serum concentrations of these important physiologically active cations can affect entities such as vasculature, synaptic transmission, and excitation-secretion coupling. By this mechanism, the authors propose magnesium and calcium fluctuations may produce the well-known premenstrual syndromes during the luteal phase, particularly in women who are somewhat deficient in magnesium or in those who have an unusually increased calcium to magnesium ratio.

425. Blum M, Kitai E, Ariel Y, et al, "Oral Contraceptive Lowers Serum Magnesium," *Harefuah*, 1991, 121(10):363-4.

The effect of an oral contraceptive on serum magnesium was assessed in a group of 32 women attending a family planning clinic. In 6 months, the contraceptive pill lowered serum magnesium from a mean of 0.82 mmol/L, to 0.61 mmol/L.

426. Seelig MS, "Increased Need for Magnesium With the Use of Combined Oestrogen and Calcium for Osteoporosis Treatment," *Magnes Res*, 1990, 3(3):197-215.

This review discusses magnesium and calcium homeostasis during estrogen and calcium treatment. Although estrogen has cardiovascular protective effects, high-dose estrogen contraceptives have caused increased thromboembolic events. The author suggest one contributing factor may be the estrogen-mediated shift of circulating magnesium to soft and hard tissues. Mechanisms by which calcium activates coagulation that are also stimulated by estrogen are discussed, along with the roles of magnesium in modulating coagulation and fibrinolysis.

427. Stanton MF and Lowenstein FW, "Serum Magnesium in Women During Pregnancy, While Taking Contraceptives, and After Menopause," *J Am Coll Nutr*, 1987, 6(4):313-9.

Based on a large survey of women in the first National Health and Nutrition Examination Survey (NHANES I), women on oral contraceptives had significantly lower serum magnesium values than other nonpregnant women of similar age. The differences were much smaller than those between pregnant women and controls. Postmenopausal women had significantly higher

FEMALE HORMONES *(Continued)*

serum magnesium values than premenopausal women. These findings are compared with findings from other studies worldwide.

428. Olatunbosun DA, Adeniyi FA, and Adadevoh BK, "Effect of Oral Contraceptives on Serum Magnesium Levels," *Int J Fertil*, 1974, 19(4):224-6.

Serum magnesium levels were determined in 224 Nigerian women attending a postpartum family planning clinic. Serum magnesium concentrations were significantly lower in women taking oral contraceptives than in the control group.

429. Seelig MS, "Interrelationship of Magnesium and Estrogen in Cardiovascular and Bone Disorders, Eclampsia, Migraine and Premenstrual Syndrome," *J Am Coll Nutr*, 1993, 12(4):442-58.

This review describes estrogen's enhancement of magnesium utilization and uptake by soft tissues and bone which may explain resistance of young women to heart disease and osteoporosis. This may also explain the increased prevalence of these diseases when estrogen secretion ceases. However, estrogen-induced magnesium shifts can be deleterious when estrogen levels are high and magnesium intake is low. The resultant lowering of blood magnesium can increase the calcium/magnesium ratio. This alteration may favor coagulation. The author expresses that calcium supplementation in the face of low magnesium intake may increase the risk of thrombosis.

Oral Contraceptives & Magnesium Depletion - Negative Studies

430. Prasad AS, Oberleas D, Moghissi KS, et al, "Effect of Oral Contraceptive Agents on Nutrients: I. Minerals," *Am J Clin Nutr*, 1975, 28(4):377-84.

Interactions of oral contraceptive agents with minerals were studied in a large population. No effect of oral contraceptive agents on plasma calcium, magnesium, and erythrocyte magnesium was observed.

Oral Contraceptives & Zinc Depletion

431. Webb JL, "Nutritional Effects of Oral Contraceptive Use: A Review," *J Reprod Med*, 1980, 25(4):150-6.

This review notes that oral contraceptives have been shown to affect a number of metabolic and nutritional processes. Oral contraceptives were shown to depress the physiologic levels of six nutrients (riboflavin, pyridoxine, folacin, vitamin B_{12}, ascorbic acid, and zinc). Levels of three others (vitamin K, iron, and copper) were elevated. Little or no change was noted in alpha tocopherol and questionable increases in vitamin A were noted. The author emphasized that females consuming oral contraceptives should pay particular attention to vitamin and mineral intake. If warranted, supplements of needed nutrients may be used.

432. Dorea JG, Ferraz E, and Queiroz EF, "Effects of Anovulatory Steroids on Serum Levels of Zinc and Copper," *Arch Latinoam Nutr*, 1982, 32(1):101-10.

Mean serum zinc and copper in women taking oral contraceptive agents were compared against mean levels observed in controls. Serum zinc was significantly lower while serum copper was significantly higher for women taking oral contraceptive agents. There was no significant correlation between serum zinc and copper levels, either in the control group or in the group taking the contraceptives.

433. Tyrer LB, "Nutrition and the Pill," *J Reprod Med*, 1984, 29(7 Suppl):547-50.

This review notes that the use of contraceptive pills has been shown to decrease the physiologic levels of six nutrients (riboflavin, pyridoxine, folacin, vitamin B_{12}, ascorbic acid, and zinc) and to increase the levels of four others (vitamin C, iron, copper, and vitamin A). The author asserts that women who take oral contraceptives and have adequate diets need little or no supplemental vitamins.

Oral Contraceptives & Zinc Depletion - Negative Studies

434. Liukko P, Erkkola R, Pakarinen P, et al, "Trace Elements During 2 Years' Oral Contraception With Low-Estrogen Preparations," *Gynecol Obstet Invest*, 1988, 25(2):113-7.

    In 17 healthy women taking oral contraceptives, iron, calcium, copper, and zinc levels were evaluated during the initial 24 months of therapy. No changes from pre-treatment levels were observed in iron, calcium, and zinc levels. The copper level was significantly increased during oral contraception and returned to baseline after discontinuation.

435. Hinks LJ, Clayton BE, and Lloyd RS, "Zinc and Copper Concentrations in Leucocytes and Erythrocytes in Healthy Adults and the Effect of Oral Contraceptives," *J Clin Pathol*, 1983, 36(9):1016-21.

    Women taking oral contraceptives showed significant increases in plasma or whole blood copper concentrations but not in leucocytes or erythrocytes. Oral contraceptives did not change the concentration of zinc in any fraction or in whole blood.

436. Vir SC and Love AH, "Zinc and Copper Nutriture of Women Taking Oral Contraceptive Agents," *Am J Clin Nutr*, 1981, 34(8):1479-83.

    A cross-sectional study of young women taking oral contraceptive agents revealed a marked increase in serum copper levels, which was significant after taking oral contraceptive agents for 3 months. No significant effect on serum zinc and hair levels of copper were observed. There was no correlation between duration of oral contraceptive agent therapy and concentrations of these minerals in serum or hair. Serum and hair concentrations of zinc or copper were not significantly correlated.

GOUT MEDICATIONS

COLCHICINE

Colchicine & Vitamin B$_{12}$ Depletion

437. Race TF, Paes IC, and Faloon WW, "Intestinal Malabsorption Induced by Oral Colchicine. Comparison With Neomycin and Cathartic Agents," *Am J Med Sci*, 1970, 259(1):32-41.

In human subjects receiving oral colchicine, widespread alteration of intestinal mucosal function and absorption were observed. Increased fecal sodium, potassium, fat, and nitrogen losses occurred. In addition, decreased absorption of D-xylose and vitamin B$_{12}$, and decreased serum cholesterol and carotene concentration were noted. Reduction of sucrase, maltase, and lactase enzyme activity of varying degrees was found in mucosal tissue. Histologic changes were variable, usually mild, and unrelated to dose. All absorptive changes were reversible upon withdrawal of colchicine.

438. Faloon WW and Chodos RB, "Vitamin B$_{12}$ Absorption Studies Using Colchicine, Neomycin and Continuous 57Co B$_{12}$ Administration," *Gastroenterology*, 1969, 56:1251.

Parenteral colchicine was shown to affect mucosal function as shown by increased fecal excretion of B$_{12}$. True blockade of B$_{12}$ absorption is produced by oral neomycin or oral colchicine, perhaps by different mechanisms, and is accentuated by the combined use of these agents.

439. Stopa EG, O'Brien R, and Katz M, "Effect of Colchicine on Guinea Pig Intrinsic Factor - Vitamin B$_{12}$ Receptor," *Gastroenterology*, 1979, 76(2):309-14.

The authors observed a dose-related, reversible reduction in the quantity of intrinsic factor-vitamin B$_{12}$ receptor in the guinea pig intestinal mucosa after 3 days of colchicine. Malabsorption of vitamin B$_{12}$ was also demonstrated. Correlation between changes in receptor quantity and B$_{12}$-absorption indicate that the receptor is a critical limiting factor in B$_{12}$ absorption.

440. Polliotti BM, Panigel M, and Miller RK, "Free Vitamin B$_{12}$ and Transcobalamin II-Vitamin B$_{12}$ Complex Uptake by the Visceral Yolk Sac of the Sprague-Dawley Rat: Effect of Inhibitors," *Reprod Toxicol*, 1997, 11(4):617-26.

Exogenous free vitamin B$_{12}$ or B$_{12}$ bound to human transcobalamin II (TCII) accumulated in the near-term rat visceral yolk sac, likely due to a saturable transport/binding process which may be rate-limiting. Uptakes were significantly decreased by trypan blue, colchicine, and low temperature but not by ouabain. It is proposed that the role of the visceral yolk sac in vitamin transfer may be related to alterations in yolk sac function associated with birth defects and diminished growth.

441. Webb DI, Chodos RB, Mahar CQ, et al, "Mechanism of Vitamin B$_{12}$ Malabsorption in Patients Receiving Colchicine," *N Engl J Med*, 1968, 279(16):845-50.

No abstract available

Colchicine & Vitamin B$_{12}$ Depletion - Negative Studies

442. Ehrenfeld M, Levy M, Sharon P, et al, "Gastrointestinal Effects of Long-Term Colchicine Therapy in Patients With Recurrent Polyserositis (Familial Mediterranean Fever)," *Dig Dis Sci*, 1982, 27(8):723-7.

Twelve patients on colchicine prophylaxis for 3 years or more were evaluated for the presence of gastrointestinal effects attributable to the drug. Serum vitamin B_{12}, calcium, and carotene levels were normal in all cases, and D-xylose absorption was normal in 11 of the 12 patients.

Colchicine & Sodium Depletion

443. Race TF, Paes IC, and Faloon WW, "Intestinal Malabsorption Induced by Oral Colchicine. Comparison With Neomycin and Cathartic Agents," *Am J Med Sci*, 1970, 259(1):32-41.

In human subjects receiving oral colchicine, widespread alteration of intestinal mucosal function and absorption were observed. Increased fecal losses of sodium, potassium, fat, and nitrogen occurred. In addition, decreased absorption of D-xylose and vitamin B_{12}, and decreased serum cholesterol and carotene concentration were observed. Reduction of sucrase, maltase, and lactase enzyme activity of varying degree was found in mucosal tissue. Histologic changes were variable, usually mild, and unrelated to the dose. All absorptive changes were reversible upon withdrawal of colchicine.

Colchicine & Sodium Depletion - No Negative Studies

Colchicine & Potassium Depletion

444. Race TF, Paes IC, and Faloon WW, "Intestinal Malabsorption Induced by Oral Colchicine. Comparison With Neomycin and Cathartic Agents," *Am J Med Sci*, 1970, 259(1):32-41.

In human subjects receiving oral colchicine, widespread alteration of intestinal mucosal function and absorption were observed. Increased fecal losses of sodium, potassium, fat, and nitrogen occurred. In addition, decreased absorption of D-xylose and vitamin B_{12}, and decreased serum cholesterol and carotene concentration were observed. Reduction of sucrase, maltase, and lactase enzyme activity of varying degree was found in mucosal tissue. Histologic changes were variable, usually mild and unrelated to the dose. All absorptive changes were reversible upon withdrawal of colchicine.

Colchicine & Potassium Depletion - No Negative Studies

Colchicine & Beta-Carotene Depletion

445. Race TF, Paes IC, and Faloon WW, "Intestinal Malabsorption Induced by Oral Colchicine. Comparison With Neomycin and Cathartic Agents," *Am J Med Sci*, 1970, 259(1):32-41.

In human subjects receiving oral colchicine, widespread alteration of intestinal mucosal function and absorption were observed. Increased fecal losses of sodium, potassium, fat, and nitrogen occurred. In addition, decreased absorption of D-xylose and vitamin B_{12}, and decreased serum cholesterol and carotene concentration were observed. Reduction of sucrase, maltase, and lactase enzyme activity of varying degree was found in mucosal tissue. Histologic changes were variable, usually mild, and unrelated to the dose. All absorptive changes were reversible upon withdrawal of colchicine.

Colchicine & Beta-Carotene Depletion - Negative Studies

446. Ehrenfeld M, Levy M, Sharon P, et al, "Gastrointestinal Effects of Long-Term Colchicine Therapy in Patients With Recurrent Polyserositis (Familial Mediterranean Fever)," *Dig Dis Sci*, 1982, 27(8):723-7.

Twelve patients on colchicine prophylaxis for 3 years or more were evaluated for the presence of gastrointestinal effects attributable to the drug. Serum vitamin B_{12}, calcium, and carotene levels were normal in all cases, and D-xylose absorption was normal in 11 of the 12 patients.

GOUT MEDICATIONS *(Continued)*

Colchicine & Calcium Depletion

447. Nassar CF, Abdallah LE, Nuwayri-Salti N, "Colchicine Inhibition of Duodenal Absorption of Calcium," *Gen Pharmacol*, 1991, 22(4):755-8.

   The effect of colchicine on calcium absorption was investigated in an animal model (rat duodenum). Colchicine (at 0.5 mM concentrations) caused a significant decrease in the rate of calcium uptake and accumulation of calcium in the duodenal cells. Colchicine resulted in a lower saturation level and decreased the average maximal flux by approximately 46%.

448. Ohya K and Ogura H, "The Effects of Colchicine or Vinblastine on the Blood Calcium Level in Rats," *Eur J Pharmacol*, 1993, 248(2):111-9.

   The authors investigated the mechanism by which microtubule inhibitors induce hypocalcemia. Histologically, the bone cells of rats injected with either drug were noted to be changed 8 hours after injection. The results were interpreted as an indication that hypocalcemia may be caused by interference with bone cell calcium homeostasis. The authors concluded destruction of microtubules may be closely related to the development of the hypocalcemia.

IMMUNOSUPPRESSANT DRUGS

(See also Corticosteroids in Anti-inflammatory Drugs)

449. Woo M, Przepiorka D, Ippoliti C, et al, "Toxicities of Tacrolimus and Cyclosporin A After Allogenic Blood Stem Cell Transplantation," *Bone Marrow Transplant*, 1997, 20(12):1095-8.

This review notes that electrolyte disturbances are a common but complex phenomenon during immunosuppression. Magnesium is a particularly common depletion, while potassium levels may be increased or decreased. Both tacrolimus and cyclosporine are implicated, although increases in potassium were more frequently associated with tacrolimus.

450. Mihatsch MJ, Kyo M, Morozumi K, et al, "The Side Effects of Ciclosporine-A and Tacrolimus" *Clin Nephrol*, 1998, 49(6):356-63.

Both cyclosporine and tacrolimus were noted to cause similar morphologic changes in kidney cells. The pattern of electrolyte loss was nearly identical, although the two agents are chemically distinct.

LAXATIVES

Laxatives & Sodium and Potassium Depletion

451. Oster JR, Materson BJ, and Rogers AI, "Laxative Abuse Syndrome," *Am J Gastroenterol*, 1980, 74(5):451-8.

   Laxative abuse syndrome (LAS) is characterized by surreptitious abuse of purgatives. Clinical findings may include sodium, potassium, and water depletion. The authors encourage healthcare providers to be aware of possible laxative abuse syndrome.

452. Fleming BJ, Genuth SM, Gould AB, et al, "Laxative-Induced Hypokalemia, Sodium Depletion and Hyperreninemia. Effects of Potassium and Sodium Replacement on the Renin-Angiotensin-Aldosterone System," *Ann Intern Med*, 1975, 83(1):60-2.

   The renin-angiotensin system of a patient with chronic hypokalemia and sodium depletion caused by laxative abuse and nutritional deficiency was evaluated. Extreme increases in serum renin concentrations were reduced with potassium replacement. Aldosterone excretion initially was low relative to the sodium-deprived state and high relative to the potassium-deprived state. These were reversed with potassium administration, but the rise was opposed by decreases in renin secretion induced by potassium and sodium administration. The results confirm a dual effect of potassium on aldosterone secretion, with renin as a mediator.

453. Chin RL, "Laxative-Induced Hypokalemia," *Ann Emerg Med*, 1998, 32(4):517-8.

   No abstract available.

454. Goldfinger P, "Hypokalemia, Metabolic Acidosis, and Hypocalcemic Tetany in a Patient Taking Laxatives. A Case Report," *J Mt Sinai Hosp NY*, 1969, 36(2):113-6.

   No abstract available.

MINERAL OIL

Mineral Oil & Beta-Carotene, Calcium, Phosphorus, and Vitamins A, D, E, and K Depletion

455. Becker GL, "The Case Against Mineral Oil," *Am J Digestive Dis*, 1953, 19:344-347.

   In this review, the author makes the following points:

   a. Mineral oil is capable of absorbing the fat soluble vitamins A, D, E, and K

   b. It also hastens the motility of the bowel content and thus prevents complete digestion

   c. Mineral oil may interfere with the process of absorption throughout the lower intestines. By partially covering the surface area of the intestines, it establishes a mechanical barrier to absorption and digestion with consequent symptoms of "indigestion".

   d. Another serious disadvantage of mineral oil is that it interferes with the utilization and retention of calcium and phosphorus. This interference is possibly of a dual nature. It interferes with the absorption of these minerals due to formation of a mechanical barrier along the gastrointestinal tract. Then, due to the inter-relationship of vitamin D and calcium-phosphorus metabolism, mineral oil actually alters the metabolic processes of calcium and phosphorus through interference with absorption of vitamin D.

e. Mineral oil also mechanically coats food particles and consequently prevents their complete absorption through the intestinal walls. This statement is borne out by the fact that the continuous use of mineral oil frequently causes a severe loss in weight.

f. Finally, because mineral oil so greatly hastens the passage of food through the intestinal tract, there is further decrease in absorption of nutrients from the intestinal tract.

456. Clark JH, Russell GJ, Fitzgerald JF, et al, "Serum Beta-Carotene, Retinol, and Alpha-Tocopherol Levels During Mineral Oil Therapy for Constipation," *Am J Dis Child*, 1987, 141(11):1210-2.

Serial monitoring of serum beta-carotene, retinol (vitamin A_1), alpha-tocopherol (vitamin A_1), and alpha-tocopherol (vitamin E) levels were performed in 25 children during mineral oil therapy. The authors concluded that a short course of mineral oil may reduce the serum level of beta-carotene, but has no adverse effect on retinol and alpha-tocopherol concentrations.

BISACODYL

Bisacodyl & Potassium Depletion

457. Ritsema GH and Eilers G, "Potassium Supplements Prevent Serious Hypokalaemia in Colon Cleansing," *Clin Radiol*, 1994, 49(12):874-6.

Hypokalemia was noted to occur in many patients receiving bowel cleansing regimens. The authors conclude that bowel cleansing with cathartics may result in a significant fall in serum potassium. This fall may be prevented by oral potassium chloride. Prophylactic replacement in patients at risk of cardiac arrhythmia is recommended.

458. Moreto M, Planas JM, and Naftalin RJ, "Effects of Secretagogues on the K+ Permeability of Mucosal and Serosal Borders of Rabbit Colonic Mucosa," *Biochem Biophys Acta*, 1981, 648(2):215-24.

A number of compounds which act as secretagogues, including the laxative bisacodyl, were found to raise the K+ efflux rate across rabbit mucosal border by 200% to 300% *in vitro*. The results suggest laxatives may increase potassium secretion into the colon by altering mucosal permeability.

SODIUM PHOSPHATE ENEMAS

Phosphate Enemas & Calcium and Magnesium Depletion

459. Soumoy MP and Bachy A, "Risk of Phosphate Enemas in the Infant," *Arch Pediatr*, 1998, 5(11):1221-3. (Article in French)

A case report involving a 14-month-old child with neonatal-repaired Hirschsprung's disease had received a pediatric phosphate enema ("Fleet® Enema") a few hours before admission. After evaluation, it was determined that the clinical symptoms and electrolyte disturbances (hyperphosphatemia, hypocalcemia) were the consequences of the enema. The authors concluded that phosphate enemas are dangerous in children with renal insufficiency or bowel dysfunction. In addition, the authors concluded phosphate enemas should be used with extreme caution in normal children 2-5 years of age, and should not be used at all in children <2 years of age.

LAXATIVES *(Continued)*

460. Post SS, "Hyperphosphatemic Hypocalcemic Coma Caused by Hypertonic Sodium Phosphate (Fleet®) Enema Intoxication," *J Clin Gastroenterol*, 1997, 24(3):192.

No abstract available.

461. Ehrenpreis ED, Wieland JM, Cabral J, et al, "Symptomatic Hypocalcemia, Hypomagnesemia, and Hyperphosphatemia Secondary to Fleet®'s Phospho-Soda Colonoscopy Preparation in a Patient With a Jejunoileal Bypass," *Dig Dis Sci*, 1997, 42(4):858-60.

No abstract available.

462. Knobel B and Petchenko P, "Hyperphosphatemic Hypocalcemic Coma Caused by Hypertonic Sodium Phosphate (Fleet®) Enema Intoxication," *J Clin Gastroenterol*, 1996, 23(3):217-9.

The authors describe an elderly woman with significant electrolyte disturbances and coma. Hyperphosphatemia, hypocalcemia, hypernatremia, hypokalemia, metabolic acidosis, and pancytopenia were noted. In addition, respiratory failure, circulatory failure, and coma were noted to be secondary to phosphate intoxication. These occurred as a result of the administration of excessive hypertonic sodium phosphate enemas.

463. Korsets A, Dicker D, Chaimoff C, et al, "Life-Threatening Hyperphosphatemia and Hypocalcemic Tetany Following the Use of Fleet® Enemas," *J Am Geriatr Soc*, 1992, 40(6):620-1.

No abstract available.

464. Grosskopf I, Graff E, Charach G, et al, "Hyperphosphataemia and Hypocalcaemia Induced by Hypertonic Phosphate Enema -- An Experimental Study and Review of the Literature," *Hum Exp Toxicol*, 1991, 10(5):351-5.

In a study to determine the hyperphosphataemic and hypocalcaemic effect of hypertonic phosphate enema, 14 patients (mean 78.5 years of age) with a mean creatinine clearance of 48.2 mL/min (+/- 17.4) were evaluated. Each received 500 mL (~7 mL/kg) of phosphate enema. The serum inorganic phosphorus level rose and serum calcium decreased significantly. The authors conclude that phosphate enemas entail potential risk in acutely ill elderly patients, and the phosphate load must be adjusted to the patient's renal function.

465. Vukasin P, Weston LA, and Beart RW, "Oral Fleet® Phospho-Soda Laxative-Induced Hyperphosphatemia and Hypocalcemic Tetany in an Adult: Report of a Case," *Dis Colon Rectum*, 1997, 40(4):497-9.

In an adult patient, administration of Fleet®'s Phospho-Soda for bowel preparation resulted in hyperphosphatemia and hypocalcemia with tetany. The patient was noted to have a partial bowel obstruction and renal failure which were believed to contribute to the development of this complication.

PARKINSON'S AGENTS

LEVODOPA

Levodopa & Potassium Depletion

466. Granerus AK, Jagenburg R, and Svanborg A, "Kaliuretic Effect of L-dopa Treatment in Parkinsonian Patients," *Acta Med Scand*, 1977, 201(4):291-97.

The influence of levodopa on renal potassium excretion was evaluated in 8 subjects (3 patients with hypokalemia and 5 normokalemic patients). Renal plasma flow, glomerular filtration rate, plasma potassium concentrations, and plasma sodium were determined. Urinary excretion of potassium, sodium, and aldosterone were also measured. Levodopa intake was found to increase potassium excretion. Sodium excretion was increased in hypokalemic patients, but not in normokalemic subjects. The authors note that levodopa's effect on renal function could be blocked by the administration of a peripheral dopa decarbodylase inhibitor. A correlation between aldosterone production and the renal effects of levodopa is suggested.

Levodopa & SAMe Depletion

467. Surtees R and Hyland K, "L-3,4-Dihydroxyphenlalanine (Levodopa) Lowers Central Nervous System S-Adenosylmethionine Concentrations in Humans," *J Neurol Neurosurg Psychiatry*, 1990, 53(7):569-72.

Increasing levodopa concentrations in the CSF of 6 children were related to decreased levels of S-adenosyl-methionine concentrations. In addition, a rise in the CSF 3-methoxytyrosine levels was observed. The authors discuss the possible relationship of these changes to the therapeutic effects of levodopa.

PSYCHOTHERAPEUTIC DRUGS

TRICYCLIC ANTIDEPRESSANTS

Tricyclic Antidepressants & Vitamin B₂ Depletion

468. Bell IR, Edman JS, Morrow FD et al, "Brief Communication. Vitamin B_1, B_2, and B_6 Augmentation of Tricyclic Antidepressant Treatment in Geriatric Depression With Cognitive Dysfunction," *J Am Coll Nutr*, 1992, 11(2):159-63.

The authors note alterations in various aspects of flavin metabolism have been observed following administration of some tricyclic antidepressant and antipsychotic agents. As an example, chlorpromazine has been shown to promote urinary riboflavin excretion in both animals and man. Structural similarities between the phenothiazine ring of chlorpromazine and the isoalloxazine ring of riboflavin are noted, as well as their potential to form a molecular complex *in vitro*. The authors note the administration of agents which enhance urinary riboflavin excretion may be of particular concern for patients who are already nutritionally compromised.

469. Tinguely D, Jonzier M, Schopf J, et al, "Determination of Compliance With Riboflavin in an Antidepressive Therapy," *Arzneimittelforschung*, 1985, 35(2):536-8.

Patients were medicated for 3 weeks with a fixed dose of amitriptyline and riboflavin. Although primarily designed to evaluate the use of riboflavin to monitor compliance, this study demonstrated enhanced urinary excretion of vitamin B_2 (riboflavin) with concurrent administration of certain tricyclic antidepressant medications.

470. Pinto J, Huang YP, and Rivlin RS, "Inhibition of Riboflavin Metabolism in Rat Tissues by Chlorpromazine, Imipramine, and Amitriptyline," *J Clin Invest*, 1981, 67(5):1500-6.

The authors concluded that imipramine and amitriptyline caused varying degrees of vitamin B_2 deficiency in laboratory animals due to metabolic inhibition.

471. Edelbroek PM, Zitman FG, Schreuder JN, et al, "Amitriptyline Metabolism in Relation to Antidepressive Effect," *Clin Pharmacol Ther*, 1984, 35(4):467-73.

In a population of 14 outpatients, the relationship between amitriptyline metabolism and clinical response was evaluated. A fixed amount of riboflavin was added to the medication to check compliance. There was great variation in the metabolic pattern between patients. After 6 weeks, concentrations of all compounds were approximately 15% lower than at 3 weeks. A modest degree of autoinduction in amitriptyline metabolism was demonstrated. The use of riboflavin as a marker supports an enhanced excretion of riboflavin (vitamin B_2) when tricyclic antidepressants are used.

472. Pinto J, Huang YP, Pelliccione N, et al, "Cardiac Sensitivity to the Inhibitory Effects of Chlorpromazine, Imipramine and Amitriptyline Upon Formation of Flavins," *Biochem Pharmacol*, 1982, 31(21):3495-9.

In rat heart tissue, chlorpromazine, imipramine, and amitriptyline each inhibited the *in vivo* formation of flavin adenine dinucleotide (FAD) from riboflavin. The structural similarity of these agents to riboflavin is discussed. Inhibition of FAD formation was noted to occur within 5 hours after a single dose of 25 mg/kg. Chlorpromazine also inhibited FAD formation in the liver, cerebrum, and cerebellum. Psychoactive agents which were structurally unrelated to riboflavin did not inhibit flavin formation. The authors concluded these data indicate an inhibitory effect of the studied medications which demonstrate organ specificity.

Tricyclic Antidepressants & Vitamin B_2 Depletion - No Negative Studies

Tricyclic Antidepressants & Coenzyme Q_{10} Depletion

473. Kishi T, et al, "Inhibition of Myocardial Respiration by Psychotherapeutic Drugs and Prevention by Coenzyme Q," *Biomedical and Clinical Aspects of Coenzyme Q*, Yamamura Y, Folkers K, and Ito Y, eds, Elsevier/North-Holland Biomedical Press: Amsterdam, 1980, Vol 2, 139-54.

In order to investigate the cardiotoxic effects of psychotherapeutic drugs, seven phenothiazines, three butyrophenones, and seven tricyclic antidepressants were evaluated for their effects on mitochondrial respiration in beef heart. The phenothiazines and tricyclic antidepressants inhibited succinoxidase, NADH-oxidase, and succinate dehydrogenase-CoQ reductase activity. The butyrophenones did not inhibit succinoxidase activity but inhibited NADH-oxidase activity in lower concentrations to a greater extent than phenothiazines and tricyclics. Analysis localized inhibition to the mitochondrial cytochrome system. Inhibition by the phenothiazines and most of the tricyclic antidepressants of succinoxidase and NADH-oxidase activities was effectively prevented by the addition of CoQ_{10}. Inhibition by the butyrophenones did not appear to be reversed by CoQ_{10}.

Tricyclic Antidepressants & Coenzyme Q_{10} Depletion - No Negative Studies

PHENOTHIAZINES

Phenothiazines & Vitamin B_2 Depletion

474. Bell IR, Edman JS, Morrow FD, et al, "Brief Communication. Vitamin B_1, B_2, and B_6 Augmentation of Tricyclic Antidepressant Treatment in Geriatric Depression With Cognitive Dysfunction," *J Am Coll Nutr*, 1992, 11(2):159-63.

The authors note alterations in various aspects of flavin metabolism have been observed following administration of some tricyclic antidepressant and antipsychotic agents. As an example, chlorpromazine has been shown to promote urinary riboflavin excretion in both animals and man. Structural similarities between the phenothiazine ring of chlorpromazine and the isoalloxazine ring of riboflavin are noted, as well as their potential to form a molecular complex *in vitro*. The authors note the administration of agents which enhance urinary riboflavin excretion may be of particular concern for patients who are already nutritionally compromised.

475. Pinto J, Huang YP, and Rivlin RS, "Inhibition of Riboflavin Metabolism in Rat Tissues by Chlorpromazine, Imipramine, and Amitriptyline," *J Clin Invest*, 1981, 67(5):1500-6.

The authors concluded that chlorpromazine caused vitamin B_2 deficiency at varying levels in laboratory animals due to inhibition of the metabolism of this vitamin.

Phenothiazines & Vitamin B_2 Depletion - No Negative Studies

Phenothiazines & Coenzyme Q_{10} Depletion

476. Kishi T, et al, "Inhibition of Myocardial Respiration by Psychotherapeutic Drugs and Prevention by Coenzyme Q," *Biomedical and Clinical Aspects of*

PSYCHOTHERAPEUTIC DRUGS *(Continued)*

Coenzyme Q, Yamamura Y, Folkers K, and Ito Y, eds, Elsevier/North-Holland Biomedical Press: Amsterdam, 1980, Vol 2, 139-54.

In order to investigate the cardiotoxic effects of psychotherapeutic drugs, seven phenothiazines, three butyrophenones, and seven tricyclic antidepressants were evaluated for their effects on mitochondrial respiration in beef heart. The phenothiazines and tricyclic antidepressants inhibited succinoxidase, NADH-oxidase, and succinate dehydrogenase-CoQ reductase activity. The butyrophenones did not inhibit succinoxidase activity but inhibited NADH-oxidase activity in lower concentrations to a greater extent than phenothiazines and tricyclics. Analysis localized inhibition to the mitochondrial cytochrome system. Inhibition by the phenothiazines and most of the tricyclic antidepressants of succinoxidase and NADH-oxidase activities was effectively prevented by the addition of CoQ_{10}. Inhibition by the butyrophenones did not appear to be reversed by CoQ_{10}.

477. Chiba M, "A Protective Action of Coenzyme Q_{10} on Chlorpromazine-induced Cell Damage in the Cultured Rat Myocardial Cells," *Jpn Heart J*, 1984, 25(1):127-37.

In cultured rate myocardial cells, the relationship between coenzyme Q_{10} (CoQ_{10}) and chlorpromazine (CPZ) was investigated. Co-incubation with chlorpromazine and CoQ_{10} led to a dose-dependent increase in ATP concentration. Indomethacin, an inhibitor of prostaglandin synthesis, blocked the protective effects of CoQ_{10}. These findings suggest that CoQ_{10} may protect myocardial cells from CPZ-induced injury, via a prostaglandin-mediated mechanism.

BUTYROPHENONES (Haloperidol)

Butyrophenones (Haloperidol) & Coenzyme Q_{10} Depletion

478. Kishi T, et al, "Inhibition of Myocardial Respiration by Psychotherapeutic Drugs and Prevention by Coenzyme Q," *Biomedical and Clinical Aspects of Coenzyme Q*, Yamamura Y, Folkers K, and Ito Y, eds, Elsevier/North-Holland Biomedical Press: Amsterdam, 1980, Vol 2, 139-54.

In order to investigate the cardiotoxic effects of psychotherapeutic drugs, seven phenothiazines, three butyrophenones, and seven tricyclic antidepressants were evaluated for their effects on mitochondrial respiration in beef heart. The phenothiazines and tricyclic antidepressants inhibited succinoxidase, NADH-oxidase, and succinate dehydrogenase-CoQ reductase activity. The butyrophenones did not inhibit succinoxidase activity but inhibited NADH-oxidase activity in lower concentrations to a greater extent than phenothiazines and tricyclics. Analysis localized inhibition to the mitochondrial cytochrome system. Inhibition by the phenothiazines and most of the tricyclic antidepressants of succinoxidase and NADH-oxidase activities was effectively prevented by the addition of CoQ_{10}. Inhibition by the butyrophenones did not appear to be reversed by CoQ_{10}.

Butyrophenones (Haloperidol) & Coenzyme Q$_{10}$ Depletion - No Negative Studies

LITHIUM

Lithium & Sodium Depletion

479. Mercado R and Michelis MF, "Severe Sodium Depletion Syndrome During Lithium Carbonate Therapy," *Arch Intern Med*, 1977, 137(12):1731-3.

Lithium carbonate, useful in the treatment of manic-depressive disorders, can produce nephrogenic diabetes insipidus. The drug, therefore, has been used to facilitate renal waste excretion when severe hyponatremia occurs in the syndrome of inappropriate antidiuretic hormone secretion. Symptomatic dilutional hyponatremia developed in a patient with pulmonary carcinoma. Lithium carbonate was administered and renal sodium wasting, hypovolemia, and hypotension occurred. Hyperkalemia was also observed, and since adrenal steroid levels were not decreased, impairment of distal tubular function was suggested. Lithium carbonate blocks antidiuretic hormone effect by decreasing collecting duct cyclic adenosine monophosphate generation. These observations suggest that more generalized inhibitory effects on renal tubular function may also result from its use.

480. Shuster J, "Lithium and Sodium Depletion," *Nursing*, 1998, 28(9):29.

No abstract available.

Lithium & Inositol Depletion

481. Agam G, Shapiro Y, Bersudsky Y, et al, "High-Dose Peripheral Inositol Raises Brain Inositol Levels and Reverses Behavioral Effects of Inositol Depletion by Lithium," *Pharmacol Biochem Behav*, 1994, 49(2):341-3.

The authors note previous data documenting lithium-induced reductions of brain inositol levels, as well as the possibility that depletion may be related to its therapeutic effect. In an animal model, the authors demonstrate a reversal of a lithium-induced CNS effect following peripheral administration of inositol. It is noted that this reversal occurs despite limited ability to penetrate the blood-brain barrier.

482. Belmaker RH, Agam G, van Calker D, et al, "Behavioral Reversal of Lithium Effects by Four Inositol Isomers Correlates Perfectly With Biochemical Effects on the PI Cycle: Depletion by Chronic Lithium of Brain Inositol is Specific to Hypothalamus, and Inositol Levels May Be Abnormal in Postmortem Brain From Bipolar Patients," *Neuropsychopharmacology*, 1998, 19(3):220-32.

Studies demonstrating chronic lithium depletion of brain inositol in the hypothalamus are reviewed. Correlation with the behavioral effects of four different inositol isomers are described. In addition, it is noted that inositol in postmortem human brain is reduced by 25% in the frontal cortex of individuals with bipolar disorder as compared with controls. The authors emphasize a complex relationship between inositol and lithium, noting the reduction in postmortem brain inositol in bipolar patients.

483. Kofman O and Belmaker RH, "Ziskind-Somerfield Research Award 1993. Biochemical, Behavioral, and Clinical Studies of the Role of Inositol in Lithium Treatment and Depression," *Biol Psychiatry*, 1993, 34(12):839-52.

Chronic lithium therapy is correlated to an inhibition of inositol-1-phosphatase in human red blood cells. Lithium is also noted to reduce brain inositol levels, due to enzyme inhibiton.

ULCER MEDICATIONS

H₂ BLOCKERS

H₂ Blockers & Calcium Depletion

484. Caron P, Gaillard J, Barousse C, et al, "Cimetidine Treatment of Primary Hyperparathyroidism," *Biomed Pharmacother*, 1987, 41(3):143-6.

   Sixteen patients with primary hyperparathyroidism were treated with cimetidine. After the fourth week of therapy, a decrease in serum calcium and urinary cAMP was observed. Parathyroid hormone levels were unchanged. The authors did not comment on the need for possible calcium repletion.

485. Hakanson R, Persson P, and Axelson J, "Elevated Serum Gastrin After Food Intake or Acid Blockade Evokes Hypocalcemia," *Regul Pept*, 1990, 28(2):131-6.

   Results of the present study suggest that exogenous and endogenous gastrin lower blood calcium. Following intraperitoneal injection of ranitidine, an increased gastrin concentration was associated with a drop in blood calcium. The ranitidine-evoked hypocalcemia could be prevented by gastrectomy. The authors conclude that gastrin evokes hypocalcemia by mobilizing gastrocalcin from the stomach.

486. Ghishan FK, Walker F, Meneely R, et al, " Intestinal Calcium Transport: Effect of Cimetidine," *J Nutr*, 1981, 111(12):2157-61.

   An *in vivo* perfusion technique was used to evaluate the net transport and lumen-to-mucosa flux of labelled calcium. A decrease in net calcium transport and lumen-to-mucosa flux was noted in rats injected with cimetidine. Adding cimetidine to the perfusate did not alter transport rates. The authors observed that the mechanism by which cimetidine affects calcium transport may be secondary to its effect on the release of parathyroid hormone or an effect on vitamin D metabolism.

H₂ Blockers & Calcium Depletion - Negative Studies

487. Line D, Sebert JL, Gregiore I, "Primary Hyperparathyroidism. Lack of Effect of Cimetidine on Plasma Levels of Parathyroid Hormone and Calcium," *Presse Med*, 1984, 13(12):727-30.

   Because of the contradictory results formerly published as regards the effect of cimetidine in primary hyperparathyroidism, the effect of cimetidine was evaluated in 14 patients with primary hyperparathyroidism. There was no significant change in both plasma concentrations of calcium and parathyroid hormone. However, a regression analysis showed that plasma calcium was negatively correlated to duration of therapy. The correlation coefficient was projected to reach a level of statistical significance if the follow-up had lasted 9 months.

488. Merenich JA, Georgitis WM, and Clark JR, "Failure of Cimetidine to Reduce Postoperative Hypocalcemia in Patients With Primary Hyperparathyroidism Undergoing Neck Exploratory Operation," *Surgery*, 1993, 113(6):619-23.

   In this randomized, double-blind, placebo-controlled trial, 20 patients with primary hyperparathyroidism were treated with either cimetidine or placebo for 10-14 days prior to exploratory neck surgery. Cimetidine treatment resulted in a modest increase in preoperative parathyroid hormone levels. No other parameter was affected, including serum calcium or renal tubular phosphate reabsorption. The authors concluded that cimetidine treatment before surgery does not diminish the frequency or severity of postoperative hypocalcemia.

489. Gluszek J, Skoluda A, Pupek-Musialik D, et al, "Effect of Intravenous Administration of Cimetidine on Renal Excretion of Calcium, Phosphates, Magnesium and Adenosine Cyclic Monophosphate," *Pol Tyg Lek*, 1990, 45(40-41):817-9.

The effect of cimetidine on parathyroid function was evaluated in healthy subjects. No significant changes in serum calcium, phosphates, and magnesium concentrations were observed.

490. Bo-Linn GW, Davis GR, Buddrus DJ, et al, "An Evaluation of the Importance of Gastric Acid Secretion in the Absorption of Dietary Calcium," *J Clin Invest*, 1984, 73(3):640-7.

Gastrointestinal absorption of calcium was determined following a single meal. A large dose of cimetidine, sufficient to reduce gastric acid secretion, did not affect calcium absorption in normal subjects. In addition, an achlorhydric patient with pernicious anemia demonstrated normal calcium absorption. The authors conclude gastric acidity does not contribute to the absorption of dietary calcium.

H₂ Blockers & Vitamin D Depletion

491. Odes HS, Fraser GM, Krugliak P, et al, "Effect of Cimetidine on Hepatic Vitamin D Metabolism in Humans," 1990, 46(2):61-4.

Nine adult patients were treated with 400 mg cimetidine orally twice daily. Serum levels of 25-hydroxyvitamin D, 24,25-dihydroxyvitamin D and 1,25-dihydroxyvitamin D were monitored before treatment, after 4 weeks of treatment, and 1 month after cessation of treatment. Although no significant increase in the level of 25-hydroxyvitamin D was observed during treatment, the level rose significantly after drug discontinuation. Other values remained normal. The data were interpreted to suggest that short-term cimetidine treatment could alter vitamin D metabolism in humans.

492. Bengoa JM, Bolt MJ, and Rosenberg IH, "Hepatic Vitamin D 25-Hydroxylase Inhibition by Cimetidine and Isoniazid," *J Lab Clin Med*, 1984, 104(4):546-52.

This *in vitro* study evaluated the effect of cimetidine and isoniazid on hepatic vitamin D 25-hydroxylase activity. Whole liver homogenates from rats deficient in vitamin D were used. Cimetidine and isoniazid both inhibited *in vitro* vitamin D 25-hydroxylase activity. The authors conclude that the long-term effect of cimetidine on vitamin D metabolism warrants further investigation.

493. Wyatt CL, Jensen LS, Rowland GN 3d, "Effect of Cimetidine on Eggshell Quality and Plasma 25-Hydroxycholecalciferol in Laying Hens," *Poult Sci*, 1990, 69(11):1892-9.

Experiments were conducted in laying hens to investigate the effect of cimetidine on vitamin D_3 metabolism and calcification. Two levels of vitamin D_3 intake were evaluated. Cimetidine significantly decreased total egg production in hens fed either level of vitamin D_3, but only at higher cimetidine dosages. Plasma calcium and inorganic phosphate concentrations were decreased in hens fed high cimetidine dosages. Cimetidine decreased plasma 25-hydroxycholecalciferol levels. Results suggest that the reduction in bone mineralization, eggshell quality, and plasma 25-hydroxycholecalciferol levels could be due to cimetidine interference with metabolism.

H₂ Blockers & Vitamin D Depletion - No Negative Studies

H₂ Blockers & Iron Depletion

494. Campbell NR, Hasinoff BB, Meddings JB, et al, "Ferrous Sulfate Reduces Cimetidine Absorption," *Dig Dis Sci*, 1993, 38(5):950-4.

ULCER MEDICATIONS *(Continued)*

A number of *in vitro* experiments were performed to examine the binding of iron with cimetidine. Additional experiments were performed to determine the effect of concurrent administration of ferrous sulfate on cimetidine absorption. At higher ferrous sulfate dosages, cimetidine absorption was completely inhibited. *In vitro* iron in its ferrous form rapidly oxidizes to the ferric form. The ferric form of iron binds to cimetidine and may be the cause of decreased cimetidine absorption. The authors advise caution when prescribing iron supplements with cimetidine. **Comment:** The bound iron/cimetidine complex is not absorbable, therefore iron absorption is reduced in conjunction with decreased cimetidine absorption.

495. Skikne BS, Lynch SR, and Cook JD, "Role of Gastric Acid in Food Iron Absorption," *Gastroenterology*, 1981, 81(6):1068-71.

Following a dose of cimetidine, radioiron absorption tests in human volunteers demonstrated a reduction in the absorption of dietary nonheme iron. More pronounced decreases were observed at higher doses. Antacids caused a decrease in iron absorption while pentagastrin had no significant effect. In usual doses, the authors believed cimetidine would not be expected to have a major effect on iron status. However, at high doses and in combination with antacids, nonheme iron absorption could be significantly impaired. **Comment:** Increased doses of H_2 antagonists affect iron absorption in patients, and potentially could affect a larger population based on individual biochemical characteristics.

496. Aymard JP, Aymard B, Netter P, et al, "Haematological Adverse Effects of Histamine H_2-Receptor Antagonists," *Med Toxicol Adverse Drug Exp*, 1988, 3(6):430-48.

Reduction of dietary iron absorption is noted as a potential adverse effect of histamine antagonists in this review. Malabsorption of dietary iron and cobalamin is proposed to result from inhibition of gastric secretion by H_2-receptor antagonists. While not considered to be of importance in short-term treatment, long-term use of H_2-receptor antagonists are proposed as possible contributors to iron or cobalamin deficiency.

H_2 Blockers & Iron Depletion - Negative Studies

497. Stewart CA, Termanini B, Sutliff VE, et al, "Iron Absorption in Patients With Zollinger-Ellison Syndrome Treated With Long-Term Gastric Acid Antisecretory Therapy," *Aliment Pharmacol Ther*, 1998, 12(1):83-98.

One hundred and nine patients with Zollinger-Ellison Syndrome without previous gastric resection were studied with respect to their iron status. Eighty-nine patients were taking omeprazole, nine patients were taking histamine H_2-antagonists and eleven patients were taking no drugs. The authors concluded that continuous treatment with any gastric antisecretory drug does not cause decreased body iron stores or iron deficiency. The authors note that their results demonstrate yearly monitoring for iron parameters is unnecessary.

498. Partlow ES, Campbell NR, Chan SC, et al, "Ferrous Sulfate Does Not Reduce Serum Levels of Famotidine or Cimetidine After Concurrent Ingestion," *Clin Pharmacol Ther*, 1996, 59(4):389-93.

A series of randomized crossover studies was performed to determine whether there was a reduction in serum levels of cimetidine and famotidine when coingested with ferrous sulfate. The authors concluded that the coingestion of ferrous sulfate with either cimetidine or famotidine failed to result in a clinically relevant reduction in serum histamine H_2-receptor blocker levels. In addition, on the basis of *in vitro* binding experiments, iron was determined to be unlikely to interact with ranitidine.

H$_2$ Blockers & Zinc Depletion

499. Sturniolo GC, Montino MC, Rossetto L, et al, "Inhibition of Gastric Acid Secretion Reduces Zinc Absorption in Man," *J Am Coll Nutr*, 1991, 10(4):372-5.

Eleven healthy volunteers were studied to evaluate the effect of cimetidine and the influence of HCl gastric secretion on zinc absorption. Zinc absorption was reduced after cimetidine administration. This suggests that gastric pH influences zinc absorption. To rule out a direct effect of the drug on zinc absorption, an effect on zinc absorption was confirmed using a different H$_2$ antagonist, ranitidine.

500. Pinelli A and Trivulzio S, "Antiprostatic Effect Associated With Zinc Depletion in Cimetidine-Treated Rats," *Pharmacol Res Commun*, 1988, 20(4):329-35.

Administration of high-dose cimetidine for 45 days decreased the weight of the prostate and lowered prostate levels of zinc metal ion in rats.

501. Pinelli P, Trivulzio S, Colombo R, et al, "Antiprostatic Effect of Cimetidine in Rats," *Agents Actions*, 1987, 22(3-4):197-201.

Based on studies in rats, the authors concluded that cimetidine interacts with zinc metal ion and androgen action by lowering zinc prostatic levels and consequently depresses the prostatic weight. Alternatively, cimetidine was speculated to bind to androgen receptors differently in the prostate and in the testicles because of differences in receptor structure.

H$_2$ Blockers & Zinc Depletion - No Negative Studies

H$_2$ Blockers & Vitamin B$_{12}$ Depletion

502. Force RW and Nahata MC, "Effect of Histamine H$_2$-Receptor Antagonists on Vitamin B$_{12}$ Absorption," *Ann Pharmacother*, 1992, 26(10):1283-6.

This article reviews the literature regarding the effect of H$_2$ receptor antagonists on vitamin B$_{12}$ absorption. The article notes that parietal cells produce gastric acid, pepsin, and intrinsic factor. Gastric acid and pepsin are required for cleavage of vitamin B$_{12}$ from food sources, while intrinsic factor is required for vitamin B$_{12}$ absorption. Although evidence demonstrating that H$_2$ receptor antagonists decrease intrinsic factor secretion are not conclusive, a significant reduction in food-bound vitamin B$_{12}$ absorption has been demonstrated in patients taking these drugs. The authors conclude that H$_2$ receptor antagonists may potentially cause vitamin B$_{12}$ deficiency. This may be particularly important in patients with inadequate diet, poor stores of the vitamin, and in patients receiving continuous therapy for more than 2 years.

503. Aymard JP, Aymard B, Netter P, et al, "Haematological Adverse Effects of Histamine H$_2$-Receptor Antagonists," *Med Toxicol Adverse Drug Exp*, 1988, 3(6):430-48.

The authors review various hematologic adverse effects of H$_2$ receptor antagonists. These are noted to be relatively uncommon and primarily associated with cimetidine. Adverse effects are reviewed under four categories; blood cytopenias, coagulation disorders, reduced absorption of dietary iron, and reduced dietary cobalamin absorption. The authors note that malabsorption of dietary iron and cobalamin appears to result from decreased gastric secretion. While this has little impact in short-term treatment, long-term use may contribute to iron or cobalamin deficiency anemia.

ULCER MEDICATIONS *(Continued)*

504. Festen HP, "Intrinsic Factor Secretion and Cobalamin Absorption. Physiology and Pathophysiology in the Gastrointestinal Tract," *Scand J Gastroenterol Suppl*, 1991, 188:1-7.

This review notes that multiple stimuli trigger secretion of gastric acid and intrinsic factor, some of which are common to both substances. H_2 receptor antagonists inhibit both intrinsic factor and acid secretion, but omeprazole has no effect on intrinsic factor despite its effects on acid secretion. Cobalamin is cleaved from protein by acid-peptic digestion in the stomach. Therefore, the author states that hypochlorhydria or achlorhydria, whether pharmacologically induced or due to medical causes, may impair cobalamin uptake. Processes within the small intestine complete the absorptive process, including cleavage of the cobalamin-R-protein complex formed in the stomach. A variety of pancreatic and intestinal abnormalities may also impair cobalamin absorption.

505. Belaiche J, Zittoun J, Marquet J, et al, "Effect of Ranitidine on Secretion of Gastric Intrinsic Factor and Absorption of Vitamin B_{12}," *Gastroenterol Clin Biol*, 1983, 7(4):381-4.

The effects of ranitidine on intrinsic factor secretion and protein-bound cobalamin absorption were evaluated in six patients with duodenal ulcer. Oral ranitidine resulted in a nonsignificant decrease of intrinsic factor secretion. This was responsible for malabsorption of protein-bound cobalamin. The observed malabsorption was reversible after ranitidine was discontinued. The authors note that cobalamin deficiency may occur during long-term ranitidine treatment. Careful monitoring in these patients is recommended.

506. Salom IL, Silvis SE and Doscherholmen A, "Effect of Cimetidine on the Absorption of Vitamin B_{12}," *Scand J Gastroenterol*, 1982, 17(1):129-31.

The effect of cimetidine on the absorption of orally administered vitamin B_{12} in either the crystalline or food-bound state was investigated in 13 patients. Cimetidine did not significantly change absorption of crystalline B_{12}. However, the uptake of food-bound B_{12} decreased in all patients by a mean of 53%. The possibility that long-term therapy with cimetidine may produce B_{12} deficiency in a manner which is similar to other hypochlorhydric states is supported. The authors note that these data indicate that malabsorption caused by cimetidine would not be detected by a standard Schilling test.

507. Steinberg WM, King CE, and Toskes PP, "Malabsorption of Protein-Bound Cobalamin but Not Unbound Cobalamin During Cimetidine Administration," *Dig Dis Sci*, 1980, 25(3):188-91.

The absorption of both unbound [57Co]cyanocobalamin and protein-bound [57Co]cyanocobalamin was evaluated in 12 patients. Patients were evaluated during and after discontinuation of cimetidine therapy. Although cimetidine did not alter the absorption of unbound cobalamin, absorption of protein-bound cobalamin decreased. This effect was reversed following discontinuation of cimetidine. The authors conclude that cimetidine causes malabsorption of protein-bound cobalamin, which may cause cobalamin deficiency during long-term treatment. In addition, this form of malabsorption is not detectable by the usual tests of cobalamin absorption, since these tests normally employ crystalline vitamin B_{12}.

H_2 Blockers & Vitamin B_{12} Depletion - Negative Studies

508. Walan A and Strom M, "Metabolic Consequences of Reduced Gastric Acidity," *Scand J Gastroenterol Suppl*, 1985, 111:24-30.

In 20 healthy volunteers, the effect of ranitidine on the absorption of food cobalamins was investigated. Subjects were randomized to treatment with ranitidine or placebo for 1 week. Radiolabelled liver cobalamins were administered orally, and the absorption of 57Co-labelled cobalamins was assessed by stool collection. There was no significant difference in the mean absorption before (47.4%) and after (50.7%) the treatment.

509. Johnson GJ, Silvis SE, Roitman B, et al, "Long-Term Treatment of Systemic Mastocytosis With Histamine H_2 Receptor Antagonists," *Am J Gastroenterol*, 1980, 74(6):485-9.

A patient with systemic mastocytosis and gastric hypersecretion with duodenal ulcer was treated with metiamide followed by cimetidine for 44 months. Complete suppression of gastric hypersecretion was documented after 33 months of treatment. Vitamin B_{12} absorption in this patient remained normal.

H_2 Blockers & Folic Acid Depletion

510. Russell RM, Golner BB, Krasinski SD, et al, "Effect of Antacid and H_2 Receptor Antagonists on the Intestinal Absorption of Folic Acid," *J Lab Clin Med*, 1988, 112(4):458-63.

The influence of antacids and H_2 receptor antagonists on folic acid absorption was studied by using tritium-labeled pteroylmonoglutamic acid. Thirty subjects were evaluated. Both cimetidine and an aluminum and magnesium hydroxide antacid reduced folate absorption from a liquid formula meal. Although ranitidine also caused a fall in folic acid absorption, the change was not statistically significant. Both cimetidine and ranitidine increased intraluminal pH in the proximal small intestine after meals. This was believed to contribute to the inhibition of folate absorption. The antacid was found to precipitate folic acid at a pH of greater than 4.0, which appeared to explain the lowered folate absorption. Although the effects were relatively small, the authors believed that reductions could become significant during long-term or intensive use of these therapies, particularly in individuals with marginal folate intake.

H_2 Blockers & Folic Acid Depletion - No Negative Studies

PROTON PUMP INHIBITORS

Proton Pump Inhibitors & Beta-Carotene Depletion

511. Tang G, Serfaty-Lacrosniere C, Camilo ME, et al, "Gastric Acidity Influences the Blood Response to a Beta-Carotene Dose in Humans," *Am J Clin Nutr*, 1996, 64(4):622-6.

A cross-over analysis evaluating the effect of gastric acidity on beta-carotene absorption was conducted in 12 normal subjects. Results demonstrated significantly higher serum trans and cis beta-carotene levels in persons with lower gastric pH. The authors suggest one possibility to explain their findings is that, at a higher pH, decreased beta-carotene concentrations could be due to slower movement of negatively charged micelles. Additional research in this area is warranted.

Proton Pump Inhibitors & Vitamin B_{12} Depletion

512. Termanini B, Gibril F, Sutliff VE, et al, "Effect of Long-Term Gastric Acid Suppressive Therapy on Serum Vitamin B_{12} Levels in Patients With Zollinger-Ellison Syndrome," *Am J Med*, 1998, 104(5):422-30.

In 131 patients treated with long-term omeprazole or histamine H_2-receptor antagonists, the effect on serum vitamin B_{12} and folate levels was evaluated. Therapy was maintained over a mean duration of 4.5 years for omeprazole,

ULCER MEDICATIONS *(Continued)*

and 10 years for H_2-receptor antagonists. Vitamin B_{12} levels decreased significantly only in patients rendered achlorhydric. Vitamin B_{12} levels were significantly lower in patients treated with omeprazole. These were particularly low in patients with omeprazole-induced hyposecretion or complete achlorhydria. The duration of omeprazole treatment was inversely correlated with vitamin B_{12} but not folate levels. Based on these data, the authors concluded that patients treated chronically with proton pump inhibitors may develop B_{12} deficiency.

513. Bellou A, Aimone-Gastin I, De Korwin JD, et al, "Cobalamin Deficiency With Megaloblastic Anaemia in One Patient Under Long-Term Omeprazole Therapy," *J Intern Med*, 1996, 240(3):161-4.

This article details the first case of cobalamin deficiency and megaloblastic anemia in a patient following long-term omeprazole therapy. The patient received omeprazole for 4 years as treatment for gastroesophagal reflux. Serum vitamin B_{12} was dramatically decreased, however a normal Schilling test was observed using crystalline [57Co] cobalamin. Hematologic status was restored after intramuscular cobalamin treatment. The authors concluded that a cobalamin deficiency due to protein-bound cobalamin malabsorption may occur during long-term omeprazole therapy.

514. Saltzman JR, Kemp JA, Golner BB, et al, "Effect of Hypochlorhydria Due to Omeprazole Treatment or Atrophic Gastritis on Protein-Bound Vitamin B_{12} Absorption," *J Am Coll Nutr*, 1994, 13(6):584-91.

The absorption of protein-bound vitamin B_{12} was examined in elderly normal and hypochlorhydric subjects. Subjects underwent protein-bound vitamin B_{12} absorption tests following ingestion with water, cranberry juice, and 0.1 N hydrochloric acid. Protein-bound vitamin B_{12} absorption was significantly lower in the omeprazole-treated group as compared to normal controls. With cranberry juice ingestion, the omeprazole-treated group showed an increase in protein-bound vitamin B_{12} absorption which was further increased after dilute hydrochloric acid ingestion. The authors concluded that omeprazole causes protein-bound vitamin B_{12} malabsorption. In addition, ingestion of an acidic drink improves protein-bound vitamin B_{12} absorption.

515. Marcuard SP, Albernaz L, and Khazanie PG, "Omeprazole Therapy Causes Malabsorption of Cyanocobalamin," *Ann Intern Med*, 1994, 120(3):211-5.

Ten healthy male volunteers were studied to determine the effect of omeprazole on vitamin B_{12} absorption. After initial testing, five patients were randomly assigned to take 1 of 2 omeprazole dosages daily for 2 weeks. Omeprazole therapy resulted in an acute, dose-dependent decrease in cyanocobalamin absorption.

Proton Pump Inhibitors & Vitamin B$_{12}$ Depletion - Negative Studies

516. Schenk BE, Festen HP, Kuipers EJ, et al, "Effect of Short- and Long-Term Treatment With Omeprazole on the Absorption and Serum Levels of Cobalamin," *Aliment Pharmacol Ther*, 1996, 10(4):541-5.

To evaluate the impact of omeprazole therapy, the absorption of unbound and protein-bound cobalamin was determined by 24-hour urinary excretion of unbound 58Co-cyancobalamin or protein-bound 57Co-cyanocobalamin following a Schilling test. Tests were performed before and during treatment with 20 mg and 40 mg omeprazole daily for 9 days. In addition, serum cobalamin levels were assessed in 25 patients before and during long-term therapy with omeprazole. The authors concluded the absorption of protein-bound, but not unbound, cyanocobalamin is decreased during treatment with omeprazole. However, the authors could not document any change in serum cobalamin levels in patients treated with omeprazole for up to 7 years.

MISCELLANEOUS DRUGS

ACETAMINOPHEN

Acetaminophen & Glutathione Depletion

517. Lores Arnaiz S, Llesuy S, Cutrin JC, et al, "Oxidative Stress by Acute Acetaminophen Administration in Mouse Liver," *Free Radic Biol Med*, 1995, 19(3):303-10.

   In an effort to study hepatic damage from acetaminophen overdose, hepatic glutathione concentrations (total and oxidized) were measured in mice at 15, 30, and 60 minutes following a single dose of acetaminophen (375 mg/kg). Total glutathione was decreased at every time point. Hepatocyte damage was observed, with severe lesions and necrosis after 60 minutes. The authors cite oxidative stress as a possible mechanism for acetaminophen-induced hepatotoxicity.

518. Richie JP Jr, Lang CA, and Chen TS, "Acetaminophen-Induced Depletion of Glutathione and Cysteine in the Aging Mouse Kidney," *Biochem Pharmacol*, 1992, 44(1):129-35.

   Since glutathione deficiency is a general property of aging tissues, including the kidney, senescent organisms have been hypothesized to be at greater risk of acetaminophen-induced renal damage. Mice at a range of ages through the life span were injected with a variety of acetaminophen dosages. The extent of glutathione and cysteine depletion was determined. In the controls, concentrations decreased about 30% in the aging mouse. Acetaminophen depleted the renal glutathione and cysteine in a dose- and time-dependent manner. The extent of depletion in old (31-month) mice was greater, and the recovery was less efficient. The authors noted that a glutathione and cysteine deficiency occurs in the mouse kidney with acetaminophen administration, which was accompanied by an impaired detoxification capacity.

METHOTREXATE

Methotrexate & Folic Acid Depletion

519. Leeb BF, Witzmann G, Ogris E, et al, "Folic Acid and Cyanocobalamin Levels in Serum and Erythrocytes During Low-Dose Methotrexate Therapy of Rheumatoid Arthritis and Psoriatic Arthritis Patients," *Clin Exp Rheumatol*, 1995, 13(4):459-63.

   Folic acid levels in patients treated with methotrexate were compared to controls. The degree of folate depletion during methotrexate therapy was found to depend on the weekly dose. Folate depletion was also postulated to be related to B_{12} deficiency in red blood cells. Folic acid levels were not related to parameters of disease severity. The authors propose that inhibition of dihydrofolate reductase by methotrexate is not a primary mechanism of action in rheumatoid arthritis, and additional folate, if necessary, should not reduce the efficacy of methotrexate.

520. Morgan SL, Baggott JE, Lee JY, et al, "Folic Acid Supplementation Prevents Deficient Blood Folate Levels and Hyperhomocysteinemia During Longterm, Low Dose Methotrexate Therapy for Rheumatoid Arthritis: Implications for Cardiovascular Disease Prevention," *J Rheumatol*, 1998, 25(3):441-6.

   In a 1-year, placebo-controlled trial of folic acid supplementation in patients receiving methotrexate therapy, folate levels were noted to decline in the absence of supplementation. The authors conclude folic acid supplementation should be considered to prevent methotrexate toxicity and to prevent or treat folate deficiency.

521. Dijkmans BA, "Folate Supplementation and Methotrexate," *Br J Rheumatol*, 1995, 34(12):1172-4.

This review discusses the influence of folate supplementation on the toxicity and efficacy of methotrexate in rheumatoid arthritis. The author concludes that folate supplementation does not appear to affect the efficacy of methotrexate but may have positive effects on toxicity.

522. Chungi VS, Bourne DW, and Dittert LW, "Competitive Inhibition Between Folic Acid and Methotrexate for Transport Carrier in the Rat Small Intestine," *J Pharm Sci*, 1979, 68(12):1552-3.

In an *in situ* rat model, folic acid absorption from the lumen of the rat small intestine obeyed Michaelis-Menten kinetics. Folic acid and methotrexate were mutual competitive inhibitors of absorption.

Methotrexate & Folic Acid Depletion - No Negative Studies

MITHRAMYCIN/PLICAMYCIN

Mithramycin/Plicamycin & Calcium Depletion

523. Thurlimann B, Waldburger R, Senn HJ, et al, "Plicamycin and Pamidronate in Symptomatic Tumor-Related Hypercalcemia: A Prospective Randomized Crossover Trial," *Ann Oncol*, 1992, 3(8):619-23.

In a randomized, crossover trial, single doses of pamidronate and plicamycin were compared in hypercalcemic patients. Both agents were noted to lower serum calcium levels significantly within 1 week. In the patients who received pamidronate, the duration of normocalcemia was significantly longer. Hypocalcemia occurred in 23% of patients in the pamidronate group and in 5% of patients in the plicamycin group. Hypocalcemia was either asymptomatic or mild, with the exception of a single pamidronate-treated patient. Overall, pamidronate was found to be more effective and better tolerated than plicamycin in the relief of the morbidity associated with tumor-related hypercalcemia.

Mithramycin/Plicamycin & Phosphorus Depletion

524. Ajlouni K and Theil GB, "Mithramycin Effects on Calcium, Phosphorus and Parathyroid Hormone in Osseous Paget's Disease," *Am J Med Sci*, 1975, 269(1):13-8.

Six patients with Paget's disease were treated with a four-day course of mithramycin. Mithramycin produced significant hypocalcemia and hypophosphatemia. Parathyroid hormone was also increased.

ORLISTAT

Orlistat & Vitamin D, Vitamin E, and Beta-Carotene Depletion

525. Melia AT, Koss-Twardy SG, and Zhi J, "The Effect of Orlistat, an Inhibitor of Dietary Fat Absorption, on the Absorption of Vitamins A and E in Healthy Volunteers," *J Clin Pharmacol*, 1996, 36(7):647-53.

In an open-label, placebo-controlled, randomized, two-way crossover study of 12 healthy volunteers (20-44 years of age), the absorption of vitamins A and E was assessed in individuals receiving orlistat. Orlistat significantly reduced the absorption of vitamin E (maximum concentrations decreased approximately 43% while AUC was decreased by 60%). Vitamin A was not affected at the dose levels studied.

MISCELLANEOUS DRUGS *(Continued)*

526. Zhi J, Melia AT, Koss-Twardy SG, et al, "The Effect of Orlistat, an Inhibitor of Dietary Fat Absorption, on the Pharmacokinetics of Beta-Carotene in Healthy Volunteers," *J Clin Pharmacol*, 1996, 36(2):152-9.

An open-label, parallel, placebo-controlled, randomized, two-way crossover study was performed in 48 healthy volunteers (ages 19-58 years) to assess the influence of orlistat on the absorption of beta-carotene. Short-term (3 to 6 days) treatment with orlistat did not alter plasma beta-carotene levels. However, orlistat decreased beta-carotene absorption by approximately one-third, and this effect was consistent for all three dose levels of beta-carotene studied. The authors concluded that two-thirds of a supplemental dose of beta-carotene will be absorbed during orlistat treatment, which may result in physiologic levels of beta-carotene being achieved.

527. Finer N, James WP, Kopelman PG, et al, "One-Year Treatment of Obesity: A Randomized, Double-Blind, Placebo-Controlled, Multicentre Study of Orlistat, a Gastrointestinal Lipase Inhibitor," *Int J Obes Relat Metab Disord*, 2000, 24(3):306-13.

A total of 228 patients were randomized to double-blind treatment with either orlistat 120 mg or placebo, in conjunction with a low-energy diet, for 12 months. To maintain normal plasma levels of fat-soluble vitamins, supplements of vitamins A, D, and E were required in 1.8%, 8.0% and 3.6% of orlistat-treated patients, respectively. The decrease in vitamin E and beta carotene was significantly greater in orlistat-treated subjects. The authors noted fat-soluble vitamin supplements may be required during chronic orlistat therapy.

528. WP James, Avenell A, Broom J, et al, "A One-Year Trial to Assess the Value of Orlistat in the Management of Obesity," *Int J Obes Relat Metab Disord*, 1997, 21 (Suppl 3):S24-30.

No abstract available.

PENICILLAMINE

Penicillamine is used in patients with Wilson's disease to lower copper levels. There are mixed reports about its ability to chelate other nutrients.

Penicillamine & Copper, Pyridoxine, Magnesium, and Zinc Depletion

529. Seelig MS, "Auto-immune Complications of D-Penicillamine - A Possible Result of Zinc and Magnesium Depletion and of Pyridoxine Inactivation," *J Am Coll Nutr*, 1982, 1(2):207-14.

The author discusses the use of supplementation in 50 patients receiving long-term penicillamine therapy. Adverse events were noted to be very low in the population studied. Zinc, magnesium, and pyridoxine were felt to be the agents which would offer the most protection.

530. Jaffe IA, "The Antivitamin B_6 Effect of Penicillamine: Clinical and Immunological Implications," *Adv Biochem Psychopharmacol*, 1972, 4:217-26.

The relationship between vitamin B_6 and penicillamine was reviewed.

531. Lu JX and Combs GF Jr, "Penicillamine: Pharmacokinetics and Differential Effects on Zinc and Copper Status in Chicks," *J Nutr*, 1992, 122(2):355-62.

The pharmacokinetics and effects of D(-)-penicillamine on the nutritional status of copper and zinc were studied in chicks. Urinary collection demonstrated that penicillamine was rapidly excreted and was associated with increased urinary excretion of both zinc and copper. The authors concluded that these results demonstrate altered tissue distribution of zinc and copper during penicillamine treatment.

532. Jepsen LV and Eggert J, "Zinc and Zinc-Dependent Enzymes in Penicillamine-Treated Patients With Generalized Scleroderma," *Acta Derm Venereol*, 1984, 64(5):424-7.

Zinc concentrations in serum, erythrocytes, and granulocytes were evaluated. No difference was found between patients receiving penicillamine and controls, however granulocyte zinc strongly tended to be decreased. The authors propose penicillamine may produce a cellular zinc depletion.

Penicillamine &Magnesium Depletion - Negative Studies

533. Dastych M, Jezek P, and Richtrova M, "Effect of Penicillamine Therapy on the Concentration of Zinc, Copper, Iron, Calcium, and Magnesium in the Serum and Their Excretion in Urine," *Z Gastroenterol*, 1986, 24(3):157-60.

In a 1-year study of copper and zinc excretion, the authors indicate zinc excretion was only moderately increased by penicillamine. Penicillamine did not influence the excretion of calcium, magnesium, and iron. Further, zinc content in patients' hair samples did not decrease. The authors concluded that treatment with penicillamine is not likely to result in zinc deficiency in liver disease.

Penicillamine & Zinc Depletion - Negative Studies

534. Dastych M, Jezek P, and Richtrova M, "Effect of Penicillamine Therapy on the Concentration of Zinc, Copper, Iron, Calcium, and Magnesium in the Serum and Their Excretion in Urine," *Z Gastroenterol*, 1986, 24(3):157-60.

Urinary copper was increased, but zinc excretion was not increased in a population receiving penicillamine. In addition, penicillamine did not influence the excretion of calcium, magnesium, or iron.

535. Teherani DK, Altmann H, Tausch G, et al, "Zinc Levels in Blood and Urine of Rheumatoid Arthritis Patients After Four Months Treatment With D-Penicillamine," *Z Rheumatol*, 1980, 39(11-12):395-400.

Ten female patients receiving penicillamine for rheumatoid arthritis were monitored to determine the effect on zinc status. Blood levels of zinc decreased distinctly until the second week, but returned to normal after 2 months of therapy.

536. Tausch G, Teherani DK, Broll H, et al, "Effect of D-Penicillamine on Zinc Levels in Blood and Urine of Patients With Chronic Polyarthritis," *Z Rheumatol*, 1978, 37(5-6):148-52.

Six female patients receiving penicillamine for rheumatoid arthritis were monitored to determine the effect on zinc status. An increase in urinary zinc excretion was noted throughout the trial. Blood values of zinc declined until the second week, but increased to a value above normal by the third week.

APPENDIX
TABLE OF CONTENTS

DRUG-INDUCED NUTRIENT DEPLETIONS

PRESCRIPTION AND NONPRESCRIPTION PRODUCTS

Drug	Brand Names	Nutrient Depletions	Potential Depletion Problems
ANTACIDS			
Magnesium and Aluminum Antacids			
Aluminum hydroxide; aluminum hydroxide and magnesium carbonate; aluminum hydroxide and magnesium hydroxide; aluminum hydroxide and magnesium trisilicate; aluminum hydroxide, magnesium hydroxide, and simethicone; magnesium hydroxide; magnesium oxide; magnesium sulfate	Various products	Calcium, phosphorus	See individual nutrient monographs
Sodium bicarbonate	Various products	Potassium	See individual nutrient monographs
ANTIBIOTICS			
General Antibiotics (Note: See individual antibiotic listings for further information)			
Aminoglycosides, cephalosporins, fluoroquinolones, macrolides, penicillins, sulfonamides, tetracyclines	Various products	*Bifidobacteria bifidum (bifidus)*, biotin, inositol, *Lactobacillus acidophilus*, vitamin B₁, vitamin B₂, vitamin B₃, vitamin B₆, vitamin B₁₂, vitamin K	Short-term nutrient depletion effects are minimal; however, alteration of gut microflora can allow dysbiosis to develop, which can further inhibit the digestion and absorption of nutrients and cause a weakening of the immune system.
Penicillins (Note: See general antibiotics listing above for further information)			
Amoxicillin, ampicillin, bacampicillin, carbenicillin, cloxacillin, dicloxacillin, nafcillin, penicillin G, benzathine, penicillin G benzathine and procaine combined, penicillin G procaine, penicillin V potassium, piperacillin, piperacillin and tazobactam sodium	Various products	Potassium	Irregular heartbeat, muscle weakness, fatigue, edema

PRESCRIPTION AND NONPRESCRIPTION PRODUCTS *(continued)*

Drug	Brand Names	Nutrient Depletions	Potential Depletion Problems
Tetracyclines (Note: See general antibiotics listing above for further information)			
Chlortetracycline, demeclocycline, doxycycline, minocycline, oxytetracycline, tetracycline	Various products	Calcium	Osteoporosis, heart/blood pressure irregularities, tooth decay
		Magnesium	Cardiovascular problems, asthma, osteoporosis, cramps, PMS
		Iron	Anemia, weakness, fatigue, hair loss, brittle nails
Aminoglycosides (Note: See general antibiotics listing above for further information)			
Neomycin	Mycifradin®; Neofradin®; Neo-Tabs®	Beta-carotene, calcium, iron, magnesium, potassium, vitamin A	Minimal problems with short-term use
Amikacin, gentamicin, tobramycin	Various products	Calcium, magnesium, potassium, sodium	
Sulfonamides (Note: See general antibiotics listing above for further information)			
Co-trimoxazole	Bactrim®; Cotrim®; Septra®; Sulfatrim®	Folic acid	Birth defects, cervical dysplasia, anemia, cardiovascular disease risk
Pentamidine	NebuPent™; Pentacarinat®; Pentam-300®	Magnesium	Cardiovascular problems, asthma, osteoporosis, cramps, PMS
Tuberculosis Drugs			
Isoniazid, INH	Laniazid®; Nydrazid®	Vitamin B₃	Skin, gastrointestinal, nervous system problems
		Vitamin B₆	Anemia, tiredness, weakness, increased cardiovascular disease risk
		Vitamin D	Osteoporosis, muscle weakness, hearing loss
Rifampin	Rifadin®; Rimactane®	Vitamin D	Osteoporosis, muscle weakness, hearing loss
Ethambutol	Myambutol®	Copper	Anemia, fatigue, cardiovascular and connective tissue problems
		Zinc	Slow wound healing, loss of sense of smell and taste, lower immunity

DRUG-INDUCED NUTRIENT DEPLETIONS *(Continued)*

PRESCRIPTION AND NONPRESCRIPTION PRODUCTS *(continued)*

Drug	Brand Names	Nutrient Depletions	Potential Depletion Problems
		ANTICONVULSANTS	
Barbiturates	Amytal®; Butalan®, Buticaps®, Butisol Sodium®; Mebaral®; Brevital®; Barbita®, Nembutal®; Luminal®; Solfoton®; Seconal™; Pentothal®; Tuinal®	Biotin	Hair loss, depression, cardiac irregularities, dermatitis
		Calcium	Osteoporosis, heart/blood pressure irregularities, tooth decay
		Folic acid	Birth defects, cervical dysplasia, anemia, cardiovascular disease
		Vitamin D	Osteoporosis, muscle weakness, hearing loss
		Vitamin K	Blood clotting and skeletal problems
Phenytoin	Dilantin®	Biotin	Hair loss, depression, cardiac irregularities, dermatitis
		Calcium	Osteoporosis, heart/blood pressure irregularities, tooth decay
		Folic acid	Birth defects, cervical dysplasia, anemia, cardiovascular disease
		Vitamin B_1	Depression, irritability, memory loss, muscle weakness, edema
		Vitamin B_{12}	Anemia, tiredness, weakness, increased cardiovascular disease risk
		Vitamin D	Osteoporosis, muscle weakness, hearing loss
		Vitamin K	Blood coagulation and skeletal problems
Carbamazepine	Carbatrol®; Epitol®; Tegretol®	Biotin	Hair loss, depression, cardiac irregularities, dermatitis
		Calcium	Osteoporosis, heart/blood pressure irregularities, tooth decay
		Folic acid	Birth defects, cervical dysplasia, anemia, cardiovascular disease risk
		Vitamin D	Osteoporosis, muscle weakness, hearing loss
Primidone	Mysoline®	Biotin	Hair loss, depression, cardiac irregularities, dermatitis
		Folic acid	Birth defects, cervical dysplasia, anemia, cardiovascular disease risk
		Vitamin D	Osteoporosis, muscle weakness, hearing loss
		Vitamin K	Blood coagulation and skeletal problems

PRESCRIPTION AND NONPRESCRIPTION PRODUCTS (continued)

Drug	Brand Names	Nutrient Depletions	Potential Depletion Problems
Valproic acid	Depacon®, Depakene®, Depakote®	Carnitine	Muscle weakness, cramps, fatigue
		Folic acid	Birth defects, cervical dysplasia, anemia, cardiovascular disease risk
Zonisamide	Zonegran®	Biotin, inositol, vitamin B₁, vitamin B₂, vitamin B₃, vitamin B₆, vitamin B₁₂, vitamin K	See individual nutrient monographs
ANTIDIABETICS			
Sulfonylureas			
Acetohexamide, glipizide, glyburide, repaglinide, tolazamide	Dymelor®, Glucotrol®, DiaBeta®, Glynase® PresTab™, Micronase®, Prandin™, Tolinase®	Coenzyme Q₁₀	High blood pressure, congestive heart failure, low energy
Biguanides			
Metformin	Glucophage®	Coenzyme Q₁₀	High blood pressure, congestive heart failure, low energy
		Folic acid	Birth defects, cervical dysplasia, anemia, cardiovascular disease
		Vitamin B₁₂	Anemia, tiredness, weakness, increased cardiovascular disease risk
ANTIFUNGALS			
Amphotericin B	Various products	Calcium	Osteoporosis, heart/blood pressure irregularities, tooth decay
		Magnesium	Cardiovascular problems, asthma, osteoporosis, cramps, PMS
		Potassium	Irregular heartbeat, muscle weakness, fatigue, edema
		Sodium	Muscle weakness, dehydration, loss of appetite, poor concentration; **Note: Replacement not recommended (depletion due to therapeutic effect)**

DRUG-INDUCED NUTRIENT DEPLETIONS *(Continued)*

PRESCRIPTION AND NONPRESCRIPTION PRODUCTS *(continued)*

Drug	Brand Names	Nutrient Depletions	Potential Depletion Problems
Salicylates			
Aspirin, choline magnesium trisalicylate, choline salicylate	Various products	Folic acid	Birth defects, cervical dysplasia, anemia, cardiovascular disease
		Iron	Anemia, weakness, fatigue, hair loss, brittle nails
		Potassium	Irregular heartbeat, muscle weakness, fatigue, edema
		Sodium	Muscle weakness, dehydration, loss of appetite, poor concentration
		Vitamin C	Weakened immune system, easy bruising, poor wound healing
Salsalate	Various products	Folic acid	Birth defects, cervical dysplasia, anemia, cardiovascular disease
Nonsteroidal Anti-Inflammatory Drugs			
Ibuprofen, naproxen, sulindac, piroxicam, diclofenac, diflunisal, etodolac, fenoprofen, ketoprofen, ketorolac, meclofenamate, nabumetone, tolmetin, mefenamic acid	Aleve®, Anaprox®, Naprelan®, Naprosyn®; Clinoril®, Feldene®; Ponstel®, Cataflam®; Motrin®, Voltaren®; Dolobid®, Lodine®; Nalfon®, Actron®, Orudis®, Oruvail®, Acular®, Toradol®, Meclomen®; Relafen®, Tolectin®	Folic acid	Birth defects, cervical dysplasia, anemia, cardiovascular disease
Indomethacin	Indochron E-R®; Indocin®	Folic acid	Birth defects, cervical dysplasia, anemia, cardiovascular disease
		Iron	Anemia, weakness, fatigue, hair loss, brittle nails

PRESCRIPTION AND NONPRESCRIPTION PRODUCTS (continued)

Drug	Brand Names	Nutrient Depletions	Potential Depletion Problems
Corticosteroids			
		Calcium	Osteoporosis, heart/blood pressure irregularities, tooth decay
		Folic acid	Birth defects, cervical dysplasia, anemia, cardiovascular disease
Betamethasone, budesonide, cortisone, dexamethasone, flunisolide, fluticasone, hydrocortisone, methylprednisolone, mometasone, prednisolone, prednisone, triamcinolone	Various products	Magnesium	Cardiovascular problems, asthma, osteoporosis, cramps, PMS
		Potassium	Irregular heartbeat, muscle weakness, fatigue, edema
		Selenium	Lower immunity, reduced antioxidant protection
		Vitamin C	Weakened immune system, easy bruising, poor wound healing
		Vitamin D	Osteoporosis, muscle weakness, hearing loss
		Zinc	Slow wound healing, loss of sense of smell and taste, lower immunity
5-Aminosalicylic Acid Derivatives			
Balsalazide, mesalamine, olsalazine, sulfasalazine	Various products	Folic acid	Birth defects, cervical dysplasia, anemia, cardiovascular disease
ANTIVIRALS			
		Calcium	Osteoporosis, heart/blood pressure irregularities, tooth decay
Foscarnet	Foscavir® Injection	Magnesium	Cardiovascular problems, asthma, osteoporosis, cramps, PMS
		Phosphorus	Stunted growth, skeletal problems, increased tooth decay
		Potassium	Irregular heartbeat, muscle weakness, fatigue, edema
Reverse Transcriptase Inhibitors			
		Carnitine	Muscle weakness, cramps, fatigue
Nucleoside: Didanosine, lamivudine, stavudine, zalcitabine, zidovudine	Various products	Copper	Anemia, fatigue, cardiovascular and connective tissue problem
		Vitamin B_{12}	Anemia, tiredness, weakness, increased cardiovascular disease risk
Non-nucleoside: Delavirdine, nevirapine		Zinc	Slow wound healing, loss of sense of smell and taste, lower immunity

DRUG-INDUCED NUTRIENT DEPLETIONS *(Continued)*

PRESCRIPTION AND NONPRESCRIPTION PRODUCTS *(continued)*

Drug	Brand Names	Nutrient Depletions	Potential Depletion Problems
		BRONCHODILATORS	
Theophylline	Various products	Vitamin B₁	Depression, irritability, memory loss, muscle weakness, edema
		Vitamin B₆	Depression, sleep disturbance, increased cardiovascular disease risk
		CANCER CHEMOTHERAPY	
	See Special Section on Nutrient Depletion and Cancer Chemotherapy on page 515		
		CARDIOVASCULAR DRUGS	
Vasodilators			
Hydralazine	Apresoline®	Coenzyme Q₁₀	High blood pressure, congestive heart failure, low energy
		Vitamin B₆	Anemia, tiredness, weakness, increased cardiovascular disease risk
Loop Diuretics			
Bumetanide, ethacrynic acid, furosemide	Bumex®, Edecrin®, Lasix®	Calcium	Osteoporosis, heart/blood pressure irregularities, tooth decay
		Magnesium	Cardiovascular problems, asthma, osteoporosis, cramps, PMS
		Potassium	Irregular heartbeat, muscle weakness, fatigue, edema
		Sodium	**Replacement not recommended (may be related to therapeutic effect)**
		Vitamin B₁	Depression, irritability, memory loss, muscle weakness, edema
		Vitamin B₆	Depression, sleep disturbance, increased cardiovascular disease risk
		Vitamin C	Weakened immune system, easy bruising, poor wound healing
		Zinc	Slow wound healing, loss of sense of smell and taste, lower immunity

PRESCRIPTION AND NONPRESCRIPTION PRODUCTS (continued)

Drug	Brand Names	Nutrient Depletions	Potential Depletion Problems
Thiazide Diuretics			
Hydrochlorothiazide, methylclothiazide, indapamide, metolazone	Aquatensen®; Enduron®; Esidrix®; Ezide®; HydroDIURIL®; Hydro-Par®; Microzide®; Oretic®; Lozol®; Mykrox®; Zaroxolyn®	Coenzyme Q₁₀	High blood pressure, congestive heart failure, low energy
		Magnesium	Cardiovascular problems, asthma, osteoporosis, cramps, PMS
		Phosphorus	Stunted growth, skeletal problems, increased tooth decay
		Potassium	Irregular heartbeat, muscle weakness, fatigue, edema
		Sodium	Muscle weakness, dehydration, loss of appetite, poor concentration
		Zinc	Slow wound healing, loss of sense of smell and taste, lower immunity
Potassium-Sparing Diuretics			
Triamterene	Dyrenium®	Calcium	Osteoporosis, heart/blood pressure irregularities, tooth decay
		Folic acid	Birth defects, cervical dysplasia, anemia, cardiovascular disease
		Zinc	Slow wound healing, loss of sense of smell and taste, lower immunity
Hydrochlorothiazide and triamterene	Dyazide®, Maxzide®	Calcium	Osteoporosis, heart/blood pressure irregularities, tooth decay
		Coenzyme Q₁₀	High blood pressure, congestive heart failure, low energy
		Folic acid	Birth defects, cervical dysplasia, anemia, cardiovascular disease
		Magnesium	Cardiovascular problems, asthma, osteoporosis, cramps, PMS
		Sodium	Muscle weakness, dehydration, loss of appetite, poor concentration
		Vitamin B₆	Depression, sleep disturbances, increased cardiovascular disease risk
		Zinc	Slow wound healing, loss of sense of smell and taste, lower immunity

DRUG-INDUCED NUTRIENT DEPLETIONS *(Continued)*

PRESCRIPTION AND NONPRESCRIPTION PRODUCTS *(continued)*

Drug	Brand Names	Nutrient Depletions	Potential Depletion Problems
ACE Inhibitors			
Benazepril, captopril, enalapril, fosinopril, lisinopril, moexipril, perindopril erbumine, quinapril, ramipril, trandolapril	Capoten®, Vasotec®	Zinc	Slow wound healing, loss of sense of smell and taste, lower immunity
Centrally-Acting Antihypertensives			
Clonidine, methyldopa	Catapres®, Duraclon®, Aldomet®	Coenzyme Q₁₀	High blood pressure, congestive heart failure, low energy
Chlorthalidone	Hygroton®, Thalitone®	Phosphorus	Stunted growth, skeletal problems, increased tooth decay
		Potassium	Irregular heartbeat, muscle weakness, fatigue, edema
		Sodium	Muscle weakness, dehydration, loss of appetite, poor concentration
		Zinc	Slow wound healing, loss of sense of smell and taste, lower immunity
Cardiac Glycosides			
Digoxin	Lanoxin®	Calcium	Osteoporosis, heart/blood pressure irregularities, tooth decay
		Magnesium	Cardiovascular problems, asthma, osteoporosis, cramps, PMS
		Phosphorus	Stunted growth, skeletal problems, increased tooth decay
		Vitamin B₁	Depression, irritability, memory loss, muscle weakness, edema

PRESCRIPTION AND NONPRESCRIPTION PRODUCTS *(continued)*

Drug	Brand Names	Nutrient Depletions	Potential Depletion Problems
Beta-Blockers			
Propranolol, metoprolol, atenolol, pindolol, acebutolol, betaxolol, bisoprolol, carteolol, carvedilol, esmolol, labetalol, nadolol, sotalol, timolol	Betachron E-R®, Inderal®; Lopressor® Toprol XL®; Tenormin®, Visken®; Sectral®, Betoptic®, Kerlone®, Zebeta®, Cartrol®, Coupress®, Coreg®, Brevibloc®, Normodyne®, Trandate®, Corgard®, Betapace®, Betimol®, Biocadren®, Timoptic®	Coenzyme Q$_{10}$	High blood pressure, congestive heart failure, low energy
CHOLESTEROL-LOWERING DRUGS			
HMG-CoA Reductase Inhibitors			
Atorvastatin, cerivastatin, lovastatin, fluvastatin, pravastatin, simvastatin	Lipitor®, Baycol®; Mevacor®; Lescol® Pravachol® Zocor®	Coenzyme Q$_{10}$	High blood pressure, congestive heart failure, low energy
Bile Acid Sequestrants			
Cholestyramine	Prevalite®, Questran®	Beta-carotene, calcium, folic acid, iron, magnesium, phosphorus, vitamin A, vitamin B$_{12}$, vitamin D, vitamin E, vitamin K, zinc	See individual nutrient monographs
Colestipol, colesevelam	Colestid®, Welchol®	Beta-carotene, folic acid, iron, vitamin A, vitamin B$_{12}$ vitamin D, vitamin E	See individual nutrient monographs
Miscellaneous			
		Coenzyme Q$_{10}$	High blood pressure, congestive heart failure, low energy
Fenofibrate, gemfibrozil	Gemcor®, Lopid®; TriCor™	Vitamin E	Greater free radical activity which weakens the immune system, increases the risk to conditions such as cardiovascular disease and cancer; accelerates the aging process

DRUG-INDUCED NUTRIENT DEPLETIONS *(Continued)*

PRESCRIPTION AND NONPRESCRIPTION PRODUCTS *(continued)*

Drug	Brand Names	Nutrient Depletions	Potential Depletion Problems
		ELECTROLYTE REPLACEMENT	
Potassium chloride (timed release)	Various products	Vitamin B₁₂	Anemia, tiredness, weakness increased cardiovascular disease risk
		FEMALE HORMONES	
Oral Contraceptives			
Estradiol and ethynodiol diacetate, ethinyl estradiol and desogestrel; ethinyl estradiol and norethindrone; ethinyl estradiol and norgestimate; ethinyl estradiol and norgestrel	Various products	Folic acid	Birth defects, cervical dysplasia, anemia, cardiovascular disease
		Magnesium	Cardiovascular problems, asthma, osteoporosis, cramps, PMS
		Tryptophan and tyrosine	Mental depression
		Vitamin B₂	Problems with skin, eyes, mucous membranes, nerves
		Vitamin B₃	Skin, gastrointestinal, nervous system problems
		Vitamin B₆	Depression, sleep disturbances, increased cardiovascular disease risk
		Vitamin B₁₂	Anemia, tiredness, weakness, increased cardiovascular disease risk
		Vitamin C	Weakened immune system, easy bruising, poor wound healing
		Zinc	Slow wound healing, loss of sense of smell and taste, lower immunity

PRESCRIPTION AND NONPRESCRIPTION PRODUCTS

Drug	Brand Names	Nutrient Depletions	Potential Depletion Problems
Estrogen Replacement (ERT) and Hormone Replacement (HRT) Therapies			
Estrogens, conjugated; estrogen and medroxyprogesterone; raloxifene; estrogens, esterified	Various products	Magnesium	Cardiovascular problems, asthma, osteoporosis, cramps, PMS
		Vitamin B$_2$	Problems with skin, eye, mucous membranes, nerves
		Vitamin B$_6$	Depression, sleep disturbances, increased cardiovascular disease risk
		Vitamin C	Weakened immune system, easy bruising, poor wound healing
		Zinc	Slow wound healing, loss of sense of smell and taste, lower immunity
GOUT MEDICATIONS			
		Beta-carotene	Lower immunity, reduced antioxidant protection
		Calcium	Osteoporosis, heart/blood pressure irregularities, tooth decay
Colchicine		Potassium	Irregular heartbeat, muscle weakness, fatigue, edema
		Sodium	Muscle weakness, dehydration, loss of appetite, poor concentration
		Vitamin B$_{12}$	Anemia, tiredness, weakness, increased cardiovascular disease risk
LAXATIVES			
Mineral oil	Various products	Beta-carotene, calcium, phosphorus, vitamin A, vitamin D, vitamin E, vitamin K	See individual nutrient monographs
Bisacodyl	Various products	Potassium	Irregular heartbeat, muscle weakness, fatigue, edema
		Sodium	Muscle weakness, dehydration, loss of appetite, poor concentration
Phosphate Enema			
Phosphate enema	Fleet®	Calcium	Osteoporosis, heart/blood pressure irregularities, tooth decay
		Magnesium	Cardiovascular problems, asthma, osteoporosis, cramps, PMS
		Potassium	Irregular heartbeat, muscle weakness, fatigue, edema
		Sodium	Muscle weakness, dehydration, loss of appetite, poor concentration

DRUG-INDUCED NUTRIENT DEPLETIONS (Continued)

PRESCRIPTION AND NONPRESCRIPTION PRODUCTS (continued)

Drug	Brand Names	Nutrient Depletions	Potential Depletion Problems
PSYCHOTHERAPEUTICS			
Lithium	Eskalith®, Lithobid®, Lithonate®, Lithotabs®	Inositol	**Replacement not recommended (may be related to therapeutic effect)**
Tricyclic Antidepressants			
Amitriptyline, desipramine, nortriptyline, doxepin, imipramine	Elavil®, Norpramin®, Pertofrane® Aventyl®, Pamelor® Adapin®, Sinequan® Zonalon®, Janimine®, Tofranil®	Vitamin B₂, coenzyme Q₁₀	Problems with skin, eyes, mucous membranes, nerves; high blood pressure, congestive heart failure, low energy
Phenothiazines			
Chlorpromazine, fluphenazine, thioridazine	Ormazine®; Thorazine®; Permitil®; Prolixin®; Mellaril®	Coenzyme Q₁₀	High blood pressure, congestive heart failure, low energy
		Vitamin B₂	Problems with skin, eyes, mucous membranes, nerves
Butyrophenones			
Haloperidol	Haldol®	Coenzyme Q₁₀	High blood pressure, congestive heart failure, low energy
ULCER MEDICATIONS			
H₂-Receptor Antagonists			
		Calcium	Osteoporosis, heart/blood pressure irregularities, tooth decay
		Folic acid	Birth defects, cervical dysplasia, anemia, cardiovascular disease
Cimetidine, famotidine, nizatadine, ranitidine	Tagamet®, Pepcid®, Axid®, Tritec®, Zantac®	Iron	Anemia, weakness, fatigue, hair loss, brittle nails
		Vitamin B₁₂	Anemia, tiredness, weakness, increased cardiovascular disease risk
		Vitamin D	Osteoporosis, muscle weakness, hearing loss
		Zinc	Slow wound healing, loss of sense of smell and taste, lower immunity
Proton Pump Inhibitors			
Lansoprazole, omeprazole	Prevacid®, Prilosec®	Vitamin B₁₂	Anemia, tiredness, weakness, increased cardiovascular disease risk

PRESCRIPTION AND NONPRESCRIPTION PRODUCTS *(continued)*

Drug	Brand Names	Nutrient Depletions	Potential Depletion Problems
		PARKINSON'S AGENTS	
Levodopa	Dopar®; Larodopa®	Potassium	Irregular heartbeat, muscle weakness, fatigue, edema
		SAMe	Unknown; possible neurotransmitter and/or nerve disturbances
		MISCELLANEOUS	
Acetaminophen	Various products	Glutathione	Decreased hepatic detoxification, decreased immunity
Edetate calcium disodium	Calcium Disodium Versenate®	Calcium	Osteoporosis, heart/blood pressure irregularities, tooth decay
Methotrexate	Folex®, Rheumatrex®	Folic acid	Birth defects, cervical dysplasia, anemia, cardiovascular disease
Orlistat	Xenical®	Beta-carotene	Weakened immunity, increased free radical damage
		Vitamin D	Osteoporosis, muscle weakness, hearing loss
		Vitamin E	Greater free radical activity which weakens the immune system, increases the risk to conditions such as cardiovascular disease and cancer; accelerates the aging process
		Copper	Anemia, fatigue, cardiovascular and connective tissue problems
		Magnesium	Cardiovascular problems, asthma, osteoporosis, cramps, PMS
Penicillamine	Cuprimine®; Depen®	Vitamin B₆	Depression, sleep disturbances, increased cardiovascular disease risk
		Zinc	Slow wound healing, loss of sense of smell and taste, lower immunity
Plicamycin	Mithracin®	Calcium	Osteoporosis, heart/blood pressure irregularities, tooth decay

HERB/NUTRIENT DEPLETIONS

Herbs are usually very safe substances to use in improving health when used responsibly. However, some herbs contain overtly toxic substances that may cause side effects and potential interactions in high dosage use or in short- and long-term therapies. Other herbs may cause interactions with pharmaceutical drugs, may be contraindicated in certain health conditions, may deplete vitamins and other nutrients from the body, or may even interact with themselves. Herbs that can have negative health consequences based on potential nutrient depletion are listed below. It should be noted that most of the herb/nutrient depletions listed are based upon evidence seen in research or reported through medical observation and scientific logic.

HERBS WITH DOCUMENTED NUTRIENT DEPLETIONS

The following herbs have been specifically reported to alter various vitamin and mineral levels in human subjects. They include:

Horsetail (*Equisetum arvense*) shoots

Horsetail may deplete thiamine (vitamin B_1) from the body due to thiaminase activity In the plant.[1] This depletion would probably occur in prolonged dosages. Always supplement with a quality multiple vitamin when recommending horsetail herb. Horsetail has also been shown to cause hypokalemia and hyponatremia in susceptible individuals based on diuretic activity.[2]

Kava kava (*Piper methysticum*) root

Kava kava root has been clinically reported to cause a yellowing of the skin in prolonged doses, attributed to a kava induced niacin deficiency. However, a clinical study reported no change in niacin levels when kava kava was administered.[3] This depletion may be dose and length of therapy dependent.

Licorice (*Glycyrrhiza glabra*) root

Licorice has glucocorticoid and mineralocorticoid properties (due to the glycyrrhizin content). Prolonged and excessive dosages can result in typical symptoms of primary hyperaldosteronism, namely hypertension; sodium, chloride, and water retention; and potassium loss.[4,5] Do not use in hypertension, hepatic or renal problems, and obesity due to the possible mineralocorticoid effects of licorice.

Tobacco (*Nicotiana tabacum*) leaf

Smoking tobacco has been reported to decrease vitamin B_{12} levels in human subjects.[6] This decrease in cyanocobalamin levels may be implicated in neurological disturbances associated with smoking. Tobacco may also increase elimination of vitamin C, thereby increasing oxidative stress on body tissues.[7,8]

DIURETIC HERBS

As with many pharmaceutical agents used for increasing diuresis, herbs with phytochemical constituents that are used as diuretic agents may potentially cause electrolyte imbalances in the body. Listed are some commonly accepted medicinal herbs that should be used with caution if the individual is currently taking pharmaceutical agents excreted renally, in individuals currently taking diuretic medications or those individuals prone to electrolyte imbalances.

Diuretic herbs include:

>Celery (*Apium graveolens*) seed
>Corn (*Zea mays*) silk
>Couchgrass (*Agropyron repens*) rhizome
>Dandelion (*Taraxacum officinale*) leaf
>Elder (*Sambucus nigra / Sambucus canadensis*) flower
>Horsetail (*Equisetum arvense*) shoots
>Juniper (*Juniperus communis*) berry
>Uva Ursi (*Arctostaphylos uva-ursi*) leaf

LAXATIVE HERBS

Laxative herbs can negatively affect nutrients, drugs, and other dietary supplements by altering their absorption, metabolism, and excretion. Whether anthraquinone-containing herbs (stimulant) or bulk-forming laxative herbs, there could be alterations in drug levels such as digitalis and antibiotics. Also, there can be a potential decrease in the absorption of and an increase in the excretion of vitamins, minerals, and other nutrients when using laxative herbs. Laxative herbs include:

>Aloe (*Aloe* sp.) leaf
>Cascara (*Rhamnus persiana*) bark
>Eyebright (*Euphrasia* sp.) whole plant
>Plantain (*Plantago lanceolata*.) leaf
>Psyllium (*Plantago* sp.) husks
>Rhubarb (*Rheum palmatum*) root
>Senna (*Cassia senna*) fruit
>Yellow Dock (*Rumex crispus*) root

TANNIN-CONTAINING HERBS

Herbs that contain tannins may alter the absorption of iron, calcium, and magnesium contained in supplements and foods. These bivalent minerals may form an insoluble complex with the tannin phytochemicals found in certain herbs. This would create a situation where the minerals may not be absorbed completely and would be partially dependent on factors such as total tannin content in the herbs and individual biochemical susceptibility. Use caution when supplementing the diet with herbs that contain high amounts of tannins concurrent with taking multiple vitamin products and other dietary supplements containing iron, calcium, and magnesium. These herbs include:

>Artichoke (*Cynara scolymus*) leaf
>Bayberry (*Myrica cerifera*) root bark
>Cascara (*Rhamnus persiana*) bark
>Corn (*Zea mays*) silk
>Elder (*Sambucus* sp.) flower
>Feverfew (*Tanacetum parthenium*) leaf
>Grape (*Vitis vinifera*) seed
>Green tea (*Camellia sinensis*) leaf
>Ground ivy (*Nepeta hederacea*) leaf
>Hops (*Humulus lupulus*) strobiles
>Horse chestnut (*Aesculus hippocastanum*) seed
>Juniper (*Juniperus communis*) berry
>Mistletoe (*Viscum* sp.) leaf
>St. John's wort (*Hypericum perforatum*) flowering tips
>Uva ursi (*Arctostaphylos uva-ursi*) leaf
>White willow (*Salix alba*) bark
>Yarrow (*Achillea millefolium*) flower

HERB/NUTRIENT DEPLETIONS *(Continued)*

EMETIC HERBS

Herbs that cause emesis can potentially cause electrolyte disturbances including hypokalemia. Many herbs in large doses will cause nausea and vomiting. The following herbs are directly associated with nausea and vomiting even in smaller doses:

> Lobelia (*Lobelia inflata*) seed
> Ipecac (*Cephalis ipecacuanha*) root

FOOTNOTES

1. Meyer P, "Thiaminase Activities and Thiamine Content of *Pteridium aquilinum, Equisetum ramosissimum, Malva parviflora, Pennisetum clandestinum* and *Medicago sativa*," *Onderstepoort J Vet Res*, 1989, 56(2):145-6.
2. Miro O, Pedrol E, Nogue S, et al, "Severe Hyponatremia and Hypopotassemia Induced by the Consumption of *Equisetum telmateia*," *Med Clin (Barc)*, 1996, 106(16): 639.
3. Ruze P, "Kava-induced Dermopathy: A Niacin Deficiency?" *Lancet*, 1990, 335(8703):1442-5.
4. de Klerk GJ, Nieuwenhuis MG, and Beutler JJ, "Hypokalaemia and Hypertension Associated With Use of Liquorice Flavoured Chewing Gum," *BMJ*, 1997, 314(7082):731-2.
5. Stormer FC, Restad R, and Alexander J, "Glycyrrhizic Acid in Liquorice--Evaluation of Health Hazard," *Food Chem Toxicol*, 1993, 31(4):303-12.
6. Halawa B and Mazurek W, "Effect of Tobacco Smoking on Vitamin B_{12} Level in Man's Blood Serum," *Wiad Lek* 1976, 29(6):469-72.
7. Hoefel OS, "Smoking: An Important Factor in Vitamin C Deficiency," *Int J Vitam Nutr Res Suppl*, 1983, 24:121-4.
8. Pelletier O, "Smoking and Vitamin C Levels in Humans," *Am J Clin Nutr*, 1968, 21(11):1259-67.

REFERENCES

These references, along with current published scientific literature, are the basis for the information in this document. It is to be noted that all of the interactions, ADRs and nutrient depletions are possible in susceptible individuals based on various factors, including biochemistry and health status, and cannot be one hundred percent predictable. Use sound professional judgment when recommending herbal medicines.

Bradley PR, ed, *British Herbal Compendium*, Vol 1, Bournemouth: British Herbal The Pharmaceutical Press, 1996.

Brinker F, *Herb Contraindications and Drug Interactions*, Sandy, Oregon: Eclectic Institute, 1997.

DeSmet P, et al, *Adverse Effects of Herbal Drugs*, Berlin, Germany: Springer Verlag, 1993, Vols 1, 2, and 3.

Leung A, et al, *Encyclopedia of Common Natural Ingredients Used in Foods, Drugs, and Cosmetics*, New York, NY: Wiley-Interscience Publication, 1996.

McGuffin M, et al, *Botanical Safety Handbook*, Boca Raton, FL: CRC Press, 1997.

Newall BA, et al, *Herbal Medicines: A Guide for Health Care Professionals*, London, England: The Pharmaceutical Press, 1996.

Schulz, et al, *Rational Phytotherapy*, Berlin, Germany: Springer Verlag, 1998.

NUTRIENT DEPLETION AND CANCER CHEMOTHERAPY

The agents used in cancer chemotherapy may have potent negative effects on an individual's nutritional status. Many individual questions with respect to nutrient depletion have not been specifically addressed in this patient population; however, the impact on general nutritional status may be profound. Cancer chemotherapy can cause nutrient depletions by five distinct mechanisms.

1. Nutrient depletions can be caused by chemotherapy due to the direct toxic effects the cytotoxic drugs have on the microvilli that line the inner surfaces of the gastrointestinal tract. This side effect of chemotherapy damages the absorptive surfaces that are responsible for absorbing nutrients into the body.

2. The damage to the lining of the gastrointestinal tract creates inflammatory changes in the protective mucous membranes (mucositis), which are particularly notable in the oral cavity (stomatitis). In these patients, the tissues in the GI tract become raw, inflamed, and highly sensitive to direct contact with digestive enzymes, acids, and partially digested foods. Because the tissues in the GI tract are raw and inflamed, eating becomes a very painful experience, causing many patients to significantly reduce their food intake, which further results in nutrient depletions. Since this form of compromise may result in

3. Many of the chemotherapy drugs cause extensive nausea and vomiting. These conditions can also result in a substantial reduction in the appetite of a cancer patient, which contributes to nutrient depletions. Many patients find it very difficult to eat when they are on the edge of nausea and fearful of another round of intense vomiting.

4. Frequently, chemotherapy causes diarrhea. Chronic diarrhea will also cause nutrient depletions due to the rapid emptying of the bowel, which reduces absorption of important nutrients.

5. Lastly, many patients undergoing chemotherapy develop dysbiosis. This is a condition characterized by an imbalance in the intestinal microbial microflora. Dysbiosis causes further disturbances in the digestion and absorption of nutrients. This can cause substantial discomfort in the form of gas, bloating, belching, as well as diarrhea and/or constipation.

The above mentioned conditions cause many cancer patients to substantially reduce their food intake to avoid pain, nausea, vomiting, etc. This form of compromise causes greater nutrient depletions, including vitamins, minerals, amino acids, and essential fatty acids. This probably results in a further weakening of the immune system and lengthens the time necessary for healing.

In addition to these primary mechanisms, certain agents may be associated with unique gastrointestinal effects. For example, asparaginase may cause pancreatitis and malabsorption, while vincristine may result in severe constipation and/or functional bowel obstruction due to a neurotoxic mechanism. Whether individual chemotherapeutic agents deplete nutrients by means other than diminished absorption has not been thoroughly evaluated. However, depletion secondary to cytotoxic effects, inflammatory responses, and effects on major organ function may be expected.

Providing these patients with intravenous nutrition during this difficult phase of cancer therapy can be very helpful. In many cases, their bodies are starving for nutrients, which can not be adequately absorbed when taken orally. Intravenous nutrients can boost the immune system and supply much needed nutrients for

NUTRIENT DEPLETION AND CANCER CHEMOTHERAPY
(Continued)

energy as well as the healing of damaged tissues. Also, numerous studies have reported that glutamine supplementation can help prevent side effects and speed up the process of healing the tissues in the gastrointestinal tract in patients undergoing chemotherapy.

CHEMOTHERAPY TABLES

For convenience, chemotherapeutic agents may be grouped into five general classes. These include alkylating agents, antineoplastic antibiotics, antimetabolites, natural source derivatives, and a miscellaneous grouping. Although there is some variability within groups, agents within these classes often demonstrate a characteristic gastrointestinal toxicity profile.

Alkylating agents: These agents are associated with moderate to high potential for nausea and vomiting but do not usually cause severe toxicity to the gastrointestinal mucosa.

Antineoplastic antibiotics: These agents are associated with moderate potential for nausea and vomiting but often cause severe toxicity to the gastrointestinal mucosa.

Antimetabolites: These agents are associated with low to moderate potential for nausea and vomiting but may cause severe toxicity to the gastrointestinal mucosa.

Natural source derivatives: These agents are associated with low to moderate potential for nausea and vomiting and may cause severe toxicity to the gastrointestinal mucosa.

Biological response modifiers: These chemotherapy agents do not have specific gastrointestinal effects. They are generally hormonal antagonists or cytokines/ immune response modifying agents. Included in this category are aldesleukin, anastrozole, bicalutamide, interferon alfa, leuprolide, megestrol, nilutamide, and tamoxifen.

The following tables list agents according to these broad classifications. Although studies of specific nutrient depletion in the setting of cancer chemotherapy are limited, the following tables may be used to identify the primary mechanism of nutritional impact an agent may have. The number in the second column corresponds to the potential of an agent to cause nausea, vomiting, and anorexia. On this scale, 1 corresponds to the lowest potential, while a rating of 5 indicates the greatest potential to cause this effect. The third column provides additional detail and highlights the extent of mucosal toxicity noted with an individual agent.

ALKYLATING AGENTS

Drug Name	Emetogenic Rating*	Mucosal Effects and Notes
Busulfan	2	Mucosal effects rare
Carboplatin	3	Emetogenic, but little mucocutaneous effect
Carmustine	4-5	Nausea and vomiting persist for 4-6 hours; few mucosal effects
Chlorambucil	1	Infrequent nausea, vomiting, diarrhea, or oral ulceration
Cisplatin	4-5	Highly emetogenic, persisting for up to 1 week; mucosal effects <1%
Cyclophosphamide	1-4	Nausea/vomiting increase with dose; stomatitis/mucositis may occur
Dacarbazine	4-5	Highly emetogenic, duration 2-4 hours; rare mucosal effects
Ifosfamide	3-4	Significant nausea and vomiting, up to 3 days; limited mucosal effects
Lomustine	4-5	Nausea and vomiting common, stomatitis and diarrhea in 1% to 10%
Mechlorethamine	5	Highly emetogenic, duration 2-8 hours; diarrhea in 1% to 10%
Melphalan	1-5	Emetogenic only at high doses; infrequent stomatitis and diarrhea
Procarbazine	4	Significant nausea/vomiting; infrequent stomatitis (1% to 2%)
Streptozocin	5	Highly emetogenic, duration 1-12 hours
Thiotepa	2-5	Mucositis frequent at doses used in bone marrow transplant (BMT)

*Emetogenic rating scale: 1 = Lowest; 5 = Highest

ANTINEOPLASTIC ANTIBIOTICS

Drug Name	Emetogenic Rating*	Mucosal Effects and Notes
Bleomycin	4	High mucosal toxicity
Dactinomycin	5	Highly emetogenic, duration 4-24 hours; high mucocutaneous toxicity
Daunorubicin	3	High mucosal toxicity
Doxorubicin	3-4	High mucosal toxicity
Idarubicin	3	High mucosal toxicity; GI hemorrhage up to 30%
Mitomycin	3	High mucosal toxicity
Mitoxantrone	3	Severe diarrhea and mucosal toxicity
Pentostatin	2	Diarrhea in >10%; stomatitis ~5%
Plicamycin	2	Moderate to high incidence of stomatitis (1% to 10%)

*Emetogenic rating scale: 1 = Lowest; 5 = Highest

NUTRIENT DEPLETION AND CANCER CHEMOTHERAPY
(Continued)

ANTIMETABOLITES

Drug Name	Emetogenic Rating*	Mucosal Effects and Notes
Cladribine	1	Low nausea/vomiting; little mucosal toxicity
Cytarabine	2-4	High mucosal toxicity
Floxuridine	4	High mucosal toxicity
Fludarabine	1	Mild nausea/vomiting; stomatitis and GI bleeding may occur
Fluorouracil	2-3	Anorexia and stomatitis; mucocutaneous toxicity may be severe
Gemcitabine	1	Stomatitis 10% to 14%
Hydroxyurea	4	Anorexia and stomatitis may be severe
Mercaptopurine	1	Moderate to high stomatitis 1% to 10%; pancreatitis
Methotrexate	2-4	High incidence of mucosal damage, also pancreatitis
Thioguanine	3	High mucosal toxicity

*Emetogenic rating scale: 1 = Lowest; 5 = Highest

NATURAL SOURCE (Plant) DERIVATIVES

Drug Name	Emetogenic Rating*	Mucosal Effects and Notes
Docetaxel	1	High mucosal toxicity; diarrhea in ~25%
Etoposide	2	Some mucosal 1% to 6%; diarrhea in 1% to 13%
Irinotecan	3	Very high incidence of diarrhea†
Paclitaxel	1	High mucositis incidence, severe at higher doses
Teniposide	3	High mucositis incidence; diarrhea up to 75%
Topotecan	2	Nausea in up to 70%, emesis <30%, diarrhea in up to 42%
Vinblastine	1	Stomatitis and diarrhea are common
Vincristine	1	High mucosal toxicity; common constipation and adynamic ileus
Vinorelbine	1	High mucositis in >44%; constipation 35%

*Emetogenic rating scale: 1 = Lowest; 5 = Highest

†Two forms: Early (within 30 minutes) due to cholinergic mechanism and late (after 6-10 days) due to direct cellular toxicity.

MISCELLANEOUS

Drug Name	Emetogenic Rating*	Mucosal Effects and Notes
Asparaginase	1	May cause pancreatitis/malabsorption but little direct mucotoxicity
Mitotane	4	May cause severe nausea, vomiting, diarrhea (occurs in ~20%)

*Emetogenic rating scale: 1 = Lowest; 5 = Highest

FOOD-DRUG INTERACTIONS, KEY SUMMARY

Drug	Food	Interaction
Acetaminophen	Watercress	Decreased levels of oxidative metabolites (mercapturate) of acetaminophen
	High pectin foods	Delayed absorption
Amoxicillin Ampicillin Aspirin Astemizole Azithromycin Captopril Cephalexin (suspension) Chlorpromazine Didanosine Erythromycin stearate Fosfomycin Isoniazid Ketoconazole Levodopa Lincomycin Mercaptopurine Methotrexate Methyldopa Nafcillin Penicillamine Penicillin G and V Phenobarbital Propantheline Rifampin (150 mg) Riluzole Tetracycline Valproic acid Valsartan Zidovudine	Any food	Decreased absorption
Aspirin Atenolol Cefaclor Cephalexin (capsule) Cephradine Cimetidine Glipizide Ibuprofen Metronidazole Piroxicam Potassium (tablet) Quinidine Sulfonamides (suspension) Tacrine Warfarin	Any food	Delayed absorption

FOOD-DRUG INTERACTIONS, KEY SUMMARY *(Continued)*

Drug	Food	Interaction
Alpha-tocopherol Carbamazepine Cefuroxime Chlorothiazide Hydralazine Hydrochlorothiazide Labetalolol Lithium Mebendazole Metoprolol Nitrofurantoin Phenytoin Propoxyphene Propranolol Riboflavin Spironolactone	Any food	Increased absorption
Cyclosporine	Many foods	Decreased absorption
Acitretin Albendazole Atovaquone Beta-carotene Cyclosporine Diazepam Dicumarol Etretinate Griseofulvin Halofantrine Isotretinoin Mefenamic acid Phenytoin Vitamin A Vitamin D Vitamin E Vitamin K	Dietary fat	Increased absorption
Biphosphonates (ie, etidronate, alendronate, tiludronate	Foods with high mineral content (ie, milk)	Reduced absorption
Griseofulvin	High-fat meal	Faster absorption; increased serum levels by 50%
Misoprostol		Reduced peak by delaying absorption
Digoxin Pilocarpine (tablets) Zidovudine		Reduced absorption

Drug	Food	Interaction
Cyclosporine Felodipine Nifedipine Nimodipine Nisoldipine Nitrendipine Verapamil	Grapefruit juice (naringen)	Increased absorption; increased oral bioavailability
Caffeine		Possibly prolongs caffeine's half-life
Coumarin		Delayed urinary excretion of 7-hydroxy-coumarin
Lovastatin		Increases lovastatin and metabolite concentrations
Midazolam (oral)		Delayed absorption; increased bioavailability
Quinidine		Delayed absorption of quinidine; inhibits metabolism of quinidine
Terfenadine		Increases terfenadine bioavailability (can increase Q-T interval on EKG); increased absorption
Erythromycin stearate	Any food	Increased or decreased absorption
Furosemide		Decreased rate of absorption, potentially decreasing effect
Mercaptopurine		Decreased bioavailability by 30%
Isoniazid	Tuna, mackerel, salmon (dark meat fish)	Increased risk for scombroid fish poisoning
Levodopa	High-protein diet	Decreased absorption
Digoxin Lovastatin	High fiber meal	Decreased absorption
Lithium	Sodium	Enhanced elimination requiring higher doses
Methyldopa	Iron	Reduced absorption
MAO inhibitors Isocarboxazid Phenelzine Procarbazine Tranylcypromine	High-protein foods that have undergone aging, fermentation, pickling, or smoking; aged cheeses, red wines, pods of broad beans and fava beans; bananas, raisins, avocados; caffeine-containing beverages, beer, ale, and chocolate	Elevated blood pressure
Phenobarbital Phenytoin	High doses of vitamin B₆ (pyridoxine) and folic acid	Decreased absorption
Levodopa	Vitamin B₆ (pyridoxine)	Reduces blood level
Diprafenone Felodipine Hydralazine Metoprolol Nitrofurantoin Propranolol	Any food	Increased bioavailability
Phenobarbital Phenytoin Theophylline Warfarin	Charcoal-broiled foods	Increased metabolism requiring higher doses
Ketoconazole	Acidic beverages (pH <2.5, ie, Coca-Cola Classic®)	Increased absorption
Phenytoin	Most foods	Absorption increased by 25%
	Pudding	Absorption decreased by 50%
Quinolones (eg, ciprofloxacin) Minocycline Tetracycline	Iron, calcium, aluminum, zinc, magnesium (eg, dairy products)	Decreased absorption

FOOD-DRUG INTERACTIONS, KEY SUMMARY *(Continued)*

Drug	Food	Interaction
Quinidine	High salt (>400 mEq/day)	Increased first-pass hepatic elimination
Warfarin	Diets rich in vitamin K such as cauliflower, spinach, broccoli, turnip greens, liver, beans, rice, pork, fish, and some cheeses	Antagonism of effect
Ace inhibitors	Potassium-containing salt substitutes	Increased serum potassium level
Bromfenac	Any food	Reduced analgesic efficacy

Reprinted with permission from Saltiel E, "Food-Drug Interactions," *New Developments in Medicine & Drug Therapy*, Glenview, IL: Physicians & Scientists Publishing Co, Inc, 1994, 3(4):61.

D'Arcy PF, "Nutrient-Drug Interactions," *Adv Drug React Toxicol Rev*, 1995, 14:233-54.

Gauthier I and Malone M, "Drug-Food Interactions in Hospitalized Patients: Methods of Prevention," *Drug Safety*, 1998, 18(6):383-93.

Parnetti L and Lowenthal DT, "How to Recognize and Prevent Dangerous Food-Drug Interactions," *J Crit Illness*, 1998, 13(2):126-33.

ALPHABETICAL INDEX

NOTES

NOTES

NOTES

Other titles offered by Lexi-Comp, Inc.

DRUG INFORMATION HANDBOOK (International edition available)
by Charles Lacy, RPh, PharmD, FCSHP; Lora L. Armstrong, RPh, PharmD, BCPS; Morton P. Goldman, PharmD, BCPS; and Leonard L. Lance, RPh, BSPharm

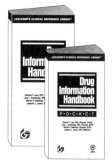

Specifically compiled and designed for the healthcare professional requiring quick access to concisely-stated comprehensive data concerning clinical use of medications.

The *Drug Information Handbook* is an ideal portable drug information resource, providing the reader with up to 29 key points of data concerning clinical use and dosing of the medication. Material provided in the Appendix section is recognized by many users to be, by itself, well worth the purchase of the handbook.

All medications found in the *Drug Information Handbook*, are included in the abridged *Pocket* edition (select fields were extracted to maintain portability).

PEDIATRIC DOSAGE HANDBOOK (International edition available)
by Carol K. Taketomo, PharmD; Jane Hurlburt Hodding, PharmD; and Donna M. Kraus, PharmD

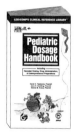

Special considerations must frequently be taken into account when dosing medications for the pediatric patient. This highly regarded quick reference handbook is a compilation of recommended pediatric doses based on current literature as well as the practical experience of the authors and their many colleagues who work every day in the pediatric clinical setting.

Includes neonatal dosing, drug administration, and (in select monographs) extemporaneous preparations for medications used in pediatric medicine.

GERIATRIC DOSAGE HANDBOOK by Todd P. Semla, PharmD, BCPS, FCCP; Judith L. Beizer, PharmD, FASCP; and Martin D. Higbee, PharmD, CGP

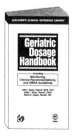

Many physiologic changes occur with aging, some of which affect the pharmacokinetics or pharmaco-dynamics of medications. Strong consideration should also be given to the effect of decreased renal or hepatic functions in the elderly, as well as the probability of the geriatric patient being on multiple drug regimens.

Healthcare professionals working with nursing homes and assisted living facilities will find the drug information contained in this handbook to be an invaluable source of helpful information.

An International Brand Name Index with names from 20 different countries is also included.

To order call toll free anywhere in the U.S.: 1-800-837-LEXI (5394)
Outside of the U.S. call: 330-650-6506 or online at www.lexi.com

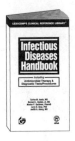
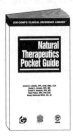
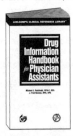

Other titles offered by Lexi-Comp, Inc.

DRUG INFORMATION HANDBOOK *for* ADVANCED PRACTICE NURSING
by Beatrice B. Turkoski, RN, PhD; Brenda R. Lance, RN, MSN; Mark F. Bonfiglio, PharmD;
Foreword by: Margaret A. Fitzgerald, MS, RN, CS-FNP

1999 "Book of the Year" — *American Journal of Nursing*
Advanced Practice Nursing Category

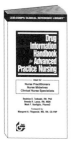

This handbook was designed specifically to meet the needs of Nurse Practitioners, Clinical Nurse Specialists, Nurse Midwives and graduate nursing students. The handbook is a unique resource for detailed, accurate information, which is vital to support the advanced practice nurse's role in patient drug therapy management. Over 4750 U.S., Canadian, and Mexican medications are covered in the 1000 monographs. Drug data is presented in an easy-to-use, alphabetically organized format covering up to 46 key points of information (including dosing for pediatrics, adults, and geriatrics). Monographs are cross-referenced to an Appendix of over 230 pages of valuable comparison tables and additional information. Also included are two indices, Pharmacologic Category and Controlled Substance, which facilitate comparison between agents.

DRUG INFORMATION HANDBOOK *for* NURSING
by Beatrice B. Turkoski, RN, PhD; Brenda R. Lance, RN, MSN; Mark F. Bonfiglio, PharmD

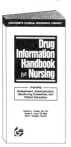

Registered Professional Nurses and upper-division nursing students involved with drug therapy will find this handbook provides quick access to drug data in a concise easy-to-use format.

Over 4000 U.S., Canadian, and Mexican medications are covered with up to 43 key points of information in each monograph. The handbook contains basic pharmacology concepts and nursing issues such as patient factors that influence drug therapy (ie, pregnancy, age, weight, etc) and general nursing issues (ie, assess-ment, administration, monitoring, and patient education). The Appendix contains over 230 pages of valuable information.

DIAGNOSTIC PROCEDURE HANDBOOK by Frank Michota, MD

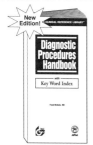

A comprehensive yet concise quick reference source for physicians, nurses, students, medical records personnel, or anyone needing quick access to diagnostic procedure information. This handbook is an excellent source of information in the following areas: allergy, rheumatology, and infectious disease; cardiology; computed tomography; diagnostic radiology; gastroenterology; invasive radiology; magnetic resonance imaging; nephrology, urology, and hematology; neurology; nuclear medicine; pulmonary function; pulmonary medicine and critical care; ultrasound; women's health.

To order call toll free anywhere in the U.S.: 1-800-837-LEXI (5394)
Outside of the U.S. call: 330-650-6506 or online at www.lexi.com

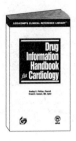
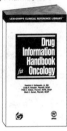
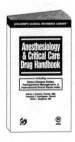

Other titles offered by Lexi-Comp, Inc.

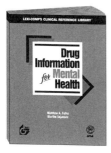
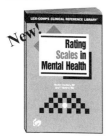
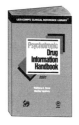

Other titles offered by Lexi-Comp, Inc.

LABORATORY TEST HANDBOOK & CONCISE version
by David S. Jacobs MD, FACP; Wayne R. DeMott, MD, FACP; Harold J. Grady, PhD;
Rebecca T. Horvat, PhD; Douglas W. Huestis, MD; and Bernard L. Kasten Jr., MD, FACP

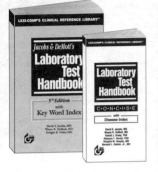

Contains over 900 clinical laboratory tests and is an excellent source of laboratory information for physicians of all specialties, nurses, laboratory professionals, students, medical personnel, or anyone who needs quick access to most the routine and many of the more specialized testing procedures available in today's clinical laboratory. Including updated AMA CPT coding, each monograph contains test name, synonyms, patient care, specimen requirements, reference ranges, and interpretive information with footnotes and references. The *Laboratory Test Handbook Concise* is a portable, abridged (800 tests) version and is an ideal, quick reference for anyone requiring information concerning patient preparation, specimen collection and handling, and test result interpretation.

CLINICIAN'S GUIDE TO LABORATORY MEDICINE—A Practical Approach
by Samir P. Desai, MD; Sana Isa, MD

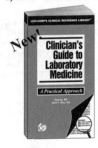

When faced with the patient presenting with abnormal laboratory tests, the clinician can now turn to Laboratory Medicine for the Clinician: A Practical Approach.

This source is unique in its ability to lead the clinician from laboratory test abnormality to clinical diagnosis. Written for the busy clinician, this concise handbook will provide rapid answers to the questions that busy clinicians face in the care of their patients. No longer does the clinician have to struggle in an effort to find this information - *it's all here.*

CLINICIAN'S GUIDE TO DIAGNOSIS—A Practical Approach Coming Summer 2001!
by Samir P. Desai, MD

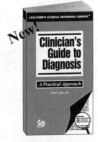

Symptoms are what prompt patients to seek medical care. In the evaluation of a patient's symptom, it is not unusual for health care professionals to ask "What do I do next?" This is precisely the question that the "Clinician's Guide to Diagnosis: A Practical Approach" provides the answer to. It will lead you from symptom to diagnosis through a series of steps designed to mimic the logical thought processes of seasoned clinicians. For the young clinician, this is an ideal book to help bridge the gap between the classroom and actual patient care. For the experienced clinician, this concise handbook offers rapid answers to the questions that are commonly encountered on a day to day basis. Let this guide become your companion, providing you with the tools necessary to tackle even the most challenging symptoms.

To order call toll free anywhere in the U.S.: 1-800-837-LEXI (5394)
Outside of the U.S. call: 330-650-6506 or online at www.lexi.com

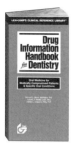
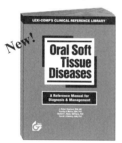
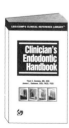

Other titles offered by Lexi-Comp, Inc.

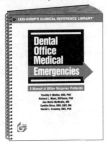
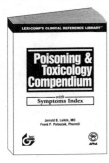
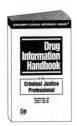

Other titles offered by Lexi-Comp, Inc.

New!
Patient Education Dental Desk Charts

A PATIENT GUIDE TO ROOT THERAPY
Contributor Thom C. Dumsha, M.S., D.D.S., M.S.

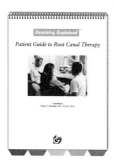

- An ideal tool used to educate and explain to your patients about root canals

- 8 1/2" x 11" colorful tabbed flip chart explaining each of the steps involved in a root canal

- Actual clinical photographs, radiographs, and diagrams

"Take home" patient education pamphlets also included.

PATIENT GUIDE TO DENTAL IMPLANTS
Contributor Marvin L. Baer, D.D.S., M.Sc.

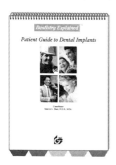

- An ideal tool used to educate and explain to your patients about dental implants

- 8 1/2" x 11" colorful tabbed flip chart explaining each of the steps involved in:

  1.) Single tooth restoration
  2.) Replacement of several teeth
  3.) Implants supported overdenture
      (4 implants/2 implants)
  4.) Screw-retained denture

"Take home" patient education pamphlets also included.

To order call toll free anywhere in the U.S.: 1-800-837-LEXI (5394)
Outside of the U.S. call: 330-650-6506 or online at www.lexi.com

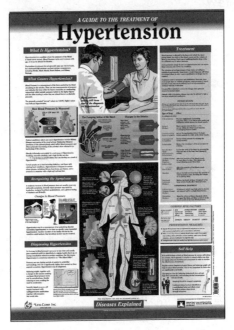

Lexi-Comp is proud to introduce Diseases Explained™, our new series of patient education material. Written in a language a patient can easily understand, each product will help the healthcare professional explain to patients about their specific medical condition.

Available now in a wall chart format and soon to be released as booklets, leaflets, and desk flip charts, this series will help you educate the patient about the cause, symptoms, diagnosis, treatment, and self-help concerning their condition.

Available now:

- Alzheimer's Disease
- Anemia
- Angina
- Asthma
- Anxiety
- Cholesterol
- COPD
- Depression
- Diabetes
- Enlarged Prostate

- Epilepsy
- Essential Tremor
- Glaucoma
- Heart Attack
- Hypertension
- Incontinence
- Insomnia
- Irritable Bowel Syndrome
- Menopause
- Migraine

- Multiple Sclerosis
- Obsessive-Compulsive Disorder
- Osteoporosis
- Otitis
- Panic Disorder
- Parkinson's Disease
- Schizophrenia
- Spasticity
- Stroke
- Thyroid Disease

**Visit www.diseases-explained.com/catalog for an updated list of products
or for more information call toll free: 1-877-837-5394**